Questions *and* Answers

A Guide to Fitness and Wellness

Second Edition

Gary Liguori
University of Tennessee, Chattanooga

Sandra Carroll-Cobb
University of Alaska, Anchorage

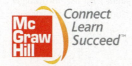

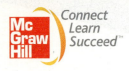

The McGraw·Hill Companies

Connect
Learn
Succeed™

QUESTIONS AND ANSWERS: A GUIDE TO FITNESS AND WELLNESS, SECOND EDITION

Published by McGraw-Hill, a business unit of The McGraw-Hill Companies, Inc., 1221 Avenue of the
Americas, New York, NY, 10020. Copyright © 2014 by The McGraw-Hill Companies, Inc. All rights reserved.
Printed in the United States of America. Previous edition © 2012. No part of this publication may be reproduced
or distributed in any form or by any means, or stored in a database or retrieval system, without the prior written
consent of The McGraw-Hill Companies, Inc., including, but not limited to, in any network or other electronic
storage or transmission, or broadcast for distance learning.

Some ancillaries, including electronic and print components, may not be available to customers outside the
United States.

This book is printed on acid-free paper.

1 2 3 4 5 6 7 8 9 0 QDB/QDB 1 0 9 8 7 6 5 4 3

ISBN 978-0-07-336926-6
MHID 0-07-336926-8

Senior Vice President, Products & Markets: *Kurt L. Strand*
Vice President, General Manager, Products & Markets: *Michael J. Ryan*
Vice President, Content Production & Technology Services: *Kimberly Meriwether David*
Managing Director: *Gina Boedeker*
Senior Brand Manager: *Bill Minick*
Director of Development: *Rhona Robbin*
Development Editors: *Emily Pecora and Sylvia Mallory*
Editorial Coordinator: *Fiso Takirambudde*
Senior Marketing Manager: *Caroline McGillen*
Marketing Coordinator: *Marcus Opsal*
Lead Project Manager: *Rick Hecker*
Buyer II: *Debra R. Sylvester*
Lead Designer: *Matthew Baldwin*
Cover Image: *Front Cover, ©Getty Images/Take A Pix Media. Back Cover, ©Getty Images/Harrison Eastwood*
Senior Content Licensing Specialist: *Jeremy Cheshareck*
Photo Researcher: *Jennifer Blankenship*
Manager, Digital Production: *Janean A. Utley*
Typeface: *10/12 Times Roman*
Compositor: *Laserwords Private Limited*
Printer: *Quad/Graphics*

All credits appearing on page or at the end of the book are considered to be an extension of the copyright page.

Library of Congress Cataloging-in-Publication Data

Liguori, Gary, 1965-
    [Fitwell]
    Questions and answers: a guide to fitness and wellness / Sandra Carroll-Cobb. —Second edition.
        pages cm
    Includes index.
    ISBN 978-0-07-336926-6 (alk. paper)—ISBN 0-07-336926-8 (alk. paper)
    1. College students—Health and hygiene—Handbooks, manuals, etc. 2. College students—United States—
Handbooks, manuals, etc. 3. Physical fitness—Health aspects. 4. Health education—Textbooks.
    5. Health—Textbooks. I. Carroll-Cobb, Sandra, 1965- II. Title. III. Title: Guide to fitness and wellness.
    RA777.3.L54 2014
    613.7'1—dc23   2012036436

The Internet addresses listed in the text were accurate at the time of publication. The inclusion of a website does
not indicate an endorsement by the authors or McGraw-Hill, and McGraw-Hill does not guarantee the accuracy
of the information presented at these sites.

www.mhhe.com

Contents

10 Stress and Its Sources   343

11 Chronic Diseases   380

Preface

Active Students / Active Learning

If students sit passively on the sidelines, how can we expect them to learn—and to change their behavior in ways that promote their health and wellness, now and in the future?

Questions and Answers empowers students to become active participants in their own fitness and wellness through a genuinely student-centered approach. This is the first fitness and wellness text to be written in direct response to students' questions about their own health and well-being. In responding to these student inquiries, authors Gary Liguori and Sandra Carroll-Cobb combine the latest science-based knowledge with practical guidance on concrete actions students can take *now* to improve their fitness and wellness. By encouraging students to be engaged participants in their learning, *Questions and Answers* also inspires them to become active shapers of their future health and happiness.

The active learning approach of *Questions and Answers* includes the following features:

FOCUS ON BEHAVIOR CHANGE: Online video case studies follow real college students attempting to change their behavior, and prompt readers to apply lessons from these experiences to their own behavior-change goals. Throughout the text itself, the use of student questions calls attention to the how and why of the content—making the real-life applications apparent. A series of lab activities provide tracking tools and self-assessment forms that can be completed in print or online.

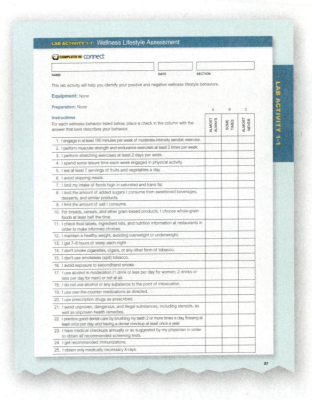

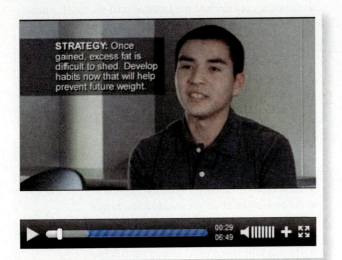

CONNECT FITNESS AND WELLNESS: Connect Fitness and Wellness is a Web-based assignment and assessment platform that promotes active learning and provides tools that enable instructors to teach the course more efficiently and effectively. Using Connect, instructors can easily assign preloaded activities, create and edit assignments, produce video lectures, upload their own articles or videos, cascade assignments, and generate reports for one or many course sections.

MEANINGFUL PEDAGOGY: The results-centered pedagogy of *Questions and Answers* ensures that every detail in every chapter works toward the larger goal of making students active participants in their own life-learning. The authors address issues that are of importance to students' daily living and well-being, such as maintaining motivation to exercise, understanding the safety of dietary supplements, and choosing the best exercise shoes. Critical thinking questions and calls to action prompt students to evaluate the content and connect it to their own experiences.

Proven and Practical Learning Features

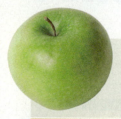

Wellness Strategies boxes offer specific approaches to and techniques for improving personal well-being.

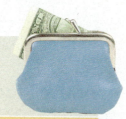

Dollar Stretcher selections provide tips to help students maximize their financial wellness.

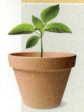

Mind Stretcher Critical Thinking Exercises challenge readers to pause, analyze, and evaluate aspects of the text discussion.

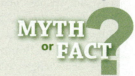

Research Brief boxes summarize recent research findings and prompt students to consider the importance of these results and their implications for their own lives.

Living *Well* with . . . selections present strategies for maintaining wellness while coping with various health issues.

Myth or Fact? callouts connect to online videos that debunk common health and wellness myths.

MYTH or FACT?

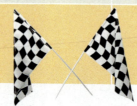

Fast Facts boxes are a go-to spot for important, high-interest statistics and other information.

What's New in the Second Edition

Chapter 1: Introduction to Health, Wellness, and Fitness

- Added new research findings in current Research Brief selection, "It's Good to Be Good"
- Added a detailed new Wellness Strategies selection, "Why Sustainability Matters—and What You Can Do"
- Integrated new information in Fast Facts selection "Driving Distracted?"
- Updated the discussion of the Healthy People initiative with new information, including details on the final progress report for *Healthy People 2010* as well as an account of the *Healthy People 2020* goals

Chapter 2: Positive Choices/Positive Changes

- Added new Fast Facts selection, "Buddy Up for Behavior Change"
- Revised SMART goals section
- Added new figure to depict SMART goals and components

Chapter 3: Fundamentals of Physical Fitness

- Updated Research Brief selection, "Exercise Keeps You Young"
- New figure, "Progressive Overload"

- New Research Brief selection, "Hate to Exercise? Think Again!"
- Updated Fast Facts selection, "Helmet Head"
- New table, "Free and Low-Cost Exercise Alternatives"

Chapter 4: Cardiorespiratory Fitness

- Streamlined and clarified the analyses of ATP's function and catabolism
- Substantially revised the treatment of the body's three energy systems—ATP-CP, glycolytic, and aerobic—for conciseness and ease of comprehension
- Extensively revised the discussion of the fat-burning effects of low-intensity exercise, for enhanced clarity
- Expanded the discussion of the challenges of sticking to an exercise program and of dealing with relapse
- New Research Brief selection, "The Effect of Acute Bouts of Exercise on Anxiety"

Chapter 5: Muscle Fitness

- New figure, "Sliding Filament Theory"
- Added material on the overload principle
- New Research Brief selection, "Strength Training and Diabetes"
- Revised the discussion of tips for joining a gym
- New Research Brief selection, "Can Being Strong Keep You Alive?"

- Clarified the text narrative on concentric and eccentric contractions
- New tables, "Training Frequency Recommendations for Resistance Training" and "Program Design Parameters for Resistance Training"
- Revised the treatment of the limited effects of spot training
- Expanded the text discussion of guidelines for putting together a muscle-fitness program and of exercise-safety recommendations

Chapter 6: Flexibility and Low-Back Fitness

- New Research Brief selection, "Heavy Backpack, Heavy Price"

Chapter 7: Body Composition Basics

- Updated Research Brief selection, "Beating the 'Fatso' Gene"
- New Research Brief selection, "You Are What You Drink"

Chapter 8: Nutrition Basics: Energy and Nutrients

- Added text on the harms of consuming sweetened soda
- New Research Brief selection, "Does Beverage Choice Make Kids Fat?"
- New Fast Facts box, "The Average American Drinker"

Chapter 9: Eating for Wellness and Weight Management

- Comprehensively revised the text, tables, and figures to reflect the USDA's MyPlate food plan
- New Fast Facts box, "Quick Tips for Avoiding Weight Gain in College"
- Revised the text on guidelines for meal planning and preparation
- New Dollar Stretcher selection on making good nutrition choices that also save time and money
- Substantially rewrote and expanded the text on making wise fast-food choices
- New Research Brief selection, "Is Whom We Eat with Just as Important as What We Eat?"
- New Research Brief selection, "How Food Cues and Portion Size Impact Eating"
- New Fast Facts box, "Mindless Eating"
- New Mind Stretcher box on weight-loss apps for smartphones

Chapter 10: Stress and Its Sources

- New Fast Facts box, "Is Your State Stressed?"
- New Research Brief selection, "Smartphone Stressing You?"
- Added material on type C and type D personality profiles
- New Wellness Strategies selection, "You Are What You Think"

- New Research Brief selection, "The Negative Consequences of Prenatal Stress"
- New Research Brief selection, "Dieting Stress: Can It Impede Weight Loss?"
- New table, "American Adults' Stress-Management Techniques"
- New Research Brief selection, "Sleep, Bad Sleep, and Really Bad Sleep"
- New Fast Facts box, "Asleep at the Wheel"
- Updated Research Brief selection, "The Stress of Setting Life Goals"

Chapter 11: Chronic Diseases

- Added information about varicose veins
- Added resources for collecting, organizing, and researching family health history
- Updated Research Brief selection, "Don't Worry, Be Happy"
- Incorporated additional resources for heart attack and stroke warning signs, as well as CPR/AED
- Integrated new information about the availability of genetic testing to screen for genes that increase the risk of CVD and diabetes, as well as other diseases and disorders
- Updated Wellness Strategies selection, "The Ups and Downs of Genetic Testing: Things to Know"
- Updated Wellness Strategies selection, "Protecting Your Skin from the Sun"
- New table, "Top Lifestyle Choices for Preventing Chronic Disease"

Chapter 12: Infectious Diseases

- New Fast Facts box, "Superbugs on the Loose"
- New Research Brief selection, "Hand Washing 101"
- New Mind Stretcher exploring issues related to annual flu immunizations
- New Fast Facts box, "STIs: The Sobering Reality"
- New Mind Stretcher selection on issues related to screening for STIs
- Updated Wellness Strategies selection, "The Dos and Don'ts of Condom Use"

Chapter 13: Substance Use, Dependence, and Addiction

- New Mind Stretcher selection probing addiction and dependence
- New Research Brief selection, "Energy Drinks and Alcohol: A Dangerous Mix"
- New Research Brief selection, "Marijuana and the Workplace"
- Added new insights on the problems associated with chewing tobacco
- New Mind Stretcher on the importance of support systems for individuals who want to quit smoking
- Added new text on electric cigarettes and water pipes
- New Dollar Stretcher selection exploring the high dollar cost of consuming alcohol

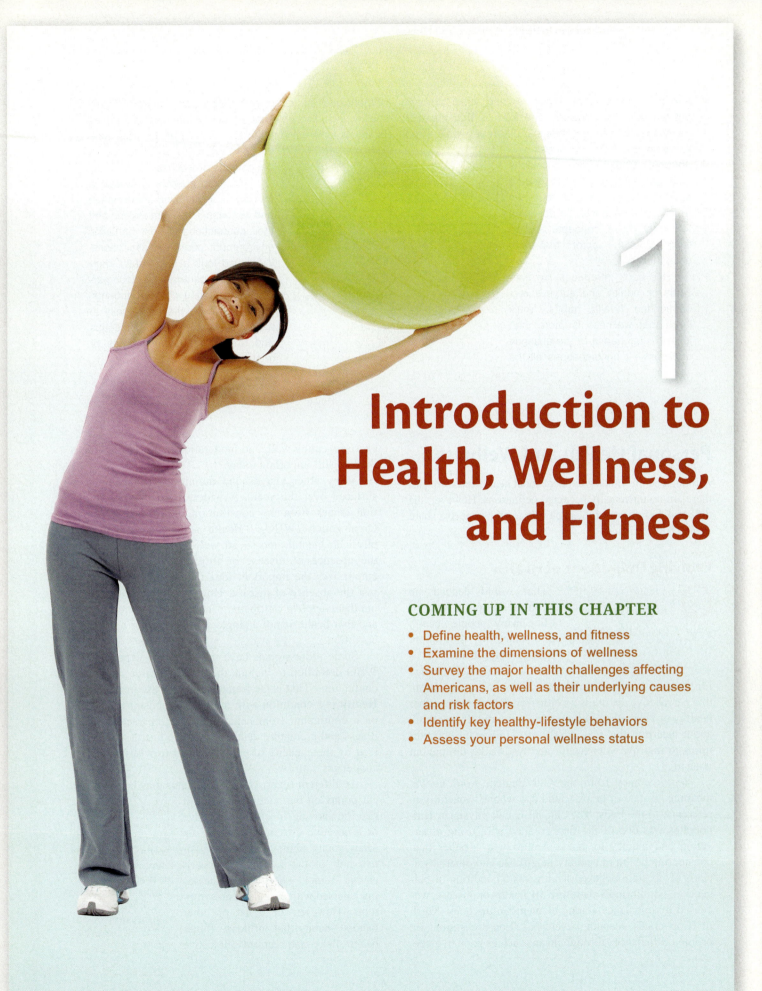

1

Introduction to Health, Wellness, and Fitness

COMING UP IN THIS CHAPTER

- Define health, wellness, and fitness
- Examine the dimensions of wellness
- Survey the major health challenges affecting Americans, as well as their underlying causes and risk factors
- Identify key healthy-lifestyle behaviors
- Assess your personal wellness status

Ask ten people what health is, and you'll probably get ten different answers. The truth is that the word *health* means different things to different people. If you throw in the terms *wellness* and *physical fitness,* the definitions may get even trickier. To gain a sound understanding of your own health and wellness, it's essential to clarify these concepts and to learn about the factors that influence them.

This book introduces the concepts of health and surveys recommended health habits. You'll learn that wellness is more than just physical health or the absence of illness—it encompasses all the dimensions illustrated in the Wellness Integrator figure below, including physical, emotional, intellectual, social, spiritual, and environmental wellness. To be truly well, you must develop and balance all the aspects of wellness.

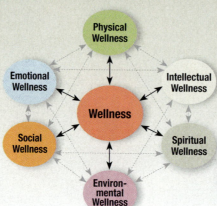

This first chapter provides a framework for thinking about health and wellness—their dimensions and their connections to your behavior, environment, goals, and aspirations. We'll also look at key health challenges, both general and those particularly affecting college students. You'll also have the opportunity to assess your own wellness status and to identify potential areas of improvement.

Personal Health and Wellness

Although people talk a great deal about health and wellness, there are no universally accepted definitions. However, the different definitions of these closely related concepts share many characteristics.

Evolving Definitions of Health

Q I haven't been sick in over a year. Can I rate myself as healthy?

That would depend on your definition of *healthy.* For many people, health is something they think about only if there is a sudden, noticeable change for the worse—for example, an illness or injury. From this perspective, health is an either-or state: You are either healthy or unhealthy, with no middle ground. If you think about health in this way, you'll miss important opportunities to improve your health and well-being throughout your life.

Health comes from the Old English word *hoelth,* meaning "a state of being sound and whole," generally in reference to the body. The ancient Greek physician Hippocrates was one of the first credited with using observation and inquiry to assess health status—rather than considering health to be a divine gift. He and other physicians of his time believed health was a condition of balance or equilibrium; therefore ill health or disease was caused by imbalance among elements in the body. Much of Hippocrates' teachings were based on prevention. He promoted "balance" through means such as good hygiene, exercise, eating well, and moderation in all things—ideas that are still important today.

Many other visions and definitions of health have surfaced over the years. A widely used modern definition comes from the constitution of the World Health Organization (WHO): "Health is a state of complete physical, mental, and social well-being, and not merely the absence of disease or infirmity."[1] This definition emphasizes the important idea that health is more than just the absence of disease. However, some critics point out that *complete* well-being is unrealistic for most people and that health is not a single state but rather a dynamic condition.

Some professionals have modified and expanded the WHO definition to include the idea of health status as a continuum.[2] That is the framework we'll use in this book: **Health** is a condition with multiple dimensions that falls on a continuum from negative health, characterized by illness and premature death, to positive health, characterized by the capacity to enjoy life and to withstand life's challenges.

At different times, your health status may be on different points on the continuum—and it may be moving in either a positive or a negative direction (Figure 1-1). Many young adults fall into the positive half of the continuum, experiencing minor, short-term illnesses interspersed with periods of no symptoms. However, in terms of other factors—habits that influence future health risks and current subjective

health A condition with multiple dimensions that falls on a continuum from negative health, characterized by illness and premature death, to positive health, characterized by the capacity to enjoy life and to withstand life's challenges.

Behavior-Change Challenge

Integrating the Dimensions of Wellness

You're juggling several college courses and a demanding job and trying to make financial ends meet. To reduce stress, you have been drinking more than you would like or perhaps indulging in salty, fatty snacks; or maybe you have been neglecting your usual exercise regimen. You want to get back on a good track but feel as if you're stuck in a rut.

Meet Erika

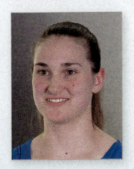

Erika is a 23-year-old student and the mother of two young children. She experienced an abusive marriage and wants to make changes in her life for herself and her children.

Erika's goal is to complete a 5K run, and while training, she hopes to return to her pre-marriage weight. View the video to learn about Erika's story and her behavior change plan and strategies. Think about how the various dimensions of wellness might influence her plan. Consider:

- How does Erika go about developing her plan? What social and environmental resources does she use? What similar types of resources are available to help you in your mission to change your behavior?
- What intellectual and other strategies does Erika use to stay motivated? What role does self-esteem play? What in Erika's experiences will help you to make positive behavior changes and improve your wellness?

VIDEO CASE STUDY   WATCH THIS VIDEO IN connect

Fast Facts

No April Fools

April 7 is World Health Day, the anniversary of the day in 1948 when the World Health Organization's constitution was adopted. On this date around the globe, thousands of events demonstrate the importance of health for happy and productive lives. Each year, World Health Day highlights a different area of WHO concern. Recent themes have included aging and health, antimicrobial resistance, and the effects of urbanization on health. Visit http://www.who .int/world-health-day/en/ to learn more.

- Choose one of the causes mentioned above in this box or on the World Heath Day site. What could you do at the local level to promote one of these campaigns?

feelings of mood, energy level, and sense of well-being—they may not feel "healthy" at all. It is in these areas that the concept of wellness can provide a useful framework for action.

Actively Working Toward Wellness

Q | Are health and wellness the same?

Health and wellness are closely related, and some people use the terms interchangeably. In this book,

![The health continuum arrow diagram: Premature death | Serious illness | Chronic disease | Minor/short-term illness | No symptoms | Optimum health]

Figure 1-1   The health continuum. At the negative end of the continuum is serious illness and premature death. At the positive end of the continuum is the capacity to enjoy life and to withstand challenges.

Sources: Adapted from Bouchard, C., Shephard, R. J., & Stephens, T. (1994). *Physical activity, fitness, and health: International proceedings and consensus statement.* Champaign, IL: Human Kinetics; *Mental health: A report of the Surgeon General.* (1999). Rockville, MD: U.S. Public Health Service.

we define the term *wellness* differently from *health.* **Wellness** is a more personalized concept than health and has several additional key characteristics:

- Wellness has multiple, clearly defined dimensions; balance is very important, but you can be at a different level of wellness for each dimension (see the next section).
- Wellness is an active process, meaning you can always work to improve your wellness status.
- Individual responsibility and choice are critical wellness components; by becoming aware of the factors that affect you and by making appropriate choices, you can significantly affect your level of wellness.
- Wellness status is a reflection of your own perceptions about your health and well-being.

Two people at similar places on the health continuum may perceive their wellness status very differently. An individual with a severe illness or impairment may still have a strong sense of well-being and may be living up to her or his full wellness potential. Wellness is determined by the decisions people make about how to live their lives with vitality and meaning.

Discovering Dimensions of Wellness

Q | Can you be physically unfit but still be happy and social at the same time?

Yes, you can. This question gets at a key aspect of wellness—that there are different dimensions, and although the dimensions are interrelated, you can be at a different level of wellness for each. A physically unfit person might not rate highly in the physical dimension of wellness but may fare much better in other dimensions, such as social and intellectual wellness. On the flip side, someone who is very fit and the picture of what we'd call physical health may rate poorly in terms of the other dimensions of wellness. True wellness requires addressing *all* the dimensions. Let's take a closer look at characteristics and behaviors associated with each of the six dimensions in our wellness model.

PHYSICAL WELLNESS. Mention physical wellness, and many will picture someone who is active and looks fit. However, physical wellness isn't only about physical fitness or appearance. **Physical wellness** is the complete physical condition and functioning of the body—both the visible aspects, such as how fit one looks, and those that are not, such as blood pressure and bone density. Throughout your life, physical wellness is reflected in your ability to accomplish your daily activities and to care for yourself.

Regular physical activity and healthy eating are the foundation behaviors of physical wellness, but they are just a beginning. Ask yourself these questions:

- Do I get enough sleep?
- Do I use alcohol and drugs responsibly?

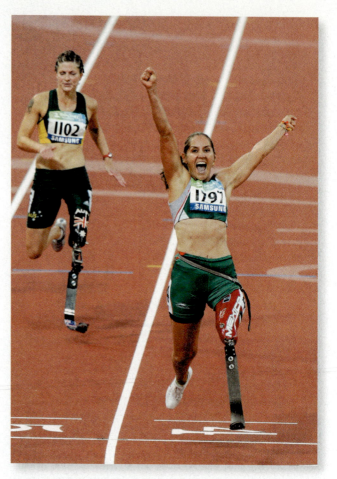

Wellness is determined by the choices people make about how to live their lives with energy and meaning. Someone with a physical impairment can achieve a high level of wellness.

- Do I make intentional and responsible sexual choices?
- Do I use sunscreen?
- Do I practice safe driving?
- Do I manage injuries and illnesses appropriately, practice self-care, and seek medical assistance when necessary?

Maintaining physical wellness means making informed health decisions on many fronts and offers many opportunities for improving your quality of life.

How does physical fitness relate to physical wellness? **Physical fitness** is the ability to carry out daily tasks with vigor and alertness, without undue fatigue, and with ample energy to enjoy leisure-time pursuits and respond to emergencies.[3] This definition ties closely with wellness and quality of life. But fitness also has

wellness An active process of adopting patterns of behavior that can improve an individual's health and perceptions of well-being and quality of life in terms of multiple, intertwined dimensions.

physical wellness Dimension of wellness referring to the complete physical condition and functioning of the body; focuses on behaviors that support physical aspects of health, including diet, exercise, sleep, stress management, and self-care.

physical fitness The ability to carry out daily tasks with vigor and alertness, without undue fatigue, and with ample energy to enjoy leisure-time pursuits and respond to emergencies.

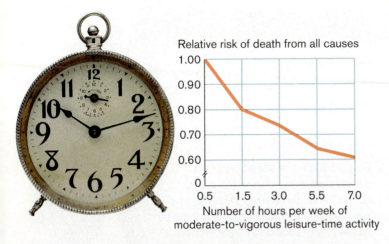

Figure 1-2 Level of physical activity and risk of death. The biggest reduction in the risk of death is at the low end of the physical activity spectrum, between people who are sedentary and people whose activity level is low or moderate; additional risk reductions accompany higher levels of physical activity.

Source: Physical Activity Guidelines Advisory Committee. (2008). *Physical Activity Guidelines Advisory Committee report, 2008.* Washington, DC: U.S. Department of Health and Human Services.

measurable components, including muscle strength and joint flexibility. Your level of fitness depends on specific physical attributes, including the functioning of your heart, lungs, blood vessels, and muscles. Importantly, good physical fitness doesn't equal good physical wellness; fitness is just one piece of physical wellness, and a person with a high fitness level can have serious risks to his or her physical health. For example, being physically fit doesn't prevent the damage that smoking does to lungs, arteries, and other body systems.

For physical wellness, you should strive for a fitness level that meets your goals for daily functioning and recreational pursuits. A certain level of fitness is needed to reap its many associated health benefits, such as reduced risk of chronic diseases like heart disease and cancer, but you don't need an extremely high level of fitness for health and wellness. Sedentary people can reap many of the benefits of fitness when they add a modest amount of activity to their daily routine (Figure 1-2).

Some individuals strive for high fitness because they have specific goals related to physical performance. For example, ballet dancers and gymnasts need a much greater degree of joint flexibility than the typical person in order to perform with excellence. Don't be discouraged from physical activity because you think you must exercise very intensely or become extremely fit in order to obtain wellness benefits. Also bear in mind that physical activity has many immediate benefits, including improved mood, reduced stress, and increased energy level.

Although all physical activity can affect wellness, not all activity builds physical fitness—for example, for most people, just walking down the hall doesn't increase measures of fitness. That usually requires **exercise**—planned,

structured, repetitive body movements specifically designed to develop physical fitness. You'll learn much more about physical activity, exercise, and physical fitness in later chapters, along with details on how to put together an exercise program that is right for you.

EMOTIONAL WELLNESS. Emotional wellness is based in your ability to carry on your day-to-day activities while understanding your feelings and expressing them in constructive and appropriate ways. It involves accepting your feelings, monitoring your emotional reactions, and recognizing your strengths and limitations. It is also exemplified by your ability to cope, manage, and adapt to normal stressors. The following qualities are associated with emotional wellness:

- Optimism
- Enthusiasm
- Trust
- Self-confidence
- Self-acceptance
- Resiliency
- Self-esteem

People with a high level of emotional wellness have a generally positive outlook and can meet challenges while maintaining emotional stability. They can deal effectively with strong feelings—they are both flexible and balanced. They can live and work autonomously while also reaching out to others. They are moreover willing to seek help for emotional problems, if needed.

INTELLECTUAL WELLNESS. Intellectual wellness is characterized by the ability to think logically and solve problems in order to meet life's challenges successfully. An active and engaged mind is vital for making sound choices related to all the dimensions of wellness. Do you relish learning new skills, solving problems, and exploring ideas? People who enjoy a high level of intellectual wellness are creative, open to new ideas, and motivated to learn new information and new skills. They actively seek ways to challenge their minds and pursue intellectual growth. They can apply critical thinking as they gather and evaluate information and use it to make sound decisions.

Every health consumer should know how to use critical thinking to evaluate the quality of online health and wellness information; see the box "Web-Surfing Safety: Finding Sound Wellness Information Online" for more information.

SOCIAL WELLNESS. Human beings are social by nature—some more than others, but all of us are social creatures.

exercise Planned, structured, repetitive body movements specifically designed to develop physical fitness.

emotional wellness Dimension of wellness that focuses on one's ability to manage and express emotions in constructive and appropriate ways.

intellectual wellness Dimension of wellness that focuses on developing and enhancing one's knowledge base and critical thinking, decision-making, and problem-solving skills.

Wellness Strategies

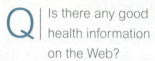

Web-Surfing Safety: Finding Sound Wellness Information Online

Q | Is there any good health information on the Web?

Yes, but it's important to examine Web sites carefully to ensure that the information is valid. Look for the following when evaluating the quality of health information on Web sites.

Consider the source: Know who is responsible for the content, and look for recognized authorities.

- Locate the "about us" page. Is the site run by a branch of the federal government, a nonprofit institution, a college or university, a professional organization, a health system, a commercial organization, or an individual?
- Use caution if the site doesn't provide a way to contact the organization or webmaster.

Focus on quality and find evidence for the claims: Ensure that information is authored by experts or reviewed and approved by an editorial board before it is posted.

- Use caution on sites that don't identify the author and that rely on testimonials and opinions rather than qualified individuals, research, or organizations.
- Look for sites with HONCode certification, meaning that they follow the code of conduct developed by the Health on the Net (HON) Foundation (http://www.hon.ch).

Be a cyberskeptic: Avoid quackery.

- Beware of claims that are too good to be true, such as a remedy that will cure a variety of illnesses, that is a "breakthrough," that will have quick and dramatic results, or that relies on a "secret ingredient."
- Avoid sites that have a sensational writing style (lots of exclamation points, for example) and those that use technical jargon or deliberately obscure—or artificially scientific-sounding—language.
- Get a second opinion. Check more than one site.

Review for currency: Look for dates on Web pages. An article on coping with the loss of a loved one doesn't need

to be current, but an article on the latest treatment of diabetes does.

Beware of bias: What is the purpose of the site? Who is funding it?

- Use caution if the site's sponsor is selling something, even if the product is only indirectly referred to on the site. Advertisements that do appear should be labeled; they should say "Advertisement" or "From our Sponsor."
- See if it is clear whether the content comes from a noncommercial source or an advertiser is providing it. For example, if a page about treatment of depression recommends one drug by name, the drug's manufacturer may have provided that information. Consult other sources to see what they say about the drug and whether others can also be used.

Protect your privacy: Health information should be confidential. Look for a privacy policy that tells you what information the site collects and what the site managers do with it. For example, if the site says "We share information with companies that can provide you with useful products," then your information isn't private.

Consult with your health professional before making any major lifestyle changes or health care decisions.

Use this information to evaluate a Web site that you consult for health and wellness information. How does the site rate on the above criteria? Is the site credible? Why or why not?

Source: Adapted from National Library of Medicine. (2006). *MedlinePlus guide to healthy Web surfing* (http://www.nlm.nih.gov/medlineplus/healthywebsurfing.html).

Social wellness is defined by the ability to develop and maintain positive, healthy, satisfying interpersonal relationships and appropriate support networks. This includes building relationships with individuals and groups both inside and outside one's family, as well as contributing to the broader community in which one lives. The ability to communicate effectively and to develop a capacity for intimacy are key elements

social wellness Dimension of wellness that focuses on one's ability to develop and maintain positive, healthy, satisfying interpersonal relationships and appropriate support networks.

of social wellness. Do you have friends or family members who you can confide in and lean on for support? Are people comfortable confiding in you and coming to you for help? Do you get along with others and communicate with respect, despite differences of opinion or values? Are you a good listener? What do you contribute to the greater community?

SPIRITUAL WELLNESS. Wellness involves more than striving for physical health; it is also a search for meaning, purpose, and fulfillment. **Spiritual wellness** means having a set of

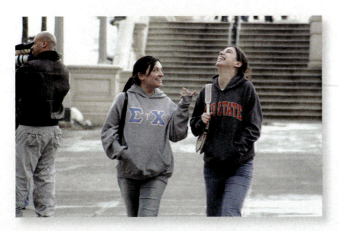

Social wellness is exemplified by positive, satisfying interpersonal relationships.

values, beliefs, or principles that give meaning and purpose to your life and help guide your choices and actions. Compassion, forgiveness, altruism (unselfish helping of others), tolerance, and the capacity for love are all qualities associated with spiritual wellness. Do the choices you make every day reflect your values and priorities? Or do you sometimes act in ways that conflict with your values?

spiritual wellness
Dimension of wellness that focuses on developing a set of values, beliefs, or principles that give meaning and purpose to life and guide one's actions and choices.

People develop and express spirituality in different ways. For some people, purpose and direction come from organized religion or the belief in a higher power in the universe; they may engage in spiritual practices such as prayer and meditation. Others may express spirituality through the arts, volunteer work, or personal relationships. See the box "It's Good to Be Good" for more information about the connection between personal wellness and volunteerism.

Spirituality is sometimes considered a controversial part of wellness models, because it touches on issues or beliefs that some people prefer to keep private and that other people feel compelled to share—or at times to press upon others. Even if talking about spirituality or specific religious issues can occasionally make people uncomfortable, spirituality is not a topic to be avoided or a less important part of personal wellness. The fact that many people become so impassioned about spiritual matters speaks to the relevance of spirituality in their lives. Regardless of the controversies and your specific beliefs, spirituality—however you may express it in your own life—is an essential part of your overall well-being. The values, beliefs, and principles you live by are an indispensable part of the whole you. As the noted neurologist and psychiatrist Viktor E. Frankl observed, "The spiritual dimension cannot be ignored, for it is what makes us human."

ENVIRONMENTAL WELLNESS. Your own wellness depends on your surroundings. Does your physical environment support your wellness or detract from it? Are there hazards in your environment—toxins such as secondhand smoke and industrial pollution, or a high degree of violence in the local community—that you should be aware

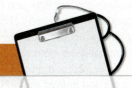

Research Brief

It's Good to Be Good

Researchers have investigated whether helping others—by participating in organized volunteer work or by providing *instrumental support* (for example, assistance with household or child-care tasks, or finances) to friends or family members—affects the health of the helper. Most studies have found clear benefits for both physical and mental health.

One recent study followed more than 7,000 older adults for eight years. The researchers found that those who were frequent volunteers had significantly reduced mortality (death from any cause). Similar benefits to health and well-being have been found for people of all ages. In another study researchers investigated the relationship between volunteering and self-reported health and happiness. Results indicate that those who volunteered reported being healthier and happier.

How does helping others improve health? The health benefits may stem from a reduction in the levels and the physiological effects of stress for people who volunteer, including changes in the levels of hormones and certain brain chemicals. Helping others may also serve to increase empathic emotions. Volunteering provides opportunities for social interaction and support as well as a distraction from one's own worries. Researchers caution, however, that helping needs to be voluntary and not overwhelming, or it won't reduce stress.

Analyze and Apply
- What lesson from the study's results can you apply to your own life?
- If you can't commit to being a regular volunteer, what random acts of kindness might you engage in each day to lighten the burden of others?

Sources: Harris, A. H., & Thoresen, C. E. (2005). Volunteering is associated with delayed mortality in older people. *Journal of Health Psychology, 10*(6), 739–752. Borgonovi, F. (2008). Doing well by doing good. The relationship between formal volunteering and self-reported health and happiness. *Social Science & Medicine, 66*(11), 2321–2334.

Wellness Strategies

Why Sustainability Matters—and What You Can Do

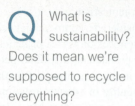

Q What is sustainability? Does it mean we're supposed to recycle everything?

Recycling is a part of sustainability, but sustainability is about more than just recycling. Sustainability rests on the idea that our very survival and well-being depend on our natural environment. Sustainability is crucial for ensuring that we have, and will continue to have, the water and other natural resources to support human health and our environment.

There are many things you can do to help the environment. Scan the following lists. Some of these practices may be beyond your ability right now, but even a few changes can make a difference.

In the dorm or at home

- Use energy-saving compact fluorescent bulbs; use natural rather than electric light when possible.
- Turn off unnecessary electrical devices when you leave a room for more than 15 minutes; unplug appliances and electronics when not in use.
- Enable your computer to go into "sleep mode" when not in use; turn your computer off overnight.
- Unplug your cell phone charger when charging is complete.
- Pull down window shades at night in the winter and during the day in the summer.
- Purchase a water filter and refill a reusable container instead of buying cases of bottled water.
- Eat locally grown foods.
- Buy inexpensive cloth napkins and washable mugs and plates rather than disposable ones.
- Turn off and defrost the refrigerator over long breaks.
- Take shorter showers; don't run the water before getting in, and turn off the water when lathering.
- Turn off the faucet while brushing your teeth and shaving.
- Report or repair leaky faucets and showerheads.
- Don't use the toilet as a garbage bin. Toss tissues and waste in trash cans.
- Only wash full laundry loads, and use cold water.
- Air-dry laundered clothing whenever possible.
- Use products containing the least amount of bleaches, dyes, and fragrances.

In the classroom or office

- Use refillable binders instead of notebooks or use a laptop.
- Recycle paper and use recycled paper.
- Take notes on both sides of paper, and use both sides when printing and photocopying.
- If it's OK with your instructor, hand in assignments by printing on both sides of the page.
- Save any single-sided pages that you've printed and use the backs to print out drafts and other things you don't have to turn in.
- Use your printer's low-quality setting to save ink.

- Bookmark Web pages instead of printing them for research.
- Edit on screen, not on paper.
- Use e-mail to minimize paper use.
- Advertise events using e-mail and by posting rather than papering the campus.

In the car

- Drive less, especially during peak traffic periods or hot days.
- Use public transportation, walk, or ride a bike.
- Shop by phone, mail, or Internet.
- Combine your errands into one trip.
- Carpool. Sharing rides reduces emissions.
- Avoid revving or idling engine over 30 seconds.
- Avoid waiting in long drive-thru lines at fast-food restaurants or banks. Park your car and go in.
- Accelerate gradually; maintain speed limit and use cruise control on the highway.
- Follow your owner's manual on recommendations for maximum economic efficiency.
- Use an energy-conserving (EC) grade of motor oil.
- Minimize air conditioning.
- Get regular engine tune-ups and car maintenance checks.
- Use EPA-certified facilities for air conditioner repairs.
- Replace your car's air filter and oil regularly.
- Keep your tires properly inflated and aligned.
- When gassing up, avoid spilling gas and don't "top off" the tank.

In the store

- Use a reusable tote bag instead of a plastic or paper bag for shopping.
- Purchase durable rather than disposable products.
- If you get a plastic bag, reuse it.
- Go vintage. Buying used clothing saves money, decreases the use of resources to make clothing, and reduces the problem of sweatshops.
- Buy used furniture and household articles.
- Buy recycled products, such as paper.
- Use environmentally safe cleaning products.

What other steps can you take to help the environment?

Adapted from United States Environmental Protection Agency—What is sustainability? http://www.epa.gov/sustainability/basicinfo.htm; Learning the Issues: Living Green http://www.epa.gov/gateway/learn/greenliving.html; and Goucher College, Tips for Students, Save the Planet—Starting With Your Little Corner of It http://www.goucher.edu/x23340.xml.

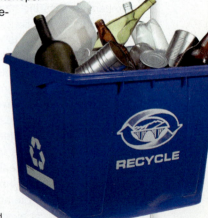

of in order to protect yourself? Are there actions you could be taking to make your world a cleaner, safer place? **Environmental wellness** recognizes the interdependence of your wellness and the condition and livability of your surroundings. You can take steps to make sure your lifestyle is respectful of the environment and helps create sustainable human and ecological communities. Do your choices reflect your awareness of the health of the planet and your place on it? See the box "Why Sustainability Matters—and What You Can Do" for some easy stops to improve your environment.

environmental wellness
Dimension of wellness that focuses on the condition and livability of the local environment and the planet as a whole.

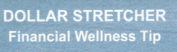

DOLLAR STRETCHER
Financial Wellness Tip

To get a handle on your finances and plan a budget, start by tracking all your income and expenses for several weeks. Many people find that by tracking expenditures, they cut back on nonessentials. Online templates are available to help you. Begin by searching for tools that are simple, free, and created for college students. If needed, you can progress to more complex models. You may also want to check out smartphone apps, many of which are free.

consider the hours, days, and years you're likely to spend at work, you can clearly see why your job choices are important to health and wellness. You want to work in environments that help you increase personal satisfaction, find enrichment and meaning, build useful skills, and contribute to your community. When you think about your potential career choices, consider your values, skills, personal qualities, and goals. Although a high-paying job may sound like the best choice, if you don't value and enjoy what you'll be doing every day, you'll gain little satisfaction from your work. Look for opportunities to learn and grow, to engage your personal interests, and to end each day feeling that your time has been well spent.

Assess your wellness status in each of these dimensions by completing Lab Activity 1-2.

OTHER WELLNESS DIMENSIONS. The wellness model in this book incorporates the six dimensions previously described—physical, emotional, intellectual, social, spiritual, and environmental. Other models may highlight different dimensions, including two we'll consider briefly here in terms of their relevance to college students: financial wellness and occupational wellness. Both can be important to wellness, and they encompass many aspects of the six dimensions we've already discussed.

Financial wellness refers to appropriate management of financial resources, a task that typically requires self-discipline and critical thinking skills. Take advantage of budgeting resources and financial planning help available on your campus and in your community (see the box "Financial Strategies for College Students"). Watch out for common financial pitfalls, including poor choices about which credit cards to get, overuse of credit cards, failure to set up a budget, and letting friends or your own unrealistic expectations pressure you into spending more than you should. Working toward wellness doesn't have to be an expensive endeavor; check the Dollar Stretcher tips throughout this book for strategies to save money while you boost your wellness.

Occupational wellness refers to the satisfaction, fulfillment, and enrichment you obtain through work. If you

Integrating the Dimensions: Recognizing Connections and Striving for Balance

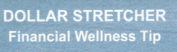

Q If you change your behavior for fitness, will that help other areas of your life too?

Absolutely. Any activity or choice that affects one dimension of wellness will directly or indirectly affect the other dimensions, and each dimension is vital in the quest for optimal wellness. For example, engaging in physical activity reduces stress and improves mood (emotional wellness) and is linked to the maintenance of cognitive functioning (intellectual wellness); it may also provide opportunities for enjoyable interaction with others (social wellness). The influence also runs in the opposite direction: strong intellectual wellness helps you plan a successful program for building fitness, and your social support system can be a huge plus as you work to change your exercise behavior.

To improve wellness, you must integrate all the dimensions of wellness with the personal choices and actions that affect your health and well-being. Balance among the dimensions is also critical for wellness. Don't focus on a few dimensions and neglect others. Doing that is like removing a few spokes from a wheel: In most ways it still looks like a wheel, but it no longer functions optimally. Figure 1-3, "Wellness Integrator," shows the close relationship among the dimensions—and with your own choices and actions. You'll also see a wellness integrator figure, tailored to each chapter's specific topic, at the start of every chapter of this book.

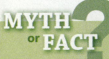

MYTH or FACT?

People spend less money when they use cash instead of a credit card.

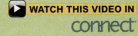

▶ **WATCH THIS VIDEO IN** connect

See page 476 to find out.

Wellness Strategies

Financial Strategies for College Students

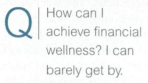

Q How can I achieve financial wellness? I can barely get by.

Financial wellness doesn't refer to being rich but rather to managing your financial resources appropriately. Money doesn't guarantee good health and happiness, but financial difficulties can strain physical, emotional, and social dimensions of wellness and thus reduce your overall well-being. A study conducted at Ohio State University's office of student affairs also correlated increased financial stress with decreased GPA. Financial security provides peace of mind and reduces stress. The big message? Live within your financial means and, when possible, save for the future.

For many traditional-age college students, money management is a relatively new experience. Unfortunately, many learn from their mistakes rather than by educating themselves up front. They build up debt while in college, not realizing the long-term implications. Although some accumulation of debt may be necessary for long-term benefit, as in the case of student loans, it's important to distinguish between necessary and unnecessary expenses and to manage resources accordingly.

Credit cards are a major financial pitfall for college students. The ease of obtaining and using credit cards can lead to unintentional and overwhelming debt. Research indicates that 84 percent of full-time undergraduate students have at least one credit card; the average number of cards is 4.6, and the average unpaid balance is nearly $3,200. As noted earlier, financial stress can negatively affect personal wellness. Research has shown a correlation between college students' credit card debt and a number of health risks, including being overweight, physical inactivity, poor nutritional habits, substance use, and violence.

Learning to develop and manage a budget is another common challenge for students. The majority of college students do not have a budget, and many who do don't stick to it. As a rule, women are more likely than men to have a budget, married students are more likely than unmarried students to follow a budget, and students over age 35 are most likely to stick to their budgets more often.

It's never too late—or too early—to make choices to improve your financial wellness. Many campuses have resources to help you develop a financial-wellness plan. If assistance is not available at your school, many reputable financial-planning tools are within reach. Your bank, credit union, or other financial institution may offer free access to Web-based financial management applications; also review the resources from the Financial Literacy & Education Commission (http://www.mymoney.gov). When you do seek financial advice, choose your sources wisely and follow up with knowledgeable individuals you trust.

Here are some specific tips to help college students stay on track financially:

- Track your income and spending carefully; you're less likely to buy on impulse when you become more aware of where your money is going.
- Be frugal: Take advantage of student discounts on everything from pizza to school supplies.
- Keep only one credit card, and use it sparingly.
- Build up an emergency fund; if you run into trouble, many colleges provide grants or emergency loans (just make sure you are using additional loan money for something related to school, like computer repair, and not an expensive spring break trip that you can't really afford).
- Develop a personal budget, and review it often.
- Use caution: Don't give out your personal account or other numbers; don't leave payments in unsecure mail boxes; and review bills and statements carefully.

Changes don't have to be huge to make a difference. What one realistic thing could you do immediately to improve your financial wellness? Are there other relatively simple steps that could have a positive impact? Visit http://www.moneymanagementtips.com/students.htm for additional tips.

Sources: SallieMae. (2009, April). *How undergraduate students use credit cards: National study of usage rates and trends 2009* (http://www.salliemae.com/about/news_info/research/credit_card_study/). Henry, R. A., Weber, J. G., & Yarbrough, D. (2001). Money management practices of college students. *College Student Journal, 35*(2), 244–249. Nelson, M., Lust, K., Story, M., & Ehlinger, E. (2008). Credit card debt, stress, and key health risk behaviors among college students. *American Journal of Health Promotion, 22*(6), 400–407.

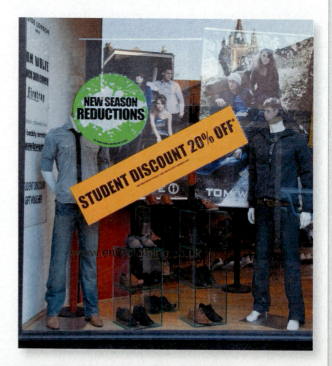

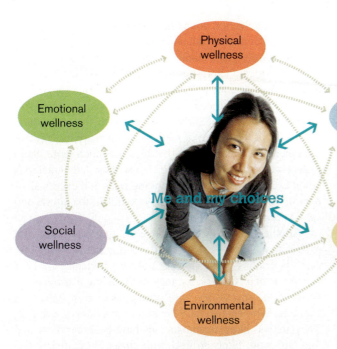

Physical wellness

Emotional wellness

Intellectual wellness

Me and my choices

Social wellness

Spiritual wellness

Environmental wellness

Figure 1-3 **Wellness Integrator.** The dimensions of wellness are linked to one another and to you and your choices.

Health in United States: The Bigger Picture

Health is an issue not only for ourselves, our family, and our friends but also for communities and the nation as a whole. A healthy population is creative and productive, the engine for economic growth. An unhealthy population raises national health care costs and lowers productivity. Tracking the health status of Americans and developing strategies for extending healthy life and reducing the burdens of illness and disability are key goals of federal health agencies.

Measures of Health and Wellness

Q | By what standards is health measured?

There is no single best measure of health. Consider the possible criteria: Is the issue how long people live? How well they live? What they die from? The rates of specific diseases and injuries? How much money people spend on health care? Different measures of health and wellness show us different things about individuals and the societies they live in.

Q | What are the chances of living to 100?

LIFE EXPECTANCY. It would depend on your age, location, and current health status. **Life expectancy** is the average number of years people born in a given year are

expected to live. Your expected life span depends on your age. A hypothetical average American born in 2007 is expected to live to age 77.9; a person who was 75 in 2007 can expect to live nearly twelve more years, to age 86.7.[4] The longer life expectancy for the 75-year-old reflects the fact that someone who has already lived to age 75 has escaped some of the causes of death common among younger individuals—and has already shown a fairly good degree of health by living to age 75.

The average life expectancy number hides some disparities. Women live longer than men (80 years versus 75 years for those born in 2007), and whites live longer than African Americans (78 years versus 73 years). And if you were wondering how life expectancy in the United States stacks up against other countries, it ranks fiftieth overall and twenty-ninth among countries with a population of 1 million or more.[5] Obviously, there's room for improvement.

Life expectancy increased dramatically in the past century. A child born in 1900 had an average life expectancy of only 47 years, compared to close to 80 years today. Much of this difference is due to decreased rates of death among infants and children. In 1900, more than 30 percent of all deaths occurred among children under age 5; today that figure is less than 2 percent.

life expectancy The average number of years people born in a given year are expected to live.

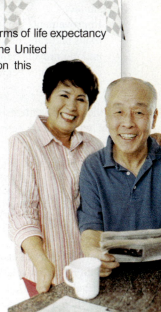

Fast Facts

Living to a Ripe Old Age

Here are the top ten countries in terms of life expectancy at birth for a child born today. (The United States ranks fiftieth, so it's not on this list.)

1. Monaco (89.73)
2. Macau
3. San Marino
4. Andorra
5. Japan
6. Guernsey
7. Singapore
8. Hong Kong
9. Australia
10. Italy (81.77)

■ Why do you think the United States is not in the top ten?

Source: Central Intelligence Agency. (2011). *The world factbook online* https://www.cia.gov/library/publications/the-world-factbook/rankorder/2102rank.html.

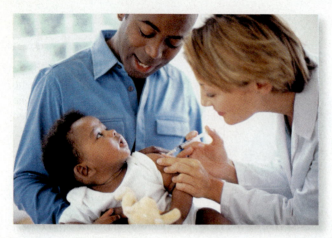

The development and use of vaccines helped increase U.S. life expectancy by dramatically reducing illness and death from infectious diseases such as smallpox, measles, mumps, diphtheria, pertussis (whooping cough), and polio.

Improvements in public health helped fuel this dramatic change in life expectancy:[6]

- Vaccinations for childhood diseases, improved sanitation, safer foods, and the development of antibiotics dramatically decreased deaths from infectious diseases like cholera, typhoid, measles, and tuberculosis.
- Better hygiene, nutrition, and health care reduced maternal and infant mortality by over 90 percent; mothers and babies are much more likely to survive and thrive today.
- Millions of smoking-related deaths were prevented by the recognition that tobacco use is a health hazard and by the subsequent anti-smoking campaigns and laws protecting nonsmokers from environmental tobacco smoke.
- Improvements in motor vehicle safety (better designed roads and cars; use of safety belts, child safety seats, and motorcycle helmets) and in workplace safety reduced motor vehicle–related deaths and occupational injuries and deaths.

Further improvements in life expectancy are possible, but they will require action by both individuals and health systems.

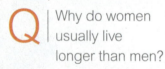

Q | Why do women usually live longer than men?

The gap in life expectancy between the sexes is due to both behavioral and biological factors. In the developing world, women do not fare as well as men due to high rates of maternal mortality (deaths related to pregnancy and childbirth). In the developed world, women live on average 5–10 years longer than men; among people over age 100 in the United States, 82.8 percent are women.[7]

One factor in men's and women's different death rates is the number of younger men who die as a result of risky and violent behavior. Young men are much more likely than young women to die from unintentional injuries (accidents), assault (murder), and suicide.[8] Is risky male behavior due to some biological factor, such as higher levels of the hormone testosterone, or does it relate to cultural norms for males? Both biological and cultural factors may play a role. With respect to suicide, the higher rate of deaths among men is a function of the choice of method: Women are more likely than men to attempt suicide, but men are much more likely to succeed because they tend to choose more lethal methods (such as a firearm). Higher smoking rates and excess alcohol consumption among men may be linked to cultural and social norms for behavior.

Another reason women have a longer average life expectancy is that they tend to develop cardiovascular disease, the leading cause of death among Americans, at a later age than men. One factor may be biological differences between the sexes—levels of hormones or iron status, for example. Women also have healthier behaviors on average: They are less likely to smoke, they have healthier diets, and they are more likely to deal with stress in positive ways, such as by seeking social support.

Both men and women can take steps to improve their lifestyle and the likelihood that they'll live a long and healthy life.

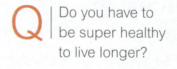

Q | Do you have to be super healthy to live longer?

QUALITY OF LIFE. Yes and no. Superior health helps, but it does not guarantee longevity—that is, a long life. A high level of health means that you are free from serious or chronic illness, at least for the moment, so you're on the positive side of the health continuum. However, many people with chronic illness live for years with symptoms of varying severity. Importantly, longevity isn't the only goal of health and wellness. You want not only *more* years but *more healthy* years, more years in which you enjoy a high quality of life.

Your overall perception of your wellness is one way to assess your quality of life. But researchers use more specific measures for research and comparative purposes. One measure is *unhealthy days,* or the estimate of the number of days of poor or impaired physical or mental health in the past 30 days. As you can see from Figure 1-4, young adults report more mentally unhealthy days, and older adults report more physically unhealthy days. It is noteworthy that young adults might be on the positive end of the health continuum because they have no symptoms, yet they rate their stress level so high that they feel unwell several days each month—a sign of definite room for improvement in several dimensions of wellness.

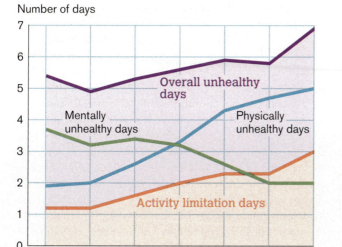

Number of days

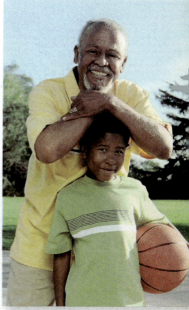

Figure 1-4 Quality of life among Americans: Unhealthy days and activity limitations during a 30-day period. Overall unhealthy days, physically unhealthy days, and days with activity limitations all increase with age, but mentally unhealthy days are highest for young adults and lowest for older adults.

Source: Centers for Disease Control and Prevention. (2005). Health-related quality of life surveillance—United States. *MMWR, 54*(SS-4).

A related measure is *years of healthy life.* The difference between life expectancy and years of healthy life is the number of years of less-than-optimal health due to chronic or acute diseases or limitations. Currently, Americans can expect an average of 68 years of life in good or better health and a life expectancy of 78 years, meaning that about 10 years will be spent in less-than-optimal health.[9] Good lifestyle choices now can help you not only to live longer but also to have more years of healthy life.

The National Healthy People Initiative

Q | Has there been any substantial improvement in physical health in the past few years in the United States, or are we all just getting less and less healthy?

Some measures of health have improved; others have worsened. For the details, check the data for Healthy People objectives. The national Healthy People initiative, sponsored by the U.S. Department of Health and Human Services, is a broad collaborative effort with the goal of improving health—the health of each individual, of communities, and of the nation. Healthy People plans, published each decade since 1990, set specific health goals framed on 10-year agendas. Progress is tracked throughout the decade, followed by the updated plan for the next 10 years.

The current plan, *Healthy People 2020,* was released in 2010. It features four overarching goals supported by

1,200 specific objectives in 42 content areas, along with national data collection strategies to track achievement. *Healthy People 2020* goals are to:[10]

- Attain high-quality, longer lives free of preventable disease, disability, injury, and premature death
- Achieve health equity, eliminate disparities, and improve the health of all groups
- Create social and physical environments that promote good health for all
- Promote quality of life, healthy development, and healthy behaviors across all life stages

The final progress report for *Healthy People 2010* was published in 2011. Here are two examples of specific objectives from *that plan* and the progress we've made—or not made:[11]

- Reduce the proportion of adults (18 and older) who engage in no leisure-time physical activity from a baseline of 40 percent to a target of 20 percent; the final figure of 36 percent means we are moving in a positive direction but have not yet met this objective.
- Reduce the proportion of college students engaging in binge drinking of alcoholic beverages (in the past month) from a baseline of 39 percent to a target of 20 percent; the final figure of 40 percent means we are farther from the target than when we started.

You can look up the *Healthy People 2020* plan or the data on all the *Healthy People 2010* objectives by visiting the Healthy People Web site: http://www.healthypeople.gov.

Leading Causes of Death

Q | How does the United States compare to other countries in terms of diseases?

We are very fortunate in this country. Consider that people in many parts of the world live in poverty and in less than desirable—sometimes even deplorable—conditions. In the developing nations, people suffer and die primarily from diseases and conditions related to the lack of necessities and basic public health measures. By comparison, people in the United States enjoy a relative abundance of resources. Yet sometimes abundance can lead to dangerous excess. Even in lower-income areas of the United

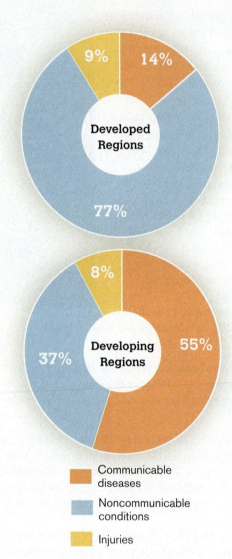

Figure 1-5 Causes of death in developed and developing regions of the world.

Source: University of California, Santa Cruz. *The UC atlas of global inequality* (http://ucatlas.ucsc.edu/cause.php).

communicable (infectious) disease
A disease that can be passed from one person to another; typically caused by a pathogen such as a bacterium or virus.

noncommunicable (chronic) disease
A disease that is not infectious or contagious; many are long-lasting or frequently recurring diseases that develop over time and are the result of the interplay of genetic, environmental, and lifestyle factors.

Communicable (infectious) diseases are those caused by a pathogen such as a bacterium or virus; they typically develop very quickly and are contagious. People who contract an infectious disease, except for serious ones like HIV infection and hepatitis, often recover completely if they receive appropriate treatment.

By contrast, **noncommunicable (chronic) diseases** are not caused by pathogens and are not contagious; they are mostly long-lasting or frequently recurring diseases that develop over time from a combination of genetic, environmental, and lifestyle factors. They include heart disease, some forms of cancer, and diabetes. People with chronic diseases must often adapt their lives to accommodate the symptoms and effects of the disease. Approximately 70 percent of the people in the United States develop and die from some form of chronic disease. (We examine chronic and infectious diseases in greater detail in Chapters 11 and 12.)

Q It seems as if everyone has some kind of cancer. Is cancer now the leading cause of death for Americans?

For many age groups, yes—but not overall (Table 1-1). Although deaths from heart disease have fallen significantly in recent decades, heart disease is still the number-one killer of Americans. Cancer tops heart disease as a cause of death for younger people, but among people age 75 and older, heart disease kills many more than cancer. As you can see from Table 1-1, these two chronic diseases—heart disease and cancer—are responsible for nearly half of all deaths in the United States each year.

Q What is the leading cause of death for young adults like most college students?

Few traditional-age college students die from heart disease or cancer, and their overall death rates are low. The top causes of death in this age group are accidents, assault (homicide), and suicide, all of which can stem from risky behaviors, violence, and depression (Figure 1-6). The chronic diseases that are the major causes of death for the population as a whole develop over many years, and their symptoms may not appear until middle or later adulthood. That doesn't mean young adults should ignore them. Your habits *now* can have a big influence on whether and when you develop a serious chronic disease.

Q What can be done to decrease the leading causes of death?

A great deal. To begin with, it's important to understand the basics about **risk factors,** which are factors that increase your susceptibility for the development, onset, or progression of a disease or an injury. Smoking is

States, the primary causes of death are linked to lifestyles. Illnesses such as diabetes and cardiovascular disease, for example, are highly correlated with lifestyle choices, including overindulgence in fat, sugar, and alcohol.

Figure 1-5 compares the general categories of leading causes of death in developing countries and developed countries. The high percentage of deaths in developing countries from communicable (infectious) diseases is similar to what was seen in the United States in 1900. In developed countries, most deaths are now due to noncommunicable (chronic) diseases.

TABLE 1-1 LEADING CAUSES OF DEATH IN THE UNITED STATES, ALL AGES

RANK	CAUSE	NUMBER OF DEATHS	PERCENTAGE OF ALL DEATHS
1	Heart disease	616,067	25.4%
2	Cancer	562,875	23.2%
3	Stroke	135,953	5.6%
4	Chronic lower respiratory diseases	127,924	5.3%
5	Accidents (unintentional injuries)	123,706	5.1%
6	Alzheimer's disease	74,632	3.1%
7	Diabetes	71,382	2.9%
8	Influenza and pneumonia	52,717	2.2%
9	Kidney disease	46,488	1.9%
10	Septicemia (systemic blood infection)	34,828	1.4%

Source: National Center for Health Statistics. (2011). Deaths: Leading causes for 2007. *National Vital Statistics Reports, 59*(8).

risk factor A behavior or a characteristic that increases susceptibility for the development, onset, or progression of a disease or an injury.

an example of a risk factor; smokers are far more likely to develop heart disease and cancer than nonsmokers. Not wearing a safety belt is another risk factor; if you don't buckle up, you are far more likely to be seriously injured in a crash than is a consistent seat belt user.

Risk factors are of two types—those that cannot be changed and those that can be changed. Age is a common risk factor for chronic disease that you can't change; for example, years of wear and tear on your joints increase the risk of developing arthritis. However, you can change other risk factors for arthritis, such as excess body weight. Most chronic diseases develop from a combination of risk factors, some of which are under your control. In short, through your own actions, you can reduce your risk for most major chronic diseases and types of injuries. Later in this chapter, we'll review the components of a wellness lifestyle that can help you both increase wellness and reduce the risk of health problems throughout your life.

Q | How many people die from obesity?

Obesity isn't on the list of leading causes of death among Americans. However, it is an important

underlying cause of many chronic diseases. Researchers have examined the lifestyle and environmental factors that contribute to the leading causes of death, and they have identified and ranked what they call the *actual* causes of death (Table 1-2). Obesity appears near the top of this list, because it contributes to heart disease, cancer, and diabetes, among other serious health conditions. Large decreases in life expectancy have been seen in obese people: Among individuals who were obese at age 40, women lost 7.1 years of life and men lost 5.8 years.[12] Being overweight, even though not obese, is also associated with reduced life expectancy.

Tobacco use (including smoking and secondhand smoke exposure) is actually the leading preventable cause of death in the United States. Individuals who are obese and subject to the effects of tobacco use may face even greater complications and lost years of life.[13] All the factors in Table 1-2 are included in the discussion of a wellness lifestyle on pp. 17–22.

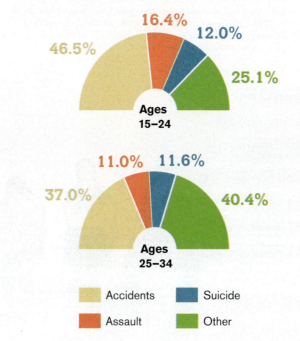

Figure 1-6 Leading causes of death among young adults. Young adults are most likely to die from causes related to risky behavior and violence.

Source: National Center for Health Statistics. (2010). Deaths: Leading causes for 2006. *National Vital Statistics Reports 58*(14).

TABLE 1-2 ACTUAL CAUSES OF DEATH AMONG AMERICANS

CAUSE	NUMBER OF DEATHS PER YEAR	PERCENTAGE OF TOTAL DEATHS PER YEAR
Tobacco	440,000	18.1%
Obesity (poor diet and inactivity)	112,000	4.6%
Alcohol consumption	85,000	3.5%
Microbial agents	75,000	3.1%
Toxic agents	55,000	2.3%
Motor vehicles	43,000	1.8%
Firearms	29,000	1.2%
Sexual behavior	20,000	0.8%
Illicit drug use	17,000	0.7%

Sources: Flegal, K., Graubard, B., Williamson, D., & Gail, M. (2005). Excess deaths associated with underweight, overweight, and obesity. *JAMA, 293,* 1861–1867. Mokdad, A., Marks, J., Stroup, D., & Gerberding, J. (2004). Actual causes of death in the United States, 2000. *JAMA, 291,* 1238–1245 [original study]. Mokdad, A., Marks, J., Stroup, D., & Gerberding, J. (2005). Correction: Actual causes of death in the United States, 2000 (letter). *JAMA, 293*(3), 293–294.

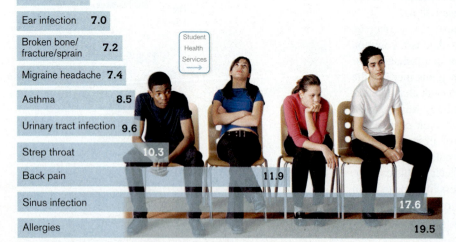

Bronchitis	6.4
Ear infection	7.0
Broken bone/fracture/sprain	7.2
Migraine headache	7.4
Asthma	8.5
Urinary tract infection	9.6
Strep throat	10.3
Back pain	11.9
Sinus infection	17.6
Allergies	19.5

Student Health Services →

Percentage of students diagnosed or treated for the problem within the last year

Figure 1-7 Most common health problems reported by college students

Source: American College Health Association. (2011). *American College Health Association national college health assessment II: Reference group executive summary spring 2011.* Baltimore, MD: 2011.

Health and Wellness on Campus

Q | What are the main health and wellness concerns of college students?

Many college students ignore their health and push their limits in terms of stress, lack of sleep, relationship strain, and poor time management. Even if the hectic life of a college student doesn't lead to illness, it can leave one feeling exhausted, overwhelmed, and generally unwell. In a recent survey in which over 80,000 college students identified health problems that affected them during the previous school year, back pain and allergies topped the list.

As Figure 1-7 shows, most health problems reported by students aren't of the chronic variety. Many are short-lived and curable. Why then should they be such a concern? The reason is that although the physical effects on the body may be short-lived, these health problems also affect other areas of life.

Are the academic, financial, time-management, and relationship effects all short term, or do some have long-term implications? Table 1-3 shows a range of common health issues that affect the academic life of college students. The high percentages of students reporting these health problems also indicate that students' health behaviors are not optimal and that there is plenty of room for improvement in multiple wellness dimensions. Students whose academic performance is being hurt by stress, sleep difficulties, depression, anxiety, relationships difficulties, or alcohol use are certainly not living up to their full wellness potential.

The truth is that when it comes to your health, any problem may produce longer-term consequences than just a missed class or two. Your finances, your relationships, and your risk for chronic conditions are among the many aspects of life that can be affected. How do you break the cycle—or at least interrupt it? It comes back to that issue of risk and responsibility. It's up to you to make good choices and to avoid risk when you can. That's where a wellness lifestyle comes into play: Make choices every day that will help boost your health and well-being now and in the future.

Factors Influencing Individual Health and Wellness

Although this book stresses the role of individual choice and behavior in health and wellness, those aren't the only factors. You have the most

TABLE 1-3 ACADEMIC IMPACT OF SELECTED HEALTH PROBLEMS*

	PERCENTAGE OF STUDENTS REPORTING AN ACADEMIC IMPACT
Stress	27.5%
Sleep difficulties	19.4%
Anxiety	19.1%
Cold/flu/sore throat	16.4%
Depression	11.9%
Concern for a troubled friend or family member	11%
Relationship difficulties	10.5%
Sinus infection/ear infection/bronchitis/ strep throat	5.7%
Alcohol use	4.4%

*Academic impacts include a lower grade on an exam or important project; a lower grade in a course; an incomplete or dropping a course; or a significant disruption in thesis, dissertation, research, or practicum work.

Source: American College Health Association. (2011). American College Health Association national college health assessment II: Reference group executive summary spring 2011. Baltimore, MD: ACHA.

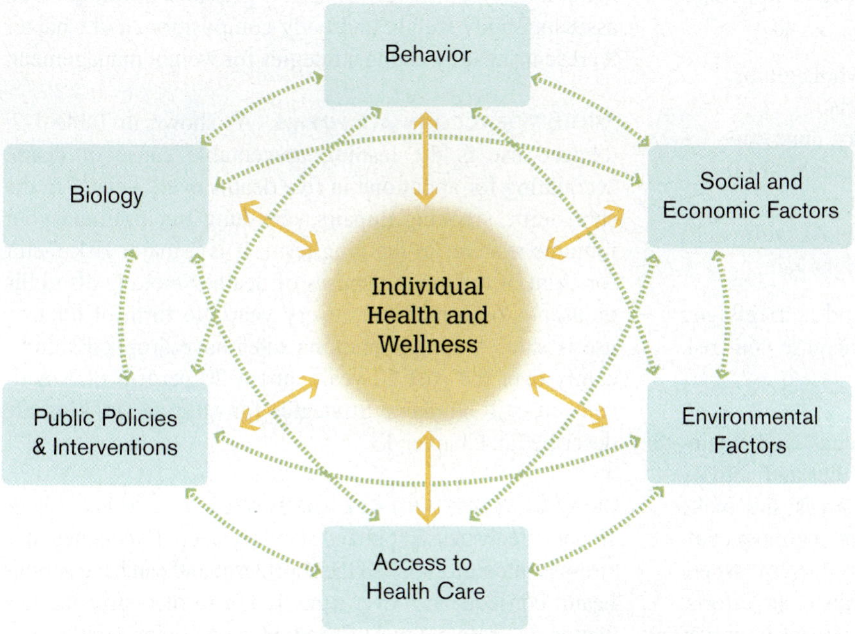

Figure 1-8 Factors determining health and wellness status.

control over your individual lifestyle choices, but it's important to be aware of all the other influences on your well-being. Even for those you can't control or change, you can make choices to help improve wellness. For example, even though a condition like high blood pressure may be common in your family—a reality that increases your personal risk of developing it—genetics isn't the only risk factor. You can make choices such as limiting the salt in your diet and getting regular blood pressure checks that can help both to reduce the risk of developing high blood pressure and to limit its adverse effects if you do develop the condition. In this section, we'll review various influences on individual health and wellness, with special attention to health-related behavior choices (Figure 1-8). Just as the dimensions of wellness interact, so do the factors that determine your health and wellness status.

Wellness Behavior Choices

Q | What basic things should I do every day or every week for a healthy lifestyle?

Your day-to-day decisions and actions affect all dimensions of wellness—physical, emotional, intellectual, social, spiritual, environmental—as well as your overall health status and risk for chronic diseases and premature death. Let's look at some best practices.

BE PHYSICALLY ACTIVE. Your body is designed to function best when it is active—and busy isn't the same thing as active. Because so much of contemporary life is tied to technologies that keep us sedentary, most people need to purposely plan time for physical activity. It's well worth the time and effort. Physically active individuals live longer and healthier lives (see Figure 1-2). And many of the benefits of physical activity are immediate: It reduces stress and anxiety, helps you sleep better, and boosts your mood and self-esteem. Chapter 3 goes into much more detail about the benefits of physical activity and physical fitness, and later chapters will guide you in putting together an exercise program that is right for you.

CHOOSE A HEALTHY DIET. Think about *diet* as your daily eating habits, not as a temporary restriction of the foods you eat. Eating well means choosing more healthful foods and fewer harmful foods, most of the time. Nutrition and dietary planning will be

Research Brief

Healthy Living Counts . . . and Every Choice Matters

A great deal of research has gone into tying specific behaviors to health outcomes—smoking to lung cancer, for example. But it's also important to consider the effects of *combinations* of lifestyle factors. For example, if you smoke, does it matter if you lose weight? If you exercise regularly, is any extra benefit gained from a healthy diet?

Researchers recently examined data on more than 20,000 adults who were tracked for an average of 8 years. They looked at healthy lifestyle factors in relation to the study participants' risk of developing a major chronic disease (diabetes, heart attack, stroke, cancer). In the analysis, participants were awarded one point for each of four healthy lifestyle factors:

■ Never having smoked
■ Engaging in physical activity for 3.5 or more hours per week
■ Having a healthy dietary pattern (high intake of fruits, vegetables, and whole grains, and low meat consumption)
■ Having a body mass index (BMI) below 30 (BMI is a single number representing weight-to-height ratio; a BMI below 30 means that the person is not obese)

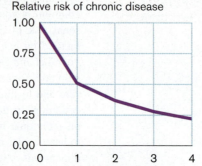

Relative risk of chronic disease

Number of healthy lifestyle factors

Researchers found that the risk of developing a chronic disease decreased progressively as the number of healthy factors increased. People with all four healthy factors had nearly an 80 percent lower risk of developing a chronic disease than participants without a healthy factor. But risk was also reduced for people with one, two, or three healthy factors. The risk reduction was most striking for diabetes, for which having one healthy factor lowered risk by more than 60 percent and having all four healthy factors lowered risk by 93 percent compared to having no healthy factors.

Analyze and Apply

■ Based on the research, what big conclusion might we draw regarding the impact of a healthy lifestyle on the risk for chronic disease?
■ What did the researchers learn about the effect of changing even one unhealthy behavior?
■ What is one unhealthy behavior that you can start changing *now*?

Source: Ford, E. S., and others. (2009). Healthy living is the best revenge. *Archives of Internal Medicine, 169*(15), 1355–1362.

---

discussed in detail in Chapters 8 and 9. General guidelines for healthy eating include the following:

■ Eat more fruits, vegetables, legumes, whole grains, fish, and low-fat or nonfat dairy products.
■ Consume fewer sugary foods and drinks, unhealthy fats, refined carbohydrates, salty foods, and full-fat dairy products, as well as less red meat.
■ Balance your overall energy (calorie) intake with your level of physical activity to prevent weight gain.

A healthy diet will give you the energy and nutrients you need today and limit the substances that increase your risk for chronic diseases in the future.

MAINTAIN A HEALTHY WEIGHT. Achieving and maintaining a healthy weight depend on your diet and activity habits—and on your ability to manage stress and make sound choices. A healthy weight is perhaps the most challenging lifestyle goal to achieve in our society, where environmental influences often work against our efforts. But even modest success at weight management improves health, reduces chronic disease risk, and makes people feel better about themselves. Chapter 7 provides information on assessing body weight and body composition, and Chapter 9 presents healthy eating strategies for weight management.

AVOID TOBACCO IN ALL FORMS. As shown in Table 1-2, tobacco use is the leading preventable cause of death, accounting for about one in five deaths every year.[14] In the short term, smoking impairs your lung function and your immune system; in the long term, it is a major risk factor for eight of the top ten causes of death. Smoking also kills thousands of nonsmokers every year. No form of tobacco use is safe. Although smoking rates have dropped significantly over the past 50 years, about 20 percent of Americans are still smokers. Strategies for quitting smoking are described in Chapter 13.

MANAGE STRESS AND GET ADEQUATE SLEEP. Many college students feel stressed out and short on sleep. Excess negative stress is uncomfortable in the short term and can have serious health consequences over time. Learn to recognize the key causes of stress in your life and develop coping strategies—time management, social support, exercise, a relaxation

Fast Facts

Too Much TV Is Harmful to Your Health

Even for people who exercise, spending too much time sitting increases the risk of dying. One study found that every hour spent watching TV each day (3 hours versus 2 hours per day, for example) increased

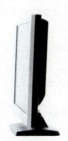

the risk of an early death from heart disease by up to 18 percent. The technologies of modern life may work against efforts to boost physical activity, but you do have control over your leisure time. Turn off that TV. Move more and sit less.

■ How many hours do you spend each day in front of the TV—or sitting and using other electronic devices? Track your screen time for a week to see how your numbers stack up.

Source: Dunstan, D. W., and others. (2010). Television viewing time and mortality. *Circulation, 121*(3), 384–391.

technique. Don't turn to alcohol, tobacco, or overeating in an effort to reduce stress; they are ineffective and harmful to your health in other ways. Adequate sleep is one of the best strategies for reducing stress and improving your ability to cope. For more on stress management, see Chapter 10.

LIMIT ALCOHOL CONSUMPTION. If you drink alcohol, do so moderately and in situations that don't put yourself or others at risk. Excess alcohol consumption damages the body, and intoxication is linked to high risk of injuries and violence. See Chapter 13 for more on the health effects of alcohol.

AVOID RISKY BEHAVIORS. Risky behaviors such as the following greatly increase the likelihood of an injury or illness:

■ Dangerous driving, including driving at high speeds, driving while distracted, and not wearing a safety belt
■ Unsafe handling of firearms
■ Unprotected sexual activity, which carries the risk of sexually transmitted infections
■ Not using appropriate safety equipment during sports and

recreational activities (for example, helmets and personal flotation devices) or during work activities (for example, goggles, gloves, helmets)
■ Drug or alcohol intoxication, which can be dangerous in itself (for example, alcohol poisoning) and can also lead to other risky behaviors, including unintentional injuries and violence

Make safety a priority for yourself and those around you. Most safety-related behaviors aren't complicated, but they can be challenging in some circumstances. Use common sense, plan ahead, and don't let peer pressure or lack of commitment get in the way of safe choices.

Behaviors related to safe driving deserve special mention. Motor vehicle crashes are the leading cause of death for Americans ages 5–34.[15] People don't think of driving as a risky behavior, but it is probably the most dangerous thing most of us do on any given day. Treat driving with the attentiveness it deserves, and always drive (or ride) safely. Pay attention, don't speed, wear your seat belt, don't tailgate, and use signals before turning or changing lanes. Just because you've previously gotten away with driving too fast—or while distracted by texting, talking, or changing the station—doesn't mean you will be so lucky next time.

LIMIT EXPOSURE TO RADIATION AND TOXINS. Exposure to pollutants and other environmental toxins is a risk factor for a number of health problems. The most common source of radiation exposure is sunlight. Always use sunscreen, and don't use tanning lamps (see Chapter 11). Have X-rays only when they are medically necessary. If you live or work in an area with high pollution levels—for example, in a building that may have high levels of radon or asbestos—take appropriate steps to protect yourself. You can boost the environmental wellness of your community through such strategies as recycling, reducing driving time, saving energy and water, and disposing of hazardous wastes properly. For more on limiting your exposure to toxins and on improving the environment, visit the Web site for the U.S. Environmental Protection Agency (http://www.epa.gov).

DOLLAR STRETCHER
Financial Wellness Tips

Reduce your spending on beverages. College students spend billions each year on beer and soft drinks. Different choices could benefit your health and your wallet.

PRACTICE GOOD SELF-CARE. To reduce your risk of infections, wash your hands frequently and limit your exposure to people who are ill with colds or the flu. Practice good dental care by brushing and flossing regularly. Use over-the-counter remedies carefully, following the label instructions. For more on avoiding and treating infectious diseases, see Chapter 12.

Fast Facts

Driving Distracted?

On average, drivers spend about 10 percent of their driving time on the phone. Here are some unsettling details about that experience:

- Drivers phone and text even at the riskiest times (in bad weather and heavy traffic, for example).
- More than 40 percent of drivers ages 18–29 text while driving, even in states with texting bans.
- People are less likely to talk on handheld phones in states that ban the practice, but the bans are frequently ignored.
- Using a hands-free phone does not reduce the risk of crashes; the mental distraction of talking on the phone is the same for every type of phone.

And it's not just calling and texting that distract the average driver. In a recent survey of 2,800 U.S. drivers, subjects reported the following activities while driving:

- 57 percent often eat or drink.
- 21 percent frequently or sometimes set/change their GPS.
- 10 percent often or sometimes read a map.
- 10 percent regularly comb or style their hair.
- 7 percent frequently apply makeup.

- 9 percent often or sometimes search the Internet.
- 7 percent say they often or sometimes watch videos.

For safety, limit all types of distractions while driving. Keep your eyes on the road, your hands on the wheel, and your mind on what you're doing. For more information, visit http://www.distraction.gov.

- What do you recommend to stop the dangerous practices of calling or texting while driving? What penalty should violators face?
- Which of the distractions mentioned in this box, if any, have you engaged in while driving? How did the experience make you feel in terms of your safety and that of other drivers? Did you ever have a close call?

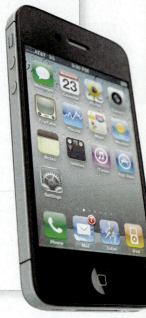

Sources: Insurance Institute for Highway Safety. (2010). Phoning while driving. *Status Report, 45*(2), 1–8. Ishigami, Y., & Klein, R. M. (2009). Is a hands-free phone safer than a handheld phone? *Journal of Safety Research, 40*(2), 157–164. Gardner, A. (2012). Most U.S. drivers engage in "distracting" behaviors: Poll. *Health Day*. Retrieved from http://www.healthfinder.gov/news/newsstory.aspx?Docid=659288&source=govdelivery.

If you have a chronic or recurring medical condition—asthma, diabetes, or migraine headaches, for example—follow your health care provider's instructions for managing it. Take preventive medications if you need them. Having a chronic condition is challenging but it doesn't mean you can't achieve optimal wellness. Take whatever actions you can to manage your condition and limit its impact on your life; see the box "Living Well with . . . Migraine Headaches" in this chapter and look for other Living Well with . . . boxes throughout the book for tips and strategies about managing common chronic conditions.

SEEK APPROPRIATE MEDICAL CARE. Don't wait to visit a health care provider until you're sick. Get recommended checkups, screening tests, and immunizations. Don't ignore symptoms that should be evaluated by a doctor; if you aren't sure, you can usually call or e-mail a doctor's office, a clinic, or your campus health center for advice. And don't neglect your mental health; if symptoms of emotional or psychological problems are interfering with your daily life, seek help. For additional advice on evaluating symptoms, treating minor medical problems, and getting appropriate tests and vaccines, visit the Web site

of the American Academy of Family Physicians (http://familydoctor.org).

APPLY CRITICAL THINKING SKILLS AS A HEALTH CONSUMER. Evaluating health Web sites (see p. 6) is only one of the ways to use critical thinking skills for health and wellness. A high level of intellectual wellness can also help you navigate the complex U.S. health care system, with its many products, services, and professionals. Other wellness-related tasks that require critical thinking skills include reading food and drug labels, considering the risks and benefits of various tests and treatments, evaluating health insurance plans, and communicating with health care providers. Keep asking questions and searching for answers. See the box "Understanding Health Headlines" to learn more about analyzing and interpreting the results of medical research studies—and their meaning for you.

CULTIVATE RELATIONSHIPS AND SOCIAL SUPPORT. Strong relationships provide emotional and material support. Spend time with the people who are important to you. Don't neglect family and friends when you are busy—make time

Living *Well* with . . .

Migraine Headaches

For those who get migraine headaches, the experience can be debilitating. These recurring, severe headaches cause pulsing or pounding pain, usually on one side of the head, often accompanied by nausea, vomiting, and sensitivity to light and sound. They can last from 6 to 48 hours. For some people, migraines are preceded by warning symptoms known as an aura—visual disturbances consisting of zigzag patterns of flashing lights, blind spots, and tunnel vision. Many people experience a "zombie phase" or "migraine hangover" of fatigue and lethargy after an attack. Migraines can be brought on by a variety of triggers, including bright lights, certain foods and food additives, stress, changes in weather, and hormonal changes (in women).

Research has revealed that migraines are related to a wave of nerve cell activity that sweeps across the brain, affecting nerve pathways and brain chemicals. Researchers are beginning to investigate gene mutations that may cause this abnormal activity in brain cells. Migraines may run in families, and they occur more frequently in women than in men.

There is no cure for migraines, but they can be managed. The goal is to identify and avoid triggers. If you get migraines, keep a headache diary for a while and record the following information:

- When you got the migraine and its severity
- What you've eaten
- How much sleep you've had
- For women, where you are in your menstrual cycle
- Other factors that may have an effect, including stress

If you start to get migraine symptoms, act quickly to treat them. You may be able to reduce or prevent further symptoms by taking these steps:

- Drink water to avoid dehydration.
- Rest in a quiet, dark room with your eyes closed. Try out some of the relaxation techniques discussed in Chapter 10.
- Place a cool cloth on your head.

Over-the-counter pain relievers and nausea medicines may help manage symptoms during a migraine. There are also prescription medications that can reduce the number of attacks, stop the headache once it starts, and treat pain and other symptoms.

The best way to prevent migraines is to modify your habits and environment to avoid triggers:

- Avoid the personal triggers you have identified through your headache diary.
- Avoid smoking, alcohol, artificial sweeteners, and other known food-related triggers.
- Get regular exercise.
- Get enough sleep.
- Learn to manage stress.

Don't let migraines stop you from living well. Further information about treatment and support is available from the American Council for Headache Education (http://www.achenet.org), the American Migraine Foundation (http://www.americanmigrainefoundation.org), and the National Headache Foundation (http://www.headaches.org).

Sources: MedlinePlus. (2009). Migraine (http://www.nlm.nih.gov/medlineplus/ency/article/000709.htm). Dodick, D. W., & J. J. Gargus. (2008, August). Why migraines strike. *Scientific American*, 56–73.

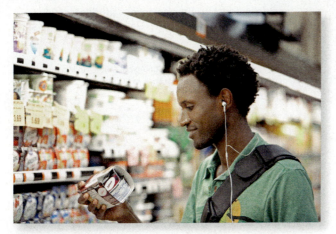

Use your critical thinking skills to read and understand the information on food, supplement, and drug labels—and to know what that information means for you.

for them. Be supportive and kind, and expect that friendships will have ups and downs. Communicate acceptance and respect.

NOURISH YOUR SPIRITUAL SIDE. Don't neglect spiritual wellness. Consider the values and principles that are important to you, and ask yourself if you need to make changes in your life to be true to them.

- When making decisions, stop and consider your options: Which choice is most consistent with your values? Don't allow expediency or peer pressure to have undue influence over your actions. Your choices and actions tell those around you what you stand for.
- Are you currently engaging in any spiritual practices or expressing your spirituality in other ways? Find an activity or organization that fits your values and your schedule.

Wellness Strategies

Understanding Health Headlines

Q | How do I know which research studies have good information?

Every day, you can find hundreds of news stories related to health. You can use your critical thinking skills to evaluate news reports about medical research findings and to determine whether the results might be important for you.

Types of research studies and findings: Studies using animals or cells in test tubes can provide important information but don't often lead directly to treatments or lifestyle advice for people. Initial studies about people are often *observational* or *correlation studies*, in which researchers track a group of people over time but don't try to change their behavior or provide special treatments. Observational studies can find associations, but they do not establish cause-and-effect relationships.

Clinical or *experimental studies* look for cause-and-effect relationships by comparing a treatment group with a control group. For example, in tests of a new drug, people in the treatment group are given the drug and those in the control group receive a *placebo* (an inactive pill) instead; then a specific health outcome between the two groups is compared. The most meaningful clinical studies have a large number of participants, are *randomized* (meaning that participants are randomly assigned to either the treatment or the placebo group), and are *double-blind* (meaning that neither the participants nor the researchers know who is receiving the treatment and who is receiving the placebo).

Research results are often reported in terms of risk

- *Relative risk* is a ratio or percentage expressing the comparative risk between two groups, such as a 50 percent reduced risk of heart attack in people who took a particular medication or engaged in a particular behavior.
- *Absolute risk* is a number expressing the incidence of a disease or event in a group, such as 25 heart attacks in every 1,000 people.

It's often important to know both numbers. Say your absolute risk of developing a disease is 8 in 1,000. If a treatment reduces the relative risk by 50 percent, it would reduce your absolute risk to 4 in 1,000—not a big change, but if the disease in question is serious or fatal, then any risk reduction might be beneficial.

Questions to ask about a new medical finding

- Was it a study in the laboratory, with animals, or with people? The results of research with people are more likely to be meaningful for you.
- Does the study include people like you? Were the participants the same age, sex, educational level, income group, and ethnic background as yourself? Did they have the same health concerns?
- Was it a randomized, double-blind, controlled clinical trial involving thousands of people? This type of study is the most expensive, but it also gives scientists the most reliable results.
- Are the results presented in a precise, easy-to-understand way? They should use absolute risk, relative risk, or some other uncomplicated number.
- If a new treatment was being tested, were there side effects? Sometimes side effects are almost as serious as the disease.
- Who paid for the research? Take special care in evaluating research that was partly or fully funded by a company that stands to gain financially from the results.
- Who is reporting the results? Is the newspaper, television station, or Web site a reliable source of medical news? Was the report written by a reporter who is trained to interpret medical findings?

Talk with your health care provider before changing your lifestyle or medications on the basis of health headlines. Progress in medical research takes years, and findings must be duplicated by other scientists at different locations before they become part of accepted medical practice.

Source: Adapted from National Institute on Aging. (2006, November). *Understanding risk: What do those headlines really mean?* (http://www.nia.nih.gov/HealthInformation/Publications/risk.htm).

HAVE FUN! Don't make a chore of your efforts to achieve good health and wellness. Wellness is about living with joy and vitality. Cultivate your sense of humor: Laughter improves health and makes you and everyone around you feel better.

How do your health habits compare with the description of a healthy lifestyle in this section? If you're like most people, you are doing well in some areas but could improve in others.

You can use Lab Activity 1-1 to identify areas of concern for you. In Chapter 2, you'll learn more about strategies and techniques for making changes in your health behaviors to improve wellness in both the short and the long term.

Fast Facts

Be a Volunteer

More than one in four Americans (26.8 percent of the population) age 16 years and older volunteer each year, for an average of about 50 hours per year. Women are more likely to volunteer than men, and rates of volunteerism also go up with education level. Popular volunteer activities are fundraising, preparing and distributing food, general labor, and supervising youth sports teams. Others include visiting homebound seniors, tutoring low-income kids, helping out at an animal shelter, and getting involved in a church.

Volunteering pays significant personal dividends. It doesn't matter what you do—just find an organization and activity you want to support and get involved. You'll boost your wellness as well as serve your community.

- What people, activities or organizations are most important to you?
- How can you get involved in helping?

Source: U.S. Department of Labor, Bureau of Labor Statistics. *Current population survey* (http://www.bls.gov).

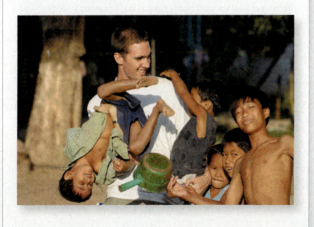

Other Factors That Influence Wellness

Q | Is my health mostly dependent on my genes and family history?

Genetic inheritance can affect your risk for certain diseases, but in most cases, your genes are just one factor in your disease risk and overall health status. Some relatively rare diseases and disorders are caused by a single gene, but most diseases stem from a complex combination of biological, behavioral, and environmental factors.

Nevertheless, it is important to know your family health history. If you are aware that you are at elevated risk for a particular condition—for example, alcoholism or high cholesterol—you can make informed lifestyle choices to reduce that risk. Someone with a family history of high cholesterol can reduce her personal risk by choosing a diet low in saturated fat and high in fiber and by getting regular exercise.

Sometimes it can be difficult to separate the effects of genetic inheritance from those of health habits; many of us have copied the eating patterns and exercise habits of our parents or caregivers. So, you might have "inherited" both a genetic predisposition for high cholesterol and an eating pattern that increases your risk. Although you can't do anything about your genes, you can change your eating habits for the better.

In the previous section of the chapter, we looked at lifestyle behaviors that affect health and wellness. Let's look next at other factors that influence wellness.

BIOLOGY. Your biology includes your genetic makeup, family health history, and any mental or physical problems you may have developed. Certain health habits, such as smoking and drinking, can "change" your biology by altering the functioning of your cells and organs. Your age and sex can also be considered part of your biology—and both have a big effect on your health and wellness. But again, lifestyle choices can help reduce the impact of biology. For example, although bone density inevitably decreases with age, a healthy diet and regular weight-bearing exercise throughout your life help maintain bone density and reduce your risk of falling.

As described on p. 12, the health differences between the sexes may be due to a mix of biological, behavioral, and cultural factors. Sex differences that have a biological basis include the following:

- Men are taller, have more muscle mass, and are more likely to store excess body fat in the abdomen; women are shorter, have relatively less muscle mass (especially in the upper body), and are more likely to store excess body fat around the hips.
- Men have denser bones than women and have lower rates of osteoporosis (loss of bone mass that can lead to fractures).
- Women have a higher risk of lung cancer than men at a given level of exposure to cigarette smoke, and they become more intoxicated at a given level of alcohol intake.
- Women have stronger immune systems than men and are less susceptible to infectious diseases, but they have higher rates of autoimmune disorders.
- Women are more likely than men to be infected with a sexually transmitted disease during intercourse and are more likely to suffer severe effects, including infertility.
- Men are more likely than women to have cardiovascular disease and classic heart attack symptoms like chest pain; women are more likely to have atypical symptoms such as difficulty breathing and extreme fatigue.

Mind Stretcher
Critical Thinking Exercise

What health habits did your parents and other family members have when you were growing up? Were family members active or sedentary? Did they smoke? What kinds of foods did they eat? How have your health habits been influenced by those of your family members and others with whom you grew up?

What about race or ethnicity? As with sex and gender, health differences among population groups usually stem from a mixture of factors—some biological/genetic and some based on lifestyle, culture, or socioeconomic factors. For example, Latinos have higher rates of diabetes than African Americans and Caucasians, and African Americans have above-average rates of high blood pressure. Just like knowing your family's health history, it's important to be aware of any health conditions for which you may be at elevated risk due to your ethnicity; in some cases, earlier or more frequent screening may be advisable. For more information, visit the Web site for the CDC Office of Minority Health and Health Disparities (http://www.cdc.gov/omhd).

SOCIAL AND ECONOMIC FACTORS. Your social environment includes all your interactions with people in your community. It also includes social institutions such as schools and law enforcement as well as factors such as the quality of housing, the availability of public transportation, and the level of violence.

The economic level of a community has a big impact on its citizens' health: Lower-income communities are likely to have a worse physical environment (more pollutants and toxins), higher rates of violence, and lower-quality health care than affluent communities. Lower-income people have higher rates of many unhealthy habits, including smoking and poor dietary choices; they are also more likely to be exposed to toxins and to be injured on the job. Income is closely tied to educational attainment. People with low incomes and a low level of education have the worst health status. See the box "The Health Burdens of Poverty and Lack of Education" for further insight into how poverty, education, and health are connected.

ENVIRONMENTAL FACTORS. The physical environment can harm health if it is high in pollutants or physical hazards. Environmental factors can also be positive, as in the case of a community that has many places to buy fruits and vegetables and an extensive network of walking trails and bicycle lanes. People with lower incomes and educational attainment are more likely to live in communities with harmful environmental factors. Look around your

Fast Facts

Smoking by the Numbers

Cigarette smoking is estimated to be responsible for $193 billion in annual health-related economic losses in the United States (for direct medical costs and lost productivity); this translates into $10.47 per pack of cigarettes. An estimated 46 million people, or 20.6 percent of all adults in the United States, currently smoke cigarettes, and smoking kills about 443,000 Americans a year. Worldwide, smoking kills about 5 million people a year, meaning that about one smoker dies every 6 seconds.

- Given that the costs and ill effects of smoking are widely known, why would someone start smoking in the first place?
- What factors might cause that individual to keep smoking?

Sources: Centers for Disease Control and Prevention. (2011). *Smoking and tobacco use* (http://www.cdc.gov/tobacco). World Health Organization. (2011). *Tobacco free initiative* (http://www.who.int/tobacco).

own community for factors or conditions that can enhance or harm health.

ACCESS TO HEALTH CARE. Access, or lack of access, to quality health care underlies many of the health disparities in the United States. Although excellent health care is

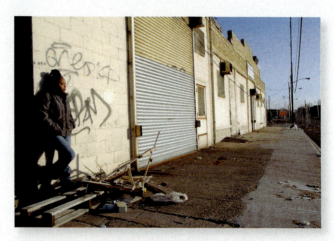

Lower-income communities are usually associated with additional health risks, including more toxins and pollutants in the physical environment, lower-quality housing and health care, and higher rates of violence.

Research Brief

The Health Burdens of Poverty and Lack of Education

Poverty and high school dropout rates pose serious social and economic challenges, but perhaps they are even more problematic in relation to health. Researchers recently analyzed the impact of selected social and behavioral risk factors on quality of life and life expectancy. They calculated the number of years of healthy life lost from smoking, low income, lack of education, obesity, and other factors. Their findings:

- Low income (below 200 percent of the federal poverty line): 8.2 years of healthy life lost
- Smoking: 6.6 years of healthy life lost
- Less than 12 years of education (high school dropout): 5.1 years of healthy life lost

- Obesity: 4.2 years of healthy life lost

Analyze and Apply

- Are you surprised by the findings of this research? Explain.
- Why do you think low income has such a negative impact on health?
- Why do you think lower education levels have a negative impact on health?

Source: Muennig, P., Fiscella, K., Tancredi, D., & Franks, P. (2010). The relative health burden of selected social and behavioral risk factors in the United States: Implications for policy. *American Journal of Public Health, 100*(9), 1758–1764.

available, some people cannot access it as easily as others. Lack of adequate health insurance and/or an inability to pay costs out of pocket keeps some people away from health care they need. In lower-income communities, health care services and availability may be very limited, and in some localities, language barriers may hinder individuals' ability to get health care.

PUBLIC POLICIES AND INTERVENTIONS. Health promotion campaigns and disease prevention services can affect health positively. Laws mandating child safety seats have increased safety for infants and children. Restrictions on smoking have had a positive effect on the health of nonsmokers and also encouraged smokers to quit. Think about it: How might you help promote positive changes to public policy that would improve people's health in your community?

Wellness is associated with vitality, joy, optimism, curiosity, empowerment, and many other characteristics exemplifying a high quality of life.

Wellness: What Do You Want for Yourself—Now and in the Future?

Q | What does it feel like to be well?

It feels great! Wellness is characterized by feelings of energy, vitality, curiosity, empowerment, and enjoyment—a high quality of life. It also means that you are consciously engaged in achieving your full potential in all the wellness dimensions.

How do you rate your own levels of health and wellness today? Are you optimally healthy and living to your full potential? Have you genuinely achieved a high level for each dimension of wellness? How does your lifestyle compare to the healthy lifestyle described in this chapter?

You probably have room for improvement, in terms of both your lifestyle behaviors and the degree to which you've developed all the dimensions of wellness. The good news is that you can decide what kind of future you want. Wellness is something everyone can work on and improve. It comes from the choices you make every day. Any improvements to your wellness behaviors will bring immediate benefits, as well as a feeling of empowerment.

Do you want to make changes but aren't sure how to get started? In the next chapter, you'll review principles of behavior change and examine strategies for making positive changes in your own life. You can apply the model of behavior change to any health-related behavior; keep the principles in mind as you work your way through subsequent chapters, each of which examines a specific area of health or health behavior.

Summary

Health is a condition with multiple dimensions that falls on a continuum from negative health, characterized by illness and premature death, to optimal health, characterized by the capacity to enjoy life and to withstand life's challenges. Wellness is an active process of adopting patterns of behavior that can improve health and perceptions of well-being and quality of life in terms of multiple, intertwined dimensions. The dimensions of wellness—physical, emotional, intellectual, social, spiritual, and environmental—are closely connected and must be developed in a balanced way for overall wellness.

Health status can be assessed through life expectancy, days and years of healthy life, and a review of the leading and underlying causes of death. Healthy lifestyle behaviors include the following:

- Be physically active.
- Choose a healthy diet.
- Maintain a healthy weight.
- Avoid tobacco in all forms.
- Manage stress and get adequate sleep.
- Limit alcohol consumption.
- Avoid risky behaviors.
- Limit exposure to radiation and toxins.
- Practice good self-care.
- Seek appropriate medical care.
- Apply critical thinking skills as a health consumer.
- Cultivate relationships and social support.
- Take time to nourish your spiritual side.
- Have fun.

Other factors include family history, income and educational attainment, the environment, access to health care, and public policies.

More to Explore

American Academy of Family Physicians (FamilyDoctor.org)
http://familydoctor.org

Centers for Disease Control and Prevention: Healthy Living
http://www.cdc.gov/HealthyLiving

Healthy People Initiative
http://www.healthypeople.gov

MedlinePlus
http://www.medlineplus.gov

National Wellness Institute
http://www.nationalwellness.org

Surgeon General's Family Health History Initiative
http://www.hhs.gov/familyhistory

U.S. Department of Health and Human Services: Prevention
http://www.hhs.gov/safety/index.html

U.S. Department of Health and Human Services: Quick Guide to Healthy Living
http://www.healthfinder.gov/prevention

COMPLETE IN connect

NAME	DATE	SECTION

This lab activity will help you identify your positive and negative wellness lifestyle behaviors.

Equipment: None

Preparation: None

Instructions

For each wellness behavior listed below, place a check in the column with the answer that best describes your behavior.

	A ALMOST ALWAYS	B SOME TIMES	C ALMOST NEVER
1. I engage in at least 150 minutes per week of moderate-intensity aerobic exercise.			
2. I perform muscular strength and endurance exercises at least 2 times per week.			
3. I perform stretching exercises at least 2 days per week.			
4. I spend some leisure time each week engaged in physical activity.			
5. I eat at least 7 servings of fruits and vegetables a day.			
6. I avoid skipping meals.			
7. I limit my intake of foods high in saturated and trans fat.			
8. I limit the amount of added sugars I consume from sweetened beverages, desserts, and similar products.			
9. I limit the amount of salt I consume.			
10. For breads, cereals, and other grain-based products, I choose whole-grain foods at least half the time.			
11. I check food labels, ingredient lists, and nutrition information at restaurants in order to make informed choices.			
12. I maintain a healthy weight, avoiding overweight or underweight.			
13. I get 7–8 hours of sleep each night.			
14. I don't smoke cigarettes, cigars, or any other form of tobacco.			
15. I don't use smokeless (spit) tobacco.			
16. I avoid exposure to secondhand smoke.			
17. I use alcohol in moderation (1 drink or less per day for women; 2 drinks or less per day for men) or not at all.			
18. I do not use alcohol or any substance to the point of intoxication.			
19. I use over-the-counter medications as directed.			
20. I use prescription drugs as prescribed.			
21. I avoid unproven, dangerous, and illegal substances, including steroids, as well as unproven health remedies.			
22. I practice good dental care by brushing my teeth 2 or more times a day, flossing at least once per day, and having a dental checkup at least once a year.			
23. I have medical checkups annually or as suggested by my physician in order to obtain all recommended screening tests.			
24. I get recommended immunizations.			
25. I obtain only medically necessary X-rays.			

	A	B	C
	ALMOST ALWAYS	SOME TIMES	ALMOST NEVER
26. I manage any chronic medical conditions (e.g., asthma, migraines, allergies, diabetes, seizure disorder) according to the advice of my health care practitioner.			
27. I abstain from sex or engage in safe-sex practices.			
28. I wash my hands frequently over the course of the day.			
29. I use sunscreen as directed and use protective clothing (e.g., a wide-brimmed hat) as needed when working or playing outside.			
30. I don't try to tan, either from exposure to the sun or through use of tanning lamps or salons.			
31. I keep my computer desk or other workspace set up in a way that allows me to maintain good posture and minimize stress on my body.			
32. I use appropriate protective equipment when participating in recreational activities that require such equipment.			
33. I use appropriate protective equipment for occupational activities that require such equipment.			
34. I am actively responsible for my personal safety by being aware of my surroundings, avoiding being alone in unprotected areas, locking doors and windows when appropriate, and so on.			
35. If I have access to a firearm, I store it securely and use it safely.			
36. I do not talk on the phone, send text messages, or engage in other distracting activities while driving.			
37. I wear a seat belt when driving or riding in a car.			
38. I avoid driving while under the influence of alcohol or other drugs or riding with others who are under the influence.			
39. I obey the rules of the road by not speeding or tailgating, by always signaling before I turn or change lanes, and by adjusting my speed and driving to road and weather conditions.			
40. I recycle paper, plastic, and other appropriate items, and I reuse items such as shopping bags.			
41. I take steps to conserve energy and water (e.g., turning off lights and faucets, carpooling).			
42. I avoid environmental toxins and areas or times of day with high pollution levels.			
43. I manage stress in positive ways (e.g., physical activity, time management, deep breathing).			
44. I have sought or would seek help for depression or another mental health concern.			
45. I maintain a group of close friends I can confide in and ask for help or support.			
46. I manage my anger in ways that are not harmful to myself or others.			
47. I resolve conflicts with family, friends, co-workers, and fellow students in positive, respectful ways.			
48. I feel a sense of connectedness with others.			
49. I accept responsibility for my own feelings.			
50. I accept responsibility for my own actions.			
51. I engage in activities that are consistent with my beliefs and values.			

	A ALMOST ALWAYS	B SOME TIMES	C ALMOST NEVER
52. I spend time each day in prayer, meditation, or personal reflection.			
53. I participate in university and/or community events, or I volunteer.			
54. I like my job.			
55. I take at least a little time each day to relax and engage in a hobby or other activity I enjoy.			
56. I make a budget, track my spending, and keep my finances under control.			
57. I manage my time well through strategies such as setting priorities, creating to-do lists, and managing my schedule using a planner.			
58. I am motivated to learn new information and skills, and I actively seek ways to challenge my mind and seek intellectual growth.			
59. I gather and evaluate information in order to make sound decisions about health and wellness.			
60. I am able to set realistic goals for myself and work toward them.			
TOTAL NUMBER OF RESPONSES IN EACH COLUMN			

Results

To calculate your score, add up the total number of responses in each column and copy them onto the appropriate lines below. Multiply the total for column A by 2, the total for column B by 1, and the total for column C by 0. Add the final three numbers together for your total score, and then find your rating on the table.

Total for column A [   ] × 2 points = [   ]

Total for column B [   ] × 1 points = [   ]

Total for column C [   ] × 0 points = [   ]

Total Score [   ]

Rating	Total score
Excellent	110–120
Good	90–109
Fair	60–89
Needs attention	Less than 60

Reflecting on Your Results

How did you score? Were you surprised by number of wellness lifestyle behaviors you currently engage in—or don't engage in? Do your results give you encouragement or cause concern?

Select two behaviors of concern for you—something for which you checked "Almost never" or something for which you checked "Sometimes" but which you know is a problem for you (for example, smoking, drinking until intoxicated, never exercising). For each behavior, make a list of how it affects the different dimensions of wellness—positively as well as negatively. For example, smoking is physically and environmentally harmful, but it may make you feel better physically and emotionally in the short term; you may enjoy smoking with certain friends, but you may miss out on other social activities due to your habit.

Behavior 1: _____

How it impacts the dimensions of wellness:

Behavior 2: _____

How it impacts the dimensions of wellness:

Planning Your Next Steps

Any behavior for which you didn't check "Almost always" is a possible candidate for change and improvement. Choose five behaviors from the assessment that you are most interested in changing and list them below. For each, give one reason you'd like to change the behavior.

Behavior 1: _____

Reason to change:

Behavior 2: _____

Reason to change:

Behavior 3: _____

Reason to change:

Behavior 4: _____

Reason to change:

Behavior 5: _____

Reason to change:

COMPLETE IN connect

NAME	DATE	SECTION

This activity will help you identify wellness strengths and the behaviors that support or detract from each dimension.

Equipment: None

Preparation: None

Instructions

For each dimension, fill in the characteristics, attributes, or abilities you currently possess that you think represent your *strengths*. Also fill in your lifestyle behaviors that support and detract from each dimension; if needed, review Lab Activity 1-1 for ideas. Because behaviors affect multiple dimensions, you can enter a particular lifestyle behavior under more than one dimension. After you complete the chart for a dimension, rate yourself for that dimension by assigning a score from 1 to 10 (1 is low, 10 is high).

Physical wellness—The complete physical condition and functioning of the body		My score: _____
Physical wellness strengths (e.g., muscular strength, healthy blood pressure)	Behaviors that support physical wellness (e.g., adequate sleep, regular exercise)	Behaviors that detract from physical wellness (e.g., binge drinking, tanning salon use)

Emotional wellness—The ability to manage and express emotions in constructive and appropriate ways		My score: _____
Emotional wellness strengths (e.g., optimism, trust, self-confidence)	Behaviors that support emotional wellness (e.g., writing in a journal every week)	Behaviors that detract from emotional wellness (e.g., using food to manage stress)

Intellectual wellness—Developing and enhancing critical thinking, decision-making, and problem-solving skills		My score: _____
Intellectual wellness strengths (e.g., common sense, curiosity, creativity)	Behaviors that support intellectual wellness (e.g., keeping up-to-date on health-related recommendations)	Behaviors that detract from intellectual wellness (e.g., getting product information from commercial Web site)

Social wellness—The ability to maintain positive, healthy, satisfying interpersonal relationships

My score: _____

Social wellness strengths (e.g., supportive, compassionate, trustworthy)	Behaviors that support social wellness (e.g., regularly contacting friends)	Behaviors that detract from social wellness (e.g., being a poor listener)

Spiritual wellness—Developing a set of values, beliefs, or principles that give meaning and purpose to life and guide your actions and choices

My score: _____

Spiritual wellness strengths (e.g., faith, tolerance, altruism)	Behaviors that support spiritual wellness (e.g., prayer, volunteer work)	Behaviors that detract from spiritual wellness (any behavior that goes against personal values)

Environmental wellness—The condition and livability of the local environment and the planet as a whole

My score: _____

Environmental wellness strengths (e.g., awareness of environmental effects of actions)	Behaviors that support environmental wellness (e.g., recycling, taking public transit)	Behaviors that detract from environment wellness (e.g., buying products with lots of packaging)

Results

Enter the scores (1–10) you assigned for each level of wellness

	SCORE (1–10)		SCORE (1–10)		SCORE (1–10)
Physical wellness		Intellectual wellness		Spiritual wellness	
Emotional wellness		Social wellness		Environmental wellness	

Reflecting on Your Results

What is your wellness status? What are your strongest and weakest dimensions, and why? When you thought about each dimension individually, were you surprised—positively or negatively—by how many strengths and supportive behaviors you were able to identify? Do you feel balanced in terms of all of the dimensions of wellness?

Planning Your Next Steps

Choose one dimension in which you'd like to improve, and describe at least three specific strategies that would help you build wellness in that area.

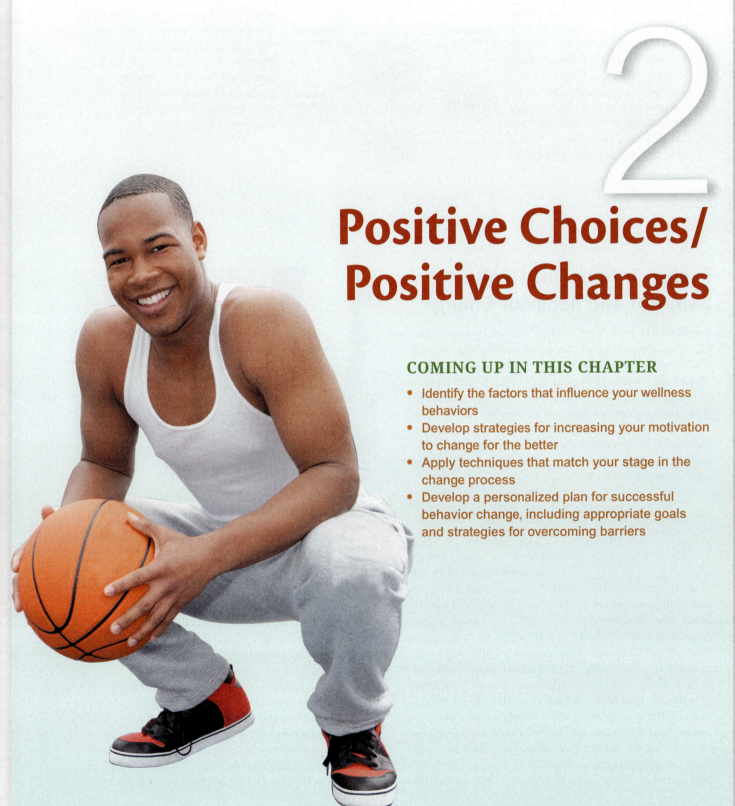

2

Positive Choices/ Positive Changes

COMING UP IN THIS CHAPTER

- Identify the factors that influence your wellness behaviors
- Develop strategies for increasing your motivation to change for the better
- Apply techniques that match your stage in the change process
- Develop a personalized plan for successful behavior change, including appropriate goals and strategies for overcoming barriers

Although almost all of us want to look and feel our best, actually doing all the things that lead to personal wellness is not so easy. Why?

Sometimes we don't have the information we need to make the best decisions and plans. Sometimes we have the knowledge, but other factors—peer pressure, social norms, emotions, motivation, environment—impede sound decision making. A good decision produces healthy behaviors and positively affects one or more components of our wellness and our collective well-being. Examples from the wellness dimensions

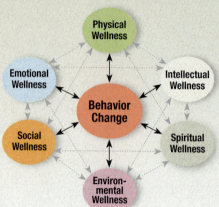

(physical, intellectual, spiritual, environmental, social, and emotional) are the decision to exercise, to wear a seat belt, to end a negative relationship, to respond appropriately when angry, to study for a test, and to recycle.

In this chapter, you'll learn about the factors that contribute to your health behaviors and your ability to sustain positive behavioral changes. Additionally, you'll review guidelines for setting appropriate goals for change, overcoming barriers to change, and developing strategies for success.

Factors Influencing Health Behavior and Behavior Change

Psychologists have long studied motivation and behavior. Why, despite all of the information about preventable chronic diseases and the importance of good lifestyle choices, do so many of us make poor choices when it comes to health and wellness? The fact is that such knowledge alone isn't enough to make us change our behavior for the better. Even knowledge coupled with good intentions will likely not be enough. Succeeding at behavior change requires a grasp of some key dimensions of behavior itself—and the factors that shape it.

Factors Inside and Outside Your Control

Q Why is behavior change so hard?

Your behavior is influenced by many factors, some of which can be difficult to recognize or control. Behavior change requires commitment and effort. If it were easy to engage in positive health behaviors, wouldn't almost everyone do so?

A *behavior* is an observable action or response. A behavior that recurs, often unconsciously, and develops into a pattern is called a *habit*. Health behaviors, or health habits, are all the actions that affect any area of your health or wellness. Your health behaviors result from a combination of influences. Some of these influences are under your control, and others are not. It's important to identify and be aware of the factors that affect your behavior—even those outside your control (Figure 2-1). You can often make adjustments in other areas to help deal with factors that

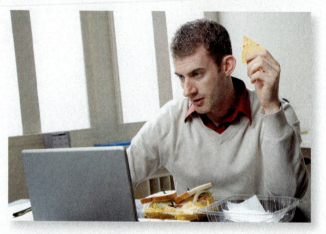

Your habits are so deeply ingrained that you often don't even notice them. A good first step in positive behavior change is to become more aware of your actions—before you eat that next chip, smoke that cigarette, or park yourself in front of the television or computer.

can't be controlled or planned for. Consider the following behavioral influences:

- *Heredity/genetic makeup:* We don't get to choose our genetic makeup, and genetically based variability makes any given health behavior or goal easier for some and harder work for others.
- *Sex:* Although there's no known biological cause, research consistently shows women are more likely than men to exhibit health-promoting behaviors and to avoid risky behaviors such as substance abuse.
- *Childhood and past experiences:* Some children are exposed to better role-modeling of healthy living and get more support for healthy choices (see the box

Behavior-Change Challenge
Breaking through the Barriers to Change

Imagine that, having dealt with a grueling course load and a challenging internship this past school term, you have let yourself go during the holidays. You have gained weight and gotten no exercise. It's winter, and you conclude that you can't work out because of all the ice and snow. You want to get back in shape and regain your sense of wellness—but where do you start?

Meet Chris

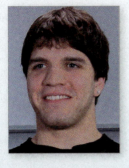

Chris is a 20-year-old student who attends classes 4 days a week and works long hours during the rest of the week. He recently injured his shoulder and feels that he is now completely out of shape. Chris hates his current condition. He wants to start a new exercise program and improve his eating habits, but he has many potential barriers to change, especially his work schedule and environment. View the video to learn more about Chris and his plans for change. As you watch, consider:

- What barriers and challenges do you (in your desire to get in shape) and Chris have in common?
- What factors work against your motivation and commitment to change?
- What strategies does Chris employ to try to overcome his barriers to change? How do these strategies reflect the wellness dimensions shown in the figure at the beginning of this chapter? What similar approaches can you use?

VIDEO CASE STUDY   WATCH THIS VIDEO IN connect

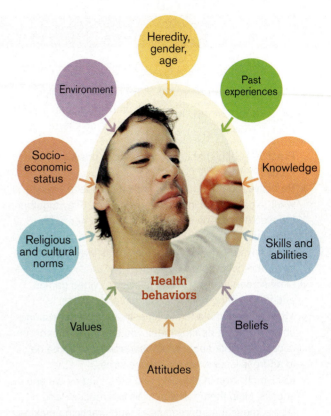

Figure 2-1 Factors that influence health behaviors.
Source: Adapted from Hayden, J. (2009). *Introduction to health behavior theory.* Boston, MA: Jones and Bartlett.

"Helping Children Develop Healthy Behaviors"). Moreover, your life experiences shape your behavior; for example, you might not have worn a bike helmet until you were injured in a crash.
- *Knowledge, skills, and abilities:* Information alone may not be sufficient to prompt you to make healthy choices, but it is necessary in shaping your behavior. You must also have the skills and abilities to act on wellness-enhancing choices.
- *Age:* Children haven't had the same opportunities as adults to develop knowledge, skills, and abilities about healthy behaviors. Additionally, they have less control and fewer choices than adults.
- *Beliefs:* Your ideas about what is real or true influence your behavior. For example, although you may know that lack of exercise is a poor health habit, you may not

believe you are susceptible to the potential consequences of a sedentary lifestyle—heart disease, for example—or that the consequences of using tanning booths will be particularly severe for you (see the box "Skin Damage from Tanning: Will It Really Happen to Me?").
- *Attitudes:* Your evaluation and judgment (opinion) of objects, people, and actions influence your behavior. For example, what is your attitude toward chewing tobacco? Toward people who are very fit or very unfit?
- *Values:* Your values help guide your choices and prioritize your activities. For health-behavior change, it can be useful to identify conflicts between your values and your behavior.
- *Religious and cultural norms and practices:* Your values, attitudes, and beliefs are shaped by religious and cultural norms as well as by your family environment. All these factors influence behavior.
- *Socioeconomic status (income, education, occupation):* Socioeconomic status affects your resources and opportunities as well as many of the other factors listed here. For example, negative health behaviors such as smoking are strongly associated with low levels of educational attainment.
- *Environment:* Environmental influences on behavior may be in or out of your control—for example, you can remove unhealthy snacks from your residence, but

Wellness Strategies

Helping Children Develop Healthy Behaviors

Q How can I help my kids develop good habits?

Try out these tips for promoting sound health habits in children.

- Practice healthy habits yourself—be a positive role model.
- Be active together but don't expect all kids to like or want to participate in the same activities. Play together but also encourage each child to pursue her or his interests.
- Don't reward kids with food. Find other ways to celebrate good behavior.
- Limit screen time, including television, video games, and Web surfing and other computer activities.
- Make dinner time a family time. In addition to ensuring children have a healthy meal, you can make dinner an occasion to talk about what happened during the day, to address issues, and to reduce stress.
- Involve children in planning and preparing meals and snacks. Help them develop skills like reading food labels, measuring portion sizes, and practicing making food choices.

- Be an advocate for daily physical education classes in school and healthy food choices in the school cafeteria.
- Be supportive and celebrate even small successes.

Sources: Adapted from American Heart Association. (2010). Help children develop healthy habits. *Healthier Kids* (http://www.heart.org/HEARTORG/ GettingHealthy/HealthierKids/HowtoMakeaHealthyHome/Help-Children-Develop-Healthy-Habits_UCM_303805_Article.jsp). U.S. Department of Agriculture. (n.d.). Develop healthy eating habits. *ChooseMyPlate.gov* (http://www.choosemyplate.gov/preschoolers/healthy-habits.html).

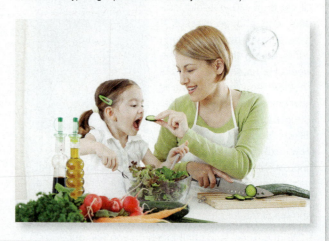

you can't change the fact that your neighborhood has twelve fast-food restaurants but no place to buy fruit. Even if you can't change certain environmental factors, you can develop strategies to minimize their impact.

The ten behavior-shaping factors illustrated in Figure 2-1 can also enhance or inhibit your ability to change your behaviors. If you completed the exercise in the "Mind Stretcher," you may have already made this connection. Although some behavioral influences are outside your control, many of them, including the most powerful ones, are under your control. And even some of the uncontrollable influences such as family role-modeling and support become much less significant as people reach adulthood and become independent. Just as some students may have to study harder than other students to get a good grade,

some people need to work harder to achieve certain wellness goals. That's reality. Fortunately, health behavior change is attainable for all of us. Our choices and plans—along with our attitudes, beliefs, and values—are factors we can control.

Predisposing, Enabling, and Reinforcing Factors

Q Is there some way I can bribe myself into making a change in my habits?

Sometimes a "bribe," or an external reward, can be a helpful support for behavior change. Just make sure it is an appropriate reward—not too expensive and not an obstacle to change. For example, allowing yourself to buy and download one song for each day or week you stick with a new healthy behavior is a more realistic and affordable reward than something like an overseas vacation.

Rewards are a form of *reinforcement*. To plan how best to use rewards for behavior change, it helps to examine behavioral influences in another way—looking beyond whether they are controllable. The factors described in the previous section can also be grouped and categorized as predisposing, enabling, or reinforcing factors (Figure 2-2).

Mind Stretcher
Critical Thinking Exercise

Examine one of your own health behaviors—positive or negative. Look at the categories of influences listed in Figure 2-1, and identify ways each factor influences that behavior.

Research Brief

Skin Damage from Tanning: Will It Really Happen to Me?

Surveys have consistently found high rates of indoor tanning booth use among college students. Most students say they tan because they want to change their appearance—they associate a tan with attractiveness and health. Do they know about the risks? More than 90 percent of college students using tanning booths report being aware that possible complications include premature skin aging and skin cancer. Why do they continue to tan? Do they believe that, somehow, they won't be affected?

In a recent study involving a group of college students who were users of tanning booths, researchers showed the 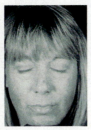 participants ultraviolet (UV) photographs of their faces. UV photographs reveal damage to facial skin caused by previous UV exposure—damage that often isn't yet visible in ordinary light. In follow-up sessions, researchers found that students who were shown their UV photographs reported less tanning booth use than the control group, who didn't see their photos. One explanation for this difference is an alteration in the students' beliefs about the consequences of tanning. The hypothetical risks became clearer and more real for those who saw their UV photos. They came to believe that they are personally susceptible to the consequences of tanning—and that those consequences are severe.

Analyze and Apply

- From this study, what do you take away regarding the strengthening of one's beliefs in the personal consequences of one's health behaviors?
- To what aspect(s) of your health behaviors can you apply these research findings?

Source: Gibbons, F. X., Gerrard, M., Lane, D. J., Mahler, H. I., & Kulik, J. A. (2005). Using UV photography to reduce use of tanning booths: A test of cognitive mediation. *Health Psychology, 24*(4), 358–363.

- **Predisposing factors** are those that you bring to the table. Your heredity, culture, age, biological sex, past experiences, beliefs, values, and attitudes are all predisposing, or preexisting, factors.

- **Enabling factors** are ones than help you change your behavior. They include your knowledge, skills, and abilities as well as various resources available to you.
- **Reinforcing factors** are ones that follow a behavior and either encourage or discourage your new behavior.

Reinforcing factors can be divided into external and internal factors. Examples of external reinforcing factors include encouragement and support from family and friends, worksite policies that make it easier for you to continue the desired behavior, and an established reward system like the downloaded songs previously described. In the early stages of changing a health behavior, external reinforcement can be very helpful. However, as you continue with a new behavior, it's important to focus on internal reinforcement, such as enjoyment of your new lifestyle or the sense of accomplishment that succeeding in your goals can bring.

External reinforcement, or bribes, can certainly help you succeed, but it is not always feasible—or necessary for success. You're the key. As you institute positive changes in your health habits, focus on your own personal reasons for change.

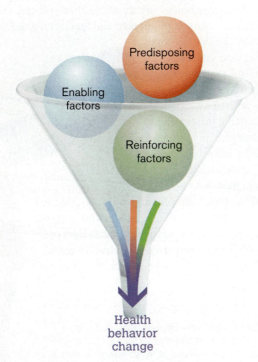

Figure 2-2 **Factors affecting behavior change.**

predisposing factors
Preexisting factors such as heredity, culture, age, biological sex, past experiences, beliefs, values, and attitudes that influence health behavior.

enabling factors
Factors, including knowledge, skills, abilities, and available resources, that make it possible or easier for an individual to change a health behavior.

reinforcing factors
Internal or external factors that encourage or discourage a new behavior.

Motivation for Behavior Change

Q | How can I find motivation?

Motivation comes from within yourself. It is one of the most challenging aspects of health behavior change, but there are many concrete strategies and techniques to help you boost motivation.

Motivation is an energized state that directs and sustains behavior. People will put out more effort and persist in the face of difficulty when their motivation is high, and they'll give up more readily or not even try at all when their motivation is low. Motivation is not something a lucky few are born with. It's a dynamic quality we all have that rises and falls because of internal and external factors, many of which we can control. For example, satisfying your hunger with a healthy snack before you shop for groceries raises your motivation to resist buying the wrong foods. Increasing factors that boost motivation and decreasing factors that interfere with motivation will help you increase your effort, persistence, and success in attaining your goals. Factors affecting motivation are locus of control, self-efficacy, goal setting, and decisional balance.

Locus of Control: Do You Feel in Charge?

Q | What's the point of all the effort? Practically everyone in my family gets diabetes about when they hit age 40.

You can do many things to reduce your risk of diabetes and other chronic diseases, regardless of your family history. How much control you feel you have over your life and behavior affects whether you will be motivated to change. Researchers investigating perceived control distinguish between people who exhibit an internal locus of control and those who exhibit an external locus of control.[1] People with an **internal locus of control** believe that their personal outcomes largely depend on what they do and how hard they try. They are higher in their perception of personal control. Conversely, those with an **external locus of control** believe that factors outside their control largely determine the outcomes of what they do. They are lower in their perception of personal control.

motivation An energized state that directs and sustains behavior.

internal locus of control Belief that the source of power or control in one's life resides in oneself—in one's own hard work, attributes, actions, and choices.

external locus of control Belief that the source of power or control in one's life resides outside oneself—in chance, fate, and the actions of others.

DOLLAR STRETCHER
Financial Wellness Tips

Rewards in a behavior-change program don't need to be elaborate or expensive. Think of free things that you enjoy, such as taking a study break to talk to a friend, watching a favorite TV show, or spending some time on a video game. Inexpensive rewards—a song download, a rented movie, a favorite book or magazine—are also effective.

The extent to which individuals take and perceive personal control affects both their success in their endeavors and their sense of well-being. Researchers have found that people who believe that how well they do in life is mostly up to them have better health, better health habits, greater happiness, less stress, greater resiliency to setbacks, and overall better mental health.[2]

How does locus of control affect health decisions and behaviors? Consider the student with several older relatives who have diabetes. A person with an external locus of control may believe she is fated by her genes to get diabetes and that nothing she does will make any difference—and therefore she takes no action to reduce her risk. A person with an internal locus of control, on the other hand, may believe that she can control her risk for diabetes, and she therefore engages in many positive practices to reduce her risk, such as regular physical activity, healthy diet, and control of body weight.

As with motivation, your locus of control may vary over time and in different situations. To boost your sense of personal control, take the time to examine your beliefs about the situations you encounter, especially the frustrating ones. Evaluate each situation realistically, and don't think in absolutes ("nothing I do will make any difference"). It may be that no good choices are available, but you can brainstorm actions that you might take and then act according to your own choices. If nothing else, you can change and control your attitude.

Also, act based on facts—or at least on the best available information. For example, in surveys asking people to identify major causes of cancer, many more individuals list air pollution than diet or excess body fat as cancer risk factors.[3] This finding indicates that it's easier to believe that things outside our control, like air pollution, pose more risk than factors over which we have some personal control. In reality, air pollution contributes to only about 2 percent

Motivation for behavior change must come from within you, but there are many strategies that will help you boost your level of effort and persistence and increase your chance of achieving your goals.

of cancer deaths, whereas diet and obesity contribute to 30 percent.[4] It's important to recognize and accurately evaluate the risks you can influence—and to take personal control of your related health behaviors.

Self-Efficacy: Do You Anticipate Success?

Q | I start a workout program for 2 weeks, and then I just stop. How do I keep motivated?

Do you begin your program expecting to succeed or to fail? Your personal expectations have a big effect on your motivation level. Expecting a positive outcome leads to greater effort and persistence.[5] When it is looked at as a personality trait, expecting success is referred to as *optimism.* Optimism combines a positive focus with positive expectations for how things will turn out.

Although optimism is associated with trying harder and being more effective in changing behavior, no one is optimistic about everything. People who are optimistic about most things can still lack confidence in their ability to lose weight or quit smoking, for example. For this reason, measuring people's tendency to be optimistic versus pessimistic may not predict their success in losing weight or quitting smoking. A more accurate predictor would be to ask them whether they specifically expect to succeed at losing weight or quitting smoking.

SELF-EFFICACY EXPECTATIONS. A person's expectations regarding his or her ability to perform a task leading to a specific outcome is called **self-efficacy.** Self-efficacy is a control-related concept formalized by psychologist Albert Bandura that has helped clarify the influence of expectations on behavior.[6] People high in self-efficacy for a particular behavior are confident they can execute it successfully—they believe they can achieve that particular goal. People low in self-efficacy lack confidence in their ability to execute a particular behavior leading to an outcome they want. In general, someone with high self-efficacy views difficult tasks as challenges rather than as things to be avoided, sets high goals and stays committed to them, perseveres when the going gets tough, and bounces back quickly from setbacks and failures. On the other hand, a person with low self-efficacy avoids challenges, sets the bar low when choosing goals and shows little commitment to reaching them, doubts his or her abilities, gives up quickly in the face of difficulties, and recovers slowly from failures.[7]

Self-efficacy is different from belief. You might believe that losing weight will improve your self-confidence and want to lose weight very much. Yet, if your personal expectations for successfully losing weight are low, you may not even try. If you don't have confidence that your efforts to achieve a particular health goal will

self-efficacy Belief in one's capability to perform a task that leads to a specific outcome.

be successful (low self-efficacy), your motivation—and with it, your effort level—goes down.

This is how self-fulfilling prophecies are formed. People who expect to succeed tend to try harder and persist longer than people who aren't sure they can succeed. So, people with strong expectations of succeeding tend to be more successful partly because they try harder—and they make their prediction of success come true. Conversely, by not trying as hard and giving up more easily, people with lower self-efficacy can make their prediction of failure come true.

See the box "Self-Efficacy for Health Goals" to gauge your level of self-efficacy for your targeted health-behavior change, whether it is to increase physical activity, improve your diet, quit smoking, or modify another behavior you identified. If your score is 90 percent or more, then you rate very highly in self-efficacy. But don't worry if your score is lower; there are many strategies you can try to boost your self-efficacy.

HOW SELF-EFFICACY DEVELOPS—AND CAN BE INCREASED. You can build up your self-efficacy, and with it your motivation and odds of success. Self-efficacy expectations develop from a combination of past performance, observational learning, verbal persuasion, and cognitive processing of cues such as emotional and physiological arousal.[8]

PAST PERFORMANCE. Direct experience is the strongest influence on self-efficacy expectations.[9] If you've successfully controlled a similar behavior or outcome in the past, your self-efficacy will be higher for the current behavior. Conversely, past failures to control relevant specific outcomes will lower your self-efficacy. Success breeds success, and failure breeds failure.

Direct experience is not only the most powerful influence on self-efficacy expectations, but it is also the factor over which you have the most control. Set a series of small, realistic goals that build toward your final goal. For example, if you are currently sedentary and your goal is to add 30 minutes of physical activity to each day, start off with a less ambitious goal—10 minutes of walking three times a week. Keep a written record of your progress. By succeeding at small initial steps, you build your confidence for the next step—and then the next.

Success breeds success. Your past experiences in changing a similar behavior have the most powerful influence on your self-efficacy. Start with a small change and build your confidence for the next step.

Wellness Strategies

Self-Efficacy for Health Goals

Q I'm discouraged because I have failed at my exercise goals in the past. Is there a way to improve my chances of success?

Having been previously unsuccessful might shake your confidence, but it doesn't mean you're condemned to fail again. Two key steps are to examine the factors that may have contributed to your past shortcomings and then to plan for future confidence and success.

Circle a number between 0 and 100 on the scale below to rate your degree of confidence for reaching your specific health goal. If you're not highly certain (score of 90 or more) that you can reach your health-behavior-change goal, ask yourself why. Identify the barriers and other controllable factors that could possibly get you off track in terms of your goal pursuit.

Here are some tips for boosting self-efficacy:

- Set realistic final and interim goals for behavior change.
- Monitor your behavior with a journal, log, or other tracking method.
- Identify potential obstacles to change and plan how to overcome them.
- Find a role model—someone similar to yourself who engages in your target behavior.
- Ask friends and family to support you and encourage your efforts.
- Make a mental picture of success by imagining yourself engaging in your target behavior.
- Recognize and celebrate your successes; attribute them to your own efforts.

Take charge. Develop a behavior-change plan that you have confidence in.

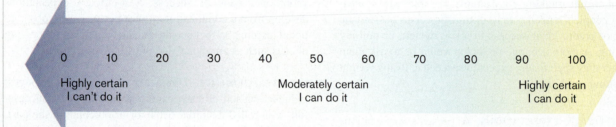

| 0 | 10 | 20 | 30 | 40 | 50 | 60 | 70 | 80 | 90 | 100 |

Highly certain
I can't do it

Moderately certain
I can do it

Highly certain
I can do it

OBSERVATIONAL LEARNING. Watching other people's actions—and thereby vicariously experiencing those actions and their outcomes—also influences self-efficacy, though not as strongly as direct experience.[10] You might see someone walking on the school track between classes and realize that you could do that, too. Or you might observe someone packing a lunch and say to yourself, "Hey, that doesn't look so hard." Seeing someone else do something successfully can increase your own expectations for success—your self-efficacy. When contemplating or starting out on a behavior change, observe people similar to yourself. For example, if you are a beginning exerciser, make your model another beginning exerciser taking a short walk rather than an elite athlete running in a marathon.

PERSUASION. Under some circumstances, people can be persuaded that they're going to do well, and this persuasion can increase their self-efficacy expectations. Generally though, persuasion is a less powerful influence on self-efficacy than either direct or vicarious experience. Someone's ability to persuade us that we really can do something rests on the degree to which we see their comments as true. When someone we view as sincere and credible believes in us—that we can do something—it can increase our self-efficacy.

INTERPRETING INTERNAL CUES. In uncertain situations, people actively look for clues about how something will go. For example, if you have never worked out in a gym in front of people, you might feel anxious when thinking about exercising at a gym. The images you create and the thoughts you entertain about how you are going to do influence your emotions and motivation. Imagining yourself failing can increase your anxiety and lower your self-efficacy; on the other hand, imagining yourself succeeding can decrease your anxiety and heighten your self-efficacy.[11]

Goal Setting: What Are You Trying to Achieve?

Q How do I come up with a good goal that fits me as an individual?

An appropriate goal is essential to successful behavior change. One strategy for developing a goal is to apply the SMART principle—the idea that your goal should be specific, measurable, achievable, realistic, and time-bound (see Figure 2-3).

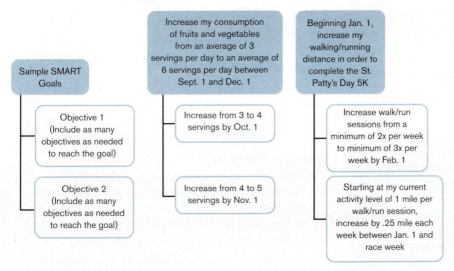

Figure 2-3 Sample SMART goals. Goals should be s̲pecific, m̲easurable, a̲chievable, r̲ealistic, and t̲ime-bound.

SPECIFIC GOALS. What *exactly* are you going to do? Cut back on smoking, exercise more, and eat better are all goals, but they aren't specific enough to be the basis of a behavior-change program. Reframe your goal with specific numbers; for example:

- Reduce cigarette smoking from 2 packs per day by 2 cigarettes every other day until I reach zero, and then keep it at zero.
- Increase my current activity level from no exercise to walking for 30 minutes per day, 5 days per week.
- Increase my consumption of fruits and vegetables from an average of 3 servings a day to an average of 6 servings a day.

Notice that these goals have both a starting point and an endpoint. If you haven't already done so, monitor your current behavior to obtain a baseline measure. How many minutes of physical activity do you currently engage in? How much sleep do you average a night? How many fast-food meals do you buy each week?

MEASURABLE GOALS. Your goal must be *measurable* in order for you to monitor your progress and see if you are on track. Develop a measure or standard for your progress, such as the number of cigarettes smoked, minutes of exercise completed, or servings of vegetables consumed. Tracking is also a great motivational tool, because it allows you to chart your progress. Many people also find that recording their behavior improves it—for example, you pass up a donut because you don't want to confess in your food journal that you ate it—and self-monitoring does increase the likelihood of successfully changing health behavior.[12] Many free tracking tools are available online and as smartphone apps. Pick a simple tool that works well for you.

ACHIEVABLE GOALS. Your goal should be meaningful and inspiring but also something that you can actually do.

Consider your limitations—such as your physical condition and available and affordable resources—when setting your goal. For example, improving skiing ability might not be an achievable goal for a man with a knee injury who lives a long distance from ski facilities and who could not easily afford the travel and ski rentals. Likewise, losing weight to wear a size 2 is not an achievable goal for a woman with an average body type.

REALISTIC GOALS. Goals should also be realistic. Your goal should be ambitious and challenging but not impossible. You want to stretch yourself, but you should also be confident that you can reach your goal. Don't set yourself up to fail: Goals that aim too high or require too much, too quickly are unrealistic and cause frustration. Realistic goals allow steady progress, which is what you want. Build on your success to increase self-efficacy and motivation.

TIME-BOUND GOALS. A time-bound goal has a time frame for action. Your plan for behavior change should have a start date and a goal completion date. You should also break up your goal into several steps, each with its own date.

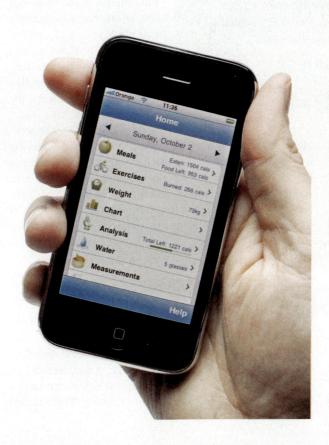

Research Brief

New Year, New You: Do New Year's Resolutions Work?

The arrival of a new year often inspires people to want to begin anew. Almost half of Americans make resolutions at the beginning of a new year. Do such resolutions work?

A study followed two groups of people for 6 months; the two groups were similar in demographics, histories, and goals, and all wanted to make changes in their lives. The first group, called *resolvers,* made New Year's resolutions. The second group, called *nonresolvers,* desired to make changes in their lives but not by way of New Year's resolutions.

After 6 months, almost half (46 percent) of the resolvers had maintained their resolutions. Research indicated these participants used more positive behavior-change strategies than the nonresolvers. Only 4 percent of the

nonresolvers were successful at the six-month mark. Although longer studies are needed, this research supports the importance of specific goals and start dates for implementing specific behavior-change strategies.

Analyze and Apply

- What is one behavior-change resolution—for New Year's Day or at some other time—you have made in the past?
- Did you succeed in meeting your goal? Based on the study results, what might explain how you did?

Source: Norcross, J., Mrykalo, M., & Blagys, M. (2002). Auld lang syne: Success predictors, change processes, and self-reported outcomes of New Year's resolvers and nonresolvers. *Journal of Clinical Psychology,* 397–405.

As previously described, a series of smaller, achievable steps/objectives can give you opportunities for success and help keep you motivated. If, for example, your goal is to increase servings of fruits and vegetables from 3–6 per day over the course of 12 weeks, set short-term objectives, evenly spaced throughout your target time frame. Objectives can also be other actions that help you reach your goal, such as selecting a tracking system or finding a workout partner.

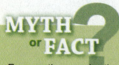

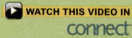

Frequently reevaluating and changing goals is a clear indication that a behavior-change program is failing.

▶ **WATCH THIS VIDEO IN connect**

See page 476 to find out.

Once you have spelled out a goal that meets the SMART criteria, take a second look at it. Does it accurately reflect what you want to accomplish? Will achieving it give you the desired outcome? Does your goal make you feel challenged but motivated to get to work? A good goal should inspire you to take action (see the box "New Year, New You: Do New Year's Resolutions Work?"). Lab Activity 2-1 will help you create a personal SMART goal.

Decisional Balance: What Are the Pros and Cons of Change?

Q What if I don't have any motivation to do anything?

No motivation to do anything at all? That's unlikely. If you feel that way about health-behavior change, it may be that you don't perceive the benefits of change as significant or that the obstacles to change seem overwhelming. There is also

the problem of behaviors that seem like good choices in the short term but are unhealthy in the long run.

Self-defeating behaviors are those that accomplish one goal (usually a short-term goal) but interfere with the chances of reaching more important goals (usually longer-term goals).[13] Examples abound. Avoiding premature death from smoking is a more important goal than reducing the short-term discomforts of the effort to quit smoking. Yet many people who are struggling to quit give in to the short-term benefit of decreasing the discomfort caused by nicotine cravings, at the expense of the more important benefit of a longer and healthier life. Similarly, wanting to lose weight commonly runs up against the desire to satisfy a craving for a favorite food when we're hungry or tired. And just like giving in to nicotine cravings, sometimes the immediate desire wins out over the more important plans to maintain a healthy weight. Doing what we know is best for us is often difficult.

One strategy that can help focus your energies and boost your motivation is to analyze the pros and cons of the change you want to make. You'll find guidelines for doing so later in the chapter. First, it is vital to understand the behavior-change process.

The Behavior-Change Process: The Transtheoretical Model

There are many models and theories about how people change their behaviors. A well-known model, one that combines various processes and principles of change from different theories, is the transtheoretical model, or TTM. Developed in the early 1980s, TTM was originally used to

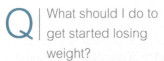

Wellness Strategies

What's My Stage?

Q | What should I do to get started losing weight?

For any behavior change, it's important first to determine your stage of change. Begin by identifying which of the following statements best describes you in terms of your target behavior:

- I do not intend to take action to change my behavior within the next 6 months.
    Your stage = precontemplation
- I do intend to change my behavior within the next 6 months.
    Your stage = contemplation

- I intend to take action within the next month and have already taken steps to make changes.
    Your stage = preparation
- I have taken action and made changes in my behavior within the past 6 months.
    Your stage = action
- I have maintained my targeted behavior change for more than 6 months.
    Your stage = maintenance

Source: Adapted from Prochaska, J. O., Redding, C. A., & Evers, K. E. (2008). The transtheoretical model and stages of change. In K. Glanz, B. K. Rimer, & K. Viswanath (Eds.), *Health behavior and health education: Theory, research, and practice* (4th ed.). San Francisco: Jossey-Bass.

---

study people who were trying to quit smoking. It has since been applied to a broad range of health and wellness behaviors. TTM is sometimes referred to as the *stages of change model* because one of its main ideas is that people must go through stages as they work to change a habit or adopt a new behavior. Let's review these stages and the processes and techniques that can help you move forward to change your behavior successfully.

Stages of Change

Q | How do I get organized, motivated, and focused to change my behavior?

First, find out where you stand. Once you determine which stage of change you are currently in for your target behavior, you can choose appropriate strategies to move forward (see the box "What's My Stage?"). The stages in the transtheoretical model each have unique attributes and build on one another (Figure 2-4). Because slips and relapses between stages of change are common, the model can be viewed as a spiral rather than a straight line.

PRECONTEMPLATION. The first stage of change in the transtheoretical model is *precontemplation*. People in this stage engage in a problem behavior and aren't yet actively thinking about change. They may be rationalizing their behavior, or they may be afraid of change, unsure of their ability to change, or unaware of the full consequences of their behavior and the need for change. Or they may have tried and failed to change and now avoid thinking about their high-risk behavior.

CONTEMPLATION. *Contemplation* is the "thinking" stage. Here individuals recognize and acknowledge a problem and have begun to think about change. Many things can

lead to the recognition that there's a problem, including new medical information, communication with others, and media messages. In this stage people must weigh the pros and cons of taking action and then decide whether to proceed with trying to change a behavior. Notably, some

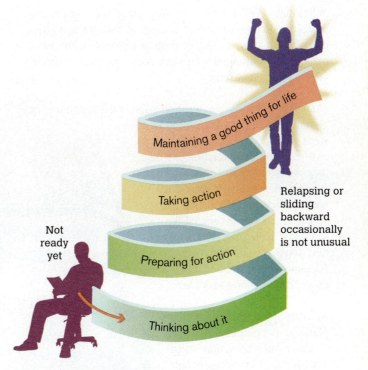

Figure 2-4 Stages of change in the transtheoretical model of behavior change.

Source: Adapted from Centers for Disease Control and Prevention / The Cooper Institute. (n.d.). *Personal Empowerment Plan (PEP) kit: Physical activity precontemplation.* Dallas, TX: The Cooper Institute.

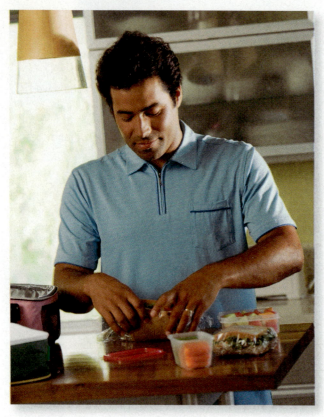

For people in the maintenance stage, their new healthy behavior is well established and serves as its own reward.

individuals spend longer in this "thinking" stage than others. In fact, some never get out of this stage. Others, though, just need sufficient time to process all the information. An individual who does decide to make a change moves to the next stage.

PREPARATION. The *preparation* stage is the "planning and getting ready" part of change. In this stage individuals take a realistic look at where they are in relation to where they want to be and then make a specific plan to reach their destination. Accurate information and appropriate tools are crucial for setting a plan. The preparation stage is a turning point for many people—when they move from thinking to doing.

ACTION. Once the preparation or planning is complete, it's time to move into the *action* stage. This is the point when people implement the plan and behavior change begins. They start increasing their fruit and vegetable consumption or the number of steps they take daily, or they start cutting back on the number of cigarettes they smoke. If they continue with their goal behavior for about 6 months, they advance to the next stage.

MAINTENANCE. For most behaviors, *maintenance* is the final stage. In this stage, people continue to work to maintain their new behavior and to avoid relapse. It is similar to the action stage, but because people have already been successful at maintaining their behavior for a while, they typically don't have to apply as many techniques and strategies to keep going. They are increasingly confident in their ability to maintain their new healthy behavior, no matter what comes along. External rewards are less important than they were earlier, because the new behavior (and all its benefits) is the true reward of behavior change.

Once you successfully change one behavior, your chance of success in making other changes increases significantly. If you make it to the maintenance stage, ask yourself what other positive changes you could undertake. Keep on working to improve wellness!

Q | Is it possible to modify behavior beyond the point of relapse?

Possibly—but only for a small number of people and only for certain types of behaviors. Researchers studying health-behavior change have found that few people ever reach a condition of zero temptation and total self-efficacy.[14] The transtheoretical model includes a final stage called *termination,* but its criterion of zero chance of relapse isn't realistic for most people and most health behaviors, including exercise and diet.

It may be best to consider yourself in a lifetime state of maintenance: You are confident in your ability to maintain your behavior, but you are also ready to apply new strategies and work to overcome any lapses that might occur in response to changes in your life. An example is someone who has been a regular exerciser for 8 years but then gets a new job that completely changes his schedule. He can continue to be active, but he'll likely need to cycle back and use strategies from the preparation and action stages to develop his new exercise plan.

This example brings up an important point about the transtheoretical model. Lapses and relapses are common—so don't get discouraged if you experience one. In most cases, people who lapse don't fall all the way back to the initial stage of precontemplation, and they can move more quickly back up through the other stages. Moving

DOLLAR STRETCHER
Financial Wellness Tip

For a behavior change that will save you money, such as quitting smoking or cutting back on eating out, consider setting aside all the money you save and buying yourself something special once you reach the maintenance stage. Have a friend hold the money or keep it in a special bank account.

through the stages gives you a taste of a success, thereby raising your self-efficacy, motivation, and chances of success when you try again.

Processes and Techniques of Change

Q | According to the questionnaire, I'm in the contemplation stage. Now what?

Your stage represents how far you've progressed in making a change. Now it's time to take a look at the processes and techniques that can help you move forward to the next stage. The transtheoretical model includes ten general change processes or strategies, each associated with a number of specific techniques.[15]

- *Consciousness raising:* Increase your knowledge about the unhealthy habit and its causes and consequences, including learning more about your status in regard to the behavior and how its consequences relate to you personally. Ask yourself what things you do that are unhealthy—and why you do them.

- *Emotional arousal (dramatic relief):* Experience the worry, fear, and other strong negative emotions that go along with an unhealthy behavioral risk (see the box " 'Super Size' Your Behavior-Change Effort"). Techniques for dramatic relief include observing an individual's personal testimony or reading the vivid case history of someone who has experienced a problem due to the target behavior—or someone who has made the change you want to make.

- *Self-reevaluation:* Look at yourself with and without the unhealthy habit and evaluate the differences cognitively (by thinking) and affectively (through feelings). Imagine the consequences that are most meaningful to you. What will your life be like as a more active person, for example? What will it be like if you continue as a couch potato? Also think about whether your current behavior is in line with your values. Highlight the benefits of change for yourself—emphasize the reasons it will be a step worth taking.

- *Environmental reevaluation:* Look at yourself with and without the unhealthy habit and imagine the effects on your environment, both physical and social. For example, think about how smoking hurts air quality and the health of people you care about—and then consider the effects of quitting. What kind of role model do you want to be for your family, friends, and community?

- *Commitment (self-liberation):* Believe in your ability to change a behavior and make a firm commitment to that change. Refer to the final section of the chapter for more on developing a plan for change that you are confident in.

- *Helping relationships:* Seek out and use social support for your behavior change. Think about how the people with whom you spend time can support your efforts. The box "Dealing with an Unsupportive Roommate or Significant Other" offers advice to encourage support from the people closest to you.

- *Countering:* Substitute healthy behaviors for the unhealthy behavior. For example, use a relaxation

---

Research Brief

"Super Size" Your Behavior-Change Effort

Would you watch a movie to get information and motivation for behavior change? Researchers tested a group of young adults on their knowledge of fast food and certain psychosocial measures, including their stage of change, self-efficacy, and locus of control for healthy weight. They then showed part of the group the film *Super Size Me,* which provides information about fast food and recounts the filmmaker's experience of eating only fast food for all meals for 30 days. The control group watched an unrelated film.

The two groups had similar scores to start. But follow-up testing showed that the group who watched *Super Size Me* scored higher on knowledge of fast food and on nearly all the psychosocial measures, including stage of change. The experience of watching the film worked as a technique for two stage-of-change processes—consciousness raising and emotional arousal.

Analyze and Apply
- Even if fast food isn't related to your target behavior, how might you use ideas from this study to identify techniques for change? To what sources might you turn?

Source: Cottone, E., & Byrd-Bredbenner, D. (2007). Knowledge and psychosocial effects of the film *Super Size Me* on young adults. *Journal of the American Dietetic Association, 107*(7), 1197–1203.

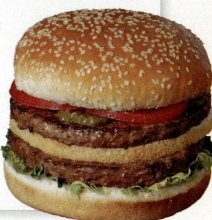

Wellness Strategies

Dealing with an Unsupportive Roommate or Significant Other

Q What if I live with someone who sabotages my efforts to be healthier?

Everyone wants a supportive roommate or significant other. Behavior change is difficult enough without having to face negativity or lack of support at home. If you find yourself without support, try these steps.

1. Share your plans. People can't help you if they don't know what you're trying to do. (If it's appropriate, invite them to join you. You may be just the motivation they need.)

2. If those close to you still aren't helpful, the reason may be that they don't know how to help. Say specifically what you would find helpful—whether it is something you need them to do or to stop doing.

3. Remember that the responsibility for your behavior ultimately lies with you. If your roommate or significant other can't or won't help, decide how to adjust your plans or environment so that you're still moving toward your goal.

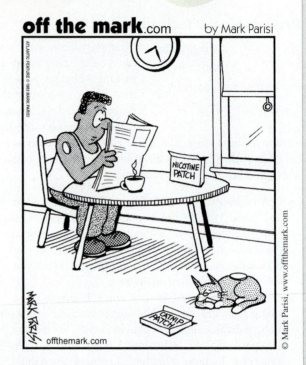

off the mark.com   by Mark Parisi

offthemark.com

© Mark Parisi, www.offthemark.com

---

technique instead of a cigarette to combat stress. Countering also includes substituting more positive thinking patterns. Instead of "I'm too tired to exercise," try "I'm tired, but I'll feel better after my workout."

- *Reinforcement management (rewards):* Enforce the consequences for behavior by increasing the rewards for the desired behavior and decreasing the rewards for the unhealthy behavior. You can set up a formal system of rewards for reaching program milestones as well as punishments for unhealthy behaviors. As a rule, rewards work better than punishments, and they work best when associated with positive changes—choosing to adopt a healthy behavior as opposed to discontinuing an unhealthy one. Also use positive self-talk for reinforcement; congratulate yourself for every program success, and think about what you enjoy about your new, healthier behavior.

- *Environment control:* Remove cues and triggers that prompt the unhealthy behavior and add new cues and triggers to encourage the healthy behavior. For example, if you are trying to cut back on big, unhealthy snacks after work, remove those foods from your home to avoid the temptation. Keeping small, healthy snacks at work to reduce hunger will also help. By restructuring your environment, you can support your new healthy behavior and reduce the risk of relapse.

- *Social liberation:* Seek different or additional social alternatives to the unhealthy behavior. Recognize when social norms and public policies provide support for healthy behavior change—such as smoke-free buildings, bike lanes, and workplace health-promotion programs.

Certain processes lend themselves to particular points in the stages of change and can make your efforts at change more effective, as Table 2-1 illustrates.

Mind Stretcher
Critical Thinking Exercise

Think about the last time you did something you knew to be unhealthy primarily because those around you were doing it. How could you have restructured the situation or changed the environmental cues so that you could have avoided the behavior? Identify several possible actions that will help you avoid the unhealthy behavior the next time you're in a similar situation.

TABLE 2-1 PROCESSES AND TECHNIQUES OF CHANGE

PROCESS OF CHANGE	EXAMPLES OF TECHNIQUES OF CHANGE
	PRECONTEMPLATION
CONSCIOUSNESS RAISING Increasing knowledge about the behavior and its causes and consequences	■ Do research about the behavior in reputable sources; look especially for information on the immediate benefits of change. ■ Examine your attitudes and self-talk about the behavior; ask yourself if you minimize the consequences of your behavior, rationalize reasons for not changing, or avoid thinking about it. ■ Ask other people about how they perceive your behavior and its consequences; also ask if they notice defense mechanisms that block change.
EMOTIONAL AROUSAL Experiencing negative emotions associated with an unhealthy behavior	■ Watch a film or read a story related to the behavior; observe personal testimony or read a case history. ■ Create personally relevant propaganda; for example, blow smoke from a cigarette into a white cloth, have someone film you while sitting on the couch eating, pile up all the junk food you eat in a week or month (but take care not to overwhelm yourself with negative messages).
ENVIRONMENTAL REEVALUATION Imagining the effects of behavior on the physical and social environment	■ Link the benefits of change to your values and priorities in terms of how your behavior affects other people and your physical environment. ■ Ask yourself what kind of role model you are and what kind you want to be.
	CONTEMPLATION
SELF-REEVALUATION Imagining the effects of current and goal behavior on your life cognitively and affectively	■ Link the benefits of change to your values and priorities in terms of what you want for yourself. ■ Create a new self-image by imagining your life in detail after you've made the change. ■ Keep a journal of your current behavior. ■ Think before you act—ask yourself if you really want to smoke a cigarette, eat a cookie, or sit instead of working out. ■ Work on your pros-and-cons list, incorporating what you've learned about yourself and your behavior.
	PREPARATION
COMMITMENT Making a firm commitment to change	■ Obtain the information and tools you need. ■ Develop a detailed plan for change that includes small intermediate steps toward your final goal. ■ Create and sign a contract. ■ Tell friends and family about the change you're making.

(continued)

TABLE 2-1 PROCESSES AND TECHNIQUES OF CHANGE (continued)

PROCESS OF CHANGE	EXAMPLES OF TECHNIQUES OF CHANGE
ACTION AND MAINTENANCE	
HELPING RELATIONSHIPS Seeking out and using social support	▪ Find a buddy to work with on the same behavior change. ▪ Arrange for supportive meetings, calls, or e-mails from a friend; ask people for the type of support you want. ▪ Join a formal support group or meet with a counselor; if face-to-face support isn't available, consider an online support group.
COUNTERING Identifying healthy behaviors that can substitute for unhealthy behaviors	▪ Divert your attention when temptation arises; exercise and relaxation are good countering strategies for many behaviors. ▪ Brainstorm ideas for overcoming obstacles to change. ▪ Refocus your energy on positive behavior change. ▪ Examine your thinking patterns for self-defeating and negative thoughts; substitute rational and positive self-talk.
REINFORCEMENT MANAGEMENT (REWARDS) Enforcing consequences for behavior to increase the reward for the desired behavior	▪ Develop a formal system of rewards for reaching milestones; build them into your program plan. ▪ Track your behavior. ▪ Engage in positive self-talk for sticking with the program.
ENVIRONMENT CONTROL Changing cues and triggers so that they prompt the healthy behavior and not the unhealthy behavior	▪ Avoid temptations (objects, places, people) and add cues and reminders to trigger your healthy behavior. ▪ Check your residence and workspace for triggers and make appropriate changes (for example, remove junk food and place healthy snacks in plain sight, put exercise shoes by the door). ▪ Examine your daily routine for triggers and make adjustments (for example, go for a walk after dinner instead of smoking a cigarette or having a big dessert).
NOT TIED TO ANY PARTICULAR STAGE	
SOCIAL LIBERATION Seeking social alternatives to the unhealthy behavior	▪ Look for social norms or public policies that can support you (for example, bike lanes, smoke-free zones). ▪ Look for enabling conditions in your environment (such as free access to the campus gym or a stress-management workshop, availability of fruits and vegetables at local stores, self-help groups sponsored by your school or online).

Sources: Adapted from Prochaska, J. O., Redding, C. A., & Evers, K. E. (2008). The transtheoretical model and stages of change. In K. Glanz, B. K. Rimer, & K. Viswanath (Eds.), *Health behavior and health education: Theory, research, and practice* (4th ed.). San Francisco, CA: Jossey-Bass. Prochaska, J., Norcross, J., & Diclemente, C. (1994). *Changing for good.* New York, NY: Morrow.

Overcoming Common Barriers to Change

Q What is the greatest obstacle to overcome in dealing with behavioral change?

The biggest obstacle to change is different for each person and her or his particular target behavior. Is lack of time your problem in working toward a behavior change? Are stress and a negative outlook holding you back? This section describes common barriers to health-behavior change and offers strategies for overcoming them.

Changing health habits isn't easy, especially because you want your change to last a lifetime, not just a few weeks or months. If you are like many people, you might go through all the work of quitting smoking, losing weight, or getting in shape, only to revert to where you started. It's a common and frustrating scenario. You can greatly improve your chances for success, however, both in the short and the long term, by having a sound plan. Starting out with a SMART goal improves your chances, as many failures are due to unrealistic or poorly defined goals. Developing a plan that anticipates common barriers to success likewise improves your odds. Identify barriers and plan how you will address them—put yourself in control.

I Don't Have Enough Time

Complaints about lack of time are most relevant for goals that require time—for example, cooking more meals at home and getting more exercise. Everyone has the same 24 hours in a day, but some people have more commitments and obligations than others. Time management skills are critical—and the more commitments you have, the more essential effective time management becomes. By managing your time well, you'll have more opportunities to relax and have fun.

The purpose of time management is not to pack more into your schedule. It's about planning and prioritizing so that you spend your time wisely. Give priority to activities that are important to your core values and long-term well-being. Scheduling and making time for important activities and goals allows you to meet your overall needs better and to achieve a healthy life balance.

Start by tracking your current activities and then take a close look at where your time goes. Identify activities and demands on which you can cut back to make time for activities that should have a higher priority. Use a calendar—paper or electronic—that has room for writing in plans and reminders. Writing things down and making a schedule are basics of good time management. Just writing something down increases the likelihood you will do it.

Ask people who engage in the healthy behavior you are trying to adopt how they make time (see the box "Self-Control Can Be Contagious"). Also look for ways to combine activities. For example, can you combine physical activity with your commute to school or with time you spend with friends or family? See Chapter 10 for more information on time management.

I Can't Get Motivated

If you're not sure that you really want to make a change or that the health goal is really worth all the effort, your motivation will suffer. To address this issue, review the discussion of motivation presented earlier in the chapter. Write out a pros-versus-cons analysis, focusing on your reasons for wanting to make this change. Behavior change is a lot of work, and you need to be clear about why you're doing it. If the cons still outweigh the pros of change, work through some of the processes and techniques associated with contemplation and planning in the stages-of-change model. If you decide that you really want to change this health habit *now,* then you can make use of all the suggestions in this chapter for planning and for overcoming barriers to keep motivated and moving forward.

Remember that your goal needs to be personal and realistic. If it is not, your motivation will suffer. Consider the example of a young woman whose doctor told her that

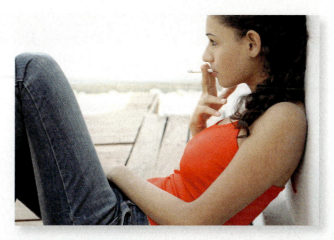

Don't wait to change your behaviors for the better. Although change at any age is beneficial, not all the effects of negative health behaviors are reversible. Many young smokers believe that they'll quit "later" and won't suffer any ill effects from smoking. But quitting is very difficult, and some risks from smoking may be permanent.

she should lose at least 50 pounds. She'd like to do that, but it seemed like such an unreachable target that she felt discouraged before she even started. After all, she'd tried before and failed. She lacked motivation to try to lose that much weight. After reading about goal setting and behavior-change strategies, she changed her goal. Instead of focusing on weight loss, which is an outcome and not a behavior, she planned to change several specific behaviors, and she felt more confident about succeeding.

She decided to keep only healthy foods in her home, as well as to eat a healthy snack before shopping for groceries and before leaving her work so that she wouldn't be too hungry to be disciplined when she got home. She scheduled times and ways to do more walking, including some laps around the campus track before her first class. She also signed up for a free cooking class with a friend to learn how to prepare her favorite foods with fewer calories. By starting out with small, manageable steps that she was confident she could accomplish (high self-efficacy), she found that her motivation was much better. She used SMART goals and built on success.

I'll Get Around to Changing—Later

Is procrastination your problem? Have you decided you'll start to exercise once your life is less busy? That you'll quit smoking when you're 30 (or 50)? That you don't need to improve your diet until you're older—and only when you eventually develop health problems?

Procrastinating, rationalizing, and minimizing the effects of your behavior are hallmarks of the precontemplation stage of behavior change. Refer to Table 2-1 for suggestions and techniques that can help you make progress in behavior change. Don't fool yourself into thinking that your

Research Brief

Self-Control Can Be Contagious

Study after study has confirmed the effects of social networks and peer groups on poor health behaviors—meaning that people copy the unhealthy behaviors of those around them. But what about the influence of others on healthy behaviors and self-control?

Researchers recently completed a series of studies with college students that looked at whether thinking about or watching someone with good self-control might make an individual more likely to exert self-control. Here are brief descriptions of three of those studies:

- Students were randomly assigned to two groups and observed people they were told were taste testing; the taste-test actors were presented with a plate of cookies and a plate of carrot sticks. One group watched people who ate carrots and not cookies; the other group observed people who ate cookies and not carrots. The group that watched the carrot eaters scored higher on a later test of self-control.
- Participants were asked to make a list of friends that included a person with very good self-control and a person with very bad self-control. The students were then given a computer-based test that measures self-control. Prior to the presentation of each test item on the screen, the participants were subliminally primed with the name of the person they identified as either very good or very bad at self-control (that is, the name flashed on the screen very briefly). The participants who were primed with the name of their friend who had good self-control scored better.
- Students were divided into three groups and were asked to write about a friend with good self-control, a friend with bad self-control, or a friend who is a moderate extrovert (an outgoing person). On a follow-up test

of self-control, those who wrote about a friend with good self-control did best, those who wrote about a friend with bad self-control did worst, and those who wrote about an extroverted friend scored in the middle.

These study results suggest that self-control is indeed contagious. If you want to make positive health behavior changes, surround yourself with people who have good self-control. Anyone you observe—not just the friends you hang out with—can have an impact (remember the study with the carrot eaters). And it doesn't matter what the context or behavior: Thinking about or watching someone exhibit self-control related to one behavior can affect your actions related to a different behavior.

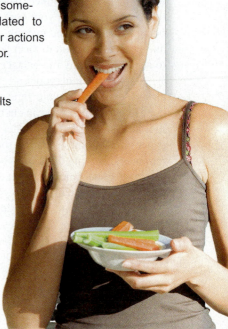

Analyze and Apply

- What do these study results say about the effects of your actions on the people around you?
- In terms of health and wellness, what do you do well? How might you use your strengths to influence others to do well?

Source: van Dellen, M. R., & Hoyle, R. H. (2010). Regulatory accessibility and social influences on state self-control. *Personality and Social Psychology Bulletin, 36*(2), 251–263.

---

life will get less busy or that your current unhealthy behaviors won't have an effect. Talking yourself into maintaining unhealthy behaviors doesn't help you. There's no better time to improve your health habits than right now.

I Don't Know How

If you're reading this text and attending college, you're in the perfect position to learn not only what to do but how to do it and how to find support for doing it. Your text provides up-to-date information on a wide variety of wellness goals and behaviors; refer to Chapter 1 for suggestions for quality health information online. Once you've clarified what you want to change, you then can use the information and the step-wise process described in this chapter to

create your behavior-change plan. Your instructor and student health service may have additional advice and help to offer. If you have specific health concerns, speak with your health care provider.

I Don't Have Enough Money

Joining a health club can be expensive, and a healthy meal in a restaurant can cost significantly more than a burger and fries from the dollar menu at one of the fast-food chains. However, getting in shape doesn't require belonging to a health club, and packing a lunch can provide you with a healthy, low-cost meal.

The fact is that healthy lifestyles are generally less expensive, not more expensive, than unhealthy ones.

Smoking is a perfect example. Not smoking is much healthier—and dramatically cheaper. In the same vein, walking and biking are free and can even save money on gas and transit fare. Likewise, cooking healthy meals from scratch at home is generally far less expensive than eating out or buying prepackaged meals. If your money is tight, look for ways to improve your health habits that don't stretch your budget—or that even save you money. Check the "Dollar Stretcher" tips throughout the text and brainstorm even more money-saving ideas.

DOLLAR STRETCHER
Financial Wellness Tip

Support for behavior change can be free. Use customizable e-cards to send a supportive message to yourself or a friend, to let others know you're trying to make a change, or to let someone know you care and would support them if they tried to make a change. Go to http://www2c.cdc.gov/ecards/

that is personally important, develop a realistic plan and build in concrete rewards for reaching program milestones. As a rule, small, positive steps are easier to accomplish and maintain than are big, quick changes. The idea that you can *never* eat your favorite foods or skip a workout is unrealistic. What matters is your behavior over the long term—if you generally eat healthy and exercise regularly, that's fine. Of course, if your goal is to never restart drinking or smoking, then it's more about planning for situations that might spark those impulses.

Activities you enjoy are easy to initiate and maintain. Therein lies yet another strategy for behavior changes: Make your new health habits pleasurable. Find ways of exercising that you enjoy—perhaps getting involved in team sports or walking with friends you wish you could spend more time with. If you hate jogging, don't jog for exercise; instead, find an activity you enjoy that provides similar benefits, whether playing tennis, rollerblading, or something else. For goals related to weight control, learn which healthy foods taste fantastic. It's much easier to get yourself to do the right thing when it's something you like.

I Lack Willpower

Some situations tempt you more than others—a fact that you can use to your advantage. For example, it's easier to resist buying unhealthy foods if you don't shop when you're hungry, and it's easier to avoid eating the wrong foods if they're not right in front of you. The key is to identify and control the situations and stimuli that trigger behaviors you want to decrease or eliminate. If an alcoholic drink triggers the desire for a cigarette at the same time it reduces decision-making capacity, then avoid drinking alcohol when cigarettes are available.

Having healthy—or healthier—alternatives available also helps us resist temptation. If you carry healthy snacks with you, you're less likely to make a bad choice if you get hungry at school, work, or home. This is an example of the strategy of relapse prevention, in which you plan ahead for challenging situations. For example, if you know you will have trouble keeping up with your exercise program when you travel, develop an alternative plan in advance. The same goes for finals week, Thanksgiving with the family, severe weather, campus or office parties, and any other challenging circumstance or situation.

You can also use some temptations—for example, to watch TV instead of exercising—as rewards. It just takes a bit of planning and effort—finish your workout without procrastinating, then watch a favorite show without guilt. Remember though, the behavior you want to increase must be done *before* you get the reward.

It's Too Hard—and No Fun

A number of factors act together to influence how difficult a behavior change seems—factors you can alter in your favor. First, remember to personalize your goal. Goals that reflect your values and choices are more motivating and yield greater persistence.[16] Once you've selected a change

I'm Too Tired

Are you a morning person or night owl? Everyone has energy rhythms, and variations in your mood and energy level will affect your motivation. Do things that require the most energy when you are at your highest energy level. If you aren't sure when that typically is, keep a log of your energy levels for a week to get an idea of your personal pattern. Also pay attention to what factors influence your energy level. If you feel tired by the time you're through with school or work, do something fun or social to get revitalized. Many times, the fatigue people feel at the end of a day is due to tension. Become one of the countless people who've discovered how exercising at the end of a long day can release tension and restore energy. Big meals also have a tendency to make people tired or sleepy. To increase energy, try a healthy snack and light exercise instead. Remember that your energy level will likely improve as you get into better physical condition.

I Can't Say "No"

We are responsible for our own choices and values. If the inability to say "no" or "not now" keeps you from sticking with your goals, work on developing a more assertive communication style. You can improve your communication

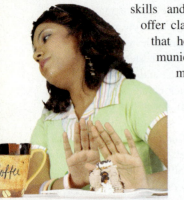

skills and assertiveness. Most colleges offer classes and other student services that help students build strong communication skills. See Chapter 10 for more on assertive communication.

I Have a Negative Outlook

Imagine two people whose fitness plan includes brisk walks. One says to himself, "I don't want to do this . . . I'm so tired . . . I need to relax." The other person thinks, "OK. Let me get this done and I'll feel better. Five minutes into this walk, I won't feel tired anymore. Once I'm done, I can relax." You don't need a psychology lesson to know which one would be more likely to do the exercising. If you approach work (and behavior change is work) thinking about how much you dislike it and how much you do not want to do it, you set up inner resistance to the task. It becomes harder and more stressful, and your focus is less productive. Approaching your goal with a positive attitude makes it easier. Starting your actions with thoughts such as "I can do this" and "I'm doing this for me" reduces inner resistance and improves effort.

If you catch yourself talking yourself out of doing something you should do, try reframing your self-talk. Consciously change what you're saying to yourself to support staying on track with your goal. You might find it helpful to write out negative thoughts so that you can examine them for their flaws. Replace inaccurate, negative self-talk with realistic, positive self-talk that will help you move toward your goal. Table 2-2 gives examples of a few common patterns of thinking. If you grow in your awareness of what makes self-talk positive, you'll likely get plenty of opportunities to practice your more positive inner dialogue in similar situations in the future. Changing mental habits isn't easy, but it has been shown to be both doable and effective in improving emotions and behavior.

TABLE 2-2   EXAMPLES OF NEGATIVE AND POSITIVE PATTERNS OF SELF-TALK

PATTERN OF DISTORTED THINKING	EXAMPLE OF DISTORTED, NEGATIVE SELF-TALK	EXAMPLE OF MORE REALISTIC, POSITIVE SELF-TALK
ALL-OR-NOTHING THINKING	Since I skipped two workouts this week, my exercise program and I are both complete failures. I give up.	I'm disappointed with myself that I skipped two workouts this week. Part of the problem was that I didn't make time for them in my schedule. I've scheduled them in my calendar next week so that I can do better.
BLAMING OTHERS	I wouldn't have eaten so much pizza if I hadn't been with those friends. It's all their fault.	I'm responsible for my own food choices. Next time, I'll suggest a different restaurant, or I'll eat just one piece. I'm a strong person and I can be in control.
OVERGENERALIZING	My roommate was so rude to me this morning. He really hates me.	My roommate was really upset this morning. He's usually in a much better mood. I'm going to talk to him about what's upsetting him.
JUMPING TO CONCLUSIONS	Our class TA asked to meet with me tomorrow. I must have done something awful on that last assignment, or maybe I'm failing the class.	Our class TA asked to meet with me tomorrow. It's the first time that's happened, but I'll just wait and see what's up.
DWELLING ON NEGATIVES	I can't believe I ate that piece of chocolate this afternoon. That's an old habit I'm supposed to be breaking. I'm such a loser.	Too bad I ate that chocolate today—that's one of my old habits. But I've done great on my eating plan all week, so I'm not going to stress about it. Next time, I'll carry a nutritious snack to have instead.

Wellness Strategies

Behavior-Change Support at Your Fingertips

Q | Do Internet support programs work?

Research findings have been mixed about the benefits of online support for behavior change, but Web-based tools seem to be improving. In general, Web-based tools have been found less effective than programs involving human interaction—but they are better than no intervention at all. If you don't have an effective face-to-face support system, or if you highly value your privacy, a Web-based program could be an option for getting started on behavior change. First, though, ask yourself if a Web-based program is a good fit for you. Will you be just as committed if your support is long distance? Will you be more or less likely to drop out?

Look for the following in online behavior-change programs:

- *A personalized or tailored approach,* based on your current behavior and situation (reflecting, for example, your stage of change and, say, your current fruit and vegetable consumption) and including some type of initial self-assessment.

- *Frequent feedback or engagement*—through e-mails, text messages, e-newsletters, and so on—plus an initial motivational interview or consultation.

- *An approach with a sound theoretical base;* look for a program based on behavior-change principles like those discussed in this chapter (such as stages of change, health beliefs, self-efficacy, and motivation).

- *Health information from reputable sources;* search for a program with recommendations from a recognized organization or government program (for example, the American College of Sports Medicine or the American Dietetic Association).

Sources: Alexander, G. L., and others. (2010). A randomized clinical trial evaluating online interventions to improve fruit and vegetable consumption. *American Journal of Public Health, 100*(2), 319–326. Norman, G., Zabinski, M., Adams, M., Rosenberg, D., Yaroch, A., & Atienza, A. (2007). A review of e-health interventions for physical activity and dietary behavior. *American Journal of Preventive Medicine,* 336–345. Spittaels, H., De Bourdeaudhuij, I., & Vandelanotte, C. (2007). Evaluation of a website-delivered computer-tailored intervention for increasing physical activity in the general population. *Preventive Medicine,* 209–217.

I Don't Feel Supported

Interested students can generally find a range of campus programs that support personal wellness, including health services, fitness programs, activity clubs, and intramural events. Unfortunately, not enough students make use of them. Many of them are funded in part—if not fully—by student fees, so take advantage!

There are also support groups and programs available in many communities, hospitals, and churches. Weight Watchers and Alcoholics Anonymous, for example, have helped countless people attain their health goals. If you can't find support locally, look online (see the box "Behavior-Change Support at Your Fingertips" for helpful guidelines).

In addition to campus and community resources, the support of family and friends is a key variable. Goals supported by important people in our lives tend to produce more satisfaction and more sustained effort.[17] In contrast, pursuing goals that are not socially supported or that result in relationship conflict decreases goal satisfaction and makes goals harder to achieve. This does not mean that unsupported goals should never be pursued, but simply that attaining goals is harder without the support and encouragement of significant others.

Let friends and family know what you're trying to accomplish with your health behavior change, and ask for their support. Doing so will also likely heighten your motivation, because your goals are now public. If, for example, friends know you've quit smoking, they will be less likely to offer you a cigarette and you'll be less tempted to accept if one is offered.

I Do OK at First and Then Backslide

Remember, there are stages to behavior change, and lapses are a normal part of the process. Maintaining positive changes is the final stage of the transtheoretical model. Without consciousness and planning for this final stage, it is easy to slide back into old habits. Schedule check-ins with yourself periodically to assess whether your goals and

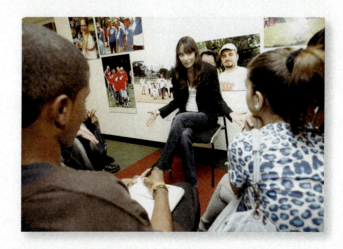

your behavior changes are still on track. Are you exercising as much as you were when you started your fitness plan? Is your consumption of junk food creeping up? For some people, the maintenance phase is the easy part: They are enjoying their new lifestyle and wouldn't go back to their old ways if you paid them. For others, maintenance takes conscious renewal. Things that are important should not be taken for granted. It's true for romantic relationships, and it's true for long-term health.

Developing a Personalized Behavior-Change Program

Q | What is the best way to start if I am trying to change a behavior?

If you've identified a behavior to change and are thinking about how to go about it, you've already started. If you haven't chosen a behavior on which to focus, review the information on wellness lifestyle behaviors in Chapter 1, your results for Lab Activity 1-1, or the ideas in the box "Top New Year's Resolutions." Select a behavior change that will enhance your health and wellness, such as increasing physical activity, reducing fast-food consumption, augmenting fruit and vegetable intake, quitting smoking, or getting more sleep.

To keep your behavior-change efforts efficient and on track, this section describes a step-by-step method for developing and implementing a plan that will help focus your attention, time, and energy. A good plan is like a good map; it gets you where you want to go reliably. Clear, specific plans improve motivation because they give you confidence that you can succeed—your fear of failure goes down, and your expectations for success go up.[18]

The steps outlined here reflect the principles and theories described in the chapter, and they can be used again and again. The general steps are the same whether we're talking about the goals of individuals or of corporations seeking to solve a companywide problem. Indeed, the steps are identical whether the goal is developing a good career, improving grade performance, maintaining a healthy weight, raising self-esteem, mending a relationship, or enjoying life more.

1. Complete a Pros-Versus-Cons Analysis

Write up a detailed analysis of the pros and cons of changing your behavior. Take into account the effects of both your current behavior and the new health habit you'd like to adopt. Your pros list should include the benefits you want to enjoy by changing your behavior; this list will help keep you motivated while you work to make a change. Your cons list should incorporate barriers to change—the factors and issues you think most keep you from changing. Think in both the short term and the long term when developing your

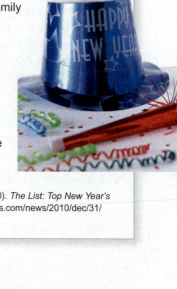

Fast Facts

Top New Year's Resolutions

1. Stop smoking.
2. Drink less.
3. Exercise more.
4. Lose weight.
5. Find a soul mate.
6. Spend more time with family and friends.
7. Get more organized.
8. Find a job.
9. Travel more.
10. Help others/do charity work.

■ Which of the listed goals have you resolved to change at some point in your life? How did you do?

Source: The Washington Times. (2010). *The List: Top New Year's Resolutions* http://www.washingtontimes.com/news/2010/dec/31/list-top-new-years-resolutions/

lists. Also consider the effects of changing your behavior (and not changing it) on both yourself and on others. If needed, do additional research on your target behavior to flesh out your analysis. Refer to the sample pros-versus-cons analysis in Figure 2-5. Consider keeping a journal with your pros-versus-cons analysis and descriptions of the techniques for change that you try. Take note of what works best for you. As you work your way forward through the cycle of change, you'll notice that the pros on your list start to outweigh the cons.

2. Monitor Your Current Behavior

Track your current behavior—for example, your food choices or activity habits—to learn more about it and the factors that influence it. Getting more detailed information about your behavior will also help you to personalize your goal and to develop appropriate strategies for change. You'll want to identify both your helpful and your counterproductive behavior. Monitor other relevant factors, too, such as whom you were with when you overate and how hungry you were.

If you're trying to add a new behavior, such as increased physical activity, you might keep a daily activity record for a week to help you identify times for exercise. For example, how much time do you spend watching TV or surfing the Web? How often do you drive or take an elevator when you could walk or take the stairs? A general activity log is also important for successful time management.

Benefits I want to enjoy:

- Feel better in body, mind, and spirit
- Reduce feelings of stress and tension
- Feel less tired
- Sleep better
- Maintain a healthy weight
- Shed abdominal fat
- Feel better about my body
- Reduce my risk of heart disease, diabetes, and osteoporosis
- Become stronger
- Try new activities and participate in more activities
- Set a good example for my family

Pros

Barriers to change:

- Difficulty finding time for activity
- Not wanting another challenge
- Feeling too tired
- Having other things I'd rather do during the time
- Had a bad experience with exercise in the past
- Sometimes find that exercise is difficult and boring
- Don't want to spend money on a gym or special equipment
- Don't want to work out in front of other people
- Don't like getting sweaty
- Feel unmotivated
- Afraid of failure

Cons

Increasing physical activity

Figure 2-5 Sample pros-versus-cons analysis for behavior change.
Source: Adapted from Centers for Disease Control and Prevention / The Cooper Institute. (n.d.). *Personal Empowerment Plan (PEP) kit: Physical activity precontemplation.* Dallas, TX: The Cooper Institute.

Track your behavior during a usual week or longer, if appropriate—rather than, say, during spring break or finals week—so that your record represents your typical behavior. That said, it's possible that some of your planning strategies may relate to atypical weeks, because relapse prevention is important. If a relapse is likely, then tracking during these weeks may make sense. Otherwise, it's important to gather information about your *typical* behavior—particularly if you're just getting started.

People sometimes find this behavior-monitoring step monotonous and time consuming and are tempted to skip it. Although it can be a little tedious, it's a very important step.

Mind Stretcher
Critical Thinking Exercise

How do you feel about the idea of putting together and carrying out a plan for changing some part of your behavior? Have you ever taken this kind of deliberate action before? Do you feel uneasy about the idea? Or is it exciting and motivating? Why?

Many people think they already know their habits and behaviors but discover surprising truths when they take the time to track their actions and thoughts. Done well, this step makes the next steps easier and potentially much more effective.

3. Set SMART Goals and Plan Rewards

Next, it's time to set your goal. Use the information you gained by tracking your current behavior as a baseline measure. Refine your goal until it meets all the SMART criteria—specific, measurable, achievable, realistic, and time-bound. Once you've refined your goal, give it another check to ensure that it accurately reflects what you really want to achieve.

When you develop the target time frame for your program, be sure to include several milestones, each with an associated reward. Your rewards should be meaningful to you and relatively inexpensive. Also consider giving yourself small rewards for each day or week you stick with your program, as well as lots of positive self-talk.

4. Develop Strategies for Overcoming Obstacles and Supporting Change

After you've completed your pros-versus-cons analysis and tracked your current behavior, you should have a pretty good idea about the obstacles and challenges to changing your behavior. Next, you want to brainstorm all of the possible things that might help you overcome these obstacles and reach your goal. When you brainstorm, you don't have to decide if the ideas you generate are good or bad. Instead, be open and creative to give yourself lots of options. Your list of strategies might include the following:

- Continue or increase things you are already doing that help your goal pursuit.
- Remove cues and triggers that prompt your unhealthy behavior.
- Add new cues and triggers that prompt your new, healthy behavior.
- Make changes in habits that are linked to your unhealthy behavior.

Recheck the list of barriers you identified to ensure you've developed strategies for all the major ones. Think about

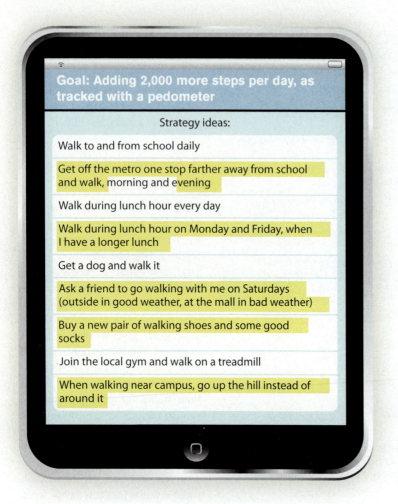

Goal: Adding 2,000 more steps per day, as tracked with a pedometer

Strategy ideas:

Walk to and from school daily

Get off the metro one stop farther away from school and walk, morning and evening

Walk during lunch hour every day

Walk during lunch hour on Monday and Friday, when I have a longer lunch

Get a dog and walk it

Ask a friend to go walking with me on Saturdays (outside in good weather, at the mall in bad weather)

Buy a new pair of walking shoes and some good socks

Join the local gym and walk on a treadmill

When walking near campus, go up the hill instead of around it

Figure 2-6 Brainstorming strategies for change. After identifying as many strategies as possible, select those you think are most realistic and helpful for you.

potential obstacles in both your physical and your social environment. Also identify circumstances most likely to cause lapses, and plan ahead.

Next, look at your list and make some choices. Pare down the possible strategies to a list of actions that reflect what you personally want to do and can do—in essence, what you *will* do. This final list will reflect your knowledge of your personal likes and dislikes, as well as your abilities and resources. For example, someone wanting to be more physically active might make plans to walk more but reject the option of joining a gym (for now) because of costs or logistics; another person with different concerns might decide that joining a gym is the way to go (see the sample in Figure 2-6). The options you choose should reflect your appraisal of what is most realistic and most likely to work for *you*. We're not all alike, and a plan that is too demanding and unrealistic will fail.

5. Identify Helpers and Resources

Think about the people in your life. Who can help you with behavior change, and how can they help? Is there someone

trying to make the same change who can act as a "buddy" and participate in your program? Is there someone who has already successfully made a change who can serve as a role model and offer advice? Is there a friend or family member who can provide daily or weekly support (phone chats, e-mails)?

Tell people about the change you are trying to make, and ask for their support in specific ways. If someone acts in ways that sabotage your efforts—by pushing you to skip your workout, snack on midnight pizza, or smoke—ask him or her to stop. Remember to use assertive communication and make clear, constructive requests. If needed, avoid problem people temporarily until you are farther along in the cycle of change and better able to resist their influence. As a last resort, consider avoiding the problem people permanently if your health or safety is compromised.

In addition to helpers, also check your resources. Do you have all the information you need? All the equipment? Have you checked your campus and community for resources—a free stop-smoking program, reduced-cost gym time, a stress management workshop, and so on? Gather all the tools you need, and take advantage of the available resources.

6. Put Together Your Program Plan

Using all the information you've gathered, put together a specific program plan. Write out your plan—your goals and rewards, the strategies and techniques you've identified, the helpers and resources that will help you succeed, and so on. See Lab Activity 2-2 for a sample program plan format.

7. Make a Commitment . . . and Act on It

Mentally commit yourself to your behavior-change program and goal. Tell people about the change you are trying to make. If you find it helpful, sign a formal contract with yourself. Then get started on change. When the start date of your program arrives, give your plan the time and energy it needs to be successful.

8. Track Your Progress and Modify Your Plan as Needed

As we considered earlier in this chapter, monitoring your behavior and your progress are key strategies for success. Track your behavior to assess your progress, to keep your motivation high, and to modify your plans as needed. Use whatever form of log, journal, or graph works for you. Carry a small paper journal, create a spreadsheet, or find an app for your phone. See the example in Figure 2-7.

Fast Facts

Buddy Up for Behavior Change

For behavior change, the social environment can be instrumental. A recent Internet-based study suggests that if you want to adopt better health and wellness habits, you might just look for a buddy—and make it someone like yourself. A Massachusetts Institute of Technology researcher worked from the idea that people tend to have friends like themselves. Individuals in the study were matched in an online social network either with randomly assigned buddies or with health buddies similar to themselves in the following aspects:

- Body mass
- Age
- Dietary preferences
- Fitness level

The study participants who were matched with someone similar to themselves in these health characteristics were much more likely to maintain a diet diary and to participate in other healthy behaviors than participants with randomly assigned buddies.

- What does this study indicate about the importance of one's social environment in behavior change?

Source: D. Centola (2011). An experimental study of homophily in the adoption of health behavior. *Science* 334(6060):1269–1272.

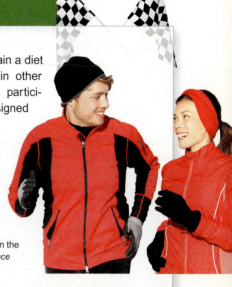

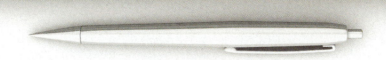

My aerobic activities this week

My goal is to do aerobic activities for a total of __2__ hours this week.

What I did	Effort	When I did it and for how long							Total hours or minutes
		Mon	Tue	Wed	Thu	Fri	Sat	Sun	
Walking outside	Moderate	20			35				55
Treadmill walking (class)	Mod/vig		25						25
Bicycling	Vigorous							35	35

Strategies used that worked:

Riding bike the long way home from the library!

Asking friend to walk with me before dinner

Using a walk as a de-stressor after a bad day at school

Reminders in my computer calendar

Weekly total | 1 hr 55 min

Figure 2-7 Sample behavior-change log.

Source: Adapted from Department of Health and Human Services. (2008). *2008 physical activity guidelines for Americans: Keeping track of what you do each week.* ODPHP Pub No. U0050. Rockville, MD: Office of Disease Prevention and Health Promotion.

Don't be discouraged by small slips and lapses—those are normal. Not every problem or snag can be anticipated, and change may require more time than you initially anticipated. You may need to break your overall goal into smaller, more manageable chunks. You may need to revise your timeline. As long as your goal feels important and attainable, make whatever modifications you need to stay on track. Most plans need to be adjusted or revitalized along the way. When it comes to personal wellness, the goal is always a permanent lifestyle change, not a temporary change in habits.

Q | How much can I say or do to encourage a family member to quit smoking or lose weight?

Helping others change health habits is difficult: You alone can't make someone else change his or her behavior. A good first strategy is to determine what stage of change the friend or family member is in with respect to the unhealthy habit. If he or she is thinking about, planning on, or working on making a change, you can offer concrete support or practical help. If your family member is in the precontemplation stage, it's trickier, because you don't want to push the person to act if he or she isn't ready.

Strategies for helping people in the precontemplation stage include:[19]

- Encourage their inclination to change, but don't push them to act.
- Recommend change frequently but not too frequently. Don't nag, but don't give up—be patient.
- Try discussing specific past instances of the problem behavior and its consequences (for example, being unfit meant skipping a fun outing with friends; remarks made while drunk hurt someone's feelings).
- Acknowledge any positive instances of healthy behavior.

Remember, your own healthy behaviors can be a role model to the people in your life and in your community. Wellness for all!

Summary

Each of us is responsible for our own choices and behaviors. Our behaviors develop over time, based on many contributing factors. When you want to change a behavior, it's important to understand what influences your ability to change—including predisposing, enabling, and reinforcing factors. Motivation directs and sustains your effort for behavior change, and it is influenced by locus of control, self-efficacy expectations, the goals of your program, and how you evaluate the pros and cons of change. For successful change, it's also important to identify your stage in the cycle of change and to apply appropriate processes and techniques of change to overcome key barriers and challenges. Steps in a successful behavior-change program include monitoring your behavior, setting SMART goals, and putting together a detailed plan for change that includes strategies, helpers, rewards, and a firm commitment.

More to Explore

America on the Move
http://americaonthemove.org
Centers for Disease Control and Prevention: Healthy Living
http://www.cdc.gov/HealthyLiving
Department of Health and Human Services Physical Activity Guidelines
http://www.health.gov/paguidelines
United States Department of Agriculture: SuperTracker
https://www.choosemyplate.gov/SuperTracker/default.aspx
Small Step: Improving the Health and Well-Being of America
http://www.smallstep.gov
SmokeFree
http://www.smokefree.gov
See also the resources listed in chapters covering the behavior you plan to change.

LAB ACTIVITY 2-1 Goals and Strategies for Change

⊡ **COMPLETE IN** connect

NAME	DATE	SECTION

Developing a clear goal for your behavior-change program is critical for success. You should also identify specific strategies and techniques to support your efforts at change.

Equipment: None

Preparation: None

Part 1: Goals

Instructions

Begin by writing out your general goal for behavior change; if you still need to choose a behavior to focus on, review the results of the assessments in Chapter 1.

Briefly explain why you've chosen this behavior and this goal for your change program. Why is this goal meaningful to you? What benefits do you expect to enjoy when you achieve this goal?

Next, apply the SMART principle to your goal. Below, work on refining your goal, and explain how it meets each of the SMART criteria:

☐ Specific   Explain: _____
☐ Measurable   Explain: _____
☐ Achievable   Explain: _____
☐ Realistic   Explain: _____
☐ Time-bound   Explain: _____

As you refine your goal and develop a time frame for your program, break your final, overall goal into several smaller short-term objectives, each with its own target start and completion dates. If your plan includes rewards, choose a reward for each short-term objective and your overall final goal.

Final goal:

Start date: _____   End date: _____   Reward: _____

Short-term objective 1:

Start date: _____   End date: _____   Reward: _____

Short-term objective 2:

Start date: _____   End date: _____   Reward: _____

Short-term objective 3:

Start date: _____   End date: _____   Reward: _____

Reflecting on Your Goal

On a scale of 0–100, how confident are you that you can achieve your goal as you set it out? [   ]

Explain:

Part 2: Pros Versus Cons of Change

Instructions

Based on the goal you've set, complete an analysis of the pros versus cons of making a change. You can use the pros as a source of motivation; the cons will help you identify barriers to change that you'll need to overcome in order to be successful.

PROS: BENEFITS I WANT TO ENJOY	CONS: BARRIERS TO CHANGE

Reflect on Your Analysis

Do you think the pros of change outweigh the cons? If so, what benefits of change are most important to you? If not, what do you think you could do to overcome some of the cons and tip the decisional balance in favor of change?

What is your current stage of change (see p. 43 in the chapter)? [   ]

Part 3: Strategies and Techniques for Change

Instructions

Start by brainstorming—think of as many strategies and techniques as you can that would support your behavior-change program. Consider your current actions and environment as well as the suggested techniques for the processes appropriate for your stage of change. What can you do to restructure your physical and social environments to help support change? What can you do to overcome key barriers to change? Use your pros-versus-cons analysis and the following categories to help you brainstorm. Just let your ideas flow.

Increase current actions that support the healthy behavior:

Decrease, eliminate, or manage cues and triggers that prompt the unhealthy behavior; include strategies for countering and for preventing lapses in challenging situations:

Add or increase cues and triggers that prompt the new, healthy behavior:

Strategies to overcome key barriers—consider what you learned by tracking your current behavior and by reviewing the list of common barriers in the chapter; check off your key barriers and brainstorm strategies for them:

☐ Lack of time   ☐ Lack of willpower   ☐ Lack of support

☐ Lack of motivation   ☐ Lack of enjoyment   ☐ Problems with maintenance

☐ Procrastination   ☐ Lack of energy   ☐ Other: _____

☐ Lack of information   ☐ Inability to be assertive ☐ Other: _____

☐ Expense   ☐ Negative self-talk   ☐ Other: _____

Reflecting on Your Strategies Lists

Next, go back and identify (circle) the strategies that you will use—select those that best fit you and your needs and preferences. You'll use these strategies when you complete your program plan in Lab Activity 2-2.

LAB ACTIVITY 2-2 Program Plan for Behavior Change

COMPLETE IN connect

NAME	DATE	SECTION

Complete this program plan with details on your specific plan for behavior change.

Equipment: None

Preparation: None

Target Behavior (the behavior you want to change) ______________________

Your Final Goal and Your Short-Term Objectives (see Lab Activity 2-1)

Final goal: ______________________

Start date: __________ End date: __________ Reward: __________

Short-term objective 1: ______________________

Start date: __________ End date: __________ Reward: __________

Short-term objective 2: ______________________

Start date: __________ End date: __________ Reward: __________

Short-term objective 3: ______________________

Start date: __________ End date: __________ Reward: __________

Your Key Strategies and Techniques for Change (see Lab Activity 2-1)

Your Helpers and Resources

Who will help with your program and how will they help?

What campus or community resources will support your program?

Your Commitment (Sign the statement below to make your plan a formal contract, or describe your own plan for making a firm commitment to change.)

I, _____, commit to achieving the following goal: _____
          (name)

_____

Signature: _____ Date: _____

OR describe your plan for making your commitment (telling others, sending e-cards, etc.):

Plan for Monitoring Behavior and Tracking Progress

Describe the journal, log, or other tracking method you plan to use:

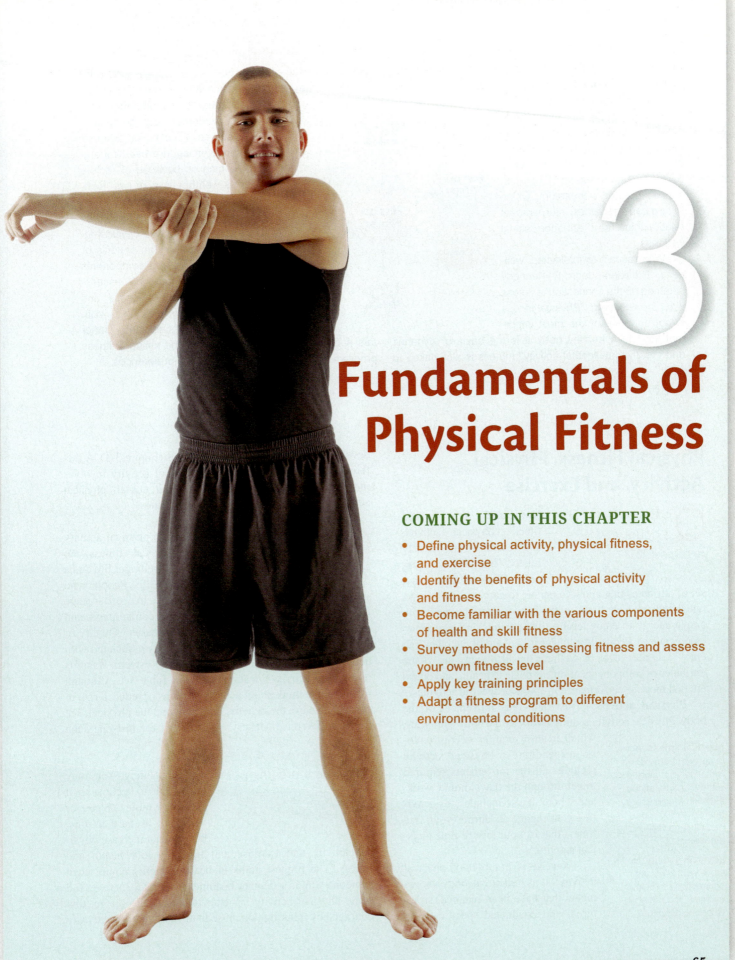

Fundamentals of Physical Fitness

3

COMING UP IN THIS CHAPTER

- Define physical activity, physical fitness, and exercise
- Identify the benefits of physical activity and fitness
- Become familiar with the various components of health and skill fitness
- Survey methods of assessing fitness and assess your own fitness level
- Apply key training principles
- Adapt a fitness program to different environmental conditions

How does fitness relate to your overall wellness? The relationship to physical wellness is clear—physical activity and physical fitness are critical to a long, healthy life. In terms of emotional wellness, exercise elevates your mood, decreases stress, and enhances your well-being. Furthermore, increased fitness can lead to greater self-esteem, which in turn can strengthen interpersonal relationships and enhance social wellness.

With respect to intellectual wellness, President John F. Kennedy summed up the connection to fitness when he observed, "Physical fitness is not only one of the most important keys to a healthy body, it is the basis of dynamic and creative intellectual activity." Fitness is also linked to spiritual wellness—to your beliefs and values—and spiritual beliefs may in turn influence your choice of activities.

Finally, there is environmental wellness: Environment can be a wonderful source of motivation, whether you can exercise in a beautiful outdoor setting or, because of factors such as weather, in a secure, high-quality indoor fitness facility.

This chapter presents the basics of physical activity and physical fitness. We'll examine the benefits of activity, the types and components of fitness, methods of assessing individual levels of fitness, and important training principles. With this foundation established, Chapters 4–6 will focus on designing and fine-tuning a fitness program that fits individuals' needs and preferences.

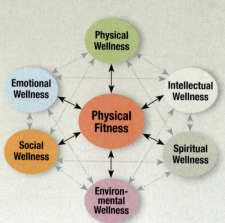

Physical Fitness, Physical Activity, and Exercise

Q | Does all activity count as exercise?

Not exactly, no. Physical fitness, physical activity, and exercise are closely related but distinct concepts. **Physical fitness** is a set of attributes that allows a person to carry out daily tasks with vigor and alertness, without undue fatigue, and with ample energy to enjoy leisure-time pursuits and respond to emergencies.[1] People live longer if they are fit, and they can enjoy a higher level of wellness in all dimensions. Some attributes or components of fitness relate to health, and others are tied more to performance in sports or specific activities.

Physical activity is just that—any movement of the body. Physical activity requires work by the body's muscles, which in turn requires energy (calorie expenditure). Physical activity includes all the movements required to get through the day at home, work, and school. It also includes any activities you engage in during your free time—that is, your leisure-time physical activity.

Exercise is a subset of physical activity; it is repetitive body movements that have been planned, structured, and conducted specifically to develop components of physical fitness (Figure 3-1). A difference to remember is that all physical activity involves movement and energy expenditure, but not all physical activity develops or increases physical fitness.

Q | Will I really lose years of my life if I'm unfit?

Yes. Both physical activity and physical fitness are linked to a longer life and a healthier life. People who are active live on average several years longer than their sedentary counterparts, and they have lower rates of many major diseases.[2] Quality of life is also improved, with physical activity associated with better mood, better sleep, and greater self-esteem. Benefits of physical activity are summarized in Table 3-1. Although many people think about activity in terms of reduced risk of chronic disease, the benefits range beyond the physical; see the box "Exercise Makes You Smarter" for just one such example.

Q | Is there any point in exercising if I can't become super-fit?

Yes, absolutely. You may not be able to become as fit as an Olympic athlete, or work out as hard as one, but you can increase physical activity and exercise and improve your health and fitness. The biggest gains in health benefits come when someone who is sedentary becomes moderately active. And some physical activity is better than none. Don't get discouraged by thinking you must do difficult or high-intensity

physical fitness Ability to carry out daily tasks with vigor and alertness, without undue fatigue, and with ample energy to enjoy leisure-time pursuits and respond to emergencies.

physical activity Bodily movement involving contraction of skeletal muscles and requiring calorie expenditure.

Behavior-Change Challenge
Targeting Physical Fitness

You're beginning your second year of college, and those freshman 15 (or more?) are right there in the mirror, staring you in the face. As a freshman, you'd gotten lax about sticking to a fitness routine, opting instead to spend your leisure time hanging out and watching sports with your new friends. Now you want to lose those pounds and get back into your high school form. Working out and staying fit were a top priority for you back then.

Meet Greg

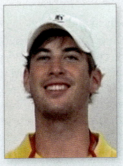

Greg is a 21-year-old college sophomore who lives in a fraternity. Greg considers himself inactive compared to his high school days. He wants to start an exercise program to try to get back into shape and to avoid the weight gain he has seen in family members. View the video to learn more about Greg, his behavior-change goals and plan, and his success over the initial weeks of his program. As you watch, consider:

- How realistic are Greg's goals and his starting program plan? How would you modify Greg's objectives and routine to fit the needs of your fitness program?
- Does Greg have enough motivation and environmental support for his program? What do you think his biggest barriers and challenges will be? What will your greatest obstacles be?
- What worked for Greg, and what parts of the program caused difficulties for him? What can you learn from Greg's experience that will help you in your behavior-change efforts?

VIDEO CASE STUDY   WATCH THIS VIDEO IN   connect

physical activity compares with that of the nation as a whole and of different population groups.

Types of Fitness

So, how do you add more physical activity, especially exercise to boost physical fitness, to your life? The first step is to learn more about types of fitness and the training principles that will help you make the best use of your time and energies.

Fitness components are typically divided into two major categories: health-related fitness and skill-related fitness. **Health-related fitness** components have a direct effect on your health status, disease risk, and day-to-day functioning. **Skill-related fitness** components or attributes influence your performance level in various activities and are less directly related to health. This section of the chapter provides a brief introduction to the different components of fitness. The health-related components are discussed in much more detail in Chapters 4–7.

exercise Planned, structured, repetitive body movements conducted specifically to develop components of physical fitness.

health-related fitness Components or areas of fitness that have a direct effect on overall health and disease risk.

skill-related fitness Components or areas of fitness that contribute to the ability to function in a skilled and efficient way and don't have a direct effect on overall health; also called performance-related fitness.

activities. Set realistic goals for improvement and gradually increase the amount of exercise you do.

Q Isn't the "couch potato" thing overblown? I seem to see more people exercising all the time.

Despite the many wonderful benefits of physical activity, most American adults don't engage in much activity during their leisure time. And rates of activity have been holding steady or dropping—not what public health officials want to see. Figure 3-2 will give you insight into how your level of

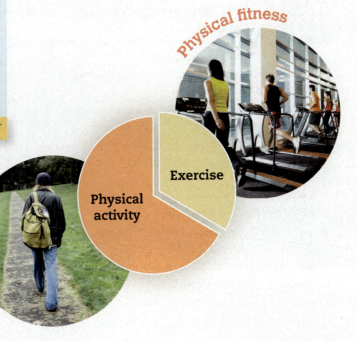

Figure 3-1 Physical activity, exercise, and physical fitness. Exercise is a subset of physical activity specifically designed to develop physical fitness.

Research Brief

Exercise Makes You Smarter

Exercise doesn't just make you feel and look better. Research suggests that exercise may also make you smarter by stimulating the production of new brain cells. It was once believed humans were born with a finite number of brain cells that died over the life span, but there is now definitive evidence that the human brain can continue to produce new brain cells throughout life.

A recent study focused on the hippocampus, a brain area that is critical for memory and learning. Using magnetic resonance imaging (MRI) to create maps of the brain and blood flow, researchers followed a group of adults as they completed a 3-month exercise program; participants also took fitness and cognitive tests. The study found that exercise increased markers for the production of new brain cells. In addition, the participants improved their scores on cognition tests, and the amount of cognitive improvement was tied to the degree of improved fitness. Other studies have shown similar effects of exercise for other age groups.

Multiple studies in recent years confirm that both aerobic and resistance-training exercises can have a positive effect on the brain and cognition. More research is needed to determine what personal factors may enhance or detract from the benefits of exercise, and to what extent. But there is already ample evidence to support the importance that physical activity and fitness play in intellectual wellness.

Analyze and Apply

- Do you think one type of exercise (aerobic or resistance training) benefits you more in terms of your ability to think clearly? Why do you think that one works better for you than the other—or that they both work equally, if that's the case?
- The Research Brief states, "More research is needed to determine what personal factors may enhance or detract from the benefits of exercise, and to what extent." What sorts of personal factors might researchers investigate in follow-up research?

Sources: Pereira, A. C., and others. (2007). An *in vivo* correlate of exercise-induced neurogenesis in the adult dentate gyrus. *Proceedings of the National Academy of Sciences, 104*(13), 5638–5643. Voss, M. W., and others. (2011). Exercise, brain and cognition across the lifespan. *Journal of Applied Physiology, 111,* 1505–1513.

TABLE 3-1   BENEFITS OF PHYSICAL ACTIVITY

- Lower mortality from all causes—that is, active people have lower overall death rates
- Better cardiorespiratory functioning and less risk of heart disease and stroke
  - Lower blood pressure, in some cases enough to reduce or eliminate the need for medication
  - Better blood fat levels—higher levels of high-density lipoprotein ("good cholesterol") and lower levels of triglycerides
  - Lower resting heart rate and blood pressure
  - Stronger heart and lungs, better blood flow
- Less risk of cancer, especially colon cancer and breast cancer
- Less risk of type 2 diabetes
  - Better control of body fat
  - Better blood sugar and insulin levels
  - Less need for insulin by people with type 2 diabetes

- Less risk of osteoporosis and related fractures
  - Better bone density
  - Less risk of falls
- Lower risk of gallbladder disease
- Better body composition
  - Less total body fat, particularly abdominal fat
  - Prevention of weight gain
  - Maintenance of weight after weight loss
- Better mental well-being
  - Better quality of sleep (active people fall asleep more quickly and sleep more deeply)
  - Higher self-esteem and better mood
  - Improvement of mild-to-moderate depression and anxiety
- Better performance in work, leisure, and sport activities
- Better quality of life and increased ability to live independently for older adults

Sources: American College of Sports Medicine. (2009). *ACSM's resources manual for guidelines for exercise testing and prescription* (6th ed.). Baltimore, MD: Lippincott Williams & Wilkins. U.S. Department of Health and Human Services. (2008). *2008 physical activity guidelines for Americans.* ODPHP Pub. No. U0036. Rockville, MD: Office of Disease Prevention and Health Promotion. Haskell, W. L., and others. (2007). Physical activity and public health: Updated recommendations for adults from the American College of Sports Medicine and the American Heart Association. *Circulation, 116,* 1081–1093.

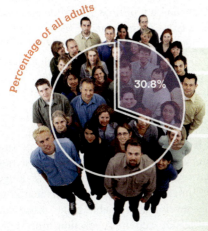

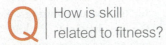
Percentage of all adults

30.8%

Percentage engaging in regular physical activity*	
All adults	30.8
Gender	
Men	32.9
Women	29.0
Age (in years)	
18–24	37.1
25–44	33.3
45–64	30.0
65 and over	21.6
Education	
No high school diploma or GED	46.7
High school diploma or GED	21.8
Some college or more	38.0
Income relative to poverty level	
Below 100%	19.7
100% to less than 200%	23.0
200% or more	34.6

*Regular leisure-time physical activity means three or more sessions per week of vigorous activity lasting at least 20 minutes or five or more sessions per week of light or moderate activity lasting at least 30 minutes.

Figure 3-2 Rates of regular leisure-time physical activity among Americans.
Source: National Center for Health Statistics. (2009). *Health, United States, 2008, updated trend tables* (http://www.cdc.gov/nchs/hus/updatedtables.htm).

Skill-Related Fitness

Q | How is skill related to fitness?

Skill-related fitness, sometimes referred to as *motor fitness* or *performance-related fitness,* includes fitness components or attributes that contribute to your ability to function in a more skilled and efficient way. They can result in an increased desire to participate in physical activities. In this indirect way, increased skill-related activity can affect your health.

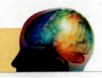

Mind Stretcher
Critical Thinking Exercise

Why are rates of leisure-time physical activity so low given its many benefits? What do you think are the key reasons for sedentary behavior? If you were a public health or campus official, how would you promote physical activity in your community or at your school?

Skill-related fitness components include agility, balance, coordination, power, reaction time, and speed. Unless you are a skilled athlete wanting to improve a particular skill, you may not even think about these components of fitness. Skill-related fitness is often taken for granted because, through normal development, we typically acquire enough balance, coordination, and so on for daily living. Although not everyone develops to the same level for each component, most people—unless they are ill or have a disability or other limitation—develop adequate levels of skill-related fitness. Typically, the levels of these components are inadequate only at the beginning of life and again in later years. As very young children, we learn these skills through trial and error and continued practice. The natural aging process, often along with decreased use, can take its toll on these skills. Older adults become susceptible to difficulties with balance, reaction time, coordination, and other skill-related abilities.

AGILITY. **Agility** is the ability to change the direction and position of the body in a quick and precise manner. Agility is important in many sports. Quick, controlled changes in direction are needed for successful performance in individual activities, such as gymnastics and diving, as well as in individual and team sports such as tennis, basketball, and football. Agility is partly determined by heredity; however, agility can be improved through practice.[3]

BALANCE. **Balance** is the ability to maintain equilibrium when sitting, standing, or moving. Maintenance of equilibrium while in a stationary position such as sitting or standing is known as *static balance;* maintenance of equilibrium during movement is known as *dynamic balance.* Each type of balance is important for many specialized activities as well as for routine daily activities.

Balance is controlled by the *semicircular canals* in the inner ear, musculoskeletal-system sensors known as *proprioceptors,* and the eyes. The inner ear is very sensitive and has the ability to detect motion and gravity. Proprioceptors in the muscles, tendons, and joints detect a limb's position in space by interpreting muscle contractions and joint angles. Your brain uses signals from each of these sensory organs as well as your ability to see and interpret

agility Ability to change the direction and position of the body in a quick and precise manner.

balance Ability to maintain equilibrium when sitting, standing, or moving.

POWER. **Power** is the ability to exert a maximum amount of force in a minimum amount of time. It is often described in terms of explosive types of movements, such as the vertical jump. Power requires both strength and speed and therefore typically is greater in those with greater muscle mass. Because strength is one of the contributors, power is sometimes included on the list of health-related fitness components.

REACTION TIME. **Reaction time** is the amount of time between a stimulus and your response to it. As a rule, young children have very slow reaction times (a longer time between the stimulus and response), but neurological changes during development enable faster processing time. In sports and leisure activities, reaction time shows up in starting a sprint or moving to block a goal in soccer or hockey. In day-to-day activities, you need good reaction time for tasks such as braking when the car in front of you stops suddenly.

SPEED. **Speed** is the ability to perform a movement in a short period of time—the shorter the time, the greater the speed. The movement may be of a single body part or your entire body. Like reaction time, speed develops during childhood. Increases in speed level off for most girls between ages 8 and 12, but boys may continue to increase speed throughout adolescence due to their increasing body size and levels of testosterone.

Health-Related Fitness

Q | I'm terrible at sports and have no interest in them. Are there other ways to be fit and healthy?

You don't have to be an athlete to be healthy and fit. Instead of focusing on the development of skill-related fitness components, you can concentrate on the health-related fitness components—things that have a direct effect on your overall functional health.[5] Health-related fitness components include:

- Cardiorespiratory endurance
- Muscular strength
- Muscular endurance
- Flexibility
- Body composition

Without a sufficient level of fitness in each of these areas, your health—and your ability to function at capacity in your day-to-day life—may be inhibited. Additionally, you may be at greater risk for some chronic diseases as well as for early onset of diseases. Conversely, adequate levels help to protect against illness and disease and contribute to a better quality of life—more years of healthy life. See the box "Exercise Keeps You Young."

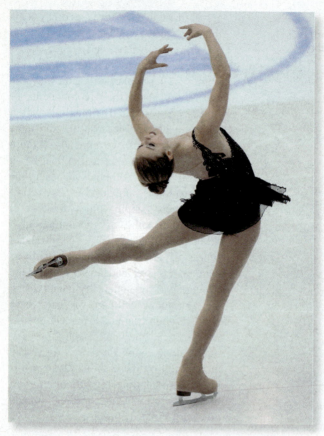

Balance is the ability to maintain equilibrium. It depends on the functioning of the inner ear, sensors in the musculoskeletal system, and vision. Although considered a skill-related fitness component, balance is necessary for many daily tasks.

images to assess any imbalance. The brain sends the data needed for correction back to the appropriate muscles—thus helping you to regain balance. Maintaining equilibrium requires this constant messaging. Balance can be trained by simple movements, such as standing on one leg and reaching forward, or by specialized exercises and equipment such as balance boards.

COORDINATION. **Coordination** is the ability to synchronize multiple movement patterns into sequenced, efficient, controlled movement. An example is throwing a ball: Multiple movement patterns (arm action, stepping action, hip rotation, and so on) are coordinated to produce a sequenced, efficient movement. Any movement patterns that require hand-eye or foot-eye transactions utilize coordination; the more complex the patterns, the greater the amount of coordination needed. Coordination includes the use of, and is therefore somewhat dependent on, balance, agility, speed, and reaction time.[4]

coordination Ability to synchronize multiple movement patterns into sequenced, efficient, controlled movement.

power Ability to exert a maximum amount of force in a minimum amount of time.

reaction time Amount of time between a stimulus and one's response to that stimulus.

speed Ability to perform movement in a short period of time.

Research Brief

Exercise Keeps You Young

Research suggests that exercise not only helps to delay the onset of age-related diseases but may also affect the aging process itself. Recent studies have examined the length of *telomeres* (the protective caps at the end of chromosomes). Telomeres typically shorten progressively over time as we age, but multiple studies have found that telomere length in individuals who participate in aerobic exercise activities was significantly longer than in the nonactive individuals. In several cases, the active individuals had telomere lengths equivalent to those of sedentary individuals several years younger. Research is ongoing, but these results suggest that people who are physically active are "biologically younger" than people who are sedentary.

Analyze and Apply

■ Could you be "biologically younger" than your number of years based on your *current* aerobic activity? Explain.

■ How might you use this information to motivate yourself—or others you care about—to exercise regularly?

Sources: Cherkas, L., and others. (2008). The association between physical activity in leisure time and leukocyte telomere length. *Archives of Internal Medicine,* 154–158. LaRocca, T. J., and others. (2010). Leukocyte telomere length is preserved with aging in endurance exercise-trained adults and related to maximal aerobic capacity. *Mechanisms of Ageing and Development, 131*(2), 165–167.

Let's now define the health-related fitness components. We'll examine each in greater detail—including contributing factors, benefits, assessment, and appropriate exercises—in Chapters 4–7.

CARDIORESPIRATORY ENDURANCE. **Cardiorespiratory endurance** is the ability of the circulatory and respiratory systems to sustain physical activity by supplying oxygen to working muscles. The heart, lungs, and entire network of blood vessels work together to provide oxygen to the muscles in order for them to continue working. The lungs take in oxygen, which blood cells pick up and deliver to muscles throughout the body as the blood is pushed through blood vessels via the pumping action of the heart. The same systems carry carbon dioxide, a by-product of the chemical reactions that produce energy for physical activity, in the reverse direction, eliminating it from the body. Cardiorespiratory endurance thus depends on the capacity of the lungs to take in oxygen, the ability of the circulatory system to carry and transport the oxygen, and the force of the heart's pumping action. The terms *cardiorespiratory fitness, cardiovascular endurance, cardiovascular fitness, aerobic endurance,* and *aerobic fitness* are often used interchangeably.

Cardiorespiratory fitness is developed by what are called *aerobic* (with oxygen) activities. This category includes activities like brisk walking, jogging, swimming, and cycling that put stress on the cardiorespiratory system but that can be maintained for a long time. Chapter 4 describes cardiorespiratory fitness training in detail.

MUSCULAR STRENGTH. **Muscular strength** is the ability of a muscle or group of muscles to generate or apply force. If, when you hear the phrases *muscular strength* or *ability to apply force,* you think only of someone with huge, bulging muscles, you need to reshape your thinking. Muscular strength is something *everyone* needs. No matter what your

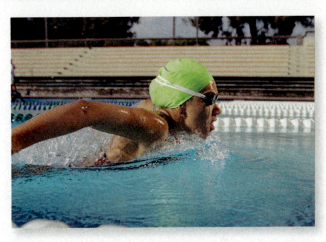

Cardiorespiratory endurance depends on the functioning of the heart, lungs, and blood vessels. It is developed through aerobic activities such as swimming and running.

size or your typical activities, a certain amount of strength is necessary for day-to-day living—thus the inclusion of this component in the health-related fitness category. For example, it requires a certain amount, maybe even a significant amount, of muscular strength to lift your book bag or backpack safely and without injury.

Activities that increase muscular strength involve the application of force against resistance. Weight training is often the chosen means of developing muscular strength, but calisthenics—exercises performed with no added weight—and other activities that use the body's own weight as resistance can also be effective strengthening exercises.

cardiorespiratory endurance Ability of the circulatory and respiratory systems to sustain physical activity by supplying oxygen to working muscles; also called cardiorespiratory fitness.

muscular strength Ability of a muscle or group of muscles to generate or apply force, often by contracting against resistance.

MUSCULAR ENDURANCE. Muscular endurance is the ability of a muscle or group of muscles to sustain an effort for an extended time; it may take the form of a single continuous exertion or repeated exertions. Muscular endurance is related to strength. For example, lifting your book bag, like many other daily tasks, requires a certain amount of muscular strength. However, simply being able to lift your bag isn't enough. You need to carry it to class, the library, your residence, and so on. Lifting the bag or backpack (exerting force) requires strength; carrying it with you (continued exertion) requires muscular endurance. Both are necessary for your daily activities. Together, muscular strength and muscular endurance, as well as some other muscle attributes, are often referred to collectively as *muscle fitness.*

Like strength, endurance improvement requires resistance exercises. However, how you perform these exercises will differ depending on whether you want to emphasize strength or endurance in your training program. Chapter 5 describes muscle-fitness training in detail.

FLEXIBILITY. Flexibility is the ability of a joint to move through its full range of motion. A certain amount of flexibility is needed for day-to-day activities and to help prevent injuries that can be caused by a restricted range of motion. Flexibility of the lower back and hamstrings (the muscles that form the back of the thigh) may be particularly important for some people to help prevent low-back pain and other related problems. For this reason, flexibility is most commonly tested in the lower back. Flexibility is best maintained or improved through stretching exercises. Chapter 6 has more on flexibility training and lower-back care.

muscular endurance
Ability of a muscle or group of muscles to sustain an effort for an extended time.

flexibility Ability of a joint to move through its full range of motion.

body composition
Relative amounts of muscle, fat, bone, and other vital tissues of the body.

BODY COMPOSITION. Body composition is the makeup of your body. How much of each of the various types of tissues make up your body? Body composition is usually defined as the relative amounts of muscle, fat, bone, and other vital tissues of the body and is stated in terms of a percentage.[6] Too much or too little fat can negatively affect your health, including putting you at an increased

Fast Facts

Survival of the Fittest
Would you believe . . .

- Gibbons have greater *agility* than other animals?
- A cat uses it ears and tail for *balance?*
- Hibernating animals lose *coordination?*
- A wolverine is more *powerful* than a moose?
- A star-nosed mole can *react* to eat its prey faster than a human can hit the brakes of a car?
- An ostrich is the *speediest* bird on land?
- A yak has great lung capacity and *oxygen-carrying capacity?*
- Certain horses have greater *endurance* than other animals?
- The rhinoceros beetle is the *strongest* creature on earth?
- Otters are very *flexible?*
- Ringed seal pups have more *body fat* than whales?

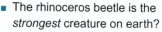

risk for various diseases. For this reason, when assessing body composition, fat is typically separated out, and all the other tissues are grouped under the heading of fat-free mass. Body composition testing reports the percentage of body weight that is fat.

Body composition can be affected by diet as well as various types of physical activities. Both aerobic and resistance types of exercise can change overall body composition. Chapter 7 provides more information on body composition.

Assessing Physical Activity and Fitness

Before beginning a fitness program, it's important to know your current fitness status. If you are healthy enough for fitness testing, then you should determine your fitness level in each of the health-related fitness components and in all the skill-related components you plan to train. This assessment will help you develop an appropriate training program and check your progress after you've trained for a while.

Medical Clearance

Mind Stretcher
Critical Thinking Exercise

When you think about exercise, do you think about developing all the components of health-related fitness? Do you rate some components as more important than others? What has informed these thoughts or beliefs—media, peers, family, other? How have these thoughts and beliefs affected your exercise habits in the past?

 Is it safe for anyone to exercise?

Starting or gradually increasing physical activity is safe for most people. If you are between the ages of 15 and 69

Living *Well* with . . .

a Disability

More than 50 million Americans have some type of chronic disability, including those from injury or illness and those present at birth. Here are a few examples among adults age 18 and older:

- Number with vision trouble: 25.2 million
- Number unable (or able only with great difficulty) to walk a quarter mile: 16.0 million
- Number with any physical functioning difficulty: 33.1 million

Assistive and adaptive technologies can help people with disabilities to perform daily tasks and to enjoy recreational pursuits. If you have a disability and want to be more active, first check with your health care provider about the amounts and types of physical activity that are appropriate for you. The Department of Health and Human Services' *2008 Physical Activity Guidelines for Adults* includes a special section for adults with disabilities:

- Adults with disabilities, who are able to, should get at least 150 minutes a week of moderate-intensity, or 75 minutes a week of vigorous-intensity aerobic activity, or an equivalent combination of moderate- and vigorous-intensity aerobic activity. Aerobic activity should

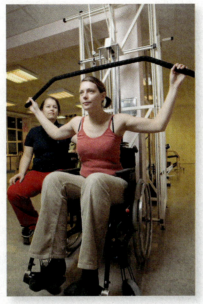

be performed in episodes of at least 10 minutes, and preferably, it should be spread throughout the week.

- Adults with disabilities, who are able to, should also do muscle-strengthening activities of moderate or high intensity that involve all major muscle groups on 2 or more days a week, because these activities provide additional health benefits.
- When adults with disabilities are not able to meet the guidelines, they should engage in regular physical activity according to their abilities and should avoid inactivity.

For more information on physical activity and disability, visit the ACSM's Web site *Your Prescription for Health,* which provides informational flyers on many health conditions: http://exerciseismedicine.org/documents/PublicAction GuideLQ.pdf. Additional information is available from the National Center on Physical Activity and Disability: http://www.ncpad.org.

Sources: National Center for Health Statistics. (2009). *Disability and functioning (Adults)* (http://www.cdc.gov/nchs/fastats/disable.htm). U.S. Department of Health and Human Services. (2008). *2008 physical activity guidelines for Americans.* ODPHP Publication No. U0036. Rockville, MD: Office of Disease Prevention and Health Promotion.

---

with no complicating health factors, you should be fine. Completing the **Physical Activity Readiness Questionnaire (PAR-Q)** in Lab Activity 3-1 will help you to be sure. If you answer yes to any of the questions, if you are not used to being very active, or if you are outside the age range listed, you should check with your doctor before starting a new activity program or significantly increasing your current level of physical activity. Depending on your situation, your physician may simply ask you additional questions, or she or he may want to perform additional tests. Your doctor's goal will not be to keep you from participating but rather to help you participate in the safest manner possible. Physical activity is a key strategy for managing or treating many chronic diseases.

Q My mother-in-law has arthritis in her knees. Is she supposed to do any exercise?

Yes, although she may need to modify a basic exercise program to be appropriate for her. Physical activity can

be beneficial for many people with arthritis and other chronic health conditions that affect mobility, cardiorespiratory functioning, and strength. According to the National Center on Physical Activity and Disability, exercise is for everyone. People with disabilities typically lead less active lifestyles, although appropriate physical activity can help prevent secondary conditions and boost overall wellness. For arthritis, physical activity can reduce joint pain and swelling, improve overall functioning, and help maintain a healthy weight, which reduces pressure on the joints. Anyone with a chronic condition or health concern should check with her or his health care provider about designing an activity program that maximizes the benefits and minimizes the risks; see the box "Living Well with . . . a Disability" for more information.

Physical Activity Readiness Questionnaire (PAR-Q) A widely used assessment tool that guides people in determining whether to seek medical clearance prior to beginning or increasing an exercise program.

Assessing General Physical Activity Levels

Q What do *sedentary* and *active* actually mean? I'm busy all the time, so I feel really active.

Unfortunately, busy and active aren't the same. Many people feel as though they are rushing around all day, but all this hurrying doesn't necessarily mean they are *physically* active.

There is no technique that is both simple and precise to judge your overall level of physical activity. One technique that can provide an approximate measure, as well as some motivation, is to wear a pedometer and record the number of steps you take each day. Pedometers provide a rough measure of activity, although they can't differentiate between types of activity (jogging versus walking or walking on a flat surface versus up hills or stairs). There are about 2,000 steps in a mile, and walking at a pace of about 100 steps per minute is considered moderately intense for many adults.[7]

The frequently promoted goal of 10,000 or more steps per day is reasonable for most healthy adults (Table 3-2). However, you need to consider your current activity level in setting goals. For example, if you are currently taking 5,000 steps per day, you'll want to set a more modest goal, at least initially. On the other hand, if you are already averaging 10,000 steps a day, then you'll need to set a higher goal in order to increase your level of physical activity. Lab Activity 3-2 takes you through the steps of determining your baseline activity level and setting appropriate goals for improvement. Figure 3-3 summarizes a simple program for increasing physical activity using a pedometer.

Assessing Fitness

Q What types of fitness assessments are available?

There are many types of fitness tests to assess and evaluate each component of fitness. Some are simple and require little equipment. Others require more specialized equipment, a lab, and a skilled administrator. Chapters 4–7 include a variety of tests you can perform to assess your fitness for each of the components of health-related fitness. Skill-related fitness components are not addressed in depth, but your instructor can refer you to appropriate tests.

Principles of Training

Understanding the different types and components of fitness is only the first step to improving your fitness. It's also important to know some of the basic principles of fitness

Aim to increase physical activity.

Clip the pedometer to your waistband midway between your side and the center crease line of your pants.

Reset the counter to zero at the beginning of each day.

Walk for a week, counting steps, to establish your baseline.

Set Goal for stepping that takes your baseline into account; see Table 3-2.

Add to your daily steps; increase every two weeks by an average of 500–1,000 per day until you reach your final goal.

Track your progress toward your goal by keeping a log of your daily steps.

Figure 3-3 A basic pedometer-based stepping program for increasing physical activity.

Sources: National Institutes of Health. (2010). General guidelines for pedometer use. *Division of Nutrition Research Coordination* (http://dnrc .nih.gov/move-health/pedometer-use.asp). Anders, M. (2006). Do you do 10K a day? *American Council on Exercise Fitness Matters, 12*(4). American College of Sports Medicine. (2011). *Selecting and effectively using a pedometer.* (http://www.acsm.org/docs/brochures/selecting-and-effectively-using-a-pedometer.pdf).

and training. These principles relate to all the fitness components, and understanding and applying them will help you reap the greatest benefits from your training.

TABLE 3-2 PHYSICAL ACTIVITY LEVEL BASED ON PEDOMETER TRACKING

AVERAGE STEPS PER DAY	ACTIVITY LEVEL
Less than 5,000	Sedentary
5,000–7,499	Low active
7,500–9,999	Somewhat active
10,000–12,500	Active
Over 12,500	Highly active

A pedometer can do more than count your steps; it can motivate you to be more active. For best results, set a step goal and keep a step diary.

Sources: Bravata, D., Smith-Spangler, C., Sundaram, V., and others. (2007). Using pedometers to increase physical activity and improve health: A systematic review. *JAMA, 298*(19), 2296–2304. Tudor-Locke, C., Hatano, Y., Pangrazi, R. P., & Kang, M. (2008). Revisiting "How many steps are enough?" *Medicine and Science in Sports and Exercise, 40*(7 Suppl), S537–S543.

Progressive Overload

Q | How do I improve my fitness level?

To improve in any area of fitness, the body must do more than it's used to doing. This principle, shown in Figure 3-4, is known as **progressive overload.** The body must be exposed to a greater amount of activity than normal. For example, if your current activity limit is walking half a mile in 10 minutes, then to improve fitness, you would need to walk farther or faster, or both. If you can currently do ten push-ups, then you would need to increase that number in order to improve muscular strength and endurance. The amount of overload or stress you place on the body is important—too little, and fitness won't improve; too much, and you may be injured.

The "progressive" part of progressive overload means that the amount of overload needs to be increased gradually. As your fitness improves, you will reach a new norm—say, 15 push-ups—and you'll need to do more to continue to improve fitness. Once you reach a goal fitness level, you can maintain it by continuing to train at that level—say, 25 push-ups. To avoid injury, you shouldn't add too much stress or overload at once; gradual increases are best for training. If you are not currently active, start slowly and progress gradually.

The amount of overload needed is specific to the individual. Someone who has high muscle fitness in the arms isn't going to improve strength or endurance by doing 10 push-ups. However, this may be a good level of overload for someone who hasn't done any muscle-fitness training. Individual differences also have a genetic component—some people can achieve higher levels of strength and endurance because of physiological characteristics they inherited. When you develop your fitness program, it's important to determine and use an amount of overload appropriate for your own fitness level and goals. Later in this section, we'll look specifically at the components of overload, including intensity and frequency of training.

Q | Is there a limit on how fit a person can be?

Yes. You can improve fitness significantly, but there is a limit. Human physiology has limits, and people's fitness limits are influenced by genetics and training. Most people don't need to train to an extremely high fitness level, because many of the health benefits from physical activity occur at lower levels of training (see Figure 3-4). Also, doing lots of very intense training increases the risk for injury. For safe improvement of fitness, you should slowly increase the amount you train until you reach a desired level of fitness—one that helps ensure good health—and then maintain that level. In Chapters 4–6, you'll learn how to set a starting level of training for each component that is right for you and how to adjust your program over time to increase fitness safely and effectively. These program adjustments follow the principle of progressive overload.

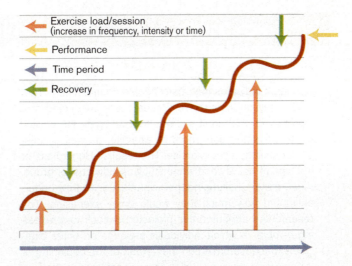

← Exercise load/session (increase in frequency, intensity or time)
← Performance
← Time period
← Recovery

Figure 3-4 Progressive overload. Over time, performance is increased by gradually increasing the overload. The amount of overload is specific to the individual and the activity.

Reversibility

Q | If I stop exercising for a while, will I lose fitness?

Unfortunately, yes. "Use it or lose it" is true when it comes to fitness. Just as an increase in activity will improve fitness levels, a decrease in activity or a period of inactivity causes a decline in fitness levels. This is known as the principle of **reversibility.** It is the opposite of the overload principle. Though declines are typically slow at first, it is possible to return to pretraining levels of fitness within a couple of months.[8]

Recovery

Q | Is it harmful to my fitness if I work out every day?

It can be, depending on the type of training you do. With the increase in activity (overload) comes the need for rest and **recovery**—the time the body needs to rebuild and improve tissues weakened from overload. When the body is overloaded, tissues break down. The body then adapts by repairing and improving the tissues—increasing strength, endurance, and so on (see Chapters 4 and 5 for more information). Without a recovery period, there is no time for rebuilding and improving.

This recovery period should not be confused with the inactivity described in answer to the previous question. Fitness declines or reverses as a result of sustained periods of inactivity. Recovery is much

progressive overload The principle that the body will respond to a gradual application of increasing amounts of stress (load) during exercise training by increasing fitness.

reversibility The principle that a decrease or discontinuance of activity will cause a decline in fitness.

recovery The time needed by the body to rebuild and improve tissues weakened from increased activity (overload).

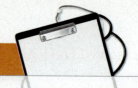

Research Brief

Hate to Exercise? Think Again!

Research indicates that many people underestimate how much they enjoy exercise. Researchers conducted four studies with 279 adult subjects to investigate the participants' predicted enjoyment of exercise, as well as their actual feelings after exercise. The results? Regardless of the type of activity and whether it was individual or group, moderate or challenging, participants significantly underestimated how much they would enjoy exercising. The researchers attributed this projected outlook to *forecasting myopia,* in which individuals prejudge an entire exercise experience based on their dread of the beginning of the exercise session, which most considered to be less enjoyable than the remainder of the session.

The good news is that researchers also demonstrated individuals' ability to control or conquer their "myopia" in order to increase their enjoyment of exercise. Equally important, they determined that improving an individual's expected enjoyment of exercise can also increase his or her intention to exercise.

Analyze and Apply

- Do you sometimes dread exercising? If so, do you think you are experiencing forecasting myopia? What other factors may be at work?
- How might individuals with forecasting myopia overcome these negative thoughts?

Source: Ruby, M., and others. (2011). The invisible benefits of exercise. *Health Psychology, 30*(1), 67–74.

---

shorter—often just a day or two. In terms of training, after a tough workout, your body may need a day to fully recover and be ready to train at a high level again. Most people can do stretching and low-to-moderate intensity exercise daily, but more intense exercise requires a recovery period to maximize the benefits of training and to avoid injury. You'll find more information on program design later in the chapter.

Specificity

Q | What kinds of activities do I need to do to increase fitness?

The effects of training are directly related to the types of activities in which you participate and the specific amount of stress placed on your body. This is known as the principle of **specificity.** For example, you will not achieve cardiorespiratory fitness by performing stretching exercises; instead, you need to perform exercises that stress the cardiorespiratory system. Similarly, you will not see any significant changes in flexibility if you are working to build muscular strength.

Specificity also applies *within* particular fitness components. Pull-ups build strength in specific muscles in the upper body only, not general strength. The most effective skill training is to practice what you want to perform—play basketball to improve your basketball skills. A complete exercise program should include exercises to build all the health-related components of fitness and, for muscle fitness and flexibility, all the major muscle groups and joints. Depending on your goals, you may also need to include activities to develop skill-related fitness.

Individuality

Q | Could everyone be as fit as, say, Lance Armstrong, if they worked hard enough?

Unfortunately, no. Everyone can improve, and some could no doubt become highly fit and highly skilled. But not everyone can be Lance. In fact, no one can be exactly like Lance. Many factors play a role in our ability to achieve and maintain various levels of fitness. Our overall health, past activities, body type, genes, and a number of other factors determine what we can accomplish physically and physiologically. The factors having the greatest effect on each component of health-related fitness are addressed in Chapters 4–7.

The FITT Formula

The **FITT formula**—an acronym for the training principles frequency, intensity, time, and type—can be applied to the different fitness components. FITT principles can form the foundation for any exercise program. This section introduces the basics of the FITT formula. Look for more on applying FITT to each fitness component in Chapters 4–6.

Q | How many times per week should I work out?

FREQUENCY: HOW OFTEN. How often, or how frequently, you should exercise depends on the component you are training, your goals, and your current fitness level. The optimal frequency of exercise is also affected by the other parts of the FITT formula. For example, if you exercise at a high intensity, a lower frequency is appropriate to allow your body to recover. Also, when starting a new program, you may need a relatively low frequency to allow your body to rest and adjust to the new level of activity. As your body becomes accustomed to the activity, or as your goals change, you may choose to increase your frequency.

Guidelines from the American College of Sports Medicine (ACSM) suggest the following frequency of exercise:[9]

- Cardiorespiratory endurance training: 3–5 days per week
- Muscle-fitness training: 2–3 days per week
- Flexibility training: at least 2–3 days per week

The guidelines from the ACSM are widely recommended. They are consistent with those from other organizations and agencies, including the *2008 Physical Activity Guidelines for Americans* from the Department of Health and Human Services.

Q | How do I know if my workout is hard enough for me?

INTENSITY: HOW HARD. In basic terms, in order to improve, you must do more than you're used to doing. How much more than normal depends on the type of fitness you're working on and what you wish to accomplish. You're trying to reach your target zone and threshold. **Target zone** is the optimal or ideal intensity for achieving maximum benefit from your activity. The **threshold** is the doorway into the target zone—it is the minimum intensity for achieving specific fitness benefits. As Figure 3-5 shows, exercising at an intensity below this threshold will burn calories and contribute to your overall activity level, but it will not cause fitness improvements. There is also an upper limit for intensity, above which fitness improvements continue but injury becomes more likely.

How is intensity measured? Many people think of target zones only in terms of measuring heart rate for cardiorespiratory training—and that is one way to measure the intensity of a cardiorespiratory workout. However, there is a target zone for exercises that address the other fitness components as well. Intensity target zones also apply to the degree of a stretch during flexibility training and to the amount of resistance during strength training. Specifics for determining the appropriate intensity for each type of fitness training are covered in Chapters 4–6.

Q | How long should I exercise, per day and per week?

TIME: HOW LONG. A training session is typically measured in number of minutes or number of exercises. The amount of time you spend in each session will depend on the fitness components and intensity you choose, the design of your program, and your goals. For example, if you exercise at a high intensity, your training session will be shorter than if you work out at a lower intensity—45 minutes of brisk walking versus 20 minutes of fast jogging. Also, if your goal includes weight loss and changes in body composition, you'll likely need to spend more time engaging in physical activity than someone who wants to maintain his or her current weight. For strength and flexibility training, the time is typically determined by the number of exercises and the number of repetitions of each exercise. A stretching program that includes eight different stretches might take 10–15 minutes.

Q | What is the best kind of exercise?

TYPE: CHOICE OF ACTIVITIES. In the FITT formula, *type* refers to the kind of activity. You'll select activities based on the fitness component as well as your goals related to that component. Remember the principle of specificity? Different activities are needed to develop each of the health-related components of fitness. That means aerobic activities like brisk walking and cycling for cardiorespiratory endurance, resistance training for muscular strength and endurance, and stretching for flexibility.

You can choose activities for your program based on your fitness level and goals, personal preferences, and environment.

specificity The principle that the body adapts to the specific types and amounts of stress placed on it.

FITT formula Acronym for the foundational components of exercise training and program design: frequency (how often), intensity (how hard), time (how long), and type (what kind of activity).

target zone Optimal intensity range for achieving maximum fitness benefits from exercise.

threshold The minimum intensity for achieving a specific fitness benefit; the doorway to the target zone.

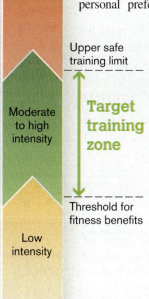

Training intensity

Very high intensity

Upper safe training limit

Moderate to high intensity

Target training zone

Threshold for fitness benefits

Low intensity

Figure 3-5 Target zone for training intensity.

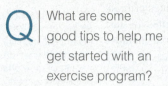

Wellness Strategies

Motivation for Physical Activity: Move More

Q What are some good tips to help me get started with an exercise program?

- Set achievable goals.
- Pick activities that you like to do and that are convenient.
- Team up with friends or family members to make activity more fun. If you work out alone, listen to music if you can do so safely.
- Work activity into your daily routine—for example, walk or bike to work and use the stairs instead of the elevator.

- Start slowly, and add activity gradually. Don't push yourself too hard and make your workouts unpleasant.
- Try a variety of activities.
- Track your time and progress to help your program stay on track.

For more specific information on motivation and goal setting, see Chapter 2.

You'll want to choose activities that are convenient and that you enjoy. For example, if you don't like exercising in a group, choose an activity you can do on your own. If you love to play tennis but have access to a court only once per week, then you'll want to choose alternative or additional activities to supplement your tennis workouts. You can stick with one activity for each component or mix things up for variety; see the box "Motivation for Physical Activity: Move More" for further suggestions.

Q What is the best fitness program?

APPLYING THE FITT FORMULA. A lot depends on you. Knowing the FITT formula is important, but the definitions alone still don't answer the questions "What should I do?" and "How much should I do?" As previously noted, the frequency, intensity, time, and type of exercise are related to what you hope to accomplish. There are as many ways to combine and vary activities as there are people. Chapters 4–6 go into detail to help you set specific goals and apply the FITT formula for each of the health-related fitness components. A summary of the ACSM FITT guidelines appears in Table 3-3.

Putting Together a Complete Workout

A safe and effective workout has several phases, and there are many ways to combine them.

Q What does a complete workout look like?

PHASES OF A WORKOUT. An exercise training session includes the following phases:

- Warm-up
- Conditioning (endurance or resistance exercise, according to the FITT formula) or sport-related activities
- Cool-down
- Stretching (after the warm-up or cool-down)

The placement of stretching exercises in your program is up to you. Stretching is a separate activity from the warm-up or cool-down. As explained in detail in Chapter 6, some types of stretching just before an activity requiring force and power may reduce performance during the activity. Therefore, if the conditioning portion of your workout includes an activity requiring significant muscular strength and if high performance is a goal, you might be better off stretching after the cool-down phase. However, if the conditioning phase of your workout includes a moderate-intensity activity like brisk walking, stretching before the workout isn't likely to have an impact.

Q Why do I sometimes feel a bit dizzy after exercise?

WARM-UP AND COOL-DOWN. It's likely that you aren't doing a proper cool-down after your workout. About 5–10 minutes each of warm-up and cool-down are essential for any training session. Both warming up and cooling down are related to exercise intensity. You can't just jump into and out of your target zone. It's important for your body to have time to adapt gradually as you make your way from a resting state to your training intensity and then again as you transition back to a resting state. **Warm-up** and **cool-down** activities prepare your body for what's coming next (see Table 3-4).

warm-up 5–10 minutes of low-intensity activity that prepares the body for exercise.

cool-down 5–10 minutes of slower-paced activity that helps the body transition to a normal or resting state after a session of exercise.

Mind Stretcher
Critical Thinking Exercise

What types of physical activity do you like best? What is it about them that you enjoy? Is it something about the activity or how it makes you feel? Does it relate to the setting or to the people you're with? Are there other activities with the same characteristics that you could try?

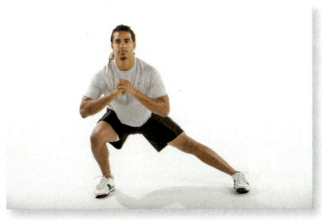

Stretching exercises are best done when muscles are warm, either after the active part of your warm-up or after your cool-down. If your conditioning activity requires significant force or power, it's best for high performance to stretch after your workout.

The dizziness you sometimes feel relates to the shift in blood flow distribution and changes in blood vessels that occur during exercise. To help working muscles get the oxygen they need, the heart pumps fast and the blood vessels widen in active muscles, including those in your legs. If you suddenly stop exercising, your heart slows quickly, but the blood vessels take more time to return to their normal size. For this reason, some blood may pool in your legs, creating a feeling of light-headedness. A cool-down will prevent this effect. If you get really dizzy, check with your physician.

MYTH or FACT?

It is best to work out in the morning, because morning workouts elevate your metabolism more than afternoon or evening workouts do.

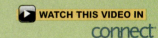 **WATCH THIS VIDEO IN** connect

See page 476 to find out.

TABLE 3-3 SUMMARY OF ACSM FITT GUIDELINES

FITNESS COMPONENT	FREQUENCY	INTENSITY	TIME	TYPE
CARDIORESPIRATORY ENDURANCE *(see Chapter 4)*	3–5 days/week (3 days if vigorous intensity, 5 days if moderate intensity)	Target heart rate zone (lower end for moderate, higher end for vigorous)	20–90 minutes/day; 60–300 minutes/week (total depends on intensity and goals)	Rhythmic, aerobic exercise of at least moderate intensity that involves large-muscle groups (brisk walking, jogging, cycling, etc.)
MUSCULAR STRENGTH AND ENDURANCE *(see Chapter 5)*	2–3 nonconsecutive days/week	Enough resistance to cause muscle fatigue after 8–12 repetitions *Note: Resistance and repetitions should be adjusted for strength training vs. endurance training*	8–12 repetitions/exercise/set; 2–4 sets/exercise	Resistance exercises that use multiple joints and target more than one muscle group (shoulder press, curl-up, squat, etc.); the program should include exercises for all major muscle groups
FLEXIBILITY *(see Chapter 6)*	2–3 days/week, at a minimum	Stretch to the point of mild tightness without significant discomfort	15–60 seconds/stretch; 4 or more repetitions of each stretch	Stretching exercises involving the major muscle/tendon groups (neck, shoulders, upper back, etc.)

Source: Adapted from American College of Sports Medicine. (2009). *ACSM's guidelines for exercise testing and prescription* (8th ed.). Baltimore, MD: Lippincott Williams & Wilkins.

TABLE 3-4 WARM-UPS AND COOL-DOWNS SUMMED UP

WARM-UP	COOL-DOWN
5–10 minutes of low- to moderate-intensity aerobic and muscular-endurance activities	5–10 minutes of low- to moderate-intensity aerobic and muscular-endurance activities
Perform before a training session	Perform after a training session
Purposes: ■ Increase core body and muscle temperature ■ Redirect blood flow to working muscles ■ Gradually increase heart and breathing rate ■ Reduce the chance of after-exercise muscle soreness or stiffness	Purposes: ■ Gradual recovery of heart rate ■ Gradual reduction of blood pressure ■ Redistribution of blood flow ■ Removal of metabolic end products such as carbon dioxide from muscles used during the conditioning phase

Putting Together a Complete Program

Q | **What is the best weekly exercise routine for health?** There are many ways to plan a routine. You can find more information and sample training routines for each health-related fitness component in Chapters 4–6. However, if you're just getting started, you may still be trying to wrap your head around how this all fits together. The examples in Figure 3-6 provide good models for incorporating recommended activities into a weekly schedule of workouts. Examples for moderate-intensity and vigorous-intensity activities are included as well as a combination of the two. If you decide to follow one of these, remember (1) that the activity minutes in Figure 3-6 do not include the 5–10 minutes of warm-up and of cool-down, and (2) these plans assume that you are incorporating stretching exercises into the warm-up or cool-down.

Q | **I don't exercise at all, and I'm crazy busy. Does any amount of activity help, even five minutes?** Yes. Any activity is better than none. Even if it's not enough to increase your fitness level, it still has benefits. If all you have is 5 minutes, be active for 5 minutes. Go for a walk. Walking is easy and inexpensive, and it can burn calories, tone muscles, strengthen bones, improve stamina, reduce stress, and lower your risk for disease. What better way to spend 5 minutes?

Then one day when you have 7 minutes, be active for 7 minutes . . . and then 10 minutes. Try doing a little more each time or adding activity on one more day during the week. In addition, look for ways to be more active during your daily activities:

■ Park your car or get off the bus some distance away from your destination and walk the rest of the way.
■ Take the stairs instead of the escalator or elevator.
■ Take a short walk during lunch or work breaks.
■ Stretch or do calisthenics while you watch TV.
■ Go for a walk when you are meeting up with a friend for a chat.
■ Do at least one active chore—such as vacuuming, laundry, or mowing the lawn—every day.

Before you know it, you may find yourself wanting to make time for more activity. See the box "Surviving a Desk Job" for additional suggestions. For help identifying and overcoming barriers to increasing activity in your life, complete Lab Activity 3-3.

Other Considerations When You're Starting a Fitness Program

You're almost ready to start your fitness program. You're familiar with the components of health-related fitness and you know how to determine your current status in each one. You're also acquainted with some essential fitness principles that will help you design a safe and successful exercise program. Before you begin, however, there are a few more things to consider. Some of the concerns addressed here may not be applicable to you at this time. Review the topics and focus on those most relevant to your personal preferences, resources, and geographic location.

Example 1: Moderate-intensity activity and muscle-strengthening activity

Sunday	Monday	Tuesday	Wednesday	Thursday	Friday	Saturday
30-minute brisk walk	30-minute brisk walk	30-minute brisk walk	Weight training	30-minute brisk walk	30-minute brisk walk	Weight training

Total: 150 minutes moderate-intensity aerobic activity + 2 days muscle-strengthening activity

Example 2: Vigorous-intensity activity and muscle-strengthening activity

Sunday	Monday	Tuesday	Wednesday	Thursday	Friday	Saturday
	25-minute jog		25-minute jog and weight training		Weight training	25-minute jog

Total: 75 minutes vigorous-intensity aerobic activity + 2 days muscle-strengthening activity

Example 3: Mix of moderate- and vigorous-intensity activity and muscle-strengthening activity

Sunday	Monday	Tuesday	Wednesday	Thursday	Friday	Saturday
30-minute brisk walk	15-minute jog	Weight training	30-minute brisk walk	Weight training	15-minute jog	30-minute brisk walk

Total: The equivalent of 150 minutes moderate-intensity aerobic activity + 2 days muscle-strengthening activity

Figure 3-6 Sample fitness program design.
Source: Centers for Disease Control and Prevention. (2011). *Physical activity for everyone: Adding physical activity to your life* (http://www.cdc.gov/physicalactivity/everyone/getactive/index.html).

Clothing and Safety Gear

Q Are some kinds of clothes really better for exercising than others, or is it all just a sales gimmick?

In most cases, special clothing is not required for exercise—especially if you're just starting out. Loose-fitting, comfortable clothing will usually suffice. However, special exercise clothes can make you more comfortable during your workout and in this way might help you stick with your program. Some people also find that a new set of exercise clothes helps motivate them to start an exercise program.

One of the benefits of new types of synthetic exercise clothing is its ability to "wick" moisture away from the skin. This means that while you sweat, the fabric will move the moisture from your skin to the outer surface of your fancy new shirt, where it can evaporate more quickly. By opting for such clothing, you avoid the icky, heavy feeling of a sweat-soaked cotton T-shirt.

If you exercise before or after school or work, you are often heading out in the dark. Use caution if you exercise alone, and avoid areas that are unlighted or suspicious or make you feel uncomfortable. Whatever your route, make it as easy as possible for others to see you. Wear light-colored clothing with as much reflective fabric as possible.

Wellness Strategies

Surviving a Desk Job

Q I sit at a desk all day for my job. How can I be less sedentary during the workday?

A desk job has some advantages, such as temperature-controlled air and pleasant surroundings, but it also has its disadvantages. Being tied to a desk not only makes you feel tired and stressed, it increases your risk for obesity and disease. According to *BizTimes.com*, 70 percent of America's workforce sits on the job, and many of us sit most of the workday. Whether you already have a desk job or you've chosen a major that will likely put you at a desk most of the time, plan for some "office activity" in your day. This added activity doesn't replace the need for regular exercise, but any activity improves circulation, decreases stress, and burns a few calories. Try these strategies.

Get ready: You're much more likely to add bits of activity if you're ready. So, wear comfortable shoes or keep a pair handy. Also, keep compact exercise equipment such as resistance bands or small weights at your desk. They don't take up much space and you'll have fun looking for creative ways to use them.

Get set: Stand whenever you can. Place items you use regularly in high places so you have to get up and reach to get them. Even if you're not reaching for objects, take the opportunity to stand regularly. Whether you stand up just for a quick stretch (try setting your timer as a reminder) or you do a few tasks while standing, you'll burn more calories and you'll already be up and ready to walk.

Get going: It's not just your computer that goes into standby mode when idle; so do the fat-burning enzymes in your body. So, take a walk:

- Hand-deliver a report or message.
- Make frequent trips to the fax or copier.
- Get a phone headset so you can stand and walk while talking.
- Take a walking break rather than a coffee break.
- Take a walk and eat your lunch outside the office.
- If practical, schedule a walking meeting instead of a sit-down meeting.

And don't forget to keep your water bottle full. You'll stay hydrated and you'll take extra steps refilling it and "unfilling" yourself. To add even more steps, use the restroom on another floor.

Sources: Brophy, A. (2007). Sitting good: Proper ergonomics reduce workplace injuries. *BizTimes.com* (http://www.biztimes.com/news/2007/10/12/sitting-good). Exercise at work. (n.d.). *Campbell's Nutrition and Wellness* (http://www.campbellwellness.com/article.aspx?id=37). Mayo Clinic staff. (2009, September 24). Office exercise: How to burn calories at work. *MayoClinic.com* (http://www.mayoclinic.com/health/office-exercise/SM00115). Hamilton, M., Hamilton D., & Zderic, T. (2007). Role of low energy expenditure and sitting in obesity, metabolic syndrome, type 2 diabetes, and cardiovascular disease. *Diabetes, 56*, 2355–2360. Mummery, W., Schofield, G., Steele, R., Eakin, E., & Brown, W. (2005). Occupational sitting time and overweight and obesity in Australian workers. *American Journal of Preventive Medicine, 29*(2), 91–97.

Some clothing manufacturers put reflective materials directly into their products. You can also purchase reflective straps to go around your lower arm or leg; small, flashing LED safety lights to wrap loosely around your upper arm or a piece of equipment; reflective stickers to place almost anywhere; and reflective vests to go over any clothing.[10]

Q Do I need different shoes for different activities? That's way too expensive.

Probably not, but it is necessary to pick a good shoe that will meet your needs. Shoes are very important because they cushion some of the impact force that occurs when your feet hit the ground. If you don't have good shoes, you increase your risk of injury. Also, poorly fitting shoes can lead to a number of other orthopedic problems, from bunions to knee, back, and hip pain. That said, fitness footwear comes in a dizzying array of choices, and knowing where to start can be a challenge.

There really isn't one best shoe. Before buying, consider the activities you'll be doing, your budget, your foot type, and the surface you exercise on. Shoes specific to running aren't very good for other activities, especially those requiring side-to-side movements. Cross-training shoes aren't ideal for running, but if you don't run much and have normal foot biomechanics, they should be fine. A large sporting goods store will have the best selection, but a specialty shoe store might provide you with the most care in determining your foot type. See the box "Put Your Best Foot Forward: Choosing the Right Exercise Shoe" for helpful guidelines.

Q Do knee pads help that much? I think they look goofy.

Yes. You'll look a lot better in the pads than you'll look if you crash without them. For some activities, you need special gear to increase your comfort and performance as well as to provide safety. Common types of safety equipment include the following:[11]

- *Elbow and wrist guards and knee pads* are often worn for in-line skating, scooter riding, and skateboarding as well as indoor activities in which there is risk for bumps and falls. Guards and pads protect you not only from cuts and scrapes but also from fractures and breaks.
- *Helmets* should always be worn when biking, skating, or engaging in similar activities. Opt for a helmet made specifically for your activity. It should fit snugly on your head, with no forward or backward slipping. Look for the sticker indicating that the helmet meets Consumer Product Safety Commission (CPSC) standards. If your helmet is quite old (perhaps bought at a garage sale or handed down), it might be time to upgrade; a good helmet doesn't have to cost much more than $35 or $40.
- *Eye protection* should be worn for contact sports and other activities with heavy or fast flying objects. Face masks are required for some activities, but goggles will suffice for many others. Most goggles are made of polycarbonate plastic. They should fit securely, with cushions above the eyebrows and over the nose. If you wear glasses, prescription goggles may be necessary. You should not rely on your regular glasses for protection.
- *Mouth guards* may be required for contact sports and other sports in which there is risk for head injury. Mouth guards protect the mouth, teeth, and tongue. They can be purchased at sporting goods stores or specially fitted by a dentist.
- *Athletic supporters* provide protection from the stresses of vigorous movement, and *athletic cups* also provide protection against direct contact. Men should wear athletic cups for contact sports, and they should wear supporters for noncontact sports. An experienced coach or a doctor can advise you if you are unsure about the appropriate type of support.
- *Sports bras* provide additional support and protection against the stresses of vigorous movement. They come in a variety of styles and can be purchased at most department and sporting goods stores.

DOLLAR STRETCHER
Financial Wellness Tip

Extend the life of your fitness shoes by using them only for exercise (don't wear them all day), and air them out between uses. Keep your "used" fitness shoes for gardening and other non-exercise tasks.

Other activities may require even more specialized gear. Check with local organizations and experienced coaches and trainers for more information on the latest and best gear for your chosen activities.

Exercise Equipment and Facilities

Q What's the best type of home exercise equipment?

The best piece of equipment is one that you will use. Home exercise equipment can be very beneficial and is an excellent choice for some exercisers. To decide if it's for you, consider both the personal and the financial factors related to such a purchase. Equipment can range from very simple and inexpensive (pedometers, jump ropes, free weights) to high-tech and expensive (treadmills, complete home gyms). If you plan to make a significant financial investment in a piece of equipment, do some research. Local sporting equipment dealers and consumer-ratings magazines and Web sites can help you sort through the specific features. The American College

Fast Facts

Helmet Head

Even if you don't ride far or fast, a bike helmet can be the difference between a brain injury and safely walking away. Consider these sobering statistics. More than 500,000 people are treated annually in U.S. hospital emergency rooms for bicycle-related injuries. About 900 people, including more than 200 children, are killed annually in bicycle-related incidents; 60 percent of the deaths involve a head injury. Importantly, a helmet can reduce the risk of head injury by up to 85 percent.

- When biking, do you always wear your helmet, no matter how short the ride or workout? If not, in what ways are you putting yourself at risk?
- What safety standards for helmets should you look for? Check out the Consumer Product Safety Commission Web site to find out: http://www.cpsc.gov/businfo/regsumbicyclehelmets.pdf

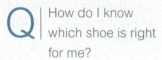

Wellness Strategies

Put Your Best Foot Forward: Choosing the Right Exercise Shoe

Q | How do I know which shoe is right for me?

With so many choices available, how do you go about selecting an exercise shoe? If you're just getting started and plan to try a variety of activities, a cross-training shoe is a good choice. A knowledgeable salesperson can help you narrow down the possibilities, and then it will be up to you to choose the best shoe for you.

When looking for and trying on new shoes, apply the **S-T-R-E-T-C-H** test.

S – Wear the same type of *socks* you will wear for your activities.

T – *Try them out.* Run or walk a few steps or simulate some of your activity movements to make sure the shoes are comfortable.

R – *Re-lace* the shoes, beginning at the toe-end and applying even pressure as you lace in a crisscross fashion.

E – Try on shoes at the *end of the day,* when your feet are at their largest.

T – Do the *toe test.* There should be three-eighths to one-half inch of space between your longest toe and the end of your shoe. You should have enough room to wiggle your toes comfortably.

C – Your shoes should be *comfortable* right away; they shouldn't require stretching out or breaking in. Choose a shoe by how it fits the shape of your foot and not by the shoe size number.

H – Make sure your *heels* are hugged snugly by the shoes. Your heels shouldn't slip as you move.

Always take the time to evaluate shoes carefully because (1) shoes and brands vary greatly, and (2) your feet change over time. Also keep in mind that there are many types of shoes for a reason—aside from sales. Shoes that are specially designed for a particular activity maximize proper functioning. If you decide you like one activity more than others and you participate in it three or more times a week, it's worth investing in a specialized shoe.

You should also evaluate your shoes regularly. If they feel or look worn, they are—and it's time for a replacement pair. Although buying a new pair can be costly, it can save you time, pain, and money in the long run. Rough guidelines for shoe replacement are every 300–500 miles of running or walking, or every 3–6 months depending on your level of activity.

For more information about specific types of athletic shoes and their recommended characteristics, visit the Web sites of the American Academy of Podiatric Sports Medicine and the American Academy of Orthopaedic Surgeons, listed below.

Sources: American Academy of Orthopaedic Surgeons. (2011). Athletic shoes. (http://orthoinfo.aaos.org/topic.cfm?topic=A00318). American Academy of Podiatric Sports Medicine. (n.d.) Selecting an athletic shoe (http://www.aapsm.org/fit_shoes.htm).

---

of Sports Medicine (http://www.acsm.org) also provides guidelines for selecting equipment.

In addition to the data gathering, you'll also want to consider personal preferences. Exercising at home is private and convenient, and you're protected from bad weather. But be sure this option is what you want. Do you like working out alone at home? Have you tried exercising at home to be sure that investing in home exercise equipment is the right choice for you? Do you have an appropriate space for the equipment—not just enough room but a place that is appealing and well ventilated? Do you know how to use the equipment properly? Improper form can hinder your results (and possibly cause injury) regardless of how much you exercise. Always try out equipment before making a purchase decision to be sure that you like

it and know how to use it.[12] Table 3-5 describes some popular home exercise equipment choices.

Q | Should I join a gym?

Deciding whether to join a health club or gym depends on your personal preferences, your environment, and your budget. If you like to exercise in public in a fitness facility, then a local health club or gym may be a good choice for you. According to the International Health, Racquet and Sportsclub Association (IHRSA), there are almost 30,000 health clubs in the United States, with more than 50 million members.[13] Not all clubs are created equal, however. Facilities range from small and quaint to large and state of the art.

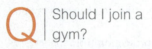

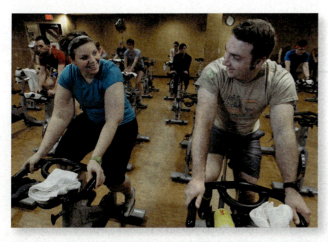

If you decide to join a fitness or health club, shop around and find one that best fits your schedule and needs. Ask for a free pass or trial membership.

Shop around to find the facility that best meets your needs. A large, flashy facility isn't necessarily the best choice or bargain if you use only a small number of its amenities. Do you want to participate in Pilates classes? Take swimming lessons? Select from a wide variety of weights and weight machines? Become a better racquetball player? Think about your goals, find facilities that meet your needs, and then do some comparison shopping. Ask around. Does each facility have a good reputation? Of those that do, how does each rate on the following characteristics?[14]

- *Location and hours:* Is the location convenient? Do the operating hours meet your needs?
- *Environment:* Is the environment friendly and welcoming? Is it clean? Is this a place you'll want to go—even when you're tired?
- *Equipment and classes:* Do the offerings meet your needs? Is the equipment well maintained? Are the classes and equipment you want available at convenient times?
- *Staff:* Is the staff friendly and knowledgeable? Do they display credentials?
- *Amenities:* Does the facility provide other services that you need (such as parking, towels, and child care)?
- *Cost and policies:* Is the price within your budget? Are convenient payment and billing methods offered?

TABLE 3-5 POPULAR HOME EXERCISE EQUIPMENT OPTIONS

MOTORIZED TREADMILL	Good for improving cardiovascular fitness and lower-body muscle tone. Most allow changes in speed and incline to change exercise intensity. Lower impact than walking or running outdoors. Cost ranges from $500 to $1,500.
STATIONARY CYCLE	Provides non-impact aerobic training. Many have devices for increasing intensity as well as measuring distance, speed, and calories burned. Some can simulate road, mountain, or racing conditions. Recumbent bikes may be more comfortable for people with back problems or those who are large. Cost ranges from $100 to $1,200.
ELLIPTICAL TRAINER	Good for improving cardiovascular fitness and upper- and lower-body muscles. Lower impact than a treadmill; may be a good choice for people with knee problems. Cost ranges from $500 to $3,000.
STAIR-CLIMBING MACHINE	Good for improving cardiovascular fitness and leg strength with less stress to knees. Many have monitors that display steps per minute, time, and calories burned. Some allow for increasing resistance. Cost ranges from $200 to $700.
CROSS-COUNTRY SKI MACHINE	Helps to develop cardiovascular fitness and muscle tone in legs and arms. Most include heart monitors. Some allow increase in incline ability to increase intensity. Cost is about $300 and up.
HOME GYM (ALL-IN-ONE WEIGHT MACHINE)	Provides a variety of strength-training options. Designed to make setup and changing of weights easier. Cost ranges from $200 to $3,000 depending on features.

Sources: American Academy of Orthopaedic Surgeons. (2007). Selecting home exercise equipment. *Your Orthopaedic Connection* (http://orthoinfo.aaos .org/topic.cfm?topic=A00415). Cardiovascular exercise machines: What's right for you. (2009, March). *UC Berkeley Wellness Letter.*

Are the membership contracts and cancellation policies unambiguous and reasonable?

- *Trial:* Does the facility offer visitor passes or trial memberships? You should try out the facility to see if it genuinely meets your needs.

Many types of equipment and facilities are available, but remember, exercise doesn't have to be expensive. Don't overlook your campus resources. Most campuses have adequate facilities, and many are available at low or no cost to students. For additional inexpensive ways to exercise, see Table 3-6.

Weather

If you choose to exercise outdoors, weather is likely to complicate your fitness program at some point. Of course, common sense tells you not to go out in a hurricane or a blizzard, but what about the average days? It's important to understand how factors such as temperature, humidity, and wind speed change your environment and affect your body.

Q Is exercising in hot and humid conditions unsafe?

HEAT. It can be, and you may need to adjust your workouts when it's hot and humid. If you're outside regularly, your body naturally acclimates as spring turns into summer. But if you haven't been outside regularly and the weather has already turned hot, you should very gradually increase exercise intensity and time. Withstanding heat is not a test of strength or toughness, and you can always choose to exercise inside on very hot days.

Exercising in the heat places extra stress on the body. The rise in external temperature increases your body temperature, potentially to dangerous levels. Elevated body temperature triggers changes, including a surge in blood circulating to the skin in an effort to cool the body, leaving less blood to flow to your working muscles. In turn, heart rate increases. Your body's natural cooling system, sweat and its evaporation, helps to alleviate some of these stresses, enabling you to acclimate to the heat. However, high humidity can make high temperatures even more difficult to adapt to. Humidity is the amount of water vapor in the air; high humidity doesn't allow sweat to evaporate as easily, so your body temperature increases and you feel hotter than the outside temperature indicates. The National Weather Service has developed the **heat index** (Figure 3-7) to help people assess the risks of the combination of temperature and humidity. When high temperatures and high humidity join forces, the risk of a serious heat-related disorder increases.

Warm temperatures don't necessarily mean you can't exercise outdoors, but it is important to take the appropriate precautions. Assuming that your doctor has not advised against it, guidelines for safely exercising in hot weather include the following:

- Check the heat index on local or national weather channels and Web sites. If the heat index is in the danger zone or higher, consider exercising inside in a location with air conditioning. If the

heat index Guide that combines outside air temperature and humidity into a single measure of perceived temperature (how hot it feels).

TABLE 3-6 FREE AND LOW-COST EXERCISE ALTERNATIVES

Don't have money to spend on a health club? Look into these free and low-cost exercise alternatives.

FREE	$	$$
Take advantage of day-to-day opportunities. Park away from buildings and walk the parking lot instead. Take the stairs, play with your kids, and step up the pace of your housework. The key is to increase your heart rate. Take a daily walk or run. See Chapters 5 & 6 for some exercises that use your own body weight for resistance. For additional resistance, try canned goods, milk jugs filled with sand or water, or bags of potatoes.	Try dumbbells. They come in a variety of sizes and are relatively low in cost. Use resistance bands and tubes to achieve a variety of resistance levels for low cost. Try jumping rope for a "blast from the past" and a great workout. Purchase or borrow exercise videos, which cater to many interests and fitness levels. You can save money by trading videos with your friends.	Explore your local recreation department. Many offer classes and programs at cheaper rates than do health clubs. Buy used equipment, especially if you're just experimenting with an activity. Some sporting goods stores sell used equipment. You can also often find items for sale in your local newspaper.

Adapted from Mayo Clinic. (2010). Fitness for less: Four low-cost ways to shape up. Retrieved from http://mayoclinic.com/health/fitness/HQ00694_D.

Temperature (°F)

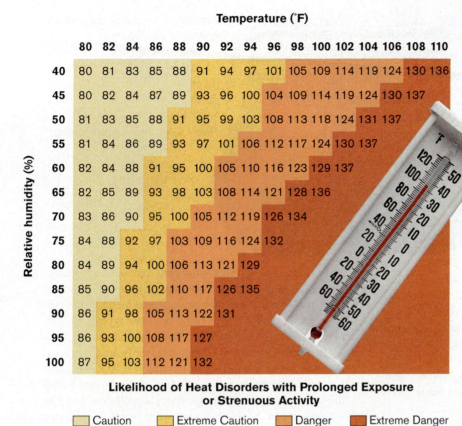

Relative humidity (%)	80	82	84	86	88	90	92	94	96	98	100	102	104	106	108	110
40	80	81	83	85	88	91	94	97	101	105	109	114	119	124	130	136
45	80	82	84	87	89	93	96	100	104	109	114	119	124	130	137	
50	81	83	85	88	91	95	99	103	108	113	118	124	131	137		
55	81	84	86	89	93	97	101	106	112	117	124	130	137			
60	82	84	88	91	95	100	105	110	116	123	129	137				
65	82	85	89	93	98	103	108	114	121	128	136					
70	83	86	90	95	100	105	112	119	126	134						
75	84	88	92	97	103	109	116	124	132							
80	84	89	94	100	106	113	121	129								
85	85	90	96	102	110	117	126	135								
90	86	91	98	105	113	122	131									
95	86	93	100	108	117	127										
100	87	95	103	112	121	132										

Likelihood of Heat Disorders with Prolonged Exposure or Strenuous Activity

☐ Caution   ☐ Extreme Caution   ☐ Danger   ☐ Extreme Danger

Figure 3-7 Heat index.
Source: NOAA, National Weather Service. (2011). *Heat: A major killer* (http://www.nws.noaa.gov/om/heat/index.shtml).

heat index is below the danger zone but still very high, you should still take appropriate precautions.

- Work out in the cooler morning or evening hours, if possible. Consider lowering your intensity or duration of exercise.
- Wear appropriate clothing. Lightweight, loose-fitting clothes allow sweat to evaporate more easily and air to pass through more freely for extra cooling. Choose light-colored clothing rather than dark colors, which absorb the sun's heat. A shirt made of moisture-wicking material will likely keep you cooler than a cotton shirt (or no shirt).

- Wear a light-colored hat to shade your face and help to keep your head cool; also wear sunglasses.
- Don't skimp on safety gear; if it's very hot, you may want to limit activities that require heavy or tight-fitting gear.
  - Use plenty of sunscreen. Reapply it often, because even waterproof and sweat-proof formulas dissipate quickly. Sunburn not only damages your skin but also decreases your body's ability to cool itself.[15]
- Keep yourself well hydrated to replace the moisture you lose through sweating.
- Take frequent breaks, preferably in the shade.

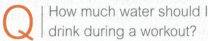

Q | How much water should I drink during a workout?

Proper hydration is always important but particularly so during exercise—not only for performance but also for health. The loss of body fluids causes a drop in blood volume, which makes the heart work harder to circulate the blood. Inadequate fluid intake, excessive sweating, length of exercise session, weather, and altitude can all affect your hydration. General guidelines for hydration appear in Table 3-7. It's best to develop a hydration plan that fits your personal sweat rate and intensity of exercise as well as the environmental conditions. The risk of dehydration increases with length and intensity of exercise.

Q | Are sports drinks a good option? Sports drinks can help replace losses of sodium, potassium, and other electrolytes. However, electrolytes are usually not significantly depleted during a typical workout. Additionally, many sports drinks are high in sugar.

TABLE 3-7 HYDRATION RECOMMENDATIONS FOR EXERCISE

HYDRATION BEFORE EXERCISE	HYDRATION DURING EXERCISE	HYDRATION AFTER EXERCISE
■ Drink about 17–20 fluid oz 2–3 hours before exercise ■ Drink about 7–10 fluid oz 10–20 minutes before exercise	■ Drink enough fluids to prevent dehydration ■ Customize fluid replacement rate by monitoring body weight changes during workouts	■ Weigh yourself before and after exercise and replace fluid losses ■ Drink 20–25 fluid oz for every 1lb lost

Sources: American College of Sports Medicine. (2007). Exercise and fluid replacement. *Medicine and Science in Sports and Exercise, 39*(2), 377–390. Casa, D. J., and others. (2000). National Athletic Trainers' Association position statement: Fluid replacement for athletes. *Journal of Athletic Training*, 35(2), 212–224.

For workouts lasting less than an hour, water is an adequate fluid replacement. For longer or particularly intense workouts, you can consider using a sports beverage for hydration. Choose one with about 4–8 percent carbohydrates, because higher concentrations can slow the absorption of fluid.

DOLLAR STRETCHER
Financial Wellness Tip

Don't buy bottled water. Water from the tap is safe—and free. Carry a reusable bottle, and you'll always have water when you are exercising or on the go. It's a good choice for the environment, too; bottled water produces over a million tons of plastic waste each year.

Q Is it bad for you to run in cold air?

indoor activities until the outside weather warms up.[17]

When it comes to weather, safety is paramount. Prolonged exposure to extreme temperatures of any kind can cause short- and long-term problems. See Table 3-8 for more information.

Air Quality

Q Can I exercise on smoggy days?

COLD. For most people, exercising in cold weather is safe. However, it can be a problem for people with health concerns such as high blood pressure or other heart-related problems. Because the cold puts extra strain on the heart, it's important to follow your doctor's advice if you have these conditions. If you are otherwise healthy, you should be fine exercising in cold temperatures, provided that you dress appropriately and follow basic safety guidelines.

When exercising in cold weather, dress in layers. A bottom layer made from synthetic material such as polypropylene helps draw sweat away from the body; synthetic layers are safer than cotton, which can quickly chill you if it becomes wet. Top the synthetic layer with one or more warming layers, such as fleece or wool. These midlayers should be snug but not too tight and should have the ability to wick moisture. If needed, top your warming layers with a final breathable, waterproof layer. Wearing a hat and gloves is also essential for maintaining warmth; the best kinds are windproof and water resistant and have wicking capabilities. Covering your mouth with a scarf will help warm the air you breathe. Choose footwear that will aid in traction. And, as always, wear sunscreen on sunny days and other safety gear appropriate to the activity.[16] Avoid going straight into the wind if you can. In contrast to hot weather, in cold weather, it is often best to wait until midday to exercise, when the temperature is at its peak.

As on hot days, the thermometer doesn't tell the full story. On cold days, high winds carry heat away from the body very quickly, causing skin temperature to drop. The temperature your body perceives, known as the **wind chill index** or **wind chill factor,** is lower than the actual temperature. Figure 3-8 shows how air temperature and wind speed combine to give you that chill. You can find information about the wind chill in your area on local or national weather channels and Web sites.

Last, keep in mind that sometimes it's just too cold to exercise outdoors. If the temperature is far below zero or the wind chill is below –20, it's best to stay inside. Select

Often you can, but special precautions may be necessary depending on the level of smog and on whether you have any health conditions that are adversely affected by smog or other types of pollution. Similar to the wind chill and heat indexes, there is an **air quality index (AQI)** that rates daily air quality and indicates if there is a risk to health. The AQI measures five major air pollutants, including ground-level ozone (the key component of smog), particle pollution, and carbon monoxide. These pollutants can irritate or inflame airways, as well as increase the production of mucus. Breathing may be more difficult, and the body's oxygen-carrying capacity may decrease. Exposure to unhealthy air can aggravate asthma and other respiratory conditions, and it can be dangerous to people with cardiovascular and other diseases.

There are six levels in the AQI, each with an associated health risk (see Figure 3-9). If pollution is a concern where you live, check the AQI (visit http://www.airnow.gov) and adjust your exercise program as needed. Some tips for exercise in areas with poor air quality include the following:

- Avoid congested streets and heavy traffic, especially heavy bus and truck traffic.
- Work out in the early morning or later in the evening, when it is cooler and smog levels are lowest.
- Avoid combinations of high temperature, high humidity, and a high AQI level.
- Exercise indoors if possible; keep outdoor workouts short.
- Exercise at a lower intensity if needed. Mouth breathing during intense exercise bypasses the nasal passages, which filter air for the body, thereby increasing contact with pollutants.
- Stop exercising immediately and seek medical attention you have difficulty breathing or experience other symptoms.

wind chill index (wind chill factor) Guide that combines outside air temperature and wind speed into a single measure of perceived temperature (how cold it feels).

air quality index (AQI) Guide that rates the quality of the air at a given location and indicates if there is a health risk; calculated with the ratings of five major air pollutants.

Temperature (°F)

Wind (mph)	Calm	40	35	30	25	20	15	10	5	0	−5	−10	−15	−20	−25	−30	−35	−40	−45
	5	36	31	25	19	13	7	1	−5	−11	−16	−22	−28	−34	−40	−46	−52	−57	−63
	10	34	27	21	15	9	3	−4	−10	−16	−22	−28	−35	−41	−47	−53	−59	−66	−72
	15	32	25	19	13	6	0	−7	−13	−19	−26	−32	−39	−45	−51	−58	−64	−71	−77
	20	30	24	17	11	4	−2	−9	−15	−22	−29	−35	−42	−48	−55	−61	−68	−74	−81
	25	29	23	16	9	3	−4	−11	−17	−24	−31	−37	−44	−51	−58	−64	−71	−78	−84
	30	28	22	15	8	1	−5	−12	−19	−26	−33	−39	−46	−53	−60	−67	−73	−80	−87
	35	28	21	14	7	0	−7	−14	−21	−27	−34	−41	−48	−55	−62	−69	−76	−82	−89
	40	27	20	13	6	−1	−8	−15	−22	−29	−36	−43	−50	−57	−64	−71	−78	−84	−91
	45	26	19	12	5	−2	−9	−16	−23	−30	−37	−44	−51	−58	−65	−72	−79	−86	−93
	50	26	19	12	4	−3	−10	−17	−24	−31	−38	−45	−52	−60	−67	−74	−81	−88	−95
	55	25	18	11	4	−3	−11	−18	−25	−32	−39	−46	−54	−61	−68	−75	−82	−89	−97
	60	25	17	10	3	−4	−11	−19	−26	−33	−40	−48	−55	−62	−69	−76	−84	−91	−98

Frostbite times   □ 30 minutes   □ 10 minutes   □ 5 minutes

Figure 3-8 Wind chill index.
Source: NOAA, National Weather Service (2009). *NWS wind chill index* (http://www.weather.gov/os/windchill/index.shtml).

TABLE 3-8   TEMPERATURE-RELATED PROBLEMS, SIGNS, AND TREATMENTS

HEAT PROBLEMS		
WHAT IT IS	**WHAT IT LOOKS LIKE**	**WHAT TO DO**
HEAT CRAMPS		
Muscle pains and spasms due to loss of moisture and salt caused by heavy sweating; an early signal that the body is having difficulty with the heat.	Moderate to severe muscle pains and spasms, typically in the abdomen, arms, or legs.	**Help the heated person:** Have the person rest in a cool place in a comfortable position. The person should lightly stretch cramped areas and rehydrate by slowly drinking water—½ glass every 15 minutes. Avoid alcoholic and caffeinated beverages.
HEAT EXHAUSTION		
A mild form of shock, which usually occurs upon heavy exertion in hot, humid places where body fluids are lost through heavy sweating. Blood flow to the skin increases, causing a decrease in blood flow to vital organs. If left untreated, may lead to heat stroke.	Cool, moist, pale, or flushed skin; heavy sweating; headache; nausea or vomiting; dizziness; and exhaustion. Body temperature near normal.	**Help the heated person:** Get the person out of the heat and to a cooler place to rest. Remove or loosen tight clothing and apply cool, wet cloths. The person should rehydrate by slowly drinking water—½ glass every 15 minutes. Avoid alcoholic or caffeinated beverages. Rest in a comfortable position and watch for changes in condition.

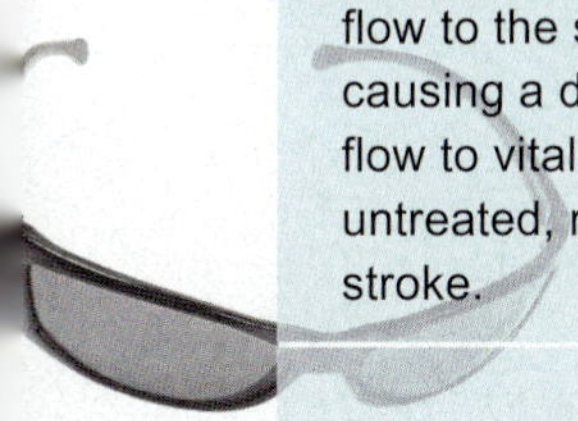

(continued)

	HEAT PROBLEMS (continued)	
WHAT IT IS	**WHAT IT LOOKS LIKE**	**WHAT TO DO**
HEAT STROKE		
A life-threatening condition that occurs when the body's temperature-control system stops working and sweat (which cools the body) is no longer produced. High temperatures can lead to brain damage and death.	Hot, red skin; changes in consciousness; rapid, weak pulse; rapid, shallow breathing. Body temperature can be as high as 105°F. Skin may feel dry, unless there is sweating from heavy work or exercise.	**Call 9-1-1 and help the heated person:** Move the person to a cooler place to lie down; quickly cool the body by immersing in a cool bath, by wrapping in cool wet sheets and fanning the body, or in any other way possible. **Also:** Watch for signs of breathing difficulties. Do not give anything to drink if there is vomiting or changes in consciousness.

	COLD PROBLEMS	
WHAT IT IS	**WHAT IT LOOKS LIKE**	**WHAT TO DO**
HYPOTHERMIA		
Abnormally low body temperature due to prolonged exposure to cold, causing the body to lose heat faster and eventually to use up the body's stored energy; likely in very cold temperatures but can occur at cool temperatures above 40°F if the person is chilled from rain or sweat or submerged in cold water. 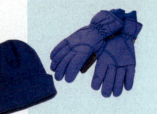	Shivering, exhaustion, confusion and memory loss, fumbling hands, slurred speech, and drowsiness. In severe cases, unconsciousness, weak pulse, and faint breathing. A body temperature below 95°F indicates an emergency requiring immediate medical attention.	**Seek medical help. If medical care is not available, help the chilled person:** Get the person to a warm room or shelter; remove any wet clothing; warm the center of the body first—including the chest, neck, head, and groin—using an electric blanket, skin-to-skin contact, layers of clothing and blankets, or any means possible. The person should drink warm beverages except those containing alcohol or caffeine. **Also:** Keep the person wrapped warmly, including the head and neck, even after temperature begins to rise, and get medical attention as soon as possible. If the person is unconscious, check for breathing and pulse. Perform CPR if warranted while warming.
FROSTBITE		
Injury caused by freezing, most often affecting the nose, ears, cheeks, chin, fingers, or toes; causes a loss of feeling and color in the affected area and can lead to permanent damage; severe cases may require amputation. **Note:** Hypothermia is a more serious medical condition and should be treated prior to any suspected frostbite.	First signs are redness or pain; additional signs include white or grayish-yellow skin, firm or waxy-feeling skin, and numbness.	**Seek medical help. If medical care is not available, help the chilled person:** Get the person to a warm room or shelter. The person should avoid walking on frostbitten feet and toes if possible; do not rub them with snow or massage; warm the affected area by immersing in warm—not hot—water or by using body heat; avoid warming with heating pads, lamps, or the heat from stoves, fireplaces, or radiators as this may unintentionally burn numbed skin.

Sources: Adapted from Centers for Disease Control and Prevention. (2011). Extreme cold: A prevention guide to promote personal health and safety (http://womenshealth.gov/health-topics/a-z-topic/details.cfm?pid=8988). American Red Cross. (2009). Be Red Cross ready: Heat wave safety checklist. Washington, DC: American Red Cross.

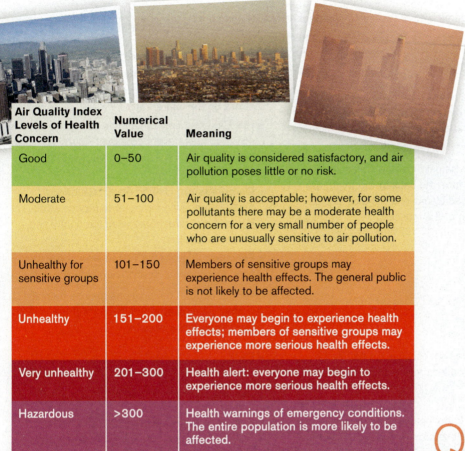

Air Quality Index Levels of Health Concern	Numerical Value	Meaning
Good	0–50	Air quality is considered satisfactory, and air pollution poses little or no risk.
Moderate	51–100	Air quality is acceptable; however, for some pollutants there may be a moderate health concern for a very small number of people who are unusually sensitive to air pollution.
Unhealthy for sensitive groups	101–150	Members of sensitive groups may experience health effects. The general public is not likely to be affected.
Unhealthy	151–200	Everyone may begin to experience health effects; members of sensitive groups may experience more serious health effects.
Very unhealthy	201–300	Health alert: everyone may begin to experience more serious health effects.
Hazardous	>300	Health warnings of emergency conditions. The entire population is more likely to be affected.

Figure 3-9 Air quality index.
Source: AIRNow. (2010). *Air Quality Index (AQI)* (http://www.airnow.gov).

Injury Prevention and Management

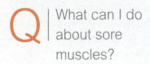 **If a person is not physically active at all but would like to be, what is the best way to start?**

It's always better to start slowly in order to reduce the risk of injury. Follow these general safety guidelines for participating in physical activity:[18]

- If you haven't been active in a while, start slowly and build up.
- Learn about the types and amounts of activity that are right for you.
- Choose activities that are appropriate for your fitness level.
- Increase your overall activity time (duration) before switching to activities that take more effort.
- Use the right safety gear and sports equipment, and make sure safety gear and shoes fit well.
- Choose a safe place to do your activity.
- See a health care provider if you have a health problem.

Q Is ice or heat better for a sprain?

Ice is often the best initial treatment—but prevention is always best. Most exercise injuries among both new and experienced exercisers are caused by overuse. Knowing the causes and treatments of the most common injuries can reduce lost activity time or prevent injury altogether (Table 3-9). Be sure to obtain medical attention for serious symptoms, such as significant pain (indicating a possible broken bone or torn ligament), chest pain, fainting, and heat illness.

Q What can I do about sore muscles?

Sore or stiff muscles are often the result of too much activity, so reducing frequency or intensity of activity might help in the future. To help reduce pain and tenderness, try the following strategies:[19]

- Massage the affected muscles gently.
- Engage in some low-intensity movement; for example, if your legs are sore, try slow walking.
- Take an over-the-counter pain medication.

Allow your body to recover fully after a tough workout. This practice will help you build additional fitness and make your exercise program more enjoyable.

TABLE 3-9 COMMON ACTIVITY-RELATED INJURIES

ANKLE SPRAIN	A sprain is a stretching or tearing of ligaments. Ankle sprain most often occurs when the foot turns inward, damaging the tissues on the outside of the ankle.	For immediate care of sprains and strains, use the PRICE method: ■ **Protection:** Protect the joint from further injury. ■ **Rest/restriction of activity:** Choose alternative activities that do not place additional stress on the injured area. ■ **Ice:** Cold reduces inflammation; use ice 15–20 minutes every couple of hours for the first 24–48 hours or until the swelling subsides. ■ **Compression:** Use an elastic bandage to apply compression in order to reduce swelling, being careful not to wrap too tightly and hinder circulation. ■ **Elevation:** Elevate the injured area above the heart (especially at night) to help reduce swelling. Over-the-counter medications may be helpful for minor pain relief. See a doctor if there is excessive swelling or pain.
GROIN PULL (STRAIN); HAMSTRING STRAIN	A strain is a stretching or tearing of a muscle or tendon. Groin strains most often occur when pushing off in a side-to-side motion causes damage to the inner thigh. Strains of the hamstrings (the collection of muscles that form the back of the thigh) are typically caused by movements that lead to overstretching of the muscles.	
SHIN SPLINTS	Pain in the shins is most often caused by the trauma of continued running on hard pavement.	■ Rest ■ Ice ■ Over-the-counter pain medication, if needed
KNEE INJURIES	A number of knee injuries can result from overuse, improper exercise, or mishaps. The most common injury is the anterior cruciate ligament (ACL) tear, which typically occurs as a result of sudden stops, sudden changes in direction, or the knee being hit from the side.	■ If an ACL tear is suspected, see a doctor. ACL tears can be serious. Complete tears require surgery.

Source: Adapted from Hoffman, M. (2007). The seven most common sports injuries. WebMD (http://men.webmd.com/guide/seven-most-common-sports-injuries).

Summary

Physical activity includes all bodily movement. Exercise is physical activities conducted specifically to develop components of physical fitness. These components may be performance/skill-related or health-related. Developing a sufficient level of health-related fitness can decrease risk of disease and mortality and increase physical functioning and quality of life.

Physical fitness is developed through planned exercise. Prior to beginning a program, you should be sure you are physically and medically ready for moderate to vigorous activity. Next, you should assess your fitness level to determine an appropriate starting point. Finally, you can establish a program by applying the FITT formula and other training principles. When implementing the program, you should also consider environmental factors, such as weather and air quality, that may affect training.

More to Explore

American College of Sports Medicine
http://www.acsm.org
American Council on Exercise: *Fit Facts*
http://www.acefitness.org/fitfacts
Department of Health and Human Services: *Physical Activity*
http://www.cdc.gov/physicalactivity/index.html
President's Council on Physical Fitness and Sports
http://www.fitness.gov
Medline Plus: *Exercise and Physical Fitness*
http://www.nlm.nih.gov/medlineplus/exerciseandphysicalfitness.html

🖱 **COMPLETE IN** connect

NAME

DATE

SECTION

Physical Activity Readiness
Questionnaire - PAR-Q
(revised 2002)

PAR-Q & YOU

(A Questionnaire for People Aged 15 to 69)

Regular physical activity is fun and healthy, and increasingly more people are starting to become more active every day. Being more active is very safe for most people. However, some people should check with their doctor before they start becoming much more physically active.

If you are planning to become much more physically active than you are now, start by answering the seven questions in the box below. If you are between the ages of 15 and 69, the PAR-Q will tell you if you should check with your doctor before you start. If you are over 69 years of age, and you are not used to being very active, check with your doctor.

Common sense is your best guide when you answer these questions. Please read the questions carefully and answer each one honestly: check YES or NO.

YES	NO		
☐	☐	**1.**	**Has your doctor ever said that you have a heart condition <u>and</u> that you should only do physical activity recommended by a doctor?**
☐	☐	**2.**	**Do you feel pain in your chest when you do physical activity?**
☐	☐	**3.**	**In the past month, have you had chest pain when you were not doing physical activity?**
☐	☐	**4.**	**Do you lose your balance because of dizziness or do you ever lose consciousness?**
☐	☐	**5.**	**Do you have a bone or joint problem (for example, back, knee or hip) that could be made worse by a change in your physical activity?**
☐	☐	**6.**	**Is your doctor currently prescribing drugs (for example, water pills) for your blood pressure or heart condition?**
☐	☐	**7.**	**Do you know of <u>any other reason</u> why you should not do physical activity?**

If
you
answered

YES to one or more questions

Talk with your doctor by phone or in person BEFORE you start becoming much more physically active or BEFORE you have a fitness appraisal. Tell your doctor about the PAR-Q and which questions you answered YES.

- You may be able to do any activity you want — as long as you start slowly and build up gradually. Or, you may need to restrict your activities to those which are safe for you. Talk with your doctor about the kinds of activities you wish to participate in and follow his/her advice.
- Find out which community programs are safe and helpful for you.

NO to all questions

If you answered NO honestly to <u>all</u> PAR-Q questions, you can be reasonably sure that you can:
- start becoming much more physically active — begin slowly and build up gradually. This is the safest and easiest way to go.
- take part in a fitness appraisal — this is an excellent way to determine your basic fitness so that you can plan the best way for you to live actively. It is also highly recommended that you have your blood pressure evaluated. If your reading is over 144/94, talk with your doctor before you start becoming much more physically active.

→

DELAY BECOMING MUCH MORE ACTIVE:
- if you are not feeling well because of a temporary illness such as a cold or a fever — wait until you feel better; or
- if you are or may be pregnant — talk to your doctor before you start becoming more active.

PLEASE NOTE: If your health changes so that you then answer YES to any of the above questions, tell your fitness or health professional. Ask whether you should change your physical activity plan.

<u>Informed Use of the PAR-Q</u>: The Canadian Society for Exercise Physiology, Health Canada, and their agents assume no liability for persons who undertake physical activity, and if in doubt after completing this questionnaire, consult your doctor prior to physical activity.

No changes permitted. You are encouraged to photocopy the PAR-Q but only if you use the entire form.

NOTE: If the PAR-Q is being given to a person before he or she participates in a physical activity program or a fitness appraisal, this section may be used for legal or administrative purposes.

"I have read, understood and completed this questionnaire. Any questions I had were answered to my full satisfaction."

NAME _____

SIGNATURE _____   DATE_____

SIGNATURE OF PARENT _____   WITNESS _____
or GUARDIAN (for participants under the age of majority)

Note: This physical activity clearance is valid for a maximum of 12 months from the date it is completed and becomes invalid if your condition changes so that you would answer YES to any of the seven questions.

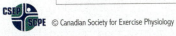 © Canadian Society for Exercise Physiology   Supported by: Health Canada   Santé Canada

General Personal Health Profile: To help further determine if you have any special exercise concerns, complete as much of the following as possible.

Results from Recent Medical Exams and Tests

Fill in any of the following that you can. Date of last physical/medical exam: ☐

Height: ☐   Weight: ☐   Any recent weight changes? If so, describe: ☐

Blood pressure: ☐   Cholesterol: ☐   Glucose: ☐

Other tests (describe):

Are your immunizations up to date (*circle*)? Yes No Not sure

Medical Conditions or Treatments

Any current acute illnesses (cold, flu, etc.):

Any current injuries (sprains, broken limbs, etc.):

Any past illnesses, injuries, surgeries that affect your health today:

Any current chronic conditions (hypertension, diabetes, allergies, depression, etc.):

Prescription medications (name, dosage, how long used):

Over-the-counter medications and supplements (name, dosage, how long used):

Current Health Habits

Activity habits (approximate level of physical activity, any regular exercise):

General eating habits or dietary pattern (e.g., vegetarian, all fast food, no breakfast):

Sleep habits (hours per night on weekdays and weekends):

Tobacco use (type and amount):

Alcohol use (frequency and amount):

Caffeine use (frequency and amount):

Use of other drugs (describe):

Reflecting on Your Results

Did the PAR-Q indicate that exercise is safe for you? Do you think there is anything in your general personal health profile that would be a special concern for starting or continuing a fitness program? If you are not currently active, do you have any additional concerns about becoming more active? (If you're unsure about whether exercise is safe for you, be sure to consult your health care provider.)

COMPLETE IN connect

NAME	DATE	SECTION

As described in the chapter, a pedometer can be helpful in tracking overall physical activity and your progress toward a goal. Pedometers can also be great motivational tools.

Equipment: Pedometer

Preparation

- Medical clearance for physical activity (if needed)
- Pedometer accuracy check: Position the pedometer according to the directions that came with it, set the counter to 0, and then take 20 steps at your usual walking pace. If the pedometer reads between 18 and 22, then it is reasonably accurate. If it is outside this range, try it in a different position. If it continues to fail this "test," consider replacing it.

Instructions

1. **Determine Your Baseline**

   Wear the pedometer all day, every day for a week, keeping your usual routine. Record the number of steps you take each day. At the end of the week, calculate your average daily step total. This average will be your baseline.

DAY 1	DAY 2	DAY 3	DAY 4	DAY 5	DAY 6	DAY 7	AVERAGE
Date:	Date:	Date:	Date:	Date:	Date:	Date:	
Steps:	Steps:	Steps:	Steps:	Steps:	Steps:	Steps:	Steps:

2. **Set Step Goals**

   Next, you'll need to set a final goal and then some interim goals. The frequently promoted goal of 10,000 or more steps per day is a reasonable one for most healthy adults (see the table). However, you need to consider your current activity level in setting your goal. For example, if you are currently taking 4,000 steps per day, you'll want to set a more modest goal, at least initially. On the other hand, if you are already averaging 10,000 or more steps a day, then you'll need to set a higher goal in order to increase your level of physical activity. Plan to increase your steps by an average of 500–1,000 per day, every 2 weeks, until you reach your final goal.

First step goal: _____   Target date: _____

Second step goal: _____   Target date: _____

Third step goal: _____   Target date: _____

Include additional interim step goals as needed for your program.

Final daily step goal: _____   Target date: _____

PHYSICAL ACTIVITY LEVEL BASED ON PEDOMETER TRACKING

AVERAGE STEPS PER DAY	ACTIVITY LEVEL
Less than 5,000	Sedentary
5,000–7,499	Low active
7,500–9,999	Somewhat active
10,000–12,500	Active
Over 12,500	Highly active

Source: Tudor-Locke, C., Hatano, Y., Pangrazi, R. P., & Kang, M. (2008). Revisiting "How many steps are enough?" *Medicine and Science in Sports and Exercise, 40*(7 Suppl), S537–S543.

3. Make a Plan for Increasing Steps

OK, you've set your goal. What strategies will you use to increase your steps by 500–1,000 per day during each segment of your program? Can you add three 10-minute walks to your daily schedule? Can you walk instead of drive when you run certain errands? Develop at least five strategies for increasing daily steps:

1. _____

2. _____

3. _____

4. _____

5. _____

Results

Keep track of your daily steps using the chart at the end of this lab or a different tracking method.

Reflecting on Your Results

After the second week of your program, review your results to date. On average, have you achieved your stepping goal?

Goal for week 1: _____   Average steps week 1: _____

Goal for week 2: _____   Average steps week 2: _____

What strategies are working for you? What barriers have you encountered to meeting your goals?

Do you find that using the pedometer, setting a goal, and tracking your steps motivates you? Why or why not?

Planning Your Next Steps

Keep moving! If you have met your goals so far, briefly describe what you'll do in the coming weeks to keep your program on track. If you haven't met your goals, make any needed adjustments to your program plan, goals, or strategies; briefly describe what you plan to do differently over the next few weeks to improve your chances of success.

Pedometer Program Variations to Consider

1. Tracking Distance Milestones

Some people find it motivational to translate their steps into approximate distance measures. Some pedometers allow you to enter an approximate step length and then automatically estimate the distance you travel each day. You can do a similar estimate yourself by walking for a measured distance—say a quarter mile around a track—and counting the number of steps required. You can also use an online mapping site to calculate the distance you traveled during a fitness walk. Calculate the distance you travel each day and plot your path across your state—or the country.

2. Walk for Cardiorespiratory Fitness

You can use a pedometer-based walking program to improve cardiorespiratory fitness. However, just accumulating more steps over the course of the day won't necessarily increase cardiorespiratory fitness—you must incorporate FITT considerations. The following advice from the U.S. Department of Health and Human Services *2008 Physical Activity Guidelines for Americans* can help you create a walking program to build cardiorespiratory fitness:

- Episodes of brisk walking that last at least 10 minutes count toward meeting the Guidelines.
- People generally need to plan episodes of walking if they are to use a pedometer and step goals appropriately.
- As a basis for setting step goals, it's preferable that you know how many steps you take per minute of a brisk walk. A person with a low fitness level, who takes fewer steps per minute than a fit adult, will need fewer steps to achieve the same amount of walking time. One way to set a step goal is the following:
  1. Determine baseline activity level (see above). Suppose the average is about 5,000 steps a day.
  2. While wearing the pedometer, the person measures the number of steps taken during 10 minutes of an exercise walk. Suppose this is 1,000 steps. Then, for a goal of 40 minutes of walking for exercise, the total number of steps would be 4,000 (1,000 × 4).
  3. To calculate a daily step goal, add the usual daily steps (5,000) to the steps required for a 40-minute walk (4,000), to get the total steps per day (5,000 + 4,000 = 9,000). Each week the person gradually increases the time walking for exercise until the step goal is reached.

(continued)

TRACKING LOG

					Steps				
WEEK	GOAL	SUN	MON	TUES	WED	THURS	FRI	SAT	WEEKLY AVERAGE
1									
2									
3									
4									
5									
6									
7									
8									
9									
10									
11									
12									

SOURCES: U.S. Department of Health & Human Services. (2008). *2008 Physical activity guidelines for Americans.* ODPHP Publication No. U0036. Rockville, MD: Office of Disease Prevention and Health Promotion. Division of Nutrition Research Coordination of the NIH. (2010). *General Guidance for Pedometer Use* (http://dnrc.nih.gov/move-health/pedometer-use.asp). Anders, M. (2006). Do you do 10K a day? *American Council on Exercise Fitness Matters, 12*(4). American College of Sports Medicine. (2011). *Selecting and effectively using a pedometer.* (http://www.acsm.org/docs/brochures/selecting-and-effectively-using-a-pedometer.pdf) .

LAB ACTIVITY 3-3   Overcoming Barriers to Physical Activity

COMPLETE IN connect

NAME	DATE	SECTION

"Not enough time." "Bad weather." "I don't want to embarrass myself." What's your reason for not being active—or more active? Complete this quiz and critical thinking activity to help identify and overcome your personal barriers to physical activity.

Equipment: None

Preparation: None

Instructions

Listed below are reasons people give for not getting as much physical activity as they think they should. Please read the following statements and indicate how likely you are to say each of them:

How likely are you to say?	Very likely	Somewhat likely	Somewhat unlikely	Very unlikely
1. My day is so busy now, I just don't think I can make the time to include physical activity in my regular schedule.	3	2	1	0
2. None of my family members or friends like to do anything active, so I don't have a chance to exercise.	3	2	1	0
3. I'm just too tired after work to get any exercise.	3	2	1	0
4. I've been thinking about getting more exercise, but I just can't seem to get started.	3	2	1	0
5. I'm getting older so exercise can be risky.	3	2	1	0
6. I don't get enough exercise because I have never learned the skills for any sport.	3	2	1	0
7. I don't have access to jogging trails, swimming pools, bike paths, etc.	3	2	1	0
8. Physical activity takes too much time away from other commitments—time, work, family, etc.	3	2	1	0
9. I'm embarrassed about how I will look when I exercise with others.	3	2	1	0
10. I don't get enough sleep as it is. I just couldn't get up early or stay up late to get some exercise.	3	2	1	0
11. It's easier for me to find excuses not to exercise than to go out to do something.	3	2	1	0
12. I know of too many people who have hurt themselves by overdoing it with exercise.	3	2	1	0
13. I really can't see learning a new sport at my age.	3	2	1	0
14. It's just too expensive. You have to take a class or join a club or buy the right equipment.	3	2	1	0
15. My free times during the day are too short to include exercise.	3	2	1	0
16. My usual social activities with family or friends do not include physical activity.	3	2	1	0
17. I'm too tired during the week and I need the weekend to catch up on my rest.	3	2	1	0
18. I want to get more exercise, but I just can't seem to make myself stick to anything.	3	2	1	0
19. I'm afraid I might injure myself or have a heart attack.	3	2	1	0
20. I'm not good enough at any physical activity to make it fun.	3	2	1	0
21. If we had exercise facilities and showers at work, then I would be more likely to exercise.	3	2	1	0

Results

To score yourself, enter the circled number in the spaces provided, writing your number for statement 1 on line 1, statement 2 on line 2, and so on. Add the three scores on each line. The barriers to physical activity fall into one or more of seven categories; a score of 5 or above in a category shows that it is an important barrier for you to overcome.

| ___ | + | ___ | + | ___ | = | _____ | | ___ | + | ___ | + | ___ | = | _____ |
| 1 | | 8 | | 15 | | Lack of time | | 5 | | 12 | | 19 | | Fear of injury |

_____ + _____ + _____ = _____
1   8   15   Lack of time

_____ + _____ + _____ = _____
2   9   16   Social Influence

_____ + _____ + _____ = _____
3   10   17   Lack of energy

_____ + _____ + _____ = _____
4   11   18   Lack of motivation or willpower

_____ + _____ + _____ = _____
5   12   19   Fear of injury

_____ + _____ + _____ = _____
6   13   20   Lack of skill

_____ + _____ + _____ = _____
7   14   21   Lack of resources

Reflecting on Your Results

What are your biggest barriers to physical activity? Are they what you expected?

Planning Your Next Steps

Now that you've identified your key barriers, your next step is to develop strategies to overcome them. Refer to the chart of suggestions and brainstorm strategies that might work for you. Choose one of your barriers, and list three strategies for addressing it.

Barrier:

Strategies:

1.

2.

3.

SUGGESTIONS FOR OVERCOMING PHYSICAL ACTIVITY BARRIERS	
Lack of time	Identify available time slots. Monitor your daily activities for 1 week. Identify at least three 30-minute time slots you could use for physical activity.
	Add physical activity to your daily routine. For example, walk or ride your bike to work or shopping, walk the dog, exercise while you watch TV, park farther away from your destination, etc.
	Select activities requiring minimal time, such as walking, jogging, or stairclimbing.
Social influence	Explain your interest in physical activity to friends and family. Ask them to support your efforts.
	Invite friends and family members to exercise with you. Plan social activities involving exercise.
	Develop new friendships with physically active people. Join a group, such as the YMCA or a hiking club.
Lack of energy	Schedule physical activity for times in the day or week when you feel energetic.
	Convince yourself that if you give it a chance, physical activity will increase your energy level; then, try it.
Lack of motivation	Plan ahead. Make physical activity a regular part of your daily or weekly schedule and write it on your calendar.
	Invite a friend to exercise with you on a regular basis and write it on both your calendars.
	Join an exercise group or class.
Fear of injury	Learn how to warm up and cool down to prevent injury.
	Learn how to exercise appropriately considering your age, fitness level, skill level, and health status.
	Choose activities involving minimum risk.
Lack of skill	Select activities requiring no new skills, such as walking, climbing stairs, or jogging.
	Take a class to develop new skills.
Lack of resources	Select activities that require minimal facilities or equipment, such as walking, jumping rope, or calisthenics.
	Identify inexpensive, convenient resources available in your community (community education programs, park and recreation programs, worksite programs, etc.).

Source: CDC Division of Nutrition and Physical Activity. (2010). *Promoting physical activity: A guide for community action* (2nd ed.). Champaign, IL: Human Kinetics.

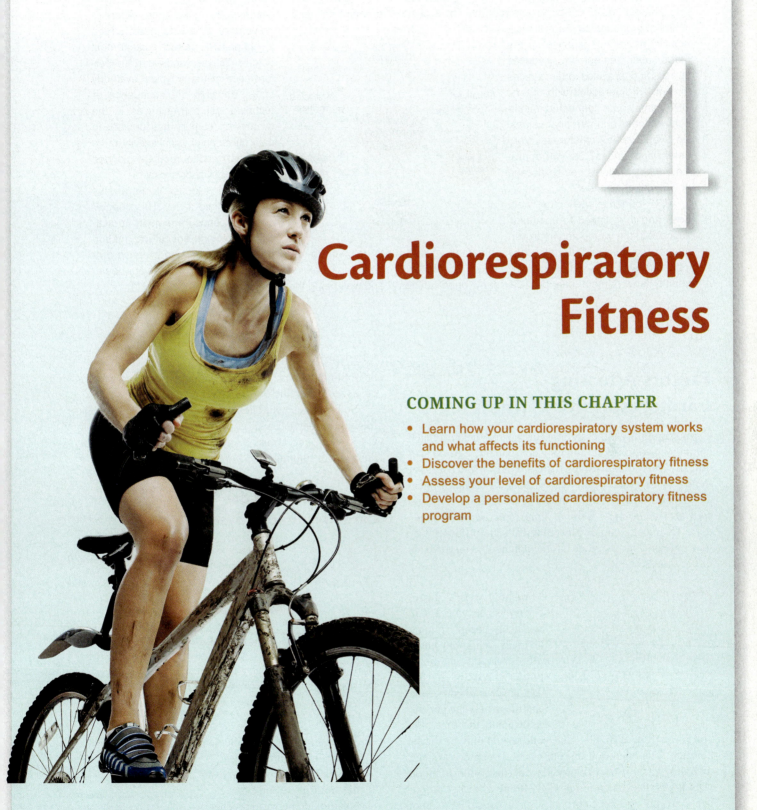

Cardiorespiratory Fitness

How does cardiorespiratory fitness relate to overall wellness? A fit heart, lungs, and circulatory system—the hallmarks of cardiorespiratory fitness—are keys to good health and boosting longevity. Moreover, cardiorespiratory fitness (CRF) and the activities that build it are linked to emotional and social wellness: Endurance exercise raises mood and self-esteem, reduces stress, and provides opportunities for positive interaction with others. CRF can also be connected to spiritual wellness and personal values. Do you value cardiorespiratory health and fitness? Do you appreciate what it allows you to do and how it makes you feel?

CRF benefits intellectual wellness, too: It is linked to academic success in the young and improved memory in the old. Finally, environmental wellness influences, and is influenced by, CRF. A safe and healthy environment can provide many opportunities for endurance activities, as well as a variety of activity options.

The *2008 Physical Activity Guidelines for Americans* (http://www.health.gov/paguidelines) is the latest government document confirming the importance of cardiorespiratory fitness to health. High levels of CRF protect against most chronic diseases and aid in the performance of many typical everyday tasks. Because the abundance of technological conveniences in the twenty-first century has decreased daily utilitarian physical activity, there is a great need for regularly planned physical activity or exercise.

Regular exercise is not always easy to fit into a day. This chapter provides encouragement, practical advice, and critical information to help you to understand how to start an exercise program, enjoy exercise, and ultimately improve your health and well-being through exercise.

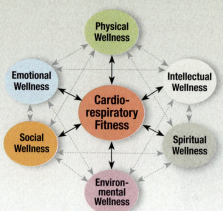

Factors Affecting Cardiorespiratory Fitness

Cardiorespiratory fitness is one of the five health-related components of physical fitness (see Chapter 3). More specifically, **cardiorespiratory fitness (CRF)** is the ability of the circulatory and respiratory systems to sustain physical activity. Cardiorespiratory fitness is also called *cardiorespiratory endurance, aerobic fitness,* or *aerobic endurance.* CRF is a complex physiological state influenced by many factors, but everyone has the potential to improve his or her fitness.

Q | I have a friend on the track team. I tried running with her once and felt like I was going to die. Why is it so easy for her?

It probably wasn't always so easy, since your friend has likely been training for many years and has a well-developed cardiorespiratory system. If you have never trained before, regardless of your genetic endowment, the first time you run will be difficult—and your results may be disappointing. The condition of your cardiorespiratory system, including each of the primary players (heart, lungs, blood vessels), is the foundation of CRF. If any of these components are not working optimally, then your CRF cannot be optimal. Disease, genetics, biological sex, and age also have a considerable overall effect on CRF.

So how does your friend make it look so easy? She has likely been blessed with good genes, no diseases, a strong CR system, and access to nutritious food—and probably done lots of training.

The Condition of the Cardiorespiratory System

Q | What are the parts of the system that make my muscles go?

The major components of the **cardiorespiratory (CR) system** are the heart, the lungs, and a vast network of blood vessels, collectively called the **vascular system** (Figure 4-1). They each play a role in cardiorespiratory fitness:

- The heart acts as a muscle pump to keep blood circulating.
- The lungs take in oxygen from the atmosphere and expel carbon dioxide (a waste product of

cardiorespiratory fitness (CRF) Ability of the respiratory and circulatory systems to provide the necessary oxygen to skeletal muscles to sustain regular physical activity; also known as cardiorespiratory endurance, aerobic endurance, and aerobic fitness.

cardiorespiratory (CR) system The heart, lungs, and network of blood vessels.

vascular system The body's network of blood vessels (arteries, veins, capillaries); blood travels in the vascular system throughout the body, delivering oxygen and nutrients and picking up carbon dioxide and other waste products.

Behavior-Change Challenge
Pursuing Cardiorespiratory Fitness

In high school you were an avid bicyclist and participated in the annual Pan Mass Challenge (PMC), which raises millions of dollars for cancer research. Now that you're well into your college courses, your heavy class and lab schedule has wiped out your free time and your opportunities to bike. You feel totally out of shape. You want to regain your cardiorespiratory fitness so that you can ride in next summer's PMC.

Meet Jessica

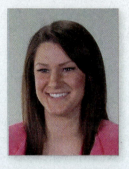

Jessica is a 21-year-old college student who wants to be a physical education teacher. While in high school, Jennifer was quite active; in fact, she completed a half-marathon during her senior year. Now Jessica is finding it harder and harder to stay active. College classes, a part-time job, and volunteering in an after-school youth program keep her very busy, and lately she hasn't been exercising much. She wants to get back into running to improve her cardiorespiratory fitness and hopes to run another half- (or even a full) marathon. Jessica's challenge to stay active is nothing new or unique, yet it is a challenge nonetheless. View the video to learn more about Jessica and her training program. As you watch, consider:

- How realistic are Jessica's goals and program? What obstacles does she encounter, and how does she deal with them?
- What aspects of Jessica's plan might you adopt for your cardiorespiratory fitness program? What major obstacles will you likely encounter, and how will you overcome them?
- What main lesson can you learn from Jessica's experience that will help you in your behavior-change efforts?

VIDEO CASE STUDY   WATCH THIS VIDEO IN connect

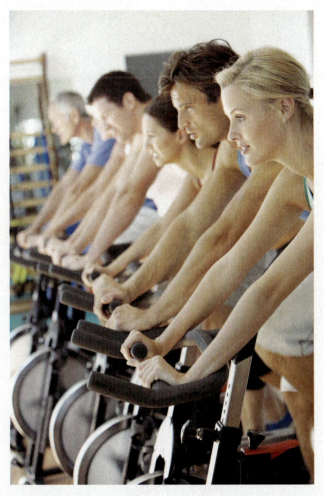

Your cardiorespiratory fitness is influenced by your age, sex, heredity, health status, and especially the degree to which you regularly engage in aerobic activities.

metabolism); this exchange of gases takes place in the **alveoli,** tiny sacs deep in the lungs that are covered by blood vessels. Together, your air passages, lungs, and breathing muscles are called the **respiratory system.**

- The vascular system circulates blood to the lungs as well as around the body; it consists of **arteries,** which carry blood away from the heart; **veins,** which carry blood toward the heart; and **capillaries,** tiny blood vessels with walls so thin that substances can pass

between the blood they carry and the surrounding cells and tissues.

Your ability to sustain physical activity, or CRF, depends on the availability of oxygen to the working muscles. Therefore, your cardiorespiratory system does its best to get oxygen from the atmosphere, circulate it through the body and into the skeletal muscles, and then move it back out (Figure 4-2). First, your lungs must bring oxygen into your body, which you do by breathing. At the same time, your heart pumps oxygen-deficient blood to your lungs, where the blood picks up the newly delivered oxygen. Next, this oxygenated blood returns to the left side of your heart and is pumped out and circulated throughout your body, where it can deliver the oxygen to the active skeletal muscles.

alveoli Tiny sacs in the lungs covered by blood vessels, where oxygen is exchanged for carbon dioxide.

respiratory system The lungs, air passages, and breathing muscles; enables gas exchange, with the body taking in oxygen and eliminating carbon dioxide.

arteries Elastic vessels throughout the body that carry oxygen-rich blood away from the heart to the muscles.

veins Elastic vessels throughout the body that store most of the blood at rest and return blood to the heart.

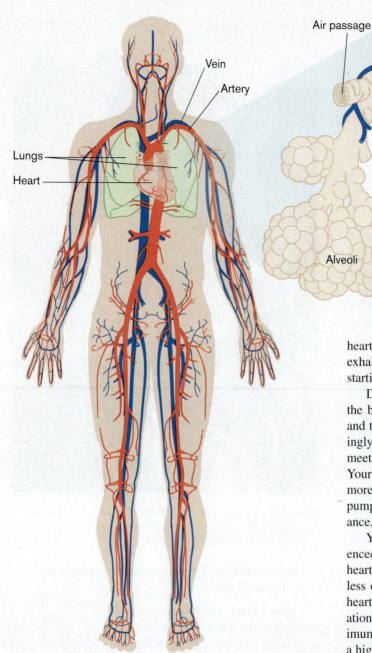

Figure 4-1 **The cardio-respiratory system.** The cardiorespiratory system consists of the heart, air passages, lungs, and a vast network of blood vessels. The exchange of oxygen and carbon dioxide takes place in the alveoli in the lungs. Capillaries are tiny blood vessels that can deliver oxygen from arteries to surrounding tissues and pick up waste products that are carried away by veins.

heart on its way to the lungs, where the carbon dioxide is exhaled and more muscle-enriching oxygen is in inhaled, starting the cycle over again.

During exercise and other types of physical exertion, the body's demand for oxygen can increase dramatically, and the cardiorespiratory (CR) system must adjust accordingly. Your exercising muscles demand more oxygen, and to meet the demand, your entire CR system must work harder. Your heart will therefore beat faster to get the blood around more quickly. Yet your heart has a limit as to how fast it can pump, and this maximum ultimately limits aerobic endurance, or the ability to sustain high-intensity exercise.

Your maximum heart rate is predetermined and influenced by age: Increasing age means a decreasing maximum heart rate. Generally, two people of the same age, regardless of their training status, will have the same maximum heart rate, even though there is considerable individual variation in heart rate.[1] Although training has no effect on maximum heart rate, training enables an individual to maintain a high heart rate for a longer time, which in essence is cardiorespiratory fitness.

To get from the heart to the skeletal muscles, the blood travels through smaller and smaller arteries and eventually through the capillaries. Because they are tiny and lie extremely close to muscles, the capillaries enable the transfer of oxygen (from blood to muscle) and carbon dioxide (from muscle to blood). Muscle cells use the oxygen to generate energy, a process that produces carbon dioxide as a waste product. The carbon dioxide is picked up by the blood and carried back to the heart via the veins. The carbon dioxide–rich blood then passes quickly through the

capillaries The smallest blood vessels, with walls so thin that substances can pass between the blood they carry and the surrounding cells and tissues; they are where oxygen and carbon dioxide are transferred between skeletal muscle cells and the bloodstream.

Q | When I try to run fast, why does it feel like I can't breathe?

Your breathing rate, or ventilation, must also adjust to the increased oxygen demands of exercise. As your heart rate speeds up during exercise, this increase tends to occur in a linear fashion from rest to maximum exercise. At the same time, ventilation also increases, although the increase is an upward curve, especially once you exceed about 50 percent of maximum intensity.[2] Part of the reason for the accelerated breathing rate is the buildup of excess CO_2 in the blood as a by-product of processing more carbohydrate for energy at higher relative intensities. As the exercise intensifies, CO_2 accumulates, along with,

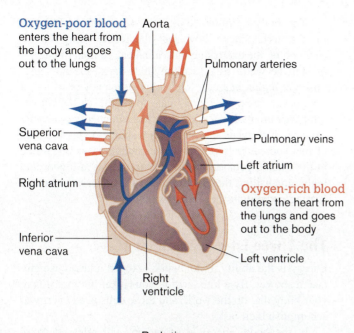

Oxygen-poor blood enters the heart from the body and goes out to the lungs

Aorta

Pulmonary arteries

Superior vena cava

Pulmonary veins

Right atrium

Left atrium

Oxygen-rich blood enters the heart from the lungs and goes out to the body

Inferior vena cava

Left ventricle

Right ventricle

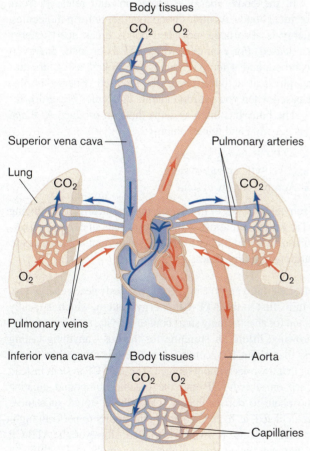

Body tissues

CO_2 O_2

Superior vena cava

Pulmonary arteries

Lung

CO_2

CO_2

O_2

O_2

Pulmonary veins

Inferior vena cava

Body tissues

Aorta

CO_2 O_2

Capillaries

Figure 4-2 Circulation of oxygen and carbon dioxide. The heart is a four-chambered pump that circulates blood to the lungs and throughout the body. The heart's right side pumps oxygen-deficient blood to the lungs, where the blood picks up oxygen. Blood returns to the heart's left side, where it is pumped out and circulated throughout the body. Oxygen is delivered to active muscles, and carbon dioxide and other waste products are picked up and returned to the heart. Carbon dioxide is eliminated when the oxygen-deficient blood is again pumped to the lungs.

lactate (lactic acid), a by-product of energy production in the body that at high levels is associated with muscle fatigue. Therefore, increased ventilation is the body's normal response to lower the level of blood CO_2 and lactic acid. In individuals who are relatively fitter, this effect is lessened due to their higher level of conditioning. Their superior condition allows them to perform at submaximum levels of exercise for a longer period of time, thereby moderating their need to breathe excessively fast.

Training to minimize this unpleasant experience requires periodic bursts (20 seconds–2 minutes) of higher intensity to increase your CRF—but more about training programs later. Just know that the increased efficiency of your CR system is a direct function of your increased training. The more you train, the better your system gets.

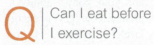

Q | Can I eat before I exercise?

It depends on the type of exercise you do. If your activity of choice is leisurely cycling, in-line skating, or walking, a recent meal will probably not affect how you perform and feel. More vigorous activity, such as running or swimming, might bring on some unpleasant feelings.

The potential issue with eating prior to exercise is that exercise redirects blood to the active muscles. Less blood goes to the gut to help you digest food still in your stomach, as the gut is

lactate (lactic acid) A chemical by-product of adenosine triphosphate (ATP) production; at low levels, it can be reconverted into ATP, but at high levels it is detrimental to performance.

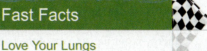

Fast Facts

Love Your Lungs

Your lungs are remarkable organs that, more than anything, allow you to breathe. Your lungs contain tens of thousands of branches—1,500 miles of airways—and up to 600 million alveoli. The total surface area of your lungs is about the size of one side of a tennis court!

You breathe in about 8,000–9,000 liters of air each day. Adults breathe about 14–16 times per minute at rest and up to 60 times per minute during vigorous exercise.

- What other functions do your lungs provide besides breathing?
- What are some things you can do to keep your lungs healthy?

Sources: National Geographic. (2010). *Lungs* (http://science.nationalgeographic.com/science/health-and-human-body/human-body/lungs-article). Franklin Institute. (2010). Respiratory system. *The Human Heart* (http://www.fi.edu/learn/heart/systems/respiration.html).

the primary area from which blood is redirected. One result of this redirection may be the dreaded "side stitch,"[3] which can have a detrimental effect on your performance—and for sure on your comfort.

Therefore, gauge the eat/exercise issue based on how much you plan to eat and how intensely you plan to exercise. Easy-to-digest foods, such as bananas, apples, and oatmeal, can usually be much better tolerated in a short time than high-protein sources like steak, chicken, and hamburger and high-fat foods such as fast foods.

Energy Production

Q | I feel tired all the time. What can I do to get more energy?

There is a difference between your energy level and your body's ability to produce energy. Your energy level—a measure of how much pep or tiredness you feel—mostly depends on sleep, diet, and stress (see Chapters 3, 8, and 10). Your body's ability to produce energy, on the other hand, depends on your fitness level, cellular efficiency, and food intake; this type of energy production is critical for the overall performance of the CR system.

Adenosine triphosphate (ATP) is the fuel for the muscles and as such is the body's key source of energy. ATP is formed when the foods you eat are catabolized—broken down. **Catabolism** is a metabolic process in which complex substances (proteins, carbohydrates, and fats) are broken down into to simple molecules. These molecules then take part in chemical reactions that release energy in the form of ATP, the fuel for almost every energy-requiring activity of the body.

For ATP production to occur, carbohydrate, protein, or fat must be present, though carbohydrate is the most readily converted to ATP. Both blood carbohydrates (**glucose**) and stored carbohydrates (**glycogen** in the liver and skeletal muscle) are convertible to ATP. However, there is a limit on how much carbohydrate can be stored. In contrast, fat, another energy source, has almost unlimited storage potential. But that potential comes with drawbacks: Not only is carrying too much fat a health risk and a detriment to exercise performance, but fat is also slower than carbohydrate to catabolize into ATP. Protein is even more inefficient than fat for energy conversion, and it, like carbohydrate, has limited storage capacity, so protein is a distant third choice for energy. Thus, carbohydrates are the body's preferred energy source for ATP.

adenosine triphosphate (ATP) A complex chemical compound formed with the energy released from food; produced in the mitochondria of cells, it is the main energy source of most cellular functions.

catabolism The breakdown of large, complex molecules into simpler compounds through a chemical process; the simpler compounds can be oxidized, releasing energy.

glucose A form of carbohydrate (simple sugar) circulating in the blood; used by the body for energy (ATP) production; derived from food sources.

glycogen A form of stored blood sugar (glucose) typically derived from food; stored in limited amounts in skeletal muscle, the liver, and the brain.

The body's limited ability to store carbohydrates is itself a disadvantage, however—the reality being that, at some point, the exercising individual can run out of energy, or "hit the wall." Since carbohydrates are especially preferred at higher exercise intensities, efficiency at using fat for energy (*beta-oxidation*) can spare the carbohydrates until they are really needed. In effect, an energy consumer can switch between the two energy sources. This toggling of fuel sources between fat and carbohydrate is magnified in the trained person, who is able to use fat at higher and higher intensities, thereby extending his or her exercise and sparing carbohydrates as long as possible.

The Three Energy Systems

Energy is the ability to do "work"—to lift a heavy weight, take a shower, fly a kite, or ride your bike. It's the cells in your body that do the work, and those cells need energy to accomplish their tasks.

In the body, energy is stored in, and released from, chemical bonds. As atoms bond together to form molecules, energy is absorbed, and when bonds break apart, energy is released. For example, when ATP is created, energy is absorbed, and when ATP bonds are broken, as occurs during physical activity, energy is released. Energy is also released when you eat food and its molecules break down.

The body has three systems that can produce ATP and thus generate and release energy:

- ATP-CP energy system
- Glycolytic energy system
- Aerobic energy system

Each energy system involves a unique means of producing ATP, yet all can assist with energy needs under certain circumstances and all are ultimately important contributors to cardiorespiratory fitness.

ATP-CP ENERGY SYSTEM. When your body needs energy fast, it turns first to the **ATP-CP energy system,** which is ideally suited for an extremely short bout of activity, such as jumping, throwing, lifting, or sprinting for the bus—anything lasting less than about 10 seconds. This system is **anaerobic,** meaning that it works without oxygen. The ATP-CP system instead relies on stored ATP and the organic compound creatine phosphate to deliver energy. Once these stored substances are depleted, as happens quickly, the ability to perform high-intensity exercise is severely curtailed. However, the ATP-CP system can replenish itself almost as rapidly, and with just a few minutes' recovery, you should be ready to go again.

Stored creatine is critical for the ATP-CP energy system. The best source of this compound is red meat, which tends to be plentiful in the typical American diet.

GLYCOLYTIC ENERGY SYSTEM. For the many activities that last longer than 10 seconds, the **glycolytic energy system** takes over. This system relies on an abbreviated

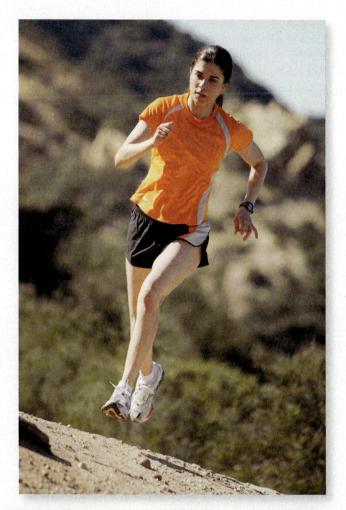

The body's three energy systems for producing ATP are called into action under different circumstances. The aerobic energy system is most important for cardiorespiratory fitness.

chemical pathway that breaks down glucose to produce ATP molecules, in a process known as **glycolysis.** Glycolysis can sustain exercise for 90–120 seconds, still in the absence of oxygen.

Although glycolysis doesn't require oxygen, it also doesn't produce much ATP. In fact, glycolysis requires two ATP molecules to get started and in the end produces just four ATP molecules—a net gain of only two ATP molecules. However, there is a second end product of glycolysis, **pyruvate (pyruvic acid),** which is important for further energy production.

Under some conditions, pyruvate is converted into lactate. Although lactate can be converted by the liver to a source of fuel for exercise, it can also accumulate in the muscles and produce excessive fatigue. Well-trained athletes can offset this effect, however, as they are able to convert pyruvate to ATP and to tolerate the uncomfortable effects of lactate accumulation. Because the glycolytic energy system has the potential to produce a lot of lactic acid and is relatively inefficient at generating ATP, glycolysis is best suited for activities that last less than about 90 seconds (Figure 4-3).

ATP-CP energy system The energy system that powers activities requiring an immediate burst of energy (no more than 10 seconds); fueled by stored adenosine triphosphate (ATP) and creatine phosphate.

anaerobic Occurring in the absence of oxygen.

glycolytic energy system The energy system that is activated for activities lasting longer than 10 seconds; it relies on an abbreviated chemical pathway that breaks down glucose to produce ATP molecules, in a process known as glycolysis.

glycolysis An anaerobic chemical reaction that converts glucose into pyruvate, yielding a small number of adenosine triphosphate (ATP) molecules.

pyruvate (pyruvic acid) An end product of glycolysis; in aerobic metabolism, pyruvate can aid in the production of ATP; in anaerobic metabolism, pyruvate can be converted to lactate.

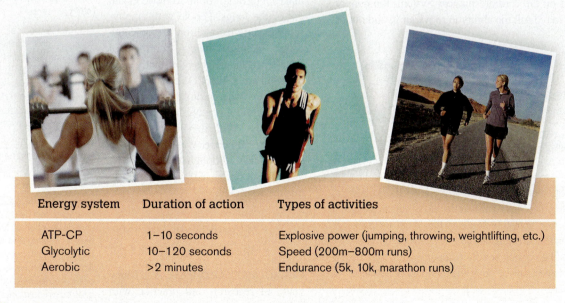

Energy system	Duration of action	Types of activities
ATP-CP	1–10 seconds	Explosive power (jumping, throwing, weightlifting, etc.)
Glycolytic	10–120 seconds	Speed (200m–800m runs)
Aerobic	>2 minutes	Endurance (5k, 10k, marathon runs)

Figure 4-3 Time span of action of the three energy systems.

Q How is aerobic exercise different, and why is it so important?

AEROBIC ENERGY SYSTEM. To build cardiorespiratory fitness (CRF), you'll need to perform activities that primarily use the oxygen-dependent **aerobic energy system**—the system that allows for longer, sustained exercise. The term **aerobic** means "occurring in the presence of oxygen."

The aerobic energy system doesn't produce ATP fast enough for a brief, all-out intense effort. However, when oxygen is present, the potential for ATP production increases dramatically. The pyruvate that was generated at the end of glycolysis is now used to start a complex series of chemical reactions for large-scale ATP production. This process takes place primarily in structures within cells called **mitochondria.** Like the glycolytic energy system, the aerobic energy system also uses up ATP. However, the net production of ATP from the aerobic system is much greater—32 ATP molecules—compared to just 2 ATP molecules from the glycolytic energy system.

Production of energy through the aerobic system depends largely on the number of mitochondria in muscle cells and the availability of oxygen. Regular physical training involving aerobic activities like brisk walking, running, and cycling helps increase the number of mitochondria and makes the cardiorespiratory system better at delivering oxygen. You also need to have enough carbohydrate present for fuel; a well-rounded diet with plenty of complex carbohydrates will ensure that this criterion is met (see Chapter 8).

Diseases Affecting the Cardiorespiratory System

Diseases of the heart, lungs, and blood vessels can all have a negative impact on the cardiorespiratory system. Pulmonary (lung) diseases may limit the ability to move air in and out of

the body, thereby decreasing the capacity for physical activity. Heart disease takes many forms, including some that decrease the pumping ability of the heart or inhibit blood flow. Although each of these conditions may be an obstacle to an active lifestyle, they need not rule it out. In fact, physical activity is an important part of the management of many chronic diseases. With a physician's clearance, careful planning and program adjustments, and possibly some supervision, most people with heart or lung disease can remain active.

Q Can you still achieve cardio fitness if you have something like asthma?

ASTHMA AND OTHER CHRONIC RESPIRATORY CONDITIONS. The most common lung diseases are asthma, chronic bronchitis, and emphysema. **Asthma** is characterized by varying and recurring symptoms affecting the air passages (bronchi). During an attack, airway inflammation and bronchoconstriction increase, and breathing becomes labored. Asthma may cause chest tightness, wheezing, shortness of breath, and a cough, so it's easy to see how it might make exercise difficult.

More and more people are being diagnosed with asthma, yet with certain precautions they can still enjoy aerobic exercise (see the box "Living Well with . . . Asthma"). Treatment usually includes making healthy lifestyle choices, avoiding triggers for asthma attacks, and taking medications.

Chronic bronchitis and **emphysema,** collectively called *chronic obstructive pulmonary disease (COPD),* are characterized by a chronic, often progressive narrowing of the airways that makes it difficult for air to move in and out of the lungs. People with emphysema experience a chronic, worsening cough, increased mucus, shortness of breath, and the need to constantly clear their airways. COPD can seriously compromise the cardiorespiratory system and limit a person's cardiorespiratory fitness. With the proper medical guidance, someone with COPD can still exercise, although the frequency, intensity, duration, and type of exercise may be restricted.

Q Is cardio exercise safe after a heart attack?

CARDIOVASCULAR DISEASE. Yes. Many years of research and practice with heart attack survivors has shown not

---

aerobic energy system The system responsible for most of the body's energy production, which takes place in the mitochondria and requires glucose and oxygen.

aerobic Occurring in the presence of oxygen.

mitochondria Structures within cells in which most of the chemical reactions in cellular (oxidative) respiration occur; these cellular "power plants" are the location for most adenosine triphosphate (ATP) production.

asthma A medical condition characterized by inflammation and constriction of air passages in the lungs, which makes breathing difficult; in some cases it can be exacerbated by exercise.

chronic bronchitis Persistent inflammation of the bronchi (air passages) in the lungs.

emphysema A condition characterized by progressive destruction of the alveoli, making breathing, especially exhalation, difficult; with chronic bronchitis, known as chronic obstructive pulmonary disease (COPD).

Mind Stretcher
Critical Thinking Exercise

Consider your daily routine. What percentage of your active time do you spend on (1) transportation, (2) planned exercise, (3) work-related activity, and (4) incidental activity (activity that occurs in the course of doing other things)? To improve your cardiorespiratory fitness, note which of the four activity categories has room for more "exercise." Also list any reasons you can think of for differences across the various activity categories. You may be surprised at how much you do in one category or how little you do in others.

Living *Well* with . . .

Asthma

People with asthma can and do exercise regularly. In fact, people with asthma can become elite athletes, as in the cases of football superstars Jerome Bettis and Emmitt Smith, Olympic gold medal swimmer Peter Vanderkaay, and recent marathon world-record holder Paula Radcliffe. Appropriate asthma management includes exercise and other physical activities as part of a healthy lifestyle. Before getting started, it is important to check with one's doctor about asthma triggers, signs and symptoms, and the correct use of medications.

Individuals with asthma generally do well with intermittent bursts of activity—as in gymnastics, volleyball, and softball, for example. Activities requiring extended exertion (such as jogging, cycling, soccer, and basketball) may be more difficult but don't need to be avoided. Cold-weather activities (ice hockey, ice-skating, skiing, and so on) may also present some problems because cold, dry air can trigger an asthma attack. Many people with asthma prefer swimming because it is done in warm, moist air.

If you have asthma, your general exercise prescription is not much different from that for anyone else. However, exercising with asthma requires some planning and precautions, including the following:

- Always use your pre-exercise asthma inhaler before beginning exercise.
- Perform an extended warm-up and cool-down.
- If the weather is cold, exercise indoors or wear a mask or scarf over your nose and mouth.
- If you have allergic asthma, avoid exercising outdoors when the pollen count or air pollution level is high.
- Limit exercise when you have a cold or other viral infection.
- Don't overdo the exercise.

If you experience asthma symptoms during exercise, stop and repeat your pre-exercise inhaled medication. If your symptoms completely go away, you may slowly restart your workout. If your symptoms return, stop, repeat your quick-relief medication, and call your health care provider.

For more information on exercise and asthma, see the American College of Allergy, Asthma, and Immunology at http://www.acaai.org/patients/resources/asthma/Pages/exercising-with-allergies-asthma.aspx.

---

only the safety of regular exercise but also its benefits.[4] Heart attack survivors who exercise regularly are much less likely to suffer a second heart attack and do not die quite as young as those who remain sedentary. Having a heart attack can kill some heart tissue (part of the muscle pump), yet exercise can still be performed, sometimes at a relatively high level. A physician's clearance is of utmost importance, but heart attacks and other forms of heart disease should not be deterrents to physical activity. See Chapter 11 for more on heart disease.

Genetics

Q | I don't like to exercise, and neither do my parents. Is my problem genetic?

How much you *like* to exercise doesn't come from your genes. However, the attitudes and beliefs of your family probably influence your likes and dislikes.

Genetics may very well play a role in your ability to get fit, though. Researchers have established that no more than about 50 percent of our ability to *improve* our cardiorespiratory fitness is inherited.[5] The other half is based on what we do—how active we are and what types of activities we engage in. These same researchers also showed that if we all did the same amount of training, a few would achieve a very high level of fitness and others would not improve much. However, the vast majority of us fall between these two extremes and can show moderate improvements in cardiorespiratory fitness with a reasonable training program. These increases in fitness in turn make us feel more energetic throughout the day, sleep better at night, and be more attentive in class.

Ultimately, regardless of your genetic disposition, regular exercise can benefit you now and in the future. Don't let others' attitudes stop you from engaging in one of the healthiest behaviors available. And don't compare yourself to others. Focus on the positive changes you experience as you increase fitness rather than how you stack up against others who may have been training much longer, competed in high school, or perhaps even have slightly better fitness genes. Go out, have fun, and get fit.

Finally, a reminder for the lucky few who appear to be naturally fit: Even though you can maintain your slender build without exercise, you miss out on all the health benefits associated with regular physical activity.

And remember that being thin is not the same as being fit. Your current fitness level and body weight may not last, because the process of aging, starting as early as 25 or 30, levels the playing field. It's best to begin a lifetime program of exercise now to improve and maintain your fitness level.

Biological Sex

Q | How do men and women differ in getting fit?

Men and women have the same ability to increase their levels of cardiorespiratory fitness, but men can typically achieve a higher absolute level of cardiorespiratory function.[6] The reason is that on average, men have larger hearts and lungs, greater blood capacity (ability to deliver more oxygenated blood), and more skeletal muscle mass than women, especially in the upper body. These differences, which are almost entirely a function of the difference in size between the sexes, usually allow men to achieve a higher level of performance. A larger heart can pump more blood, bigger lungs can bring in more oxygen, and a greater muscle mass can produce more force—all adding up to superior performance. The important message, though, is that regardless of whether you're male or female, regular physical activity will improve cardiorespiratory functioning to a level that promotes lifetime wellness.

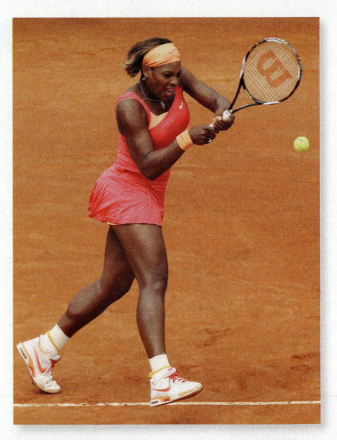

On average, men have larger hearts and lungs and can achieve a higher absolute level of cardiorespiratory fitness. However, women can and do become extremely fit, and both men and women can improve their cardiorespiratory functioning for better health and wellness.

Use and Age

Q | My dad is 58 and wants to start exercising. Is he too old?

You're only as old as you feel, and if your dad feels like exercising, he should go for it. A natural result of aging is a steady decline in the functioning of the cardiorespiratory system. However, for people who participate in regular physical activity, the rate of decline is much less than that of their sedentary counterparts. Therefore, a well-conditioned 60-year-old has the same, or better, cardiorespiratory fitness (CRF) as a sedentary 30-year-old.[7] And it's never too late to start a fitness program, as fitness can increase at any point in the life span.[8] Fortunately, there is no evidence that reaching a particular age makes someone too old to exercise.

Most people associate the phrase "use it or lose it" with muscle fitness, but it also holds true for cardiorespiratory fitness. Although it is difficult to see the CR system become less or more fit (in the way that you can observe your muscles change in size or strength), your body is constantly doing what you ask of it. If you ask little of it, then that is what it will do, making any greater physical effort difficult. Remaining sedentary offsets many of the health benefits associated with physical activity and healthy aging. Your heart doesn't pump as strongly, your lungs don't bring in as much oxygen, your overall blood volume decreases, you have fewer mitochondria, and your arteries stiffen. These harmful effects work together to keep your CRF low, a condition that increases your chance of developing heart disease, diabetes, and high blood pressure—and of dying prematurely.

Mind Stretcher
Critical Thinking Exercise

Do you have pleasant memories of exercise from your childhood? What were some things you liked the most about exercise when you were younger? Can you still do those activities today, even if you need to modify them? If your exercise memories aren't all pleasant, how can you change things now so that exercise brings you some satisfaction? Everybody has different experiences with exercise, so try to use yours to make exercise work well for you today.

If you still aren't convinced that people of all ages can exercise, check out your local Senior Olympics to see runners, jumpers, swimmers, cyclists, and others competing well into their seventies and eighties. One doesn't need to be a competitive athlete to gain benefits, though. Many activities can be enjoyed throughout the life span regardless of chronological age, and all bring numerous health and fitness benefits—as well as pleasure and an improved quality of life.

Benefits of Cardiorespiratory Fitness

Increased cardiorespiratory fitness may be one of the best investments you can make for your health and wellness. Numerous research studies have established the strong inverse relationship between CRF, chronic disease, and all-cause mortality. Even the most unfit person will reap immediate benefits from just a slight increase in cardiorespiratory fitness. What's more, increasing your fitness requires only a small financial investment and not too much of your time.

While attending college, you may have free access to a campus fitness or wellness center, safe and secure walking paths, personnel who can assist you in developing an exercise plan (exercise-science faculty, wellness-center staff), and friends with a similar interest who can help you stay motivated. College offers built-in opportunities to be more active; an example of this incidental physical activity is walking across campus several times a day. You don't plan the walking and probably don't think of it as activity, yet you reap the benefits. In fact, a residential college student typically walks 2–3 miles a day just to get around campus.

See the box "Cardiorespiratory Fitness and Academic Success" for even more on the benefits of exercise.

Improved Performance

Q | My boyfriend made me do an online fitness survey, and it said my VO_2 was 41. What does that mean?

VO_2, an abbreviation for the volume of oxygen (O_2) consumed over time, is a measure of your body's ability to take in and utilize oxygen. In fitness magazines and journals, you will see this term or VO_{2max}, which is the absolute maximum amount of oxygen you can consume during peak exercise. VO_{2max} is the term used to refer to a person's peak fitness level—or what was measured on the online fitness survey. To improve cardiorespiratory fitness, you need to increase your body's ability to take in and utilize oxygen, as is done through aerobic exercises.

What exactly does your VO_{2max} score of 41 mean? Specifically, it means that you can utilize 41 milliliters of oxygen per minute, relative to your body weight, or milliliters per kilogram per minute (ml/kg/min). The typical college female has a VO_{2max} in the high 30s, so you're on the high side of average. In comparison, college males are normally in the mid 40s, and very fit aerobic athletes on campus are in the high 60s or low

VO_2 (volume of oxygen consumed) The absolute amount of oxygen, or volume of oxygen, that can be consumed and used by an individual; usually reported in liters per minute and highly correlated to body size.

VO_{2max} (maximum volume of oxygen consumed) The maximum amount of oxygen that can be consumed and used by skeletal muscles, typically reported in terms of milliliters of oxygen consumed per minute per kilogram of body weight (ml/kg/min); considered one of the best measures of aerobic fitness.

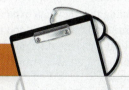

Research Brief

Cardiorespiratory Fitness and Academic Success

Research over the years has shown a link between fitness and better grades among grade school children. What about young adults?

Recently, researchers looked at the results of fitness tests and intelligence tests given to 1.2 million 18-year-old Swedish men enlisting in mandatory military service. The study found cardiovascular fitness to be positively associated with intelligence at the time of the testing and with educational achievement later in life. The researchers found no such association between muscle strength and cognitive performance. They aren't sure what underlies the correlation between cardiorespiratory fitness and intelligence, but they think that CRF affects brain function—possibly through improved blood flow to the brain.

Analyze and Apply

- What do these results mean for you with respect to the importance of cardiorespiratory exercise?
- On what *specific* areas of your life might CRF have an impact?

Source: Aberg, M. A., and others. (2009). Cardiovascular fitness is associated with cognition in young adulthood. *Proceedings of the National Academy of Sciences, 106*(49), 20906–20911.

70s. World-class endurance athletes usually have a VO_{2max} in the low to mid 70s.[9]

VO_2 is largely determined by the amount of oxygen you can bring into your lungs, so the bigger the lungs, the greater the VO_2. Therefore, to compare the fitness of people of different heights (since height is directly related to lung size), ml/kg/min is used, as this unit of measure corrects VO_2 for body size.

Q Every time I start an exercise program I feel worse! Does it ever get better?

Yes, it gets better. For some people, it takes a while before they (and their body) are comfortable with a new exercise routine—anywhere from 2 weeks to 3 months. Don't try to go from couch potato to serious jogger in 1 week. Set realistic short-term goals and ease into it. Start with slow-to-moderate walking. Then gradually mix in some more vigorous activity (brisk walking or slow jogging) during a 20- to 30-minute walk. It takes just two or three spurts, 1–2 minutes long, of more vigorous activity to stimulate and challenge your CR system. Over time, you can add more spurts or make them longer. You'll start feeling comfortable before long, and your newfound cardiorespiratory fitness will have you feeling better throughout the day. In addition, your increased CRF will bring changes to your CR system, including the following:

- Your heart muscle will grow stronger, and this greater strength allows you to pump more blood to the active muscles.
- Your lungs will become more efficient at bringing in large volumes of oxygen-rich air, which can then be transported around the body by your newly strengthened heart.
- Your blood vessels will become more elastic, meaning that they can expand to a greater degree to allow more blood to the active muscles, while at the same time quickly constricting and shunting blood away from noncritical areas during exercise.
- Your cells will develop more mitochondria, which also become more efficient, thereby increasing overall conversion of pyruvate into ATP so that you have the energy necessary to sustain aerobic exercise.

Q If the heart is a muscle, can you bulk it up?

Actually you can. Even though its properties aren't exactly the same as skeletal muscle, heart muscle can grow in size, or experience what is called *hypertrophy*. The left ventricle is the main pumping chamber, and healthy people engaged in regular aerobic exercise have a thicker left ventricle than sedentary people do. In addition, regular exercise allows the heart muscle to stay flexible or elastic, and the left ventricular cavity remains quite large. Aerobic exercise enables the heart to pump more blood per beat, or have greater **stroke volume.** A higher stroke volume leads to more blood pumped per minute, or higher **cardiac output.**

Both stroke volume and cardiac output are signs of the heart's strength and fitness. Having a high stroke volume usually results in a lower resting heart rate, sometimes even in the mid 30s in elite endurance athletes. In essence, if the heart can pump as much blood in one beat as a sedentary person's heart can in two beats, the overall resting heart rate can be twice as slow. A low resting heart rate is an indicator of cardiorespiratory fitness and is also linked to a reduced risk of several types of chronic disease.

stroke volume The amount of blood pumped by the heart in each beat.

cardiac output The amount of blood pumped by the heart per minute.

Reduced Risk of Disease

Q My mom's doctor told her to walk every day to help lower her blood pressure. Does just walking really work?

Regular physical activity can lower resting blood pressure by as much as 5–7 points, or millimeters of mercury (mmHg), in people with high blood pressure,[10] which may be enough to minimize the need for medication. However, anyone with high blood pressure, also known as hypertension, should check with his or her doctor before starting an exercise program. Daily walks are a great way to begin lowering blood pressure, but no one should stop medication without consulting with a physician. For people whose blood pressure is currently in the healthy range, regular exercise can keep it from rising with age.

According to *2008 Physical Activity Guidelines for Americans,* daily physical activity can reduce the risk of chronic diseases and improve many other conditions.[11] Here is a brief summary of the positive results physical activity can bring:

- *Improved blood pressure:* Physical activity leads to a more efficient heart muscle and more elastic blood vessels.
- *Improved cholesterol levels:* Physical activity increases HDL, or "good cholesterol," and lowers LDL, or "bad cholesterol."
- *Reduced risk of type 2 diabetes:* Physical activity makes the skeletal muscles more efficient at using blood sugar, helping to keep blood sugar levels in the healthy range.
- *Reduced risk of certain cancers:* Physical activity affects sex hormone levels, cellular metabolism, and the rate of digestion, and it helps control body fat; these changes reduce the risk of cancers of the colon and breast and possibly other sites.

- *Reduced risk of osteoporosis:* Exercise that is weight bearing (such as walking) increases bone density and reduces the risk of fractures.
- *Reduced risk of cardiovascular disease (CVD):* Elevated blood pressure, unhealthy cholesterol levels, and type 2 diabetes are all major risk factors for CVD, so by improving these, physical activity reduces overall CVD risk.

Figure 4-4 summarizes the benefits and effects of cardiorespiratory fitness. See Chapter 11 for more on preventing chronic diseases.

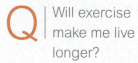

Q | Will exercise make me live longer?

Although nothing is guaranteed to make you live longer, plenty of evidence suggests that, yes, regular cardiorespiratory exercise may increase longevity and quality of life. Data collected for more than 20 years by the Cooper Institute of Aerobics Research in Dallas, Texas, indicates that people who have at least a moderate level of cardiorespiratory fitness (CRF) have almost *half* the rate of premature death from any cause ("all-cause mortality") compared to those who are just barely fit.[12] The Aerobic Center Longitudinal Study (ACLS) researchers divided participants into five fitness categories (Figure 4-5) and found the most dramatic difference in all-cause mortality, almost 50 percent, between category 1 (least fit) and category 2 (minimally fit). This means that engaging in even a small amount of physical activity has huge health benefits, especially compared to remaining sedentary. Therefore, if

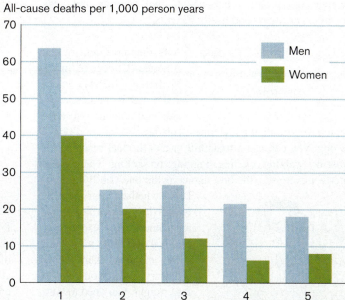

Figure 4-5 Cardiorespiratory fitness and all-cause mortality. Analysis of mortality rates during 10-year follow-up of Aerobics Center Longitudinal Study (ACLS).

Source: Blair, S. N., & Wei, M. (2000). Sedentary habits, health, and function in older women and men. *American Journal of Health Promotion, 15,* 1–8.

you want to minimize your risk of dying prematurely, get out and get fit—even if just a little fit.

Healthier Body Composition

Q | How much exercise do I need if I want to lose some serious weight before spring break?

Well, if spring break is next week, you're out of luck. The healthiest weight loss (that is both safe and sustainable) averages about 1 or 2 pounds a week. Do you consider this "serious weight"? Added up over time, it can be significant, but weight loss is difficult to maintain. A 1-pound change in body weight represents a change of 3,500 calories through diet, exercise, or both. If you want to lose 1 pound, you must consume fewer calories or burn more calories, for a net loss of 3,500 calories. (Flip the equation if you want to gain a pound—increase your caloric intake and reduce your caloric expenditure.) Walking and jogging burn around 80–110 calories per mile, so it takes a while to lose weight through exercise alone. For weight loss, many people find it easier initially to make dietary changes. However, weight loss either plateaus quickly or becomes difficult to maintain. Therefore, a combination approach is usually most successful.[13] Including exercise in your

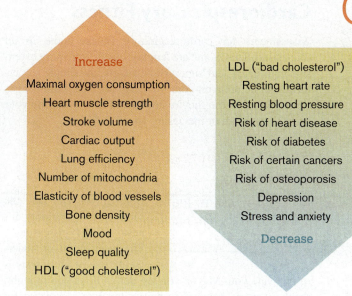

Figure 4-4 Summary of the effects and benefits of cardiorespiratory exercise.

Source: U.S. Department of Health and Human Services. (2008). *2008 physical activity guidelines for Americans,* Chapter 2 (http://www.health.gov/paguidelines/guidelines/default.aspx#toc).

weight-loss program burns additional calories and adds many other fitness and health benefits.

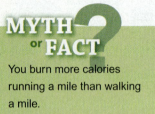

Q | **What is the best weight-loss exercise?**

A former president of the American College of Sports Medicine (ACSM) joked that a dog is the best exercise equipment because you have to walk it a few times each day.[14] If you don't have a dog, you can use a treadmill or an elliptical machine, or just try walking, cycling, jogging, or skating. There is no perfect exercise—the best choice is the one you'll do regularly, whether your goal is weight loss or cardiorespiratory fitness. Any exercise or physical activity will burn more calories than being sedentary, and if you want to lose weight, you need to burn some additional calories. The ACSM recommends that initial weight-loss goals be no more than 10 percent of current body weight and that a healthy diet be combined with regular exercise to achieve this goal.[15] See the discussion of program planning later in this chapter for more information on selecting appropriate exercises for weight loss. For much more on achieving and maintaining a healthy weight, refer to Chapter 9.

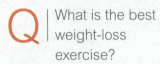

MYTH or FACT?

You burn more calories running a mile than walking a mile.

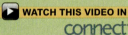

WATCH THIS VIDEO IN connect

See page 476 to find out.

Stress Management and Improved Emotional Wellness

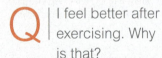

Q | **I feel better after exercising. Why is that?**

Exercise or almost any type of physical activity can cause feelings of elation, particularly when it is moderate in duration and intensity. Plenty of research indicates that people who exercise regularly are less prone to depression, have greater self-efficacy and more self-confidence, suffer fewer acute illnesses, and manage stress more effectively.

Although the reasons are difficult to pinpoint, several mechanisms have been proposed to explain how exercise affects emotional wellness:

- *Distraction:* Exercise is a distraction from whatever has been making us feel sad, mad, blue, or depressed. By engaging in this healthy, distractive behavior, we put aside our worries, and our mood lifts, at least temporarily.
- *Increased temperature:* Endurance exercise, even at low levels, increases the body's core temperature, thereby allowing our muscles, and in essence our whole being, to relax.

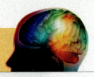
- *Changes in brain chemistry:* Exercise increases the circulation of certain mood-enhancing chemicals (neurotransmitters and endorphins) that make us feel better.

It is likely that a combination of all these factors and others not yet known provide the positive emotional benefits of exercise for mood. Benefits have been documented both after a single bout of activity (immediate short-term mood enhancement) and among people who regularly exercise (much lower rates of depression).

Self-efficacy benefits from regular physical activity (see Chapter 1), but it's difficult to determine whether the increase in self-efficacy or the regular exercise behavior occurs first. Regardless, being regularly active seems to enhance how people feel about themselves. If you feel overwhelmed when you think about exercise, try adding little bursts of 10–15 minutes of activity at a couple points during your day. The mood-enhancing effects will provide immediate benefits, and you'll likely be inspired to be more active.

Assessing Your Cardiorespiratory Fitness

Assessments for cardiorespiratory fitness come in all shapes and sizes. Some are lengthy, costly, or require extensive equipment and supervision; others are simple to perform, can be done on your own, and are free. Fitness tests can be valuable, but they're not critical before starting your exercise program or increasing your CR fitness.

Types of Cardiorespiratory Fitness Tests

Q | **How do my friend and I figure out who is more fit?**

Both of you can take the same cardiorespiratory fitness (CRF) assessment. The usual point of undertaking one of these tests is to motivate you. Maybe you are not as fit as you thought; maybe you are required to have your fitness assessed for a college course; or maybe you want to know where your fitness level is today, to see if it improves over time as you exercise more regularly. In this section we consider several types of CRF tests.

Research Brief

The Effect of Acute Bouts of Exercise on Anxiety

It has long been documented that acute bouts of aerobic exercise are associated with reduced anxiety. However, two aspects of this positive effect remain unclear: (1) the exercise intensity that is necessary to elicit this benefit and (2) the post-exercise point at which the benefit begins to occur.

Researchers at the University of Missouri asked 24 adults to participate in either treadmill or stepping exercises for 30 minutes at 50 percent and 75 percent of predicted VO_{2max}. The participants answered questions about their anxiety level at baseline and at 5, 30, and 60 minutes post-exercise so that the researchers could assess when, if at all, the exercise lessened the anxiety. Comparing baseline anxiety scores with the post-exercise scores revealed significant differences between baseline and the 30- and 60-minute measures. There was no difference in anxiety scores between baseline and the 5-minute measure, however.

Analyze and Apply

- What are some times in your day in which you could use exercise to reduce anxiety?
- Have you ever tried to use exercise specifically to relieve anxiety? How successful were you?

Source: Cox, R. H., Thomas, T. R., , and Davis, J. E. (2000). Delayed anxiolytic effect associated with an acute bout of aerobic exercise. *Journal of Exercise Physiology, 3*(4):59–66.

LAB TESTS. Some college exercise science departments have highly specialized equipment designed to measure VO_2 accurately. The equipment includes a device called a *metabolic cart,* which can precisely measure the amount of oxygen and carbon dioxide that are breathed in and out for each breath. The metabolic cart is typically used in a *maximal VO_2 test,* in which the individual exercises for 8–15 minutes progressively harder until the point of complete exhaustion (*volitional fatigue*). For people who are already fit and active, this can be a fun challenge, but for sedentary individuals, it may be unpleasant to push the body to an absolute limit.

FIELD TESTS. Although less accurate than lab tests, there are several field tests that are easier and less expensive to administer. They provide results that may be compared to those of others of similar age and sex, and establish norms for measuring individual fitness levels. Examples:

- The *Rockport walk test* estimates cardiorespiratory fitness (CRF) based on heart rate after one walks a mile as quickly as possible. A faster time and a lower heart rate indicate higher fitness. This simple test requires only a timing device and a measured track.
- The 1.5-mile *run/walk test* is similar to the Rockport test. CRF is estimated based on the time it takes to complete the distance by either running or walking.
- The 3-minute *step test* involves stepping up and down on a 16.25-inch step for 3 minutes at a constant rate. At the completion of the stepping, heart rate is measured for 15 seconds. The lower the heart rate, the better the ability to recover from an aerobic task, which is a sign of better CRF.

See Lab Activity 4-1 for more information on completing one of these field tests.

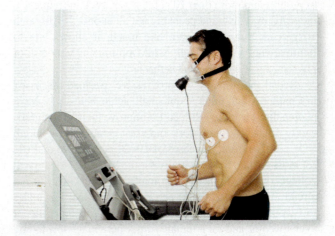

A metabolic cart measures the amount of oxygen and carbon dioxide that are breathed in and out with each breath, as captured by the face mask.

RESTING HEART RATE. A final method for assessing cardiorespiratory fitness doesn't involve exercise at all; instead, it is simply a measure of true resting heart rate (RHR). Generally, trained people have a much lower RHR than untrained individuals, so those with the lowest resting heart rates are likely to be the most fit. For reference, normal RHR is considered to be 60–100 beats per minute (bpm) for both sexes, though women's heart rates are typically about 10 bpm higher than men's. Very fit male athletes have a RHR in the low 40s or even the high 30s, and well-trained females are about 10 bpm higher. Because genetics plays a role in determining fitness, RHR may not be an extremely accurate assessment of fitness, but it is simple to determine, easy to track, and generally reliable.

To measure true RHR accurately, count your heart rate for 1 full minute after you've quietly woken in the morning from a restful night's sleep. If you sleep poorly or are awakened by an alarm clock, your heart rate will be higher than in true resting. Heart rates taken at other times of the day, even if you have been inactive, will also be noticeably higher than true resting rate.

Evaluating Assessment Results and Setting Goals

Q | How much can I improve? How much do I really *need* to improve?

Improvements in cardiorespiratory fitness (CRF) vary for everyone. The type of training you do, your diet, and your genetic heritage are among the variables that determine your rate and level of improvement. Aerobic capacity can increase by about 10–30 percent over the course of a fitness program, depending on factors such as the starting level of fitness.[16]

The previous sections have discussed the physiology of CRF and how it improves. In terms of manipulating the FITT equation (see Chapter 3), science tells us that it's best to progress no more than 10 percent per week in frequency, intensity, or time—and probably not all at once.[17] Although 10 percent might not seem like much, it allows you to improve your VO_2 gradually while minimizing your risk of physical and psychological setbacks.

Recall the principle of progressive overload discussed in Chapter 3, and think about small, achievable steps. Most people don't want to—or can't—improve their VO_2 significantly. It takes a lot of work and great genes to have a high VO_{2max}. Therefore, increases of 10–20 percent are realistic for most people. Strive initially for the VO_{2max} of the typical college female (high 30s) or male (mid 40s). If you are already there, try to go 10 percent beyond that. For males this would mean shooting for a VO_{2max} in the upper 40s or even low 50s, and for a female somewhere in the low to mid 40s. To see how you compare with others, use the tables in Lab Activity 4-1 for nationally representative norms.

Q | How often should I do an assessment to check for improvement in my cardio fitness?

Although the rate of progress varies from person to person, reassessing fitness can be done 4–6 weeks after starting a new program. This should be a short enough

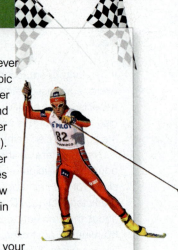
window to provide positive feedback quickly and help keep motivation high. After the initial period, you can push back the assessment schedule to every 8–12 weeks. For a reliable comparison, be sure to use the same fitness test every time.

Q | Can I judge my fitness without taking a test?

If you haven't had a fitness test or simply don't want one, no problem. You can just use your exercise performance as your guide. If you can currently jog for 10 minutes, then that is your baseline. Can you swim four lengths of the pool? Does it take you 15 minutes to walk a mile? Can you not quite yet cycle to the top of the big hill in town? These are examples of baseline measures of fitness. As you run farther or faster, swim more laps, or cycle farther up the hill, you are improving your cardiorespiratory fitness. Are these baseline measures scientific evidence of improvement? Yes and no. They certainly are evidence of physiological changes occurring, but they don't provide any basis for comparison to anyone but you.

Creating a Cardiorespiratory Fitness Program

A successful cardiorespiratory fitness program applies the FITT formula you learned about in Chapter 3. Equally important is that it includes activities you enjoy and will stick with over time. If you've been sedentary for a while, your first step is to fire up your motivation and make a commitment to improve your health and well-being through exercise.

Getting Started

Q | How do I learn to like exercise? Right now, I just don't.

Finding exercise you like precedes everything else concerning improved fitness. The reason is that lack of motivation, no matter what its source, will prevent you from improving your health—fitness included. Increasing CRF is not a typical goal for college students with so many activities competing for their time, among them sleep, classes, work, study, and socializing. It may seem as if there isn't time to get fit or stay fit. Recall, however, that the ACLS study found that higher levels of CRF clearly reduce the risk of disease and death (Figure 4-5).

You might be thinking, "I'm 20 years old. Disease and death are not my problem, so whatever!" If your thoughts trend this way, remember that you'll feel better *right now* if you get fitter. And you'll be more attentive in class. And sleep better at night. And meet new people in the wellness or fitness center. Further, you'll be able to keep up with your kids, today and in the future. In short, there are many physical and emotional reasons to get moving, your health being number one.

Importantly, focusing on fitness doesn't have to mean going to the gym. It can take the form of getting up and moving more throughout the day, joining a dance club, playing pick-up basketball, or navigating the campus by in-line skating. Ultimately, only you can decide what your goals are and how motivated you are to reach them. See the box "Getting Started on a Cardiorespiratory Fitness Program" for strategies to try. Once you find an enjoyable source of exercise and do it often, you'll wonder why you didn't start a long time ago.

Applying the FITT Formula

Q | How do I know I'm doing all the right things—not going too far, or too fast or too slow?

Use the FITT formula—frequency, intensity, time, and type—a simple device for remembering and applying different training variables. Following the basic FITT guidelines will make it easier to plan your program and achieve your fitness goals. The most widely referenced exercise guidelines come from the American College of Sports Medicine, the U.S. Department of Health and Human Services' *2008 Physical Activity Guidelines for Americans,*[18] and the U.S. Department of Agriculture's *Dietary Guidelines for Americans.*[19] These public health resources all have the same goal—to get Americans moving—although each has a slightly different emphasis.

Q | Is it safe to work out every day?

FREQUENCY. *Frequency* is the FITT formula term about how often you should exercise. Most exercise guidelines encourage resting 1 or 2 days a week to prevent injuries and avoid **burnout**—physical and emotional exhaustion. However, if you vary your routine and exercises and do not regularly exercise at a high intensity, you should be able to work out every day with no problems. You can do low-impact activities like walking, swimming, and cycling every day, but you should plan some days off if you mostly jog, do step aerobics, or engage in other higher-impact or higher-intensity activities.

Recommendations for exercise frequency range from 3 days a week to "most" days of the week. The variation among the recommendations is based on exercise intensity, because intensity and frequency need to balance each other. Simply put, the greater the intensity, the less frequent the exercise, and vice versa. The American College of Sports Medicine (ACSM) recommends exercising a minimum of 3 days a week for vigorous intensity (for at least 20 minutes a day) and 5 days a week for moderate intensity

burnout Physical and emotional exhaustion from exercise.

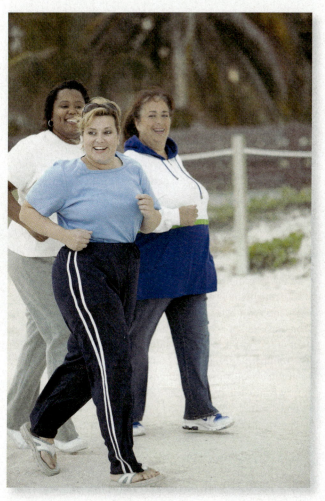

All public health recommendations for exercise share a common goal: to get Americans moving.

Wellness Strategies

Getting Started on a Cardiorespiratory Fitness Program

 Q How many types of cardiorespiratory workouts are there? What would you recommend if you are just getting back into working out?

Step I: Set Long- and Short-Term Goals: First, have a basic goal, such as to feel better about yourself, to improve your health, to lose weight, to meet more people, or to compete in intramurals. Whatever your goal, remember two basic principles to goal setting: KISS and SMART. KISS stands for Keep It Simple and Succeed. SMART is the acronym for the goal criteria you learned in Chapter 2: specific, measurable, achievable, realistic, and time-bound. Both principles emphasize the importance of small, realistic goals that can be achieved in a short time. Longer-term goals are also important, but getting there is much easier when you have something tangible to keep you going today.

Step II: Choose an Activity: Next, identify types of exercise that you enjoy most and can access easily. Never really liked jogging? Then skip it. Like to swim but your school doesn't have a pool, or the hours don't work for you? Skip it. You always liked bike riding and still have a decent bike. Go for it.

Step III: Plan Ahead: You want to start exercising, you like to ride, and you have a bike. What next? Is your bike in working condition? Do you need a water bottle, comfortable biking clothes, and a helmet? Attending to such details can take you a long way. If you are psyched to go riding, only to discover a flat tire, it can be pretty deflating. If you are out riding and get really thirsty and have no water available, it can leave you feeling hot and bothered. Planning for these little things will make that first day out much more pleasant—and make you more likely to do your preferred exercise again soon.

OK, your bike is working, you've found your gear, you've picked out a route, and you're ready to go. Are you forgetting anything? Think everything through so you can have the best experience possible. What is the weather forecast? Do you have an important appointment early in the day? Think your way through your workout and your day, and address any possible problems.

As you can see, starting and maintaining an exercise program requires planning. The more you do your workout, the more routine and easier it becomes. Ultimately, when you are done exercising each day, you will feel invigorated and proud—and ready to go at it again tomorrow.

(for at least 30 minutes a day). The ACSM also notes that additional improvements in cardiorespiratory fitness can be gained by exercising more frequently, but the intensity should be adjusted accordingly. The recommendations in the Department of Health and Human Services (HHS) *2008 Guidelines for Physical Activity for Americans* are for all adults to accumulate at least 150 minutes of moderate exercise or 75 minutes of vigorous activity each week, spread over as many days as possible.

People with a very low level of fitness might benefit from several short exercise bouts a day, because they often cannot do a lot of exercise at any one time. Bouts of 10 minutes or longer can count toward the daily activity total. Once unfit people increase their level of cardiorespiratory fitness, they find that a single bout of exercise daily is usually more practical and effective. Several short bouts can also be helpful for people with tight schedules.

 Q How hard should I exercise?

INTENSITY. You should exercise in your target intensity zone, as described in Chapter 3—hard enough to cause fitness improvements but not so hard that you risk injury or burnout. Generally,

you can exercise as hard as you want, as long as you are enjoying it. Most people don't enjoy exercising at very high intensities; it's just not that pleasant. Therefore, balance intensity with frequency and duration: The higher the intensity, the shorter the duration and the lower the frequency.

Intensity is also closely tied to your personal goals. If enjoyment is at the top of your list, then find an intensity that brings you the most joy. If you are looking to get the most out of your exercise (to get fit or to improve your health, for example), then go for a little higher intensity. And if you are training for a competitive goal, then even higher intensity may be necessary. Remember, if you exercise hard, you don't need to do it as often or for as long as when you exercise at a lower level. If you exercise at a comfortable intensity, you are less likely to run into setbacks.

Exercise guidelines typically differentiate between moderate-intensity activity and vigorous-intensity activity. There are a number of ways to define and calculate target intensity. As a frame of reference, two minutes of moderate activity confers about the same benefit as one minute of vigorous activity.

Q | What's considered moderate activity and vigorous activity?

For aerobic activities, intensity, or how hard you exercise, is usually based on your heart rate or on your perception of your level of exertion. The **talk test** is a simple method for judging exercise intensity, as it measures how well you can hold a conversation, or talk, during exercise. The HHS physical activity guidelines describe the talk test this way:[20]

- Moderate-intensity exercise: You can talk but not sing.
- Vigorous-intensity exercise: You can say only a few words before pausing to take a breath.

The **heart-rate maximum (HR_{max}) method** is one of the oldest methods for calculating exercise intensity. Simply put, this approach involves exercising at a certain percentage of your **maximum heart rate (MHR)** depending on your current fitness level. The ACSM suggests exercising at 57–94 percent of HR_{max} to ensure increases in cardiorespiratory fitness.[7] A sedentary individual might start at an intensity at the low end of the range, whereas a seasoned vigorous exerciser might work out at the top of the range.

Heart-rate maximum (HR_{max}) method:
Target heart rate = MHR × %

You can determine your maximum heart rate by performing an all-out exercise test—which is challenging and uncomfortable. Alternatively, you can use your age as a starting point. By subtracting your age from 220 (220 − age = MHR), you have a pretty good estimate of your maximum heart rate. Even with an error of +/− 15 beats per minute, this method is considered generally reliable. Therefore, a 20-year-old who is sporadically active and plans to use 70–80 percent of HR_{max} for her **target heart-rate range** would calculate her range as 140–160 beats per minute (bpm) this way:

Predicted maximum heart rate (MHR) = 220 − 20
= 200 bpm
70% exercise intensity = 0.70 × 200 = 140 bpm
80% exercise intensity = 0.80 × 200 = 160 bpm

The **heart-rate reserve (HRR) method** of calculating intensity is a more accurate means of reflecting energy expenditure during exercise.[21] However, the formula is slightly more complex: you will need your maximum heart rate (MHR) and your resting heart rate (RHR). MHR is described above; RHR can be determined by counting your pulse for a minute before you get out of bed in the morning—on a day you wake up naturally and are not startled by your alarm. Calculate your HRR by subtracting your resting heart rate from your maximum heart rate. Then multiply that value by the percentage of HRR you are aiming for. Finally, add this result to your resting heart rate (RHR). This will yield a target heart rate for you to use. The ACSM suggests a target heart-rate range based on 30–85 percent of HRR, depending on your initial fitness level.

Heart-rate reserve (HRR) method:
Target heart rate =
[(MHR − RHR) × %] + RHR

Using this method, a 20-year-old who has a resting heart rate of 64 and is somewhat active might choose a target range based on 55–80 percent of heart-rate reserve. She would calculate an exercise-intensity target range of 139–173 beats per minute (bpm).

HRR = [(200 − 64) × %] + 64
= exercise heart-rate range
55% exercise intensity: (136 × 0.55) + 64 = 139 bpm
80% exercise intensity: (136 × 0.80) + 64 = 173 bpm

talk test A qualitative assessment of exercise intensity based on the ability to talk during exercise.

heart-rate maximum (HR_{max}) method A method of calculating target cardiorespiratory-endurance-exercise intensity based on a percentage range of maximum heart rate.

maximum heart rate (MHR) The maximum number of beats per minute of a person's heart, which can be measured directly through laboratory testing or estimated according to age; the value typically starts to decrease at about 20 years of age.

target heart-rate range A range of heart rates that reflects an intensity of exercise that will result in cardiorespiratory fitness improvement.

heart-rate reserve (HRR) method A method of calculating target cardiorespiratory-endurance-exercise intensity based on a percentage range of heart-rate reserve, which is the difference between resting heart rate and maximum heart rate.

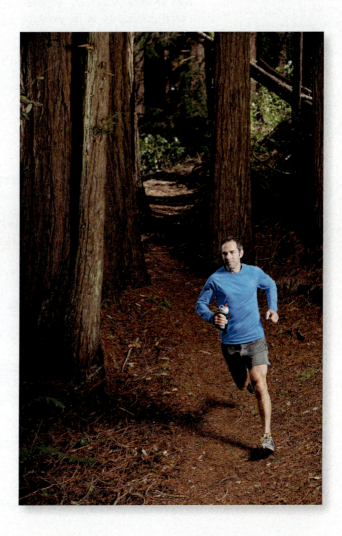

Lab Activity 4-2 will help you work through the appropriate calculations. Table 4-1 shows the ACSM recommendations for intensity based on current fitness levels. These are ranges, and there is no need to try to keep your heart rate exactly at one particular level.

The HR_{max} and HRR methods are *objective* measures of intensity, each requiring certain heart-rate values. **Rating of perceived exertion (RPE),** also called the Borg scale (after its originator, Gunnar Borg), is a *subjective* measure of exercise intensity that does not require heart-rate information. On a scale of 6 to 20, users rate their level of effort (Figure 4-6). The reason for the unusual range—starting at 6 and ending at 20—is that the levels are meant to loosely correlate to the user's current heart rate. Therefore, if the user rates intensity at 14 on the RPE scale, her or his heart rate is likely to be around 140 bpm. To achieve a moderate intensity on the RPE scale, similar to that calculated by the HR_{max} and HRR methods, the user would strive for an RPE value between 12 and 16. This moderate-exercise intensity should bring about the same increases in cardiorespiratory fitness as HR_{max}, HRR, or the talk test.

Yet another way of measuring exercise intensity is in terms of **metabolic equivalents (METs),** in which the MET level is used to estimate the amount of oxygen the body utilizes during physical activity. The MET approach provides a simple method of quantifying activity at different absolute levels. One MET is equal to the energy used by the body when sitting quietly. The harder you work during any activity, the higher the MET requirement. Moderate-intensity activity, such as a brisk walk, requires 3–6 METs; vigorous-intensity activity requires more than 6 METs, or six times the energy required at rest.[18] Because intensity can vary based on individual effort, the same activity can be classified as light, moderate, or vigorous. Figure 4-7 provides some general intensity classifications of different physical activities.

rating of perceived exertion (RPE) A scale that provides a subjective measure of exercise intensity; widely used when heart-rate monitoring is not available; also known as the Borg scale.

metabolic equivalents (METs) A physiological concept expressing the energy cost of a physical activity relative to resting metabolic rate; the value of sitting at rest is defined as 1.0 MET; more vigorous activities have higher MET requirements.

Figure 4-6 Rating of perceived exertion (RPE) scale.

6	No exertion at all
7	Extremely light
8	
9	Very light
10	
11	Light
12	
13	Somewhat hard
14	
15	Hard (heavy)
16	
17	Very hard
18	
19	Extremely hard
20	Maximal exertion

Source: Borg, G. (1970). Perceived exertion as an indicator of somatic stress. *Scandinavian Journal of Rehabilitation Medicine,* 2(2), 92–98. © Gunnar Borg, 1970, 1985, 1994, 1998.

TABLE 4-1 RECOMMENDED STARTING INTENSITY OF EXERCISE BASED ON CURRENT ACTIVITY LEVEL

ACTIVITY LEVEL	HEART-RATE MAXIMUM (HR_{MAX}) METHOD* (%)	HEART-RATE RESERVE (HRR) METHOD* (%)
SEDENTARY	57%–67%	30%–45%
MINIMAL PHYSICAL ACTIVITY	64%–74%	40%–55%
SPORADIC PHYSICAL ACTIVITY	74%–84%	55%–70%
HABITUAL PHYSICAL ACTIVITY	80%–91%	65%–80%
HIGH AMOUNTS OF HABITUAL PHYSICAL ACTIVITY	84%–94%	70%–85%

*The percentage values for heart-rate maximum and heart-rate reserve methods of calculating intensity would be multiplied according to the appropriate formula:

Heart-rate maximum (HR_{max}) = MHR × %
Heart-rate reserve (HRR) = [(MHR − RHR) × %] + RHR

Source: American College of Sports Medicine. (2009). *Guidelines for exercise testing and prescription* (8th ed.). Baltimore, MD: Lippincott Williams & Wilkins.

Beginners should start at a lower intensity. This strategy helps to improve retention and prevent injuries and leaves them eager for greater challenges. To begin, calculate target intensity using 40–60 percent HRR or an RPE of 10–12. Once you get comfortable at this intensity and can repeat it over the course of about 2 weeks, then increase the intensity gradually.

Lab Activity 4-2 has more information and help for program planning.

Q | What's the best way to take my heart rate when I'm exercising?

The easiest way is with a heart-rate (HR) monitor. HR monitors are available with a range of features and at a range of prices. The least expensive HR monitors cost around $40; the most expensive can be more than $400 and will determine calories burned, altitude climbed,

distance traveled, the ambient temperature, and more. The most reliable HR monitors are those that come in two parts: a chest strap worn around the torso and a watch or monitor worn on the wrist. A signal is transmitted from the chest strap to the monitor, with the heart rate displayed and updated about every 3–5 seconds. Most brands are relatively reliable, although interference can be a problem near strong electrical fields or when many HR monitor users are in a small place (a spinning class, for example).

Your fingers can also provide an accurate measure of your exercise HR. You simply place your fingers on the inside of your wrist (thumb side) at the radial artery, or gently on your neck by the carotid artery, and feel your heart beating. This method is cheap, but it does have minor drawbacks. First, you probably will need to stop for at least 10 seconds to take your HR. With an HR monitor, you don't need to stop—you just glance at your watch. You

Moderate Intensity Activity 3.0 to 6.0 METs (3.5 to 7 calories burned per minute)	Vigorous Intensity Activity More than 6.0 METs (more than 7 calories burned per minute)
Walking at a moderate or brisk pace of 3 to 4.5 mph on a level surface (90–110 steps per minute)	Walking at a pace of 5 mph or faster
Hiking	Waking or climbing briskly up a hill
	Jogging or running
	Wheeling a wheelchair
	Mountain climbing or backpacking
Bicycling 5 to 9 mph on level terrain	Bicycling more than 10 mph or on steep terrain
Stationary cycling using moderate effort	Stationary cycling using vigorous effort
Using a stair climber, rowing machine, elliptical, etc., with moderate effort	Using a stair climber, rowing machine, elliptical, etc., with vigorous effort
Dancing with moderate effort	Dancing energetically with vigorous effort
Tennis—doubles	Tennis—singles
	Wheelchair tennis
Swimming–recreational	Swimming—steady paced laps
Basketball—shooting baskets	Basketball—playing a game
Gardening or yard work—moderate (raking the lawn, bagging grass or leaves, digging or light shoveling [less than 10 lbs per minute], weeding)	Gardening or yard work—heavy or rapid (shoveling more than 10 lbs per minute, digging ditches, carrying heavy loads)
Pushing a power lawn mower	Pushing a nonmotorized lawn mower
Moderate housework: scrubbing the floor, sweeping outdoor areas, washing windows, general housework tasks	Heavy housework: Moving or pushing heavy furniture (75 lbs or more), carrying household items weighing 25 lbs or more up the stairs
Actively playing with children	Energetically/vigorously playing with children

Figure 4-7 Intensity levels of different physical activities.

Source: Adapted from Centers for Disease Control and Prevention, National Center for Chronic Disease Prevention and Health Promotion. *General physical activities defined by level of intensity* (http://www.cdc.gov/nccdphp/dnpa/physical/pdf/PA_Intensity_table_2_1.pdf). A complete listing of MET values for many different physical activities can be found at http://prevention.sph.sc.edu/tools/compendium.htm.

The easiest way to measure heart rate while exercising is with a heart-rate (HR) monitor. The most reliable HR monitors have a chest strap worn around the torso and a watch or monitor worn on the wrist.

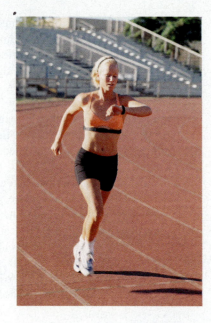

will need to count the heartbeats for between 6 seconds and 15 seconds to get a reasonably accurate heart-rate measure. If your target heart-rate range is 140–170 bpm, and you decide to count your pulse for 10 seconds, you would determine your target 10-second count by dividing your bpm goal by 6, which means 23–28 beats per 10 seconds.

If you don't want to buy an HR monitor or aren't comfortable taking your pulse, there is always the RPE option. Simply rate your perception of your effort on the RPE scale. If you use the scale properly, you'll be aware of your effort level every time out.

Q | Doesn't lower-intensity exercise burn more fat?

More fat than what? More than sitting on the couch—absolutely. More than jogging or some other higher-intensity activity? No, at least not in absolute terms. When it comes to fat loss (and weight control), what appears to matter most is the *total calories used* ("burned"). Low-intensity exercise uses about 4–5 calories per minute, and high-intensity exercise burns more than twice as much, or about 10–13 calories per minute. It is true that low-intensity exercise uses a higher percentage of fat, but a high-intensity workout uses more overall calories and more total fat than lower-intensity exercise. Therefore, interspersing brief periods of higher-intensity exercise will allow you to burn more calories per exercise session. Also, over time, you will find that the lower-intensity pace gets easier and you can maintain the higher intensity even longer, therefore using still more calories.

People who find it difficult to do high-intensity exercise shouldn't be discouraged. Many individuals lose weight and successfully keep it off by using moderate-intensity exercise, albeit for slightly longer durations. It may take a little longer to burn the same number of calories, but the long-term benefits are still pretty good.

Q | How many hours of cardiovascular activity are necessary to be healthy?

TIME. The amount of time you need to spend on cardio-respiratory exercise depends on a number of factors. In general, *time,* or duration of exercise, refers to how long each exercise session should last and should be balanced with frequency and intensity.

The balance between time and intensity applies to individual workouts as well as to a weekly exercise plan. A 60-minute exercise session tends to be lower intensity than a 20-minute session; and, generally speaking, as duration increases, intensity decreases (Figure 4-8). Recall that the ACSM recommends at least 30 minutes of moderate activity 5 days a week or 20 minutes of vigorous activity 3 days a week, while the Department of Health and Human Services (HHS) advises accumulating 150 minutes of moderate-intensity or 75 minutes of vigorous-intensity activity weekly. HHS also states that doubling those times to 300 minutes of moderate exercise or 150 minutes of vigorous exercise brings about even greater health benefits.

The law of diminishing returns also applies, though, and doing too much exercise or working out at too high an intensity may create more problems than benefits. For continued cardiorespiratory fitness improvement, the intensity, duration, and/or frequency of exercise need to increase. Ultimately, national physical activity recommendations encourage people to find activities they enjoy and to perform them at an intensity and duration that they can sustain on a regular basis. Therefore, *any exercise is better than none.* However, certain precautions do apply for pregnant women, as outlined in the box "Exercise During Pregnancy."

TYPE. Individuals may improve their cardiorespiratory fitness (CRF) through a variety of activities, including those that are aerobic, rhythmic, and involve regularly performed work by large muscle groups. (Anaerobic activities are typically used to develop strength and power.) The list of aerobic activities is long. It includes individual activities, such as walking, jogging, cycling, swimming, in-line skating, cross-country skiing, rowing, and dancing, as well as team "pick-up" activities, such as volleyball, basketball, and softball, that can be accessed through your school's intramural sports office. Try out different activities and then focus on the ones you most enjoy.

If you don't want to go outside and like the idea of a consistent routine throughout the year, the aerobic exercise machines in your campus wellness or fitness center may be the choice for you. Treadmills, ellipticals, and stationary and spinning bikes provide an opportunity for a great aerobic workout. The advantages of machines are always knowing what to expect, having a timer close at hand, and usually having the opportunity to let the

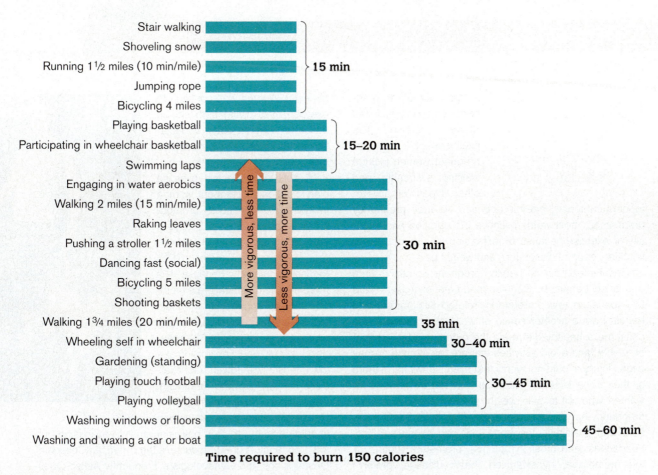

Figure 4-8 **Relationship between exercise time and intensity.** Each example on the chart is roughly equivalent to physical activity requiring 150 calories. The activities listed near the top require more effort (intensity) and less time to burn 150 calories than those toward the bottom. Therefore, 15 minutes of stair walking is the equivalent of 45–60 minutes of washing or waxing a car.

Source: Adapted from U.S. Department of Health and Human Services. (1996). At a glance. *Physical activity and health: A report of the Surgeon General* (http://www.cdc.gov/nccdphp/sgr/ataglan.htm).

machine create a workout for you. Machines also provide rough estimates of calories burned, which may be appealing.

Putting Together a Complete Workout

A complete workout should include a warm-up phase, a conditioning phase, and a cool-down phase.

Q Do I really need a warm-up just to go walking with my friends?

No, you don't need to do a formal warm-up before going for a walk. By definition, a warm-up consists of 5–10 minutes of low-intensity large-muscle activity, such as jogging before running, or slow walking before brisk walking. Because you probably start your walk with your friends slowly and then increase the tempo gradually, you are in fact warming up even though you don't call it a warm-up.

If you are planning more vigorous exercise or exercise that requires skill-dependent movement, then you do need a more formal warm-up—for all the reasons described in Chapter 3. You can include stretching exercises at the end of your warm-up, or you can choose to stretch after the more active part of your workout. Chapter 6 discusses stretching in greater detail.

The next phase of a complete workout is conditioning. See discussion earlier in this chapter.

The final phase of the complete workout is the cool-down, a time of gradual recovery from endurance activity. During the cool-down, slowly decrease your intensity from the conditioning phase. If you were taking a brisk walk, then you could add several minutes of easier walking at the end, or start slowing down a little before your endpoint. Many people enjoy doing stretching exercises immediately after aerobic activities, so do that too if you'd like. Overall, the cool-down helps your body transition to a less active state and allows you to resume your other daily tasks with ease. Figure 4-9 shows the three phases of a complete workout.

Wellness Strategies

Exercise During Pregnancy

Q | My sister is expecting a baby. What kind of exercise should she do—if any?

Almost half of all pregnant women in the United States exercise. The exercises of choice for pregnant women include walking, swimming, and other types of low-to-moderate-intensity aerobic activities. As their pregnancy progresses, most women reduce the duration and intensity of exercise because of increasing fatigue, nausea or vomiting, general discomfort, and weight gain.

Regular exercise in healthy pregnant women is safe and often beneficial. Regular moderate exercisers tend to experience fewer pregnancy-related discomforts and benefit from a greater sense of well-being. Women who consume a healthy diet, gain the recommended amount of weight, and avoid activities that are too intense or may cause injury should not worry that exercise will harm them or their baby. However, exercise may not be advised for women who fail to gain weight or have *preeclampsia* (a pregnancy-specific disorder marked by high blood pressure and protein in the urine that can cause swelling, headaches, and other symptoms), premature rupture of the membrane, hypertension, heart disease, preterm labor, second- or third-trimester bleeding, or a weak cervix.

Although regular exercise is beneficial for pregnant women, their fetuses can be harmed by overly vigorous activity in the third trimester, activities with a high risk of falling or a high level of contact, and activities in the supine position (lying on the back, face up), especially after the first

trimester. Women who continue to exercise after giving birth should notice no adverse effect on lactation in terms of milk composition, milk volume, or their health.

A safe and effective exercise plan for a healthy pregnant woman includes 30–40 minutes of moderate exercise, at least 3 days a week. Pregnant women should use rate of perceived exertion (RPE) to assess intensity, because it is more reliable than heart-rate methods during pregnancy; they should aim for an RPE of 11–13. Women who were sedentary before pregnancy should begin exercising at a low intensity with low-impact exercises like walking and swimming. Regardless of their pre-pregnancy fitness or activity level, all women should consult with their physician prior to exercising during pregnancy. A great resource is the American College of Obstetricians and Gynecologists' Frequently Asked Questions regarding exercise during pregnancy: http://www.acog.org/~/media/For%20Patients/faq119.pdf?dmc=1&ts=20120406T1403031110.

Source: American College of Obstetricians and Gynecologists. (2002). Exercise during pregnancy and the postpartum period. ACOG Committee Opinion No. 267. *Obstetrics & Gynecology, 99,* 171–173.

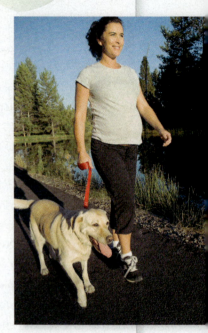

Making FITT Work for You

Q | I don't have much time to work out but I still want to get fit. What can I do?

Understanding the FITT guidelines is a first step (Table 4-2). Next, you need to consider your current level of fitness, your schedule, your activity options, your preferences, and your goals. The following examples may give you some ideas:

- *Jenna is extremely busy—school in the mornings, work*

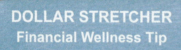

DOLLAR STRETCHER
Financial Wellness Tip

You don't need to spend much on home exercise equipment. Jump ropes, aerobic steps, exercise DVDs, and video games are inexpensive and can get you fit. Even some of today's commercial home video-based programs are cheaper than a gym membership.

in the afternoons—but she has to admit that she isn't very active physically. She doesn't have the time or inclination to go to a gym, so to get started being less sedentary, she's going to add brisk walking to her daily routine. She timed the walk between the second-closest transit stop and where she works, and walking that distance instead of riding to the closest stop would give her about 20 minutes of brisk walking time, 5 days per week. She doesn't mind getting a bit winded and sweaty on her way home from work. She arranges with one of her friends to get

Research Brief

Short Bout, Long Bout: Which Is Best?

Research indicates that short bouts of exercise may be just as effective as longer bouts for both fitness and weight control. In one study, overweight female college students were assigned to one of the following groups:

- Control group, which did no exercise
- Short-exercise group, which performed three 10-minute bouts of exercise
- Medium-exercise group, which performed two 15-minute bouts of exercise
- Long-exercise group, which performed one 30-minute bout of exercise

The primary outcome measures were VO_{2max} and weight loss. Each of the exercise groups worked out for a minimum of 3 days a week at about 75 percent of VO_{2max}, with the total volume of exercise meant to be the same across the groups. At the end of the study, women in all three of the exercise groups improved their VO_{2max} and decreased their body weight, body fat, and body circumference measures compared to the control group, which did not show any of these changes.

Analyze and Apply

- What does this study indicate about the *volume* of exercise versus the *duration* of our exercise?
- Is it possible that the observed effects of the exercise bouts occurred as a result of something other than the exercise itself? Explain.
- Looking at your typical week, what specific 10-minute, 15-minute, and 30-minute windows of opportunity are there for performing exercise bouts?
- What benefits might adding these exercise bouts have for your fitness and body weight?

Source: Schmidt, W. D., Biwer, C. J., & Kalscheuer, L. K. (2001). Effects of long versus short bout exercise on fitness and weight loss in overweight females. *Journal of the American College of Nutrition, 20*(5), 494–501.

---

together for a walk once each weekend, starting with 30 minutes and working up to an hour. They plan to walk outside in good weather and at the mall in bad weather. For added motivation, they'll wear pedometers during their walk to track their steps—trying to increase each week or two. Jenna plans to monitor intensity with the talk test and with her pedometer (tracking steps versus time), but she'll check her heart rate during activity once or twice a week.

- *Zach loves to go to the campus fitness center during the week, and he plays about an hour of fast and hard basketball with friends on most Saturdays. At the fitness center, he works out on the strength machines, and he's realized that despite feeling fairly fit, his basketball time doesn't quite add up to the recommended level of cardiorespiratory training. Because he enjoys the campus fitness center, he decides to add some cardio training on the machines there—he'll do two vigorous 10-minute bouts of training three times per week, mixed in with his strength training. He's afraid he'll get bored, so he plans to alternate on different types of cardio training machines. Zach is interested in doing some interval and high-intensity training; he likes to compete with himself, so he'll use a heart-rate monitor to track his intensity.*

Another strategy for time-crunched fitness routines is to perform *high-intensity training (HIT)*. Although this type of training carries risk, it also can produce results quickly. There are many commercial programs promoting high intensity, whether they are led by an instructor at the gym or through a video or DVD. Regardless of the particular HIT approach, it might be best to perform HIT only a few days a week since doing it every day may be asking for trouble, as the law of diminishing returns would indicate.

Mind Stretcher
Critical Thinking Exercise

Do you often have to deal with windy conditions during outdoor aerobic exercise? If so, consider starting out by going into the wind, especially if you do an "out and back" route. This way, as you get more tired and sweaty toward the end, you will have the wind at your back—a much more pleasant experience than having to push into the wind at the end. Also, if possible, choose quality wind-proof gear, especially if you run in cold and wind.

- What routes can you use to minimize wind exposure?
- Can you exercise with others and take turns blocking the wind?
- Can you exercise at different times of the day to minimize the effects of the wind? Early in the morning tends to be the calmest time of the day.

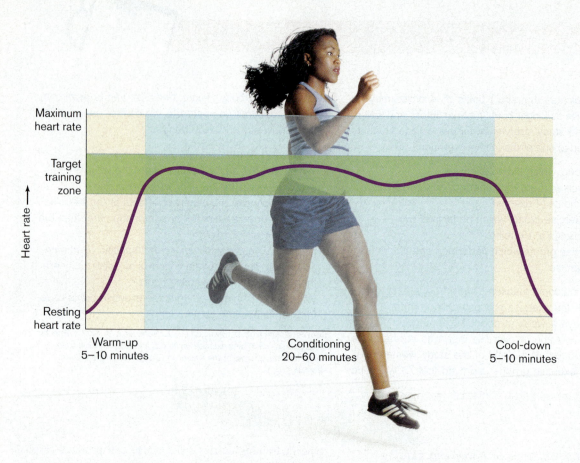

Maximum heart rate

Target training zone

Heart rate →

Resting heart rate

Warm-up
5–10 minutes

Conditioning
20–60 minutes

Cool-down
5–10 minutes

Figure 4-9 **Cardiorespiratory workout.** A workout has three stages—warm-up, conditioning, and cool-down.

TABLE 4-2 SUMMARY OF RECOMMENDED EXERCISE GUIDELINES*

	ACSM[a]	HHS[b]
FREQUENCY	3–5 days/week	Spread throughout the week, across at least 3 days
INTENSITY	57%–94% HR_{max} 30%–85% HRR	Moderate or vigorous
TIME	20–60 minutes/day, in bouts of 10 or more minutes	150 minutes/week or 75 minutes/week, in bouts of 10 or more minutes
CALORIES	≥150/day	N/A
TYPE	Aerobic activities	Aerobic activities
NOTES	Longer duration requires less intensity.	Longer duration, moderate or vigorous, brings even greater benefits.

*These are minimum guidelines for health/fitness benefits; additional health benefits are obtained by increasing activity over these levels. Additional activity is recommended for people whose goals include losing weight or maintaining weight loss.

Sources: (a) Thompson, W. R., Gordon, N. F., & Pescatello, L. S. (2009). *ACSM guidelines for exercise testing and prescription* (8th ed.). Baltimore, MD: Lippincott Williams & Wilkins. (b) U.S. Department of Health and Human Services. (2008). *2008 physical activity guidelines for Americans*.

Putting Your Personal Fitness Plan into Action

Completing your first workout is a great step, but the key to cardiorespiratory fitness is maintaining your program over time. A successful program is one in which you continue to make progress, exercise safely, and adjust to changing goals and conditions.

Making Progress Toward Your Fitness Goals

Q | How long until I can run for 5 miles?

It depends on your starting level of fitness. If you can't run around the block today, this goal might take a while. If you can already run for 30 continuous minutes, then it might occur much sooner. The aspect of training involved here is **progression**—gradual increases in frequency, intensity, and duration of exercise in order for the body to grow fitter—and each person progresses at a different rate, depending on age, previous training status, training program, goals, and other factors. Aerobic exercise progresses at a different rate for everyone, depending on a variety of factors including baseline fitness and motivation.

If you are a beginner, progression could start with up to 15 minutes of conditioning, which can be done multiple times a day over at least 3 days a week (Figure 4-10). Gentle increases in duration (5–10 minutes more) can occur every other week during the first 4 to 6 weeks of training. This is the overload principle at work. Also during this phase, it is helpful to establish individualized, attainable, short-term goals, as well as a reward system, to give yourself positive reinforcement.

After a month or two of regular conditioning, you will have a better feel for when and how much to increase frequency, intensity, and duration to achieve your fitness goals. For someone starting in a very deconditioned state, it may take up to 8 months to be able to accumulate 30 minutes of cardiorespiratory exercises on most days of the week. For many exercisers, adding a variety of routines, routes, and modes of exercise may help increase adherence and reduce the risk or injury or burnout.

Q | Do I need a special diet to increase cardio fitness?

Your diet, discussed in more depth in Chapters 8 and 9, can't directly increase your CRF, but it can go a long way toward improving your overall health. Fitness gains come from training, and your diet helps determine the quality of training you can sustain. Eating a variety of fruits and vegetables, lean meats, and low-fat dairy products will give you the energy you need, along with a rich base of vitamins and minerals. This type of diet will allow you to engage in exercise at varying intensities and frequencies without feeling unusually tired or run-down.

Making Exercise Safe

Exercise will be fun and enjoyable if you plan for potential problems. To minimize the chances of injury, overuse, boredom, and burnout, take precautions, listen to your body, and use moderation in your planning. Refer to Chapter 3 for advice on choosing exercise clothing and shoes, guidelines for proper hydration and safety equipment, and additional information on safety, including tips for exercising in hot, cold, and smoggy conditions.

Q | I have a cold. Can I still work out?

You can if you don't have a fever and your symptoms are from the neck up.[22] It might be difficult to maintain intensive exercise with a cold, so put that off for a few days, but otherwise you can work out, maybe at a slower pace or for a shorter duration.

If you think you might have the flu (fever, extreme tiredness, muscle aches, swollen lymph glands), then you should

progression Gradual increases in frequency, intensity, and duration of exercise in order for the body to adapt and increase fitness.

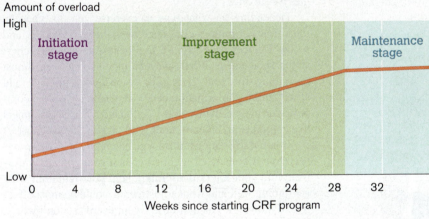

Figure 4-10 **Sample cardiorespiratory-fitness-program progression.** The initiation stage, with its short, relatively low-intensity workouts, allows you to develop the habit of exercise without getting too sore or uncomfortable. During the improvement stage, slowly and progressively increase overload until you reach your desired level of fitness (maintenance stage). Don't increase frequency, intensity, and duration during the same week, and don't increase overall exercise volume more than 10 percent a week.
Source: Adapted from American College of Sports Medicine. (2009). *Resource manual to accompany guidelines for exercise testing and prescription* (6th ed.). Baltimore, MD: Lippincott Williams & Wilkins.

take some time off from your exercise program. Wait about a week before starting back slowly and at least 2 weeks before you work out at higher intensities.

Personal Training—Online, in Person, or Somewhere in Between?

Personal trainers came into vogue in the 1950s, after Jack LaLanne popularized personal fitness. LaLanne opened the first health spa and hosted the first nationally syndicated TV exercise show. Since then, personal training as a profession has grown by leaps and bounds.

Q How do I know who is a good personal trainer?

Unfortunately, personal training is a loosely regulated field, and many organizations offer personal training certification. A handful of organizations are considered rigorous and creditable, including the American College of Sports Medicine (ACSM), the American Council on Exercise (ACE), the Cooper Institute of Aerobics Research, the National Academy of Sports Medicine (NASM), and the National Strength and Conditioning Association (NSCA). If you are in the market for a personal trainer, look for certification and a relevant degree. A degree in kinesiology, exercise science, wellness, fitness, or a related field indicates a minimal level of competency. Someone with both a degree in the field and a certification is likely to have the best background. Experience by itself is no guarantee of competency.

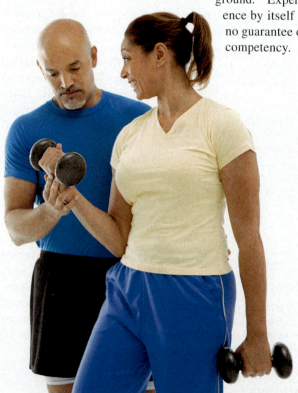

Today personal trainers can be found online just as easily as at your local gym. You should use the same care, if not more, when looking online for a personal trainer. Always ask questions, perform a Web search, and find out as much as you can about a trainer or author of a fitness Web page. If you find a fitness Web site you like but you cannot locate the author's name or credentials, proceed with caution.

Find out if personal trainers have a fitness-related college degree, an advanced degree, or no degree at all. What certifications, if any, do they have? Do they have references from people they have trained? Don't forget to check their fees—and read all the fine print. Finally, ask them what they expect of you and what you can expect of them; that will give each of you a certain level of accountability in moving toward your goals. Don't be afraid to switch if you don't like what you have.

If you have a college wellness center, it probably provides some level of personal training, usually from full-time staff or students in fitness-related majors. This service usually costs little, if anything, and a complete baseline evaluation and health screening are often available. If you seek a private trainer, you should expect the same; otherwise, look elsewhere.

Fine-Tuning Your Program to Maintain Success and Enjoyment

Q Is there anything in particular I should keep track of over time?

What to keep track of depends on your goals and interests. Some people don't want to feel tied to a fitness log, but others see keeping a diary of their exercise as a motivational tool. Research has found that setting goals and tracking the progress of your fitness routine are good strategies for success.

Depending on what type of exercise you do, you can track miles or minutes, days per week, heart rate, RPE, and so on. Devices such as GPS and heart-rate watches, chest straps, shoe inserts, iPods, and smartphones can track almost everything for you. They will record your mileage and speed, and the information can be downloaded onto a computer for later viewing. Some pedometers can also connect to a computer and record, track, and graph your progress.

If you track your exercise, you can really see your progress. And if you are struggling to reach your goal, the information in your log or diary might help you figure out what isn't going well and what adjustments would be most effective. If, however, you don't track your exercise, don't worry. As long as you are enjoying your exercise and feeling good, keep doing what works.

Q I get bored easily. Any suggestions?

So many new gadgets are available to make exercise fun that there is no reason to be bored. While walking, jogging, skating, or biking, you can carry an iPod or MP3 device and listen to music or podcasts of anything from talk radio to your class notes. Just be sure listening won't distract you from hazards while you're on the move. In many wellness centers, you can watch in-house satellite TV while you are on the cardio equipment. Video-game consoles are now available with fitness software, so you can play tennis or dance to get in your workout without ever leaving the house.

If you want to know exactly what your workout accomplished, get a GPS/heart-rate device, which will tell you the exact distance you have covered, your exact pace, your heart rate every 5 seconds of the workout, and even your real-time caloric expenditure. Some of these can even download the information onto your computer, where you can store it, make it into pretty graphs, and compare it over time as your fitness level and goals change.

Need some non-gadget ways to get around boredom? Juice up your workouts by adding faster or higher-intensity spurts, otherwise known as **interval training.** These changes will force you occasionally to break out of your comfort zone, more quickly increase your fitness, burn more calories, and show you how much more you might be capable of—all in the same amount of time you spent exercising yesterday. If your exercise is walking, add three or four bursts of 1–2 minutes of faster walking to your routine. Make sure you warm up sufficiently, and do easy walking for at least an equal amount of time between the faster bursts. Over time, you will be able to go faster for longer, and you will quickly start seeing bigger improvements in fitness, calorie expenditure, and the like.

Do you want still more variety? Consider **cross training,** which means doing a few different activities throughout the week. One "menu" could be walking, yoga, strength training, and salsa dance. Another might feature tennis, basketball, jogging, and strength training. You get the idea.

One of the main benefits of cross training is indeed reduced boredom. For some people, it may also decrease injury risk by varying the muscles used, which prevents overuse of a few muscles and provides the opportunity to build fitness in many different muscles. A drawback of cross training is that doing many different activities puts you at risk for a wider range of injuries. Other disadvantages are that cross training requires a lot of planning for the various activities, and that buying the appropriate clothing and equipment for all of them may be costly.

Many people find cross training enjoyable, however, and change their activities with the seasons.

Other types of activity to pursue include skill-related sports, which can provide as many benefits as the exercises just discussed. Ultimate Frisbee and racquetball, flag football and tennis—all these and more can deliver tremendous health benefits and add plenty of variety to anyone's exercise program.

interval training
Workouts that include periodic higher-intensity bouts of exercise in order to increase maximal oxygen consumption.

cross training
A pattern of training that alternates different activities (modes of exercise) that develop the same fitness component; may be done to improve performance or to avoid or rehabilitate injuries.

DOLLAR STRETCHER
Financial Wellness Tip

Do you like fitness DVDs? You don't need to buy them—instead, check them out from the library or rent them through Netflix or another service. Save money and enjoy the variation for your exercise routine.

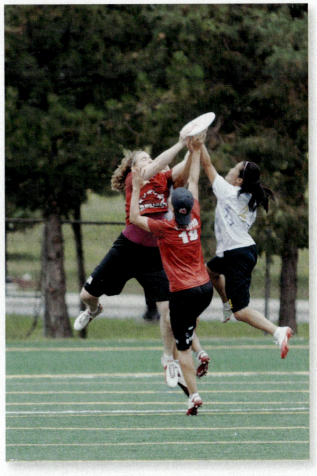

Skill-related sports can provide high-intensity, full-body workouts and can be a fun change of pace in an exercise program.

Research Brief

Cardiorespiratory Activity and Psychological Health in College Students

Suicide is the third leading cause of death among Americans ages 10–24 years, and about 1,000 college students die by suicide each year. Researchers recently explored the association between physical activity and mental health in college students. They looked at data on over 40,000 students collected from the National College Health Assessment survey and found that physical activity, especially cardiorespiratory fitness activity, was linked to a reduced risk of hopelessness, depression, and suicidal behavior among college students. Students who were not physically active were more likely to report feeling hopeless or depressed; rates of depression and thoughts about suicide decreased as the amount of time spent in aerobic activity increased. This study adds to the evidence that cardiorespiratory fitness has many positive psychological health benefits.

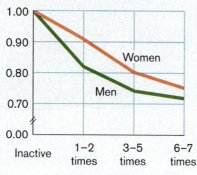

Relative risk of depression according to weekly level of aerobic activity

Analyze and Apply
- Describe a time when you felt exercise helped improved your mood.
- What is it about regular exercise that might be creating these mental health benefits?

Source: Taliaferro, L. A., Rienzo, B. A., Pigg, R. M., Jr., Miller, M. D., & Dodd, V. J. (2008). Associations between physical activity and reduced rates of hopelessness, depression, and suicidal behavior among college students. *Journal of American College Health, 57*(4), 427–435.

Sticking with Your Program—and Restarting It After a Lapse

Q | How am I supposed to stick with exercise over time? I've never had much luck.

Starting or maintaining an exercise program is no easy task for college students. Given shifting schedules and the need to balance classes with work, family, and friends, it's no wonder that many students don't have much "luck" with exercise. But careful planning and scheduling can help change your luck. Plus being active can be a real benefit to mental health, as outlined in the box "Cardiorespiratory Activity and Psychological Health in College Students."

Starting an exercise program is not too hard. Staying with it is much harder. Many things can challenge your commitment. Maybe it has been rainy for a few days, or your schoolwork is getting tougher, or you broke up with your significant other, or your child is sick. These are all real issues to deal with in terms of maintaining exercise, and sometimes it is better to skip exercise to take care of yourself or someone else. However, we've seen that chronically skipping exercise is a risk in itself, so don't make a habit of it.

Even with proper planning and goal setting, there are still likely to be bumps in the road—relapses. Having a plan to prevent relapses is important, but in truth, they are unavoidable. Therefore, being prepared to get right back to your plan is just as important as planning to prevent relapse in the first place. What will you do during finals; what if it's been raining for 40 days and 40 nights; what if you just started a new job? When you are faced with challenges, it's always better to try to do some exercise than to avoid it.

The good news is that it doesn't take long—maybe 6–12 weeks—before exercise becomes a routine. And the not-so-good news is that it takes 6–12 weeks for exercise to become routine. To get started on this new (or new again) habit, make separate lists of all the things you like and dislike about exercise, and see which list is longer. Then try to figure out how you can emphasize the items on the "like" side and deal with the items on the "dislike" side (also see the box "Tips for Exercise Motivation and Adherence").

Recall that Chapter 2 offers tips and strategies for successful behavior change. There is no one best approach, but consider using the SMART and KISS principles. Choose an activity and program plan that you think will be effective. If it turns out not to work for you, change the activity or the schedule and try again.

Q | How do I find more time to exercise?

The most common challenge that keeps people from regular exercise is the perception of too little time in the day. Those who have successfully integrated exercise often work out in the

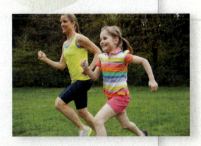

Wellness Strategies

Tips for Exercise Motivation and Adherence

 How do I get motivated to exercise—and to keep fitting exercise into my busy schedule?

1. Dedicate a regular time each day for exercise.
2. Do activities you enjoy.
3. Socialize with exercise.
4. Dance whenever you hear music.
5. Do more than one activity (spice it up).
6. Use quality clothing and equipment.
7. Set realistic short- and long-term goals.
8. Keep a diary or use a pedometer to track your progress.
9. Take walking breaks during the day.
10. Walk or bike when you can.
11. Incorporate exercise into family routines.
12. Listen to your body (don't overdo it).

early morning or just before and after work or meals. This routine is easier if you have a regular schedule but more difficult for part-time students, part-time workers, or full-time parents who don't have much "regular" in their life. One strategy to help you find the time is to keep a log of what you do throughout the day, recording in increments of 15 or 30 minutes. You may be surprised at how much time you actually have to dedicate to exercise.

For college students who face an ever-changing course schedule, these ideas may help:

- Find a time when you know you won't be working or going to class.

- Find a friend or two who can help get you out the door when you don't feel like it.
- Sign up for an exercise class in the wellness or fitness center each semester so that you have some sense of commitment to participate in exercise regularly.
- Use contracts, rewards, and goal setting (discussed in detail in Chapter 2).

If you can figure out ways to make your schedule work for you now, you will be much better off once you are out of college and face even more demands on your time. It is well documented that parents with children living at home are not likely to do much exercise—and the younger the children, the less exercise their parents get.

 I used to exercise but haven't for a while. What would you recommend for me since I'm just getting back into working out?

Restarting an exercise program can do wonders for your physical and emotional health. If your break was due to an injury or illness and has been less than 3 weeks, then start back slowly, doing about half of your previous level. Within a week or two, you should be able to progress to where you were.

If your break was longer—more than a month—then you should also start at half of where you were, but you shouldn't expect to catch up as quickly. Instead, focus on a steady progression without increasing too much or too fast. Stick with it and you will get back to where you were, or even beyond, before you know it. If your break from exercise has been a long time—more than 6 months—then resuming your workouts will be like completely starting over.

Regardless of the cause or length of any exercise breaks you experience, you should feel proud to restart your program and to take the proper steps to ensure success. With informed planning, success is well within your reach.

Fast Facts

Move to the Beat

Try listening to music during your next workout. Most research on listening to music while working out has found positive effects, including feelings of pleasant distraction and motivation to keep moving. When listening to music, people tend to work out longer and report less discomfort. A fast music tempo may be preferable for higher-intensity exercise. If your workout takes you outside, use caution when exercising in heavy-traffic areas and other locations where headphones and inattention to your surroundings could jeopardize your safety.

- What exercises that you do might be enhanced by listening to music?
- On what occasions have you exercised to music? What have been the benefits and drawbacks?

Summary

This chapter has emphasized several benefits of cardiorespiratory fitness (CRF): increased longevity, reduced risk of chronic disease, enhanced energy, and improved mental health. College provides a great opportunity to start an exercise program because you have so many resources available. If you already exercise, this is the time to cement your habits, try new activities, and find other people to exercise with you. Exercise doesn't have to be hard to do or hard to figure out. Keep it simple, and you will likely succeed: Find something you like, be active on most days, and try to mix both moderate and vigorous activities into your week. Once you have developed good exercise habits, you will find a way to keep them throughout life—and the benefits will show.

More to Explore

American College of Sports Medicine
http://www.acsm.org

American Council on Exercise: Fit Facts
http://www.acefitness.org/fitfacts

Department of Health and Human Services *2008 Physical Activity Guidelines for Americans*
http://www.health.gov/paguidelines

MedlinePlus: Exercise and Physical Fitness
http://www.nlm.nih.gov/medlineplus/exerciseandphysical
fitness.html

President's Council on Physical Fitness, Sports, and Nutrition
http://www.fitness.gov

[icon] COMPLETE IN connect

NAME	DATE	SECTION

This lab includes three field tests for assessing cardiorespiratory endurance:

1. Rockport 1-mile walk test

2. 1.5-mile run/walk test

3. 3-minute step test

These three tests provide results in terms of VO_{2max}. Choose the test that best fits your current fitness status and the equipment you have available. The 1.5-mile run/walk test is best suited for people who can jog for 15 minutes and have some experience pacing themselves. For people with lower fitness or less running experience, the walk test or the step test is probably a better choice. A partner is helpful to time you, but you can perform the tests on your own, timing yourself. The 3-minute step test is just as reliable when self-administered as it is under the supervision of trained personnel. Refer to the information about safety of exercise in Chapter 3 if you have any questions about whether CRF testing is appropriate for you.

Rockport 1-Mile Walk Test

Equipment

- A flat track or course that provides a measurement of 1 mile
- Stopwatch, clock, or watch with a second hand
- Weight scale
- Partner to time you (optional)

Preparation

Perform a general warm-up. Weigh yourself and record the result. Weight: [____] lb

Instructions

1. Walk the 1-mile course as fast as possible without breaking into a run.

Record the time it takes you to walk the mile in minutes and seconds.

Time: [____] minutes [____] seconds

2. As soon as you finish the 1-mile walk, count your pulse for 15 seconds.

15-second pulse count: [____] beats

3. Cool down after the test.

Results

1. Convert your weight in pounds to kilograms: [____] lb ÷ 2.2 = [____] kilograms

2. Convert your 1-mile walk time in minutes and seconds to a decimal value (the nearest hundredth of a minute). For example, a time of 13 minutes and 12 seconds would be $13 + (12 \div 60)$, or 13.2.

Time: [____] minutes + ([____] seconds ÷ 60) = [____]

3. Multiply your 15-second pulse count by 4 to determine your 1-minute recovery heart rate.

Recovery heart rate (RHH): 15-second pulse count [____] × 4 = [____] beats per minute (bpm)

4. Enter your values into the equation below; for sex, enter 1 if you are male and 0 if you are female.

$$VO_{2max} = 132.853 - (0.1692 \times weight \,\boxed{}\, kg) - (0.3877 \times age \,\boxed{}\, years)$$

$$+ (6.315 \times sex \,\boxed{}\,) - (3.2649 \times time \,\boxed{}\, minutes) - (0.1565 \times RHH \,\boxed{}\, bpm)$$

$$= \,\boxed{}\, ml/kg/min$$

5. Find the rating for your VO$_{2max}$ value from the table.

Rating: $\boxed{}$

MAXIMAL OXYGEN CONSUMPTION (VO$_{2MAX}$) RATINGS*

Males

AGE (YEARS)	WELL ABOVE AVERAGE	ABOVE AVERAGE	AVERAGE	BELOW AVERAGE	WELL BELOW AVERAGE
20–29	>51.1	45.8–51.1	42.3–45.7	38.1–42.2	<38.1
30–39	>47.5	44.4–47.5	41.0–44.3	36.7–40.9	<36.7
40–49	>46.8	42.4–46.8	38.4–42.3	34.6–38.3	<34.6
50–59	>43.3	38.3–43.3	35.2–38.2	31.1–35.1	<31.1
60+	>39.5	35.0–39.5	31.4–34.9	27.4–31.3	<27.4

Females

AGE (YEARS)	WELL ABOVE AVERAGE	ABOVE AVERAGE	AVERAGE	BELOW AVERAGE	WELL BELOW AVERAGE
20–29	>44.0	39.5–44.0	35.5–39.4	31.6–35.4	<31.6
30–39	>41.0	36.7–41.0	33.8–36.6	29.9–33.7	<29.9
40–49	>38.9	35.1–38.9	31.6–35.0	28.0–31.5	<28.0
50–59	>35.2	31.4–35.2	28.7–31.3	25.5–28.6	<25.5
60+	>32.3	29.1–32.3	26.6–29.0	23.7–26.5	<23.7

*In terms of percentiles, well above average = over the 80th percentile; above average = between 60th and 80th percentiles; average = between 40th and 60th percentiles; below average = between 20th and 40th percentiles; and well below average = below the 20th percentile.

Source: Cooper Institute for Aerobics Research. *Physical fitness assessment and norms.* Dallas, TX: Cooper Institute. For more information: http://www.cooperinstitute.org.

1.5-Mile Run/Walk Test

Equipment

- A flat track or course that provides a measurement of 1.5 miles
- Stopwatch, clock, or watch with a second hand
- Partner to time you (optional)

Preparation

Perform a general warm-up that includes brisk walking or slow jogging.

Instructions

Cover the 1.5-mile course as quickly as possible. Take care to pace yourself, as careful pacing can significantly affect your time; don't overexert yourself at the start. You can alternate walking with jogging or running if needed. Record the time it takes you to complete the 1.5-mile distance in minutes and seconds. Cool down after you complete the test.

Time: ☐ minutes ☐ seconds

Results

1. **Convert your 1.5-mile run/walk time in minutes and seconds to a decimal value (the nearest hundredth of a minute).** For example, a time of 11 minutes and 12 seconds would be 11 + (12 ÷ 60), or 11.2.

Time: ☐ minutes + (☐ seconds ÷ 60) = ☐

2. **Enter your time into the equation below:**

VO_{2max} = 3.5 + (483 ÷ time ☐ minutes) = ☐ ml/kg/min

3. **Find the rating for your VO_{2max} value from the table in the section on the 1-mile walk test.**

Rating: ☐

3-Minute Step Test

Equipment

- 16.25-inch step
- Stopwatch or clock with a second hand
- Metronome (these can be found at music stores; free versions are also available online)

Preparation

Warm up before taking the test. Check your equipment: Make sure the step is stable and wide enough to step up and down on comfortably and safely. Set the metronome cadence as follows:

- Women: 88 beats per minute
- Men: 96 beats per minute

Place the metronome close enough so that you can hear it throughout the test, above the sound of your stepping. Take a few practice steps. Start with both feet on the ground and then with each beat, step in this pattern: up-up-down-down. At this pace, women will complete 22 step cycles per minute and men will complete 24 step cycles per minute. You can lead with either foot and can change lead legs at any time during the test.

Practice your step technique until you are comfortable with it. During the test, you will step for 3 minutes and then stop and take your pulse for 15 seconds. As you practice your stepping technique, also practice taking your pulse; you can take your pulse at the radial artery in your wrist or the carotid artery in your neck.

Instructions

Once your equipment is set and you are comfortable with the technique, you are ready to begin. Step up and down for a total of 3 minutes. At the end of the test, remain standing and count your pulse for 15 seconds; start counting your pulse 5 seconds into the recovery period (if you keep the stopwatch running, you would count from 3:05 to 3:20). Note your 15-second pulse count. Then cool down for several minutes.

Results

1. 15-second pulse count: ⬚ **beats**

2. Convert your 15-second pulse count into a 1-minute pulse count

15-second pulse count ⬚ beats × 4 = ⬚ beats per minute (bpm)

3. Enter your 1-minute pulse count into the appropriate formula below.

Women: $VO_{2max} = 65.81 - (0.1847 \times$ ⬚ $bpm) =$ ⬚ ml/kg/min

Men: $VO_{2max} = 111.33 - (0.42 \times$ ⬚ $bpm) =$ ⬚ ml/kg/min

4. Find the rating for your VO_{2max} value from the table in the section on the 1-mile walk test.

Rating: ⬚

Reflecting on Your Results

Copy your results into the chart at the right. Are you surprised with your overall rating? Did your results match what you thought about your own cardiorespiratory fitness?

	VO₂MAX (ML/KG/MIN)	RATING
Rockport 1-mile walk test		
1.5-mile run/walk test		
3-minute step test		

Planning Your Next Steps

Cardiorespiratory fitness (CRF) is typically a function of training. If your scores were lower than you expected—or want—then it's time to change your activity routine or to start one. If you scored well, then strive to maintain your current level of fitness, or add some new or more advanced activities or training techniques to boost your results and add variety to your program. Set realistic goals for improvement and create a plan to achieve them. Then, in 6–10 weeks, repeat the same CRF tests you completed and note any improvements.

Describe your goals and the specific steps you will take to improve your cardiorespiratory fitness. If needed, refer to Lab Activity 4-2 on program planning.

What effect, if any, did your actions have on your CRF level? Was your plan effective? Why or why not?

Sources: Protocols and formulas for Rockport 1-mile walk test and 1.5-mile run/walk test: American College of Sports Medicine. (2008). *Health-related physical fitness assessment manual* (2nd ed.). Philadelphia: Lippincott Williams & Wilkins.
Formula for calculation of VO₂max for the 3-minute step test: McArdle, W. D, Katch, F. L., Pechar, G. S., Jacobson, L., & Ruck, S. (1972). Reliability and interrelationships between maximal oxygen intake, physical work capacity, and step-test scores in college women. *Medicine and Science in Sports and Exercise, 4*(4), 182–186.
Liguori, G., & Mozumdar, A. (2009). Reliability of self-assessments for a cardiovascular fitness assessment. *International Journal of Fitness, 5*(1).

▣ **COMPLETE IN** connect

NAME	DATE	SECTION

Equipment

None required; you may want to develop and track your program using a paper notebook, digital spreadsheet, smart-phone application, or online program.

Preparation: None

Instructions

1. **Set SMART goals:** Set short- and long-term goals for your cardiorespiratory fitness program. Your goals can be about training—number of minutes of cycling or steps on a pedometer—or based on the results of the fitness tests you completed in Lab Activity 4-1, or both.

Current status	Goal	Target date	Notes (rewards, special considerations)

2. **Apply the FITT principle:** Use the chart below to create a program that meets the recommended criteria for success and fitness your schedule and preferences. Use one of the sets of guidelines from the chapter to help structure your program; review Table 4-2 as needed. The basic FITT guidelines from the ACSM are as follows:

- Frequency: 3–5 days per week
- Intensity: Target heart-rate range based on 57%–94% HR_{max} or 30%–85% HRR
- Time: 20–60 minutes per day, in bouts lasting 10 or more minutes
- Type: Aerobic activities (those that are rhythmic, continuous, and involve work by large-muscle groups)

To monitor exercise intensity, you may use rating of perceived exertion (RPE) or one of the target heart-rate-range formulas; instructions for the heart-rate calculations appear after the program plan chart. Remember the relationships among frequency, intensity, and time: Higher-intensity activities can be performed for a shorter time and at a lower frequency. So, for example, three 25-minute bouts of high-intensity jogging over the course of a week would be approximately equivalent to five 30-minute bouts of brisk walking.

PROGRAM PLAN

Frequency (✓)							Intensity			Time		Type
M	T	W	TH	F	SA	SU	HEART RATE (BPM)	RPE (6–20)	TALK TEST (✓)	MODERATE INTENSITY (MIN)	VIGOROUS INTENSITY (MIN)	
✓		✓		✓				14–15		30		*Sample: Walking*
			✓			✓	148–168				15	*Sample: Jogging*

Weekly total of moderate- and vigorous-intensity activities

RECOMMENDED STARTING INTENSITY OF EXERCISE BASED ON CURRENT ACTIVITY LEVEL

ACTIVITY LEVEL	HEART-RATE MAXIMUM (HR_{MAX}) METHOD	HEART-RATE RESERVE (HRR) METHOD
Sedentary	57%–67%	30%–45%
Minimal physical activity	64%–74%	40%–55%
Sporadic physical activity	74%–84%	55%–70%
Habitual physical activity	80%–91%	65%–80%
High amounts of habitual physical activity	84%–94%	70%–85%

Source: American College of Sports Medicine. (2009). *Guidelines for exercise testing and prescription* (8th ed.). Baltimore, MD: Lippincott Williams & Wilkins.

3. **Determine Target Heart-rate Range:** Choose one of the following methods to calculate your range. Use the table to identify appropriate percentages for your level of fitness, and then use those values (in decimal form, e.g., 75% = 0.75) in the appropriate set of formulas below. You'll do the calculations twice to get a bottom and top for your target heart-rate range. You'll also calculate 10-second pulse counts by dividing the total count by 6; these 10-second pulse counts can be more easily used to monitor intensity, because you can count your pulse for 10 seconds rather than a full minute. Both methods require calculation of your maximum heart rate (MHR).

MHR = 220 − age ☐ years = ☐ bpm

Heart-Rate Maximum (HR_{max}) Method

Selected percentage range (from table): ☐

Bottom of range: MHR ☐ bpm × training % 0.☐ = ☐ bpm

Corresponding 10-second count: ☐ bpm ÷ 6 = ☐ beats

Top of range: MHR ☐ bpm × training % 0.☐ = ☐ bpm

Corresponding 10-second count: ☐ bpm ÷ 6 = ☐ beats

Full target heart-rate range: ☐ to ☐ bpm 10-second counts: ☐ to ☐ beats

Heart-Rate Reserve (HRR) Method

Selected percentage range (from table): ☐

Resting heart rate (see pp. 115–116): ☐ bpm

Heart-rate reserve (HRR) = MHR ☐ bpm − RHR ☐ bpm = ☐ bpm

Bottom of range: (HRR ☐ bpm × training % 0.☐) + RHR ☐ bpm = ☐ bpm

Corresponding 10-second count: ☐ bpm ÷ 6 = ☐ beats

Top of range: (HRR ☐ bpm × training % 0.☐) + RHR ☐ bpm = ☐ bpm

Corresponding 10-second count: ☐ bpm ÷ 6 = ☐ beats

Full target heart-rate range: ☐ to ☐ bpm   10-second counts: ☐ to ☐ beats

Results

Track your progress with a log like the one below or one you create for yourself.

WEEK: _____

Day/Date	Activity	Intensity	Time		Distance
		HEART RATE (BPM), RPE (6–20), OR TALK TEST	MODERATE INTENSITY (MIN)	VIGOROUS INTENSITY (MIN)	MILES YARDS STEPS
M Sep 30	Sample: Walking	RPE 15	30		4,835 steps
M					
T					
W					
Th					
F					
Sa					
Su					
Weekly total of moderate- and vigorous-intensity activities/Weekly total distance					

Reflecting on Your Results and Planning Your Next Steps

After several weeks of your program, consider your progress. Have you been sticking with your program plan? How have you responded to it? Has your cardiorespiratory fitness increased? How do your workouts make you feel? If you have been keeping up with your program, describe your plans going forward. If you haven't been following your plan, come up with at least three plan changes or strategies to help improve your motivation and adherence.

5

Muscle Fitness

COMING UP IN THIS CHAPTER

- Learn how your muscles work and what affects their functioning
- Discover the benefits of muscle fitness
- Assess your level of muscle fitness
- Develop a personalized muscle-fitness program

How does muscle fitness relate to your overall wellness? The physical-wellness dimension of muscle fitness is relatively obvious: Either you have the strength and endurance to perform certain tasks or you don't. Therefore, you can remain as you are, or you can train to increase your muscle fitness, and best of all is it that it doesn't have to be complicated.

Muscle fitness also affects other wellness dimensions. As you build muscle fitness, your self-esteem may rise, thereby improving your social and emotional wellness. Once you start improving selected wellness dimensions, you'll become aware of other areas in your life that you want to fine-tune, and you'll be more likely to try to make positive changes there also. In this way, developing muscle fitness can have a positive impact on your overall wellness.

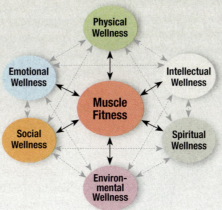

Every person, regardless of age, biological sex, or ability, can improve through physical training. Training the body to be stronger (or to jump higher or move faster) provides numerous physical and emotional benefits throughout the life span.[1] Young or old, male or female, it doesn't take much to hone your muscle fitness. And muscle fitness is essential, since muscles make your body move. Without muscles, your heart would not beat, your lungs would not inflate, and food would not pass through your digestive tract.

If you take care of your muscles, they will help you stay strong and well throughout life. This chapter provides guidance on achieving that key health and wellness goal as it explores muscle fitness, including the factors affecting it, its benefits, ways to assess it, and many of the options available to improve muscle fitness.

Factors Affecting Muscle Fitness

Q | What's muscle fitness? Is it the same as weight lifting?

As described in Chapter 3, **muscle fitness**—the ability of muscles to perform routine tasks without undue fatigue—has several components:

- **Muscle force:** The effort required to overcome resistance, such as that from a barbell or your body weight
- **Muscle endurance:** The ability to sustain an effort for a prolonged period, such as snow shoveling or leaf raking
- **Muscle strength:** The ability to generate maximal force against resistance, such as lifting something extremely heavy
- **Muscle power:** The ability to exert optimal force rapidly, such as when throwing a baseball or jumping a puddle

Although muscle fitness means more than just lifting weights, fitness can certainly be improved through weight lifting. However, gains in muscle fitness are not limited to structured weight-training programs.

Many factors can affect your muscle fitness, including age, biological sex, injuries, and training. Another key factor is your genetic makeup: Look at your parents

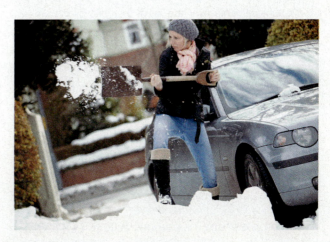

One component of muscle fitness is muscle power, which is the ability to exert force rapidly.

and siblings—what you see is usually what you get![2] This doesn't mean you don't have some control of your muscle fitness, because you do. However, if you want to be a champion powerlifter, you'll need a set of genes that puts you on that path. If, on the other hand, you simply want to improve your overall health, you don't need any special genes: You need just a few minutes a week to practice muscle-fitness exercises. The improvement will be quickly noticeable.

muscle fitness The ability of one or more muscles to perform routine tasks without undue fatigue.

Behavior-Change Challenge
Building Muscle Mass

Imagine that, as an incoming freshman, you meet your new roommate, Chuck, and his tree-trunk biceps make an instant impression. It's no surprise to learn that he was a star performer in his high school's win in the state wrestling championships last year and that his passion is working out. You, in turn, spend your free time in front of your computer, designing video game graphics—and muscle fitness has been the last thing on your mind. But you quickly decide that this has to change. You want to look more like Chuck and less like the stereotypical computer guy.

Meet Rhett

Rhett is an off-campus college student attending Georgia Southern University. Rhett considers himself scrawny and wants to start working out with weights in order to gain strength and muscle mass. View the video to learn more about Rhett, his behavior-change goals and plan, and 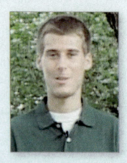 his achievements over the initial 9 weeks of his program. As you watch, consider:

- How realistic are Rhett's goals and his starting program plan? If you were to embark on a program to build your muscle fitness, how would your own goals and fitness plan differ from Rhett's?
- What types of motivation and environmental support does Rhett have? What motivation and support do you think you would need in order to succeed in your behavior-change goal?
- What can you learn from Rhett's experience that will help you in your behavior-change efforts?

VIDEO CASE STUDY WATCH THIS VIDEO IN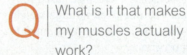

Types of Muscles

Q Is it true that there are different kinds of muscles?

Yes, it is true, and we all have some of each kind. There are three specific muscle types:

- **Skeletal muscle,** which is found throughout the body, covering and attached to the skeleton. Skeletal muscles move your bones to produce body motions.
- **Cardiac muscle,** which is found only in the heart and has its own electrical conduction system to keep your heart beating at a speed to match your body's need for oxygen.

- **Smooth muscle,** which is found in the walls of body organs like the stomach and the intestines. It typically acts to make an organ expand or contract.

Cardiac and smooth muscle are *involuntary muscles,* meaning that they contract without any conscious effort on your part. This is a good thing; otherwise, essential activities like respiration, circulation, and digestion would require conscious effort. The action of smooth muscles is controlled by the autonomic nervous system and body chemicals such as hormones, both of which function outside conscious control.

Skeletal muscles, in contrast, are *voluntary muscles,* meaning that they are mostly under your control. Skeletal muscle can be activated with conscious thought, allowing you to decide how, when, and where your body will move. Because they appear to have stripes or lines—striations—when viewed under a microscope, skeletal muscles are referred to as striated muscles.

Although both cardiac and skeletal muscle can be shaped and strengthened over time, most people are interested in training skeletal muscle, because they can see and feel when these muscles change. But they should not overlook the importance of strengthening cardiac muscle. Chapters 4 and 11 discuss the many risks of not conditioning your heart.

There are over 500 skeletal muscles in the body, or 35–45 percent of the body's weight. A typical skeletal muscle stretches from one bone to another, usually crossing a joint. Skeletal muscle attaches to bone via bands of fibrous connective tissue known as **tendons.** (Another type of connective tissue, **ligaments,** connects bone to bone.)

Q What is it that makes my muscles actually work?

Skeletal muscle is made up of many tiny **muscle fibers** (**muscle cells**), which

muscle force The speed with which a muscle can move a given object one time. The force of a muscle depends on its size, length, speed, and the joint angle. A muscle develops greater force when it is elongated, and less force when it is shortened.

muscle endurance The ability to sustain an effort for an extended time. This is often measured by determining the maximum number of repetitions of a given resistance.

muscle strength The ability of one or more muscles to exert force by contracting against resistance. This is often measured by determining the most weight lifted during one effort.

muscle power The ability of a muscle to move an object quickly and repeatedly.

skeletal muscle Muscle tissue that is connected to bones and moves them in order to produce body movement.

cardiac muscle A specialized muscle tissue found only in the heart. It has its own electrical conduction system and keeps the heart beating in response to the body's need for oxygen. Cardiac muscle is much less resistant to fatigue than other muscle types.

smooth muscle Muscle tissue in the walls of body organs such as the stomach and intestines. It controls involuntary movement and makes the organs expand and contract.

tendon The fibrous connective tissue by which a muscle attaches to a bone.

ligament A sheet or band of tough, fibrous tissue connecting bones or cartilage at a joint or supporting an organ.

are elongated and typically run the length of the muscle (Figure 5-1). The fibers stay together thanks to special connective tissue that also houses blood vessels and nerves. Each muscle fiber contains these parts:

- **Myofibrils:** Protein filaments making up muscle cells, including thin filaments known as actin and thick filaments known as *myosin*.

- **Nucleus** (plural, nuclei): A structure inside a cell that contains the cell's genetic material; muscle cells have multiple nuclei, which enhance their ability to synthesize proteins and to grow.

- **Mitochondria:** Intracellular structures containing enzymes that convert the energy in food into fuel for the muscle.

- **Sarcoplasmic reticulum:** A lacy membrane surrounding myofibrils that plays an important role in triggering muscle contraction.

For a skeletal muscle to move or contract, the contractile protein filaments actin and myosin need to slide over each other. This process is explained by the **sliding filament theory** (Figure 5-2). As we saw in Chapter 4, in order for a muscle to move, adenosine triphosphate (ATP) needs

muscle fiber (muscle cell) Each skeletal muscle consists of hundreds or thousands of tiny fibers bundled together and wrapped in a connective-tissue covering. Muscle fibers coordinate muscle contractions for movement.

myofibrils Microscopic protein filaments that make up muscle cells.

nucleus A structure in a cell that contains most of the cell's genetic material, which controls gene expression.

mitochondria Structures within cells in which most of the chemical reactions in cellular (oxidative) respiration occur; the location for most adenosine triphosphate (ATP) production.

to be present, the majority of which is produced within the mitochondria. Recall that the aerobic energy system is most important for cardiorespiratory endurance exercise, yet it can also be important for some muscular endurance activities. However, energy needed for muscle fitness doesn't usually require oxygen and can be derived from ATP-CP energy system and the glycolytic energy system (see Chapter 4).

Q | What makes my arms feel "pumped" when I'm lifting?

Your arms feel "pumped" when you lift because of the increase in blood flow to your arm muscles. As you exercise, there is a dramatic shift or redistribution of blood to the active muscles, in this case your arms, while other, noncritical areas, such as the gut, see much less blood flow. This is one reason to be cautious about eating right before exercising, because your stomach can't digest food effectively while you are working out. The result is often an uncomfortable cramping or an unpleasant feeling of food sloshing around.

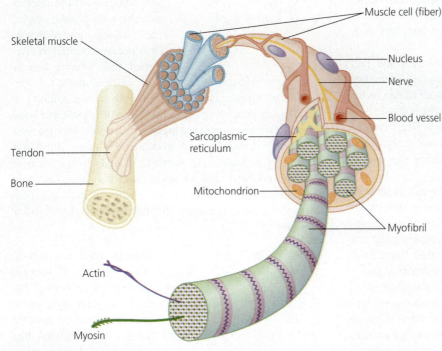

Skeletal muscle
Muscle cell (fiber)
Nucleus
Nerve
Blood vessel
Tendon
Bone
Sarcoplasmic reticulum
Mitochondrion
Myofibril
Actin
Myosin

WATCH IN CONNECT   Figure 5-1 Basic components of skeletal muscle tissue.

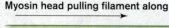

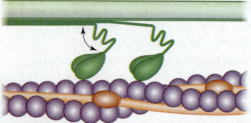

Figure 5-2 Sliding filament theory. The sliding filament theory explains that in order for a skeletal muscle to move or contract, the contractile protein filaments actin and myosin need to slide over each other. The figure shows the myosin head bending as it pulls the actin filament.

Types of Muscle Fibers

Skeletal, cardiac, and smooth muscles are the three main types of muscle. Skeletal muscle—the type that moves our bones, makes us look good, and keeps us strong—is made up of two general fiber types: **slow-twitch muscle fibers (type I)** and **fast-twitch muscle fibers (types IIa and IIx).** The slow-twitch fibers perform well in endurance events, while the fast-twitch fibers are best suited for power and sprinting.

Q How can I get more "fast" muscles?

Because the percentage of each type of muscle fiber is largely determined at birth, changing your fiber type is impossible. However, proper training can enhance what you have, though maybe not to the point that you will become an elite sprinter if you have predominantly slow-twitch fibers. Fast-twitch and slow-twitch fibers differ in level of endurance and potential for **hypertrophy,** or increase in muscle-fiber size, yet each muscle contains a mix of fiber types.

A typical person has about half fast-twitch and half slow-twitch fibers. However, there is tremendous individual variation, with elite athletes having a lot more of one or the other fiber type depending on the event in which they excel.[3]

sarcoplasmic reticulum In muscle cells, a network of vesicles and tubules that store calcium, which is released as one step in the muscle-contraction process.

sliding filament theory An explanation of how muscles shorten, or produce force. According to the SFT, thick and thin filaments within muscle cells slide past one another to shorten the muscle. This process requires the presence of ATP.

Most of us have muscle fibers that are well suited for our basic daily needs, which include improving our overall wellness.

Your fast-twitch fibers can generate force quickly, whereas your slow-twitch fibers sacrifice rapid force production for fatigue resistance, meaning that you can run farther rather than faster. Fast-twitch fibers are much better at generating short bursts of strength or speed by using anaerobic metabolism to create fuel (see Chapter 4 for more on aerobic and anaerobic energy production). Fast-twitch fibers can generate lots of force in a little time, although

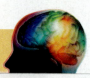

this force production lasts for only a few seconds. Fast-twitch fibers are also more prone to hypertrophy, meaning that they can grow larger more easily than slow-twitch fibers can.

Slow-twitch fibers contain more mitochondria and myoglobin than fast-twitch fibers do. This composition makes them more efficient at using oxygen, generating ATP, and maintaining muscle contractions for an extended time and thus allows for prolonged activity. Typically, postural muscles tend to be slow-twitch, and this characteristic enables us to stay erect for long periods.

So yes, muscle-fiber type plays a role in determining who reaches the dining hall first. Yet although you may not be blessed with as many fast-twitch fibers as someone else, consistent training can increase your speed and eventually get you there first.

Biological Sex

Q As a woman, do I really need to lift?

Yes, especially if you want to maintain your health, weight, and lifelong independence. Evidence has consistently confirmed that women benefit from muscle-fitness training just as much as men do. A particular benefit of muscle-fitness training is the possibility of delaying or preventing age-related loss of muscle and bone mass, to which women are highly susceptible. Women who allow their muscle strength to decrease with age often lose the ability to handle the activities of daily living (such as bathing, cooking, and shopping) and may therefore lose their independence. Women who maintain muscle fitness throughout their life span are much less likely to suffer this fate.

Q Can I get strong but not look like a guy? What can I do to get toned instead of becoming too muscular?

Women often fear getting "too big" from strength training. This is perhaps the most common myth about muscle fitness, because it is very unlikely that women will develop male-size muscles. The primary barrier women face in increasing

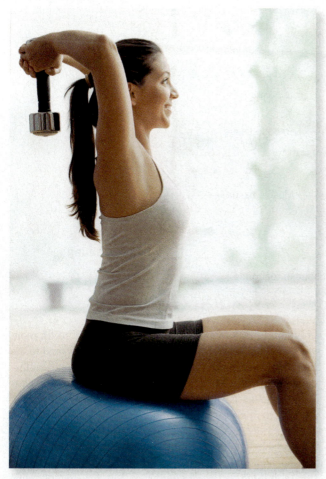

Women can increase strength and muscle size in response to training, but due to fiber-type and hormonal differences, their muscles do not become as large as men's muscles do.

their muscle mass through hypertrophy is hormone related. **Testosterone,** a hormone that helps to increase muscle-fiber size, is present to a much lesser degree in women than men. In fact, women have as much as 7–8 times less testosterone than men—a distinct disadvantage in terms of building large muscles.[4]

Another component of developing big muscles is hard work, or what is often called the *overload principle.* Basic muscle-fitness training is beneficial but not necessarily sufficient to produce hypertrophy. To increase muscle mass, training for men and women alike should consist of a moderate-to-heavy load (6–10 reps) and a relatively high volume (3–4 sets) with short rest periods (60–90 seconds), which is quite an intense level of muscle-fitness training.[5] Importantly, although the typical 3 sets of 10 reps may produce initial strength gains and will keep muscles fit, it is not likely to increase muscle mass unless the intensity is continuously boosted. Ultimately, however, given the muscle-fiber and hormonal differences between men and women, women's muscles will not get big as men's. The fitness benefits nonetheless are just as good.[6]

Q I heard that weight lifting will make me gain weight. Is that true?

It is possible but not likely. Muscle tissue is denser than fat tissue, meaning that the same amount of muscle tissue weighs more than fat tissue.[7] But on the flip side, this means that a pound of muscle tissue is smaller than a pound of fat tissue. The typical changes that occur when starting a muscle-training program include:

1. Loss of body fat due to increased exercise
2. Increased muscle mass (after a few weeks)
3. Loss of inches in some areas

The loss of body fat and the increase in muscle mass may cause a small change in body weight, or they may offset each other. However, if you lose a pound of fat and gain a pound of muscle, there will be a loss of inches because muscle's greater density takes up less space (Figure 5-3). The loss of inches, which is the most important change for many people, may not show up on a scale, but you are likely to notice a better fit in your clothes, and possibly a smaller clothes size, along with stronger muscles. A well-rounded exercise program (cardiovascular and muscle training) is most likely to result in a net *loss* of body weight. It is relatively uncommon, however, to accumulate enough muscle to offset the loss of fat unless a person is involved in fairly intense muscle-fitness training.

Age and Use

Q At what age do I start losing my strength?

Muscle mass and strength both decrease with age in men as well as women, starting around age 25 or 30.[8] This effect is largely due to the combination of decreased levels of circulating testosterone and other hormones and decreased physical activity.

Regular strength training, however, is highly effective for maintaining muscle fitness throughout the life span. Between the ages of 20 and 60, active and well-trained people can maintain most of their muscle fitness, reaching a peak around the age of 30. In untrained or sedentary people, muscle fitness begins to decline slowly and steadily at age 25 or 30, and by age 40 it is already less than it was at age 20. The typical untrained male loses about 30 percent of his peak strength by the age of 60, whereas a trained male does not lose any noticeable strength by that

slow-twitch muscle fibers (type I) Muscle fibers that have a slow rate of force generation. Slow-twitch fibers are highly dependent on oxygen and can sustain a given effort indefinitely.

fast-twitch muscle fibers (types IIa and IIx) Muscle fibers that have a fast rate of force production. Fast-twitch fibers can produce force with little, if any, oxygen, but cannot sustain an effort for very long.

hypertrophy An increase in the size of muscle fibers, typically accomplished through resistance training.

testosterone Derived from cholesterol, this anabolic steroid hormone is the principal male sex hormone and is critical for increasing muscle mass. The average male produces about 20 times more testosterone than a female, thereby allowing men to produce greater muscle mass than women.

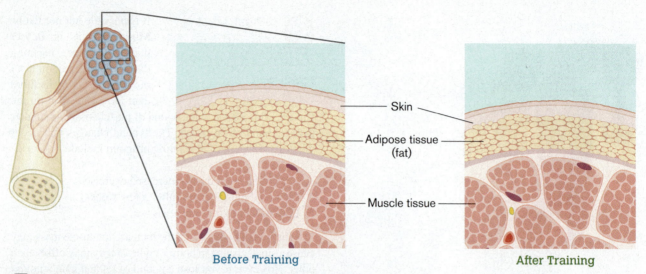

Skin

Adipose tissue (fat)

Muscle tissue

Before Training

After Training

▶ **WATCH IN CONNECT**   Figure 5-3 Changes in muscle and fat tissue in response to training. The number of muscle fibers and fat cells does not change, but muscle fibers (especially fast-twitch fibers) increase in size and fat cells decrease in size.

age. Over age 60, the noticeable reduction in testosterone and growth hormone causes a more rapid decline in muscle strength—all the more reason to continue with muscle-fitness training as you age.[9]

Q | Doesn't muscle turn to fat if you quit working out?   Muscle can be negatively affected if you are overly sedentary and as you age, but you can prevent most of the changes by staying regularly active. Muscle-fiber types (slow-twitch and fast-twitch) cannot convert from one to another, nor can muscle change into fat or vice versa, contrary to popular belief. What does occur with prolonged sedentary behavior and aging is selective atrophy of the fast-twitch muscle fibers, meaning less type II fiber surface area. However, the fast-twitch fibers do not become slow-twitch fibers.[10]

An additional age-related phenomenon is **sarcopenia,** the loss of muscle mass, strength, and function. Because there is a clear relationship between muscle mass and strength, as mass decreases, so does strength. Sarcopenia begins in the fourth decade of life and typically accelerates after the age of 75. With aging and inactivity, most atrophy occurs in fast-twitch muscle fibers. Don't be discouraged, because this atrophy can be largely offset by maintaining a muscle-fitness training program. Without training, however, aging will bring an increase of fat tissue and a decrease of muscle tissue.

Q | How long until I start getting big? How long do I stay big if I have to stop my training for some reason?   Most research shows that muscle size begins to increase after 6–8 weeks of regular training, assuming that the overload principle is being used regularly. However, an increase in *strength* is noticeable almost from the beginning of a muscle-training

program. In fact, it is not unusual for a beginner to lift more weight on the second and third training day compared to the first day. The typical reason, though, is improved neuromuscular functioning, not increased muscle size.[11] The neurological change is similar to what a child experiences when learning to ride a bike. The child's leg muscles don't become stronger right away, but the muscles and nerves get more comfortable with the movement pattern, thereby making riding much easier. This same phenomenon applies to muscle-fitness training and is largely responsible for strength gains over the first 6–8 weeks of training.

At that point, if the training has included sufficient overload, then muscle-fiber size, or mass, begins to build. This increase in muscle-fiber mass, or muscle hypertrophy, is due to muscle fibers' increasing in size rather than in number; the latter process is called *hyperplasia.* The number of human muscle fibers is largely determined at birth. Although increases in the number of muscle fibers have been noted in animals, it is yet to be determined if the same is true in humans.[12]

If muscle-fitness training ceases after hypertrophy starts, then **atrophy,** or a decrease in muscle-fiber size, begins within 4–6 weeks. It is not the case that the muscle turns to fat, as popular myth would have us believe; rather, the size of muscle fibers decreases due to sedentary behavior. At the same time, subcutaneous fat—fat just under the skin—may increase, so the individual looks and feels fatter and less muscled.

Genetics

Q | Is strength mostly genetic?

Genetics plays a clear role in overall fitness, but its influence on muscle fitness is difficult to study. Twin

sarcopenia An age-related loss of muscle fiber, muscle strength, and muscle mass.

atrophy A decrease in the size of muscle fibers, typically as a result of chronic disuse.

Muscles Lost in Space

Astronauts face many challenges during long space flights, one of which is maintaining muscle strength. Although astronauts perform plenty of physical tasks during the typical space flight, their muscles can suffer greatly due to the lack of gravity and its associated resistance. A zero-gravity environment causes a rapid decrease in muscle-fiber size, which can quickly reduce peak muscle power by as much as 50 percent. Spaceships and space stations are outfitted with treadmills and stationary bikes to help astronauts offset the lack of gravity. Although totally counteracting weightlessness effects is impossible, astronauts who regularly exercise in space show only a 13 percent decrease in muscle power compared to a 51 percent decrease for astronauts who do only a little exercise. Consider:

- How does the astronauts' experience apply to your own muscle fitness?
- If you ever have had a casted arm or leg, what was your limb like once the cast was removed? Do you imagine that the effects of wearing a cast are similar to or different from the astronauts' experience with weightlessness?

studies and family studies are the best ways to identify the contribution of genes *(heritability)* in determining muscular strength, power, and endurance. The current evidence seems to indicate that the inherited genetic influence (heritability) of muscle differs between the sexes and also varies for strength, endurance, and power. Furthermore, the role of genes in determining absolute muscle strength appears to be greater for men than for women.

The overall heritability for hand-grip *strength* is estimated to be about 50 percent. This means that your hand-grip strength is half due to your genetic makeup and half due to your day-to-day efforts to get stronger.[13] The genetic contribution to *power,* however, tends to be a bit more than 50 percent due to the influence of muscle-fiber types: Fast-twitch fibers can generate more power by means of faster contraction rates. The heritability of muscle *endurance* seems to be lowest of all. Therefore, your genes are responsible for no more than about 50 percent of any of your muscle functions (strength, power, or endurance), so if

you want to get bigger, faster, or stronger, you will need to train appropriately.

An aspect of muscle fitness that does have a strong genetic influence is muscle hypertrophy, which, as we have seen, is the ability of a muscle to increase in size.[14] Type II (fast-twitch) muscle fibers are much more likely to experience hypertrophy than type I (slow-twitch) fibers, though as previously stated, fiber type is largely determined at birth. Type II fibers can get bigger with regular muscle training—through formal strength training, heavy physical labor, or recreational activities. Cardiac muscle can also increase in size, and although less specific, this typically occurs in response to regular aerobic exercise.

Benefits of Muscle Fitness

If you keep your muscles strong throughout life, you can expect numerous benefits. These include improved control of body weight, better-fitting clothes, a greater ability to perform work and leisure tasks, a decreased risk of age-related diseases, and better psychological and emotional wellness.

Body-Weight Control

Q Will weight lifting increase my metabolism?

We seem to hear this advice all the time: Lift weights and your *metabolism*—the rate at which you burn calories—will increase. But the scientific literature is mixed on the connection between weight lifting and increased metabolism.[15] What seems clearer is that metabolic rate is closely related to the amount of fat-free mass, which can be increased through muscle-fitness training. Although muscle-fitness exercise does boost your metabolism during your workout, as well as for a limited time afterward, the overall effect may not be substantial. However, muscle is metabolically active, so your metabolism may be affected when your muscle cells grow in size. In other words, as the absolute amount of muscle in your body increases, so does your resting metabolism, and you therefore burn more calories throughout the day, week, month, and year. Generally speaking, for every pound of muscle you gain, you burn 35–50 more calories each day. Although it's not necessarily easy to build muscle mass, doing so can add up over time, all the way to the loss of about 4 pounds of body weight per year—from adding just 1 pound of muscle.

Q Which burns more calories—running or lifting weights?

Both types of exercise burn calories, and the number of calories burned is largely dependent on the intensity of the effort. Running is a continuous activity, and muscle-fitness training tends to be discontinuous (you often stop to rest between sets); therefore, running has the potential to burn more calories. However, the frequent rests in muscle-fitness training do allow for a consistently higher intensity of activity than during a run. The overall difference is not too significant given similar intensities and time. For optimal all-around physical wellness and weight management, it's best to engage in *both* types of exercise. If your time for exercise is limited, it is possible to do both types of training together, alternating a few minutes of running with a few minutes of muscle-fitness exercises.

Improved Performance

Q | What can I do to improve my sports performance?

You can train, train, and keep on training. Muscle-fitness training plays an important role in improving performance in most sports. Skiers ski better, golfers drive the ball farther, and cyclists ride faster for a longer time. Whatever sport you play, muscle training can improve overall performance by boosting speed and intensity and making you more efficient—and the results are most dramatic for beginners. Muscle training can also reduce your risk of injury.

Budding athletes often ask, "How much strength is enough?" However, optimal performance depends more on improving individual sports skills (for example, a swimming stroke or tennis swing) than on simply getting stronger, so strength without skill tends to produce less than optimal results. For most recreational athletes, training at a moderate intensity of 6–10 repetitions should suffice to achieve personal goals.

Reduced Risk of Injury and Disease

Although it may be asking a lot for any type of exercise to reduce the occurrence of injury and disease, strength training can do both. Muscle fitness can help prevent overuse injuries, improve mobility and balance, and help prevent and manage chronic diseases like diabetes, osteoporosis, and heart disease.

Q | What can I do to keep from spraining my ankle all the time?

Many factors can be involved in ankle sprains, including playing surfaces, footwear, and skill level, so there is no guarantee that you can avoid them entirely. However, muscle-fitness training can go a long way toward reducing the risk of experiencing minor aches and pains and also toward preventing common injury. Tendinitis, a common injury of overuse, can be avoided or treated with a moderate level of muscle-fitness training; balance can be improved with increased muscle strength (and improved balance reduces the risk of falls in older persons); and muscle strains, particularly in the case of the weekend athlete, can be minimized with more regular exercise, including muscle-fitness training.

Q | I thought walking and jogging were enough to prevent diseases. Do I really need to strength-train?

Muscle-fitness training is not often the first kind of exercise that comes to mind when people think about disease prevention. However, plenty of evidence supports strength training, or increased muscle fitness, as being quite beneficial for reducing the risk of certain chronic diseases.[16] Osteoporosis, back pain, arthritis, heart disease, and diabetes can all be positively affected by regular muscle-fitness training (see the box "Strength Training and Diabetes"). Muscle training obviously builds stronger bones and muscles, but did you know it also strengthens connective tissues and increases the stability of joints?

Back pain and osteoarthritis are two major health problems facing U.S. adults. Back pain is usually a result of muscle weakness, poor posture, and repetitive motions such as bending and twisting (see Chapter 6). As muscle weakens, it leads to poor posture, and poor posture can in turn cause further muscle weakness. Strength training can prevent or reverse this cycle and improve your back's health. Regular muscle training is effective 80 percent of the time in eliminating or reducing symptoms of back pain. Neck pain may also benefit from strength training, as noted in the box "Strength Training for Chronic Neck Pain."

You might be thinking, "So what—my back doesn't hurt." But at some point in their life, 80 percent of all adults miss time from work due to low-back pain, so don't wait until it is too late. Get those muscles fit now!

Osteoporosis is another condition that noticeably improves with strength training. **Osteoporosis** is characterized by the loss of bone density, which then weakens bones; it can result in hip, wrist, and ankle fractures, especially from falls. Osteoporosis can occur through the effects of aging, inactivity, and poor diet. Well over half of all women will develop this condition, but today more men are developing it as well. Strength training is one of the cornerstones for preventing osteoporosis and minimizing its debilitating effects; it helps build and maintain bone density, as well as improving balance and reducing falls.

Cardiovascular disease (CVD) and diabetes are debilitating and deadly diseases that affect many Americans, yet regular strength training can help prevent or improve both of these conditions. Strength training can lower LDL ("bad") cholesterol, raise HDL ("good") cholesterol, and decrease resting blood pressure. Strength training may also improve the body's ability to process sugar, which reduces the risk of diabetes. If improving muscle fitness can lessen the risk of CVD and diabetes, then that is a true health benefit!

osteoporosis A progressive decrease in bone mineral density that leads to an increased risk of fracture. It is more common in women than in men, especially after menopause.

Improved Emotional and Psychological Wellness

Although cardiovascular fitness and muscle-fitness training have long been accepted as a means of reducing negative

Research Brief

Strength Training and Diabetes

Aerobic-based exercise can dramatically improve diabetes, an ever more common chronic condition. Does the same effect hold true for strength training? Recently researchers compared the effects of resistance (strength-training) and treadmill (aerobic) exercises on blood sugar levels in adults with type 2 diabetes.

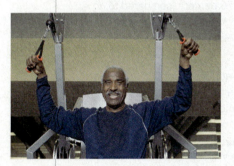

Twenty inactive, older subjects with type 2 diabetes were assigned to either a resistance or a treadmill exercise group. Each group exercised 3 times per week for 10 weeks and had their diets controlled so that both groups were eating the same amount through the study duration. Various baseline measures were taken on each participant, including diabetes markers of HbA1c and blood glucose levels, along with heart rate and blood pressure.

Both exercise groups showed a reduction in blood glucose and HbA1c values at the end of the 10 weeks compared to the beginning. However, the improvement was greater in the resistance-training group. The resistance group also showed significant differences in the daily pre-exercise plasma glucose readings between the beginning and the end of the exercise protocol. Neither group showed changes in resting blood pressure or heart rate during the course of the 10- week intervention. The researchers concluded that not only is resistance-training exercise (muscle-fitness training) effective at managing type 2 diabetes, but it is at least as effective as aerobic-based exercise, if not better.

Analyze and Apply

- Why was it important to have the study participants exercise the same number of times per week and to follow a controlled diet?
- What are some types of resistance training that a person with type 2 diabetes might implement to help manage the disorder?

Source: Bweir, S., Al-Jarrah, M., Almalty, A.-M., Maayah, M., Smirnova, I. V., Novikova, L., & Stehno-Bittle, L. (2009). Resistance exercise training lowers HbA1c more than aerobic training in adults with type 2 diabetes. *Diabetology & Metabolic Syndrome 1*(27). DOI: 10.1186/1758-5996-1-27.

emotions, recent evidence indicates that they can also enhance positive psychological states, particularly increased feelings of energy.[17] Individuals engaged in muscle training or other forms of regular exercise tend to display more positive than negative emotions, more favorable thoughts, more energy and vigor, and less anxiety and depression, all leading to greater levels of overall emotional wellness.

Q | Why does weight lifting always makes me feel better?

Scientists do not entirely understand the underlying cause for the mood-enhancing effect of exercise, but here are some possible explanations:

- Distraction—the exercise allows for a time-out from stress and negative emotions
- Release of endorphins, which are hormones linked to pain relief and elevation of mood
- Increased core temperature, which reduces muscle tension and results in a more relaxed psychological state
- Changes in brain chemistry—specifically, alterations in the levels or actions of the neurotransmitters epinephrine, norepinephrine, and dopamine

These changes are typically short term, occurring mostly after a single session of exercise. However, longer-term psychological benefits can also result from muscle-fitness training. Research supports the idea that as little as 10 weeks of muscle-fitness training can reduce clinical depression symptoms more effectively than counseling,[18] and women actively working to improve their muscle fitness commonly report feeling more confident and capable (increased self-esteem and self-efficacy), important factors in fighting depression.

Table 5-1 summarizes several specific changes and benefits related to muscle-fitness training.

TABLE 5-1 CHANGES AND BENEFITS IN RESPONSE TO MUSCLE-FITNESS TRAINING

CHANGES AND BENEFITS	MALE	FEMALE
Improved balance, stability, posture	Yes	Yes
Increased muscle endurance	Yes	Yes
Increased muscle speed, power, strength	Yes	Yes
Reduced disease risk	Yes	Yes
Weight loss or maintenance	Yes	Yes
Muscle gain	Yes	Yes

Research Brief

Strength Training for Chronic Neck Pain

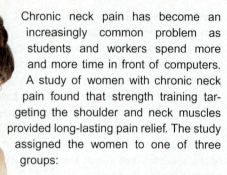

Chronic neck pain has become an increasingly common problem as students and workers spend more and more time in front of computers. A study of women with chronic neck pain found that strength training targeting the shoulder and neck muscles provided long-lasting pain relief. The study assigned the women to one of three groups:

- A group who engaged in supervised, high-intensity strength training of the neck and shoulder muscles
- A group who engaged in general fitness training

- A control group who received general health counseling

After 10 weeks, neck pain in the strength-training group decreased by over 70 percent, compared to no significant change in the neck pain for the general fitness-training and health-counseling groups.

Analyze and Apply

- What do these findings suggest about the effectiveness of strength training of the neck and shoulder in the treatment of neck and shoulder pain?
- What are you doing to minimize neck pain?

Source: Andersen, L. L., and others. (2008). Effect of two contrasting types of physical exercise on chronic neck muscle pain. *Arthritis Care and Research, 59*(1): 84–91.

Assessing Your Muscle Fitness

Q | How strong do I need to be— and how do I know how strong I am right now?

You need to be strong enough to complete your daily goals and to minimize your risk of injury and disease. As with any fitness component, you will need some type of assessment to gauge how strong you are. Measuring your current strength will help you to design an effective and appropriate training program and to check your progress periodically. First, however, you need to determine which component of muscle fitness you want to assess—strength or endurance.

Muscle strength is typically assessed by measuring or estimating the maximum amount of weight you can lift one time, which is referred to as a **1-repetition maximum (1-RM).** The bench press is the most common upper-body assessment, while the leg press, squat, deadlift, and power clean can also be used, depending on your level of expertise and available equipment. Alternatively, if the 1-RM is not feasible, you can instead perform a variety of other tests to estimate your 1-RM (see Lab Activity 5-1). Muscle endurance, on the other hand, can be measured by performing as many repetitions as possible of a given exercise, such as push-ups or curl-ups, or by doing a timed test, such as a count of how many push-ups or curl-ups you can do in 1 minute. Norms are available to compare your level of muscular fitness to that of others of your age and sex (see the tables in Lab Activities 5-1 and 5-2). If your score ranks you at the 50th percentile, that means half the people in your category can do more and half can do less than you. If you are in the 80th percentile, then 20 percent can do more than you and 80 percent can do less.

You can also use these tests to measure your progress through periodic reassessment. Assessment can play a big role in helping you achieve your muscle-fitness goals, which should be personal and realistic (see the box "Motivation for Achieving Goals").

If you've been sedentary for a long time or haven't done any muscle-fitness training in a while, don't perform an assessment on your first day of training. Instead, take a few

1-repetition maximum (1-RM) The maximum amount of weight lifted one time.

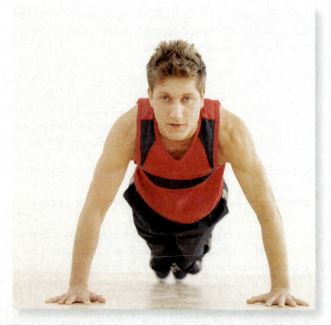

You can assess your muscular endurance by counting the number of times you can complete an exercise like a push-up with good form or the number you can do during a set period of time.

Wellness Strategies

Motivation for Achieving Goals

Q | How can I motivate myself to stay fit and healthy?

Once you have set your goals, you need to use successful techniques to make them happen. There are numerous behavior-change strategies for keeping yourself motivated to reach your goals. For fitness-related goals, try these:

- *Find an exercise partner:* Partners are great motivators and lots of fun. The best partners have similar daily schedules and goals. If your partner(s) like different types of exercise, try switching your workouts around, as variety will prevent boredom and expose you to new things.
- *Draw up a behavioral contract:* Make a contract with yourself (see Chapter 2) or have your exercise partner create one for you. Print the contract on colored paper, place it in a prominent place, and look at it frequently. Make rules you can live with ("I will do my muscle-fitness training at least twice each week"), and avoid unrealistic rules ("I will never miss another weight-training

session"). Make your short-term goal the primary focus of the contract, but also include your long-term goals. Update the contract each time you meet a goal by using a different color paper, displaying it in a different place, and letting those around you know that you have achieved a goal and you are moving on to the next one.

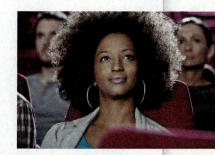

- *Give yourself a reward:* Rewards can be part of your contract or they can be stand-alone motivators. Reward yourself with new clothes, a movie, or some pampering (like a massage or a manicure)—a treat you might not otherwise indulge in. Be sure your rewards, like your goals, are realistic and achievable. Don't overspend or do something that gets you off track with your fitness goals. Save the really big reward for when you achieve your ultimate fitness goal.

days or weeks to get your muscles used to training and to familiarize yourself with the equipment. Most college-age students in good physical health should have no problem with these assessments. If, however, you have special health concerns or a family history of chronic disease (such as high blood pressure or diabetes), it is wise to check first with your physician before engaging in muscle-fitness training or assessment. See Chapter 3 for more on exercise safety.

Putting Together a Muscle-Fitness Program

Now that you are ready to improve your muscle fitness, the next step is deciding which exercises to use. Luckily, college students often have many options for types of exercises, equipment, and facilities. You can develop a muscle-fitness program that fits your individual goals, schedule, and preferences—a key to sustaining your regimen and keeping muscles strong for life.

Choosing Appropriate Equipment and Facilities

Questions abound as to what type of exercise equipment is best. The key point is that gains in muscle fitness require

overload, meaning that you have to continuously increase the resistance your muscles are working against. With the overload principle in mind, you can use your creativity—safely, of course—to come up with a variety of ways to establish resistance for your muscles. A quick Web search or a scan through a fitness magazine or therapy catalog will reveal free weights, weight machines, elastic bands, rubber balls, bars, bows, ropes, straps, and other equipment—all designed to provide muscle resistance. Which you choose depends on factors such as access, cost, physical environment, and personal preference.

Q | Aren't free weights a lot better than machines?

Although there is always debate about whether free weights or machines are better for novice weight trainers, the choice comes down to access, personal preference, and, most importantly, which you will use regularly. Free weights and machines are the most common types of training tools for increasing muscle fitness, but you probably couldn't tell the difference between someone who uses free weights and someone who uses machines. As long as you follow the overload principle, gains in muscle strength and endurance will follow, regardless of the equipment you use.

Free weights are objects or devices that can be moved freely in any direction. Common types of free weights are

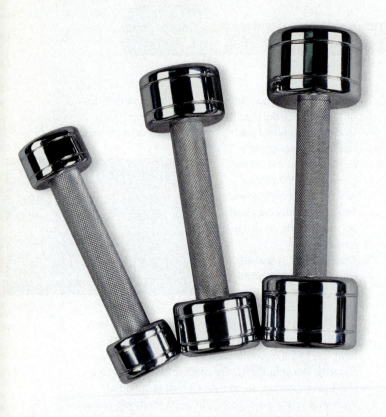

dumbbells, barbells, medicine balls, and the human body—which may be the ultimate free weight. Research has shown that free weights can promote quicker strength gains than machines, in part due to the greater demand for balance and coordination, which causes more muscle groups to be recruited. Free weights are also considerably less expensive than machines, and you can create an effective muscle-fitness program with just a few dumbbells and a little creativity. Free weights, however, require the help of a spotter and pose a higher risk of causing injury than machines. Careful instruction and training are essential for the safety and effective use of free weights. (We consider safety in greater detail later in this chapter.)

An exercise machine does not move in all directions and is usually tethered to the floor, a wall, or a heavy base. Machines are safer than free weights and are often preferred by those lifting alone, performing circuit training, or simply looking for a quicker workout.

In short, you should use the muscle-fitness equipment that suits your training needs in terms of accessibility, cost, convenience, and safety. Even world-class athletes use both free weights and machines to train their muscles, so there is no reason you can't also use both.

Q I want to work out in my dorm. What do I need?

Not much! When most people visualize training for muscle fitness, they picture a weight room full of machines, dumbbells, and barbells. But one of the most effective strength-training tools is your own body weight and gravity. Body-weight exercises are great anytime but especially appropriate if you are just starting muscle-fitness training, don't have access or a gym, want to save money, or like being creative with your exercise. Exercises like push-ups, planks, squats, lunges, and step-ups can make for a vigorous workout, and with a little tweaking they don't require any additional resistance other than your body, even for experienced strength trainers. The best part is that body-weight exercises cost nothing and can be done almost anywhere, anytime.

Push-ups, pull-ups, lunges, and squats, along with some core exercises, tend to incorporate most major muscle groups and are challenging enough for most people. The resistance (body weight and gravity) can be continuously increased as your muscle fitness increases, so the overload principle is always in play. Adding resistance balls and bands, weight vests, and unstable surfaces will provide a satisfying muscle-fitness workout. With such a regimen, you never need to step into the gym, lift an actual weight, or go near a machine.

If you need convincing that your own body weight provides enough resistance to increase your muscle fitness, look no further than the world's top gymnasts. These athletes rarely train with conventional weights. Instead, their outstanding muscular fitness is a result of pushing and pulling their bodies through various motions all day long.

Q What's the best gym to join for strength training?

The best fitness facility depends on convenience, cost, the available equipment and classes, and the feel of the place. Join a gym that you will use—that's the prime consideration. Don't overlook your campus facilities: You may already be paying a student fee to use the campus gym or wellness center.

If you are joining a gym to get expert instruction and motivation, be sure to check the qualifications of the training staff. Also look into how busy the facility is at the times you plan on going. Consider, too, that gyms can also provide many other amenities, among them a juice or coffee bar, a clothing shop, and so on. If you have no interest in these extras, be wary of joining a gym with them, as you might end up paying for them in your monthly fees. Also, many gyms today require automatic monthly payments for a minimum of 12 months. Most importantly, make sure you know what you are signing up for before you get locked into something you don't want.

Once you join the gym, don't be intimidated if you are new to strength training; ask for help in setting up an appropriate program and learning safe techniques. Private gyms may require payment for this service, which is OK if they have an expert staff. At campus gyms, personalized assistance with set-up and safety training may be a free service supported by your student fees. Also keep in mind that a little gym etiquette can help improve everyone's experience:

- Remember that you are sharing equipment, so don't sit on a machine after you've finished your set. If you're using a barbell, unload the weight plates after you finish. Return dumbbells, barbells, and weight plates to the racks or floor area designated for storage.
- Keep your sweat to yourself by sitting on a towel you carry with you or by wiping all the parts of the machines you use—or both.
- Follow the rules of the particular fitness facility.

One of the big trends in recent years is women-only gyms. Although such facilities may not be dramatically different from coed gyms, there is an emphasis on making women's workouts more pleasant. The machines are designed specifically for women (for example, they are smaller); there are more dumbbells in the range women tend to use; the staff caters to new users; and the entertainment and for-sale products are more women friendly. There even appears to be evidence that women-only workout environments produce better fitness results. Another trend in fitness gyms is 24-hour access. Although very convenient, all-day gyms tend to have limited staff available outside the traditional hours, so make sure that if you want to consult with staff experts, they will be there when you are.

Selecting Types of Muscular Training

Q | I want to get more fit, but I don't want big muscles. What type of training is right for me?

Getting fitter through muscle training is a great idea and in fact may even help extend your life, as examined in the box "Can Being Strong Keep You Alive?" As for getting big muscles, remember that muscle size is largely dependent on the muscle type and testosterone (and so for women, developing big muscles is uncommon). To get fitter, you will first need to decide what equipment to use (such as free weights, machines, body resistance) and then choose a type of muscle-training program. There are three main types of muscle training:

- Static
- Isokinetic
- Dynamic

Static (isometric) training involves a muscle contraction without any change in the length of the muscle because the resistance

is too great to move. For example, if you push against a solid brick wall, the wall isn't going to move, but you are generating great force in a very small **range of motion (ROM)**. In a short time, your strength will noticeably increase through such training. Exercises like planks, glute bridges, and side bridges are in fact excellent ways to train your core muscles, although the strength will be limited to a specific and small ROM. Also, the strength gains tend to dissipate quickly if the exercises aren't done daily. For these reasons, static training isn't widely used for general fitness training. It is, however, effective for muscular rehabilitation therapy.

The second type of training is **isokinetic training,** or exertion of a constant force at a constant speed throughout the entire ROM. Isokinetic training requires special machines that control the speed of contraction so that you move at a steady rate and apply a constant force throughout the entire exercise. This equipment is typically reserved for rehabilitation and therefore has limited utility for general fitness.

The third type of training—the most popular by far—is **dynamic (isotonic) training,** in which muscle force is exerted throughout the entire contraction. Regardless of the resistance type (free weights or machines), the speed of a dynamic contraction varies because the muscle is weakest when it is longest and shortest, and is strongest in the middle of the ROM. This is why weight rooms are full of people arching their backs and swinging their arms at the start of a biceps curl (a major safety violation). The biceps is longest and weakest when the arm is straight, so the swinging helps to get the weight past the weakest point. When the arm curl moves through the middle of the ROM, the biceps is strongest, so no swinging is needed.

Dynamic training can be performed with body weight, rubber tubing, machines, and free weights. Because of the variety, it is also accessible almost anywhere and anytime. Drawbacks to dynamic training are few, especially when it is done with machines or

static (isometric) training Resistance exercise against a stationary force. During static muscle training, force is applied to an immovable object, so the agonist muscle does not change in length. Strength gains are limited to the range of motion used.

range of motion (ROM) The full range through which a joint can move.

isokinetic training Resistance exercise in which the resistance automatically adjusts throughout the ROM, thereby ensuring a constant rate of speed. This training requires specialized equipment.

dynamic (isotonic) training Exercise in which muscle force is exerted throughout the entire contraction. Resistance may be fixed or variable; the speed of contraction varies because the muscle is weakest at its longest and shortest and strongest in the middle of the ROM.

DOLLAR STRETCHER
Financial Wellness Tip

You can develop muscle fitness at home for little or no money. A calisthenics program using body weight for resistance is free. Small dumbbells and exercise bands can be purchased at very little cost. What articles around your house, apartment, or dorm room can you use for muscle-fitness training?

Research Brief

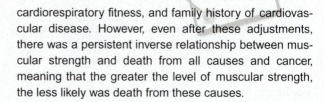

Can Being Strong Keep You Alive?

Researchers at the Cooper Institute in Dallas, Texas, followed over 8,000 men for 20 years to see if there was any association between muscular strength and all-cause mortality and death from cardiovascular disease or cancer. Each of the 8,000+ men was tested for maximal leg press and maximal bench press to categorize their muscular strength. They were each then put in one of three groups based on their strength score as low, moderate, and high muscular strength. Over the 20 years these men were followed, 503 deaths occurred—145 from cardiovascular disease, 199 from cancer, and the rest from other causes. The results were adjusted to take into account factors such as age, physical activity, smoking, alcohol intake, body mass index, baseline medical conditions,

cardiorespiratory fitness, and family history of cardiovascular disease. However, even after these adjustments, there was a persistent inverse relationship between muscular strength and death from all causes and cancer, meaning that the greater the level of muscular strength, the less likely was death from these causes.

Analyze and Apply

- How long do you hope to live?
- What exercises are you doing to increase your chances of living a long, healthy life?

Source: Ruiz, J. R., Sui, X., Lobelo, F., Morrow, Jr., J. R., Jackson, A.W., Sjöström, M., & Blair, S. N. (2008). Association between muscular strength and mortality in men: Prospective cohort study. *British Medical Journal, 12;*337(7661), 92–95. DOI: 10.1136/bmj.a439.

body weight. Free weights may require a partner to act as a spotter.

Table 5-2 compares the three basic types of training.

Q | Is it true that muscles get bigger if you go slower in your workout?

In tackling this question, let's first consider that there are two types of contractions in each "lift"—eccentric and concentric (Figure 5-4):

- In **concentric contraction,** the muscle shortens as it contracts.
- In **eccentric contraction,** the muscle lengthens as it contracts.

Muscle contraction occurs during both the shortening and the lengthening phases of a lift—and each type of contraction has different benefits. The absolute amount of force generated during muscle lengthening (eccentric) is greater than the force generated during muscle shortening (concentric). Practically speaking, this means that you can set down

a much heavier object than you can lift up, such as in performing a biceps curl.

However, the idea of going slow (or fast) has limited application, and slower contractions don't produce any more strength than other contractions. It's true that using slow eccentric contractions in your workout, especially if they are not a typical part of your routine, can increase muscle strength (as well as short-term soreness). However, this effect is a function of using the overload principle throughout the entire range of motion, not necessarily a function of the speed of movement.[19]

Faster contractions may be advantageous for certain athletes, especially those in sports requiring rapid, explosive movements (such as volleyball and basketball), because faster contractions better mimic the action needed during sport competition. For most of us, the speed of contraction in each direction should be 2–3 seconds

concentric contraction Skeletal muscle movement leading to shortening of the agonist muscle.

eccentric contraction Skeletal muscle movement leading to lengthening of the agonist muscle.

TABLE 5-2 TYPES OF MUSCULAR TRAINING

	STATIC TRAINING	ISOKINETIC TRAINING	DYNAMIC TRAINING
RANGE OF MOTION	Limited	Good	Excellent
RESISTANCE	Static	Adjusting	Fixed or variable
STRENGTH GAINS	Good*	Excellent	Excellent
COST	Inexpensive	Expensive	Inexpensive

*Strength gains are easy to come by in static training but quick to lose.

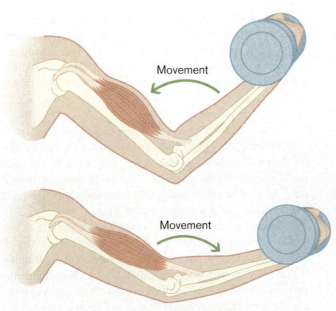

Figure 5-4 Concentric versus eccentric muscle contraction. During a concentric contraction (top), a muscle shortens as it contracts; during an eccentric contraction (bottom), a muscle lengthens as it contracts. Emphasizing the eccentric phase of an exercise usually builds more strength but may cause more muscle soreness.

initially, and more experienced exercisers can progress to a 1- to 2-second contraction.

Applying the FITT Formula: Frequency, Intensity, Time, and Type

Applying the FITT principle may be the best way to optimize your muscle fitness. Just as in cardiovascular training, the four FITT components should form the foundation of your muscle-fitness program planning. Through careful planning, you can improve your muscle strength and endurance in a reasonable amount of time, as long as the balance of intensity, duration, and frequency is set properly to meet your goals.

Q | Should I lift every day if I want to get really strong?

FREQUENCY. How frequently you perform resistance training depends almost entirely on your personal goals. If your goal is general fitness, the American College of Sports Medicine (ACSM) recommends muscle-fitness training on 2 or 3 days per week, with at least 48 hours between workouts.[20] Training on nonconsecutive days—for example, Tuesday and Friday or Monday, Wednesday, and Friday—allows your muscle fibers to recover from each training session and to work effectively. Recall that delayed-onset muscle soreness is likely to occur when you try something new in your muscle-training program—even the most experienced people encounter it occasionally.

Recovery from delayed-onset muscle pain is a further reason to give your muscles adequate rest.

Once you've moved beyond the beginner level, you can add more frequent training sessions, assuming that this change serves your goals (see Table 5-3). Although you may hear about athletes doing muscle training 4–7 days a week, it is important to note that they alternate muscle groups to ensure adequate rest and that they often have a lot riding on their athletic performance (such as a scholarship or a salary). If you are a typical college student, however, increasing your workout frequency raises your risk of injury, fatigue, and burnout. Additionally, if you already have a physically demanding job or participate in vigorous leisure activities, increasing your strength-training frequency may be ill advised. You are already doing work- or leisure-related strength training, and adding more may lead to overtraining.

Finally, there is sufficient evidence that engaging in muscle-fitness training only 1–2 days a week may be beneficial for some people.[20] For beginners, strength will almost certainly increase with just 1 day a week of muscle-fitness training, because this is a lot more than no days a week of training. However, beginners should progress to 2–3 days per week. For all other exercisers, 1 day a week is enough to maintain muscle fitness for up to 6 weeks, as long as the resistance or load is held constant. This is especially good news around the start or end of a semester when you are particularly busy and might not have as much time as usual for your preferred exercise program. The bottom line is that if you are new to muscle training, you should not feel overwhelmed. One or 2 days a week, along with your aerobic training, will have you well on your way to a new, more fit you.

Q | What's the best amount to lift to get stronger?

INTENSITY. You need to lift enough weight to overload your muscles. The overload principle indicates that in order to improve a muscle's fitness, it must be stressed beyond its present capacity. A muscle will adapt to stress by increasing in size, strength, and/or endurance capacity.

TABLE 5-3 TRAINING FREQUENCY RECOMMENDATIONS FOR RESISTANCE TRAINING

TRAINING STATUS	FREQUENCY PER WEEK
BEGINNER/OLDER/DECONDITIONED	2–3
INTERMEDIATE	3–4
ADVANCED/ELITE	4–7

According to a fable, Milo of Crotona lifted his newborn calf every day. As the calf grew, so did the boy's strength, until one day he was a strapping youth who could lift a full-grown cow. Although it is unlikely that you or I will ever lift a cow, if we repeatedly increase the amount of resistance or weight in our training program, our muscle strength will build accordingly—up to a point, of course.

For strength training, *intensity* refers to the amount of weight or resistance required to elicit a training response, or the overload principle. Intensity is often calculated as a percentage of an individual's 1-RM (one-repetition maximum). The ACSM recommends the following intensity guidelines:[20]

- 60–70 percent of 1-RM for deconditioned persons, older adults, or beginners
- 60–80 percent of 1-RM for improvement in overall strength, mass, and to some extent endurance
- 70–100 percent of 1-RM for advanced-level training

For example, if your 1-RM for the bench press is 125 pounds, a workload of 70 percent means that you would be using about 85 pounds of resistance.

Finding your 1-RM is not always practical, so working within a prescribed range of repetitions ("reps") is a useful alternative. The ACSM recommends 8–12 reps for each resistance exercise for general fitness, as this protocol will provide some level of gain in strength, endurance, and hypertrophy. Therefore, if you don't know your maximum strength or don't want to find out, start with a light weight and see how many reps you can perform while still maintaining good form. (Note: To prevent injury, it is always better to use less weight or do fewer reps with good form than to lift more weight or do more reps with poor form.) If you can easily perform 11 or 12 reps, try a slightly heavier weight next time. Your goal is to use an amount of resistance that is sufficient to fatigue your muscles when you complete 8–12 reps with good form.

Recall that many neuromuscular adaptations occur in the first few weeks of training, even in the first few days. Therefore, you may very well increase your resistance quite a bit over the first few days of training. Take your time; though, and build up slowly so that you decrease the risk of muscle soreness and injury.

In addition to the intensity and reps of your training, you also need to plan the number of sets. Reps are the number of times you lift the weight up and down. Lifting the weight 10 times is 1 set of 10 repetitions. The ACSM recommends performing 2–4 sets to fatigue (with good form), on 2 or 3 days per week, of 8–10 exercises targeting all major muscle groups.

Once you have established some comfort level with your training, met your short-term goals, and reduced the incidence of muscle soreness, you may want to consider modifications to your program. Changes in intensity, repetitions, sets, or frequency may help keep you challenged and motivated as you work toward your goals.

Remember to start slow, avoid muscle soreness, use good technique, and rest for at least 48 hours between training sessions. One of the beauties of muscle-fitness training is that even the true beginner will notice an almost immediate improvement. With some sustained effort, gains in muscle strength, endurance, and fitness will keep coming.

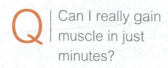

Q Can I really gain muscle in just minutes?

TIME. While there is no minimum time required to spend on muscle fitness, doing 2 sets of 8–10 exercises should take no more than 30 minutes. Using weight machines will probably be a little quicker than using free weights, and using balls, bands, body weight, and so on will be even faster.

If you don't have 30 minutes, is it possible to get benefits in, say, half the time? Possibly. As with any aspect of fitness, the law of diminishing returns applies: You can get a lot of benefit from only a small amount of workout time and smaller increments of benefit from doing more.

There are a number of ways to manipulate the time it takes to get through a muscle-fitness routine, and varying the rest interval between sets is quite common, as shown in Table 5-4. A person interested only in strength will typically employ longer rest intervals (2–5 minutes) than an individual whose goals include hypertrophy (30–90 seconds) or endurance (less than 30 seconds). A good rule is to allocate enough time between sets and exercises to allow you to perform each exercise with proper form.

TABLE 5-4 PROGRAM DESIGN PARAMETERS FOR RESISTANCE TRAINING

TRAINING GOAL	INTENSITY (% OF 1-RM)	REPETITIONS	SETS	REST BETWEEN SETS
STRENGTH	≥85%	≤6	2–6	2–5 min
POWER	75%–90%	1–5	3–5	2–5 min
HYPERTROPHY	67%–85%	6–12	3–6	0.5–1.5 min
MUSCULAR ENDURANCE	≤67%	≥12	2–3	≤30 s

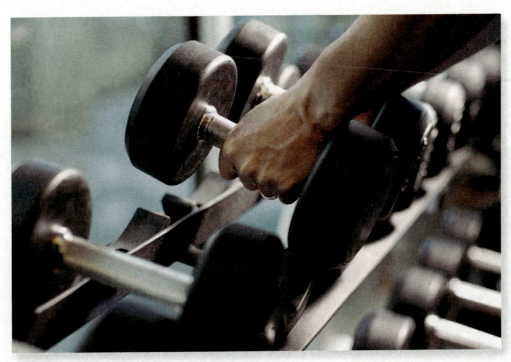

TYPE. Deciding what type of exercises to include in your muscle-fitness program can seem mind-boggling because there are so many from which to choose. Exercises can be classified in two general types: *single-joint exercises,* which use one major muscle group or joint, and *multiple-joint exercises,* which stress more than one muscle group or joint. A biceps curl is an example of a single-joint exercise (involving the elbow joint), and a squat is an example of a multiple-joint exercise (engaging the knee and hip). Both types of exercises can be included in a muscle-fitness routine, but multiple-joint exercises have certain advantages: They can use greater resistance, they mimic real-life activities, and they can make workouts more time efficient.

Time between sets should also be balanced with the muscle groups involved in the exercise. Most experts recommend alternating "push and pull" (biceps on the front of the arm and triceps on the back of the arm) or upper- and lower-body exercises. Such programs allow you to proceed from one exercise to another with very little recovery.

Of course, the number of sets will also influence the amount of time. While 2–3 sets are recommended, you can do more or less as time allows.

Q What can I do to get my arms bigger? And what is the best way to get a six-pack or burn the fat off my belly?

Spot training—doing any one exercise for a single body part—has limited effects. You may strengthen an individual muscle, but you won't selectively reduce fat in that area, and the increased strength may not be particularly functional. For example, doing lots of biceps curls will give you bigger, stronger biceps. However, other than for carrying groceries, there are very few occasions when your biceps function in complete isolation. Therefore, the recommendation is to use movements, not muscles, to produce the most effective workouts, as ultimately your fitness program should allow you to move better, not just have bigger muscles. Biceps typically work with the shoulder muscles, so chin-ups have a more overall effect than do simple biceps curls. Besides, if you do a chin-up, your biceps perform the same exact movement as in a curl; your shoulder and back muscles are included; and your workout becomes more efficient.

As for the belly fat and the six-pack, crunches might help give you strong abdominals, but unless you combine them with aerobic exercise, you might never get rid of the belly fat. Also, crunches have limited utility in daily function and should be supplemented with a variety of exercises designed to strengthen the core.

Q I like to bench and do arm curls. Is that enough?

Not really. Bench, or bench press, and biceps curls, or curls, will surely increase bicep and pectoral muscle fitness; however, an exercise program that is more inclusive of the whole body will better serve your fitness goals. For instance, every muscle has a reciprocal muscle that is important to consider. For each muscle that controls movement in one direction (an **agonist muscle**), there is a muscle that performs the opposite action (**antagonist muscle**). As an example, to bend your arm, you need to contract the biceps muscle (agonist) on the front of the arm. In order for this

agonist muscle The muscle primarily responsible for movement of a bone.

antagonist muscle The muscle opposite the agonist, which must relax and lengthen during contraction of the agonist.

MYTH or **FACT?**

Doing lots of sit-ups makes your stomach flatter.

▶ **WATCH THIS VIDEO IN** connect

See page 476 to find out.

action to occur, the triceps muscle (antagonist) on the back of the arm must relax and lengthen. To straighten your arm, the actions are reversed, and the triceps becomes the agonist while the biceps lengthens and becomes the antagonist. This reciprocal coordination of the agonist and antagonist muscles makes smooth and complex body movements possible. Individuals in strength-training programs should always perform exercises that allow for equal development of both agonist and antagonist muscles to realize their strength potential.

Q | Does it matter how I combine exercises?

PUTTING IT ALL TOGETHER. The best workout is one that you can do regularly and that lets you work toward your goals. Balancing the FITT principle with your goals and the time you can commit to exercise is sometimes the hardest part of any exercise program, muscle-fitness regimens included. In addition to the workout, you still need to include a proper warm-up and cool-down, which are important for minimizing injury and maximizing performance.

For a muscle-fitness program, there are three basic workout structures: (1) total-body workouts, (2) upper- and lower-body split workouts, and (3) muscle-group split routines. All three types can improve muscle fitness.

Total-body workouts typically feature multi-joint exercises that work the body's major muscle groups (Figure 5-5). These types of workouts are great for anyone and can be extremely time efficient. Exercises like push-ups, pull-ups, squats, and lunges can be used in a total-body workout. All are multi-joint, and all focus on movement, not muscles.

Upper- and lower-body split workouts consist of upper-body exercises on some days and lower-body exercises on other days; for example, you might do upper-body exercises on Monday and Wednesday and lower-body exercises on Tuesday and Thursday. College and professional athletes commonly use upper- and lower-body split workouts because they allow for a greater total amount of work and

are more sport specific, although this workout structure is time consuming.

Muscle-group split routines consist of exercises for specific muscle groups. An example of this type of routine is a chest and triceps workout one day, followed by a back and biceps workout the next session. This workout structure is most commonly used by bodybuilders and people whose sole goal is hypertrophy. Muscle-group split workouts are not the most practical for athletes or individuals interested in general muscle fitness, because they emphasize single-joint exercises.

Sample workout plans and descriptions of exercises are included at the end of this chapter.

Managing a Safe and Successful Muscle-Fitness Program

Starting a muscle-fitness program is great, but for maximum benefits, you must stick with it. A well-designed program based on sound training principles and good technique will not only prevent injuries but also boost both your progress and your motivation.

Weight-Training Safety and Injury Prevention

Q | What's the best way to lift weights and not get hurt?

Up to this point, we have focused on the many benefits of strength or resistance training. However, as with any exercise, there are potential risks—for example, using free weights carries the risk of dropping a weight on yourself; lifting too frequently or too heavily can lead to tendonitis or burnout; and using a machine improperly can cause injury. Basic exercise-safety recommendations apply to strength training: Warm up before exercise and cool down after, wear appropriate clothing and shoes, tie your hair back if it will fall in your eyes, and don't chew gum.

Specific strategies for safe strength training include the following:

- Warm up before you start resistance training. You should begin each workout with an appropriate warm-up consisting of at least 5 minutes of light aerobic activity to get the blood moving throughout your body; movement of your arms and legs through the full range of motion you will be using during your workout routine; and the use of light weights to move through the range of motion.
- Use proper technique during your actual workout. Common technique mistakes, which can lead to injury, include swinging your back during biceps curls, arching your back during bench press, and having poor back alignment during squats. Lift weights smoothly,

Mind Stretcher
Critical Thinking Exercise

You and your friends strength-train several times a week and consider yourselves to be in great shape. Have you ever thought about your motivation for getting fit? Is your routine just that—a routine—or are you working toward a particular goal, maybe an upcoming ski trip, a beach vacation, or the coming softball season? How is your muscle-fitness program preparing you for your mundane daily tasks, such as walking around campus, riding your bike, carrying your backpack, and working at your job? What changes can you make to your program to move it from routine to functional?

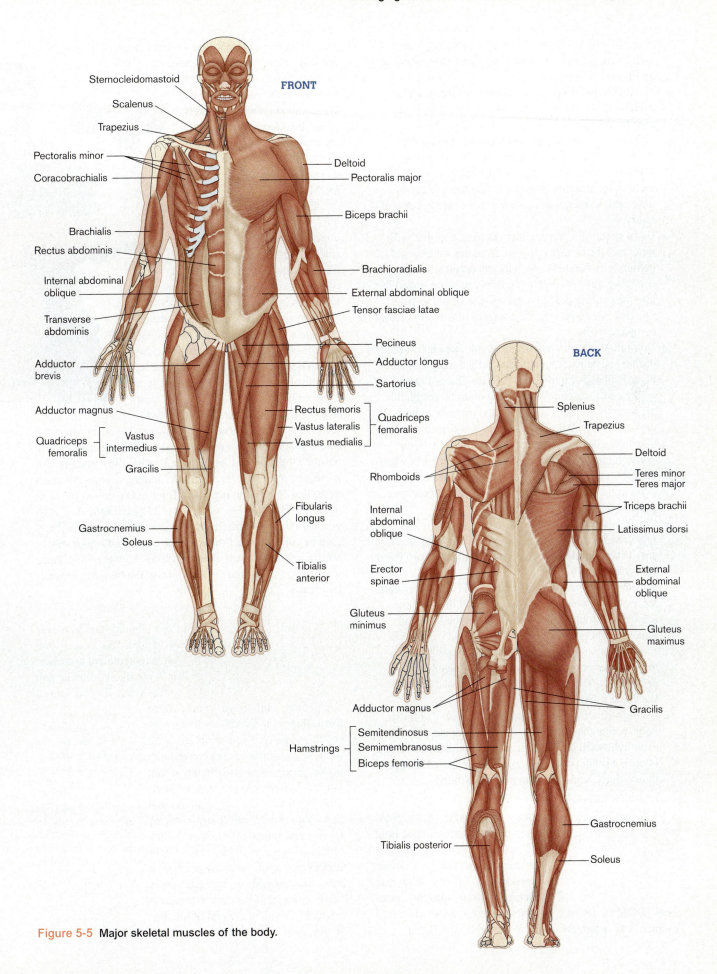

Figure 5-5 Major skeletal muscles of the body.

in a controlled fashion. Don't lift beyond the limits of your strength, and maintain good form and posture at all times.

Technique is not just a concern for free-weight exercises. Weight machines always have proper (and user-friendly) guidelines posted on them in a high-visibility spot. Although it is imperative to follow these instructions, it is not uncommon to see people applying creative techniques. This behavior not only violates the machine's warranty and the liability of the manufacturer, but it puts the user at greater risk of injury.

- Use a spotter for free weights. Having a spotter will minimize the chances of your dropping weights and getting hurt—and is especially important when you lift heavy weights. A spotter can help you move a weight into the starting position and into the finishing position and can assist you if the weight tilts or you cannot complete a lift.
- Don't hold your breath. Many people hold their breath during resistance training, especially during the contraction phase of a lift. This practice places a large load on the cardiovascular system and often forces blood pressure to skyrocket. This sudden increase in blood pressure can lead to serious injury—and even death in extreme cases. It is best to follow the exhale-on-exertion model, which encourages breathing out when the lift is most challenging. Ultimately, breathing is a good thing, and you should strive to do it all the time, especially when exercising.
- Check your equipment:
  Free weights: Are handles easy to grip? For barbells, are the weight plates secured with collars to keep them from slipping off the ends?
  Machine weights: Are you clear of all cables or weight stacks before you begin? Did you reset the machine (resistance, foot or back position, and the like) and lock everything in place?
  Elastic bands: Do the bands stretch smoothly? Are there cracks or other signs of wear and tear?
  Stability balls: Is the ball the recommended size for you? Is it inflated to the proper level?
- Cool-down after you are done. It is too easy to finish your workout and rush off to some other task. However, light stretching and flexibility exercises at the end of each workout will help reduce your risk of muscle injury. See Chapter 6 for more on flexibility.

Q | Why am I sometimes so sore the day after lifting?

GET ADEQUATE REST. Muscles can get sore after a bout of resistance training, usually within 24 hours of the exercise session. This effect is known as **delayed-onset muscle soreness (DOMS).** DOMS is a normal response to increased exertion and unfamiliar physical activities.[21,22] Therefore, if

you do an exercise that you've never done or haven't done recently, there is a good chance you will experience DOMS. Additionally, even for a seasoned weight trainer, DOMS is likely when the effort is dramatically increased. And as the eccentric emphasis of an exercise increases, so does the chance of experiencing DOMS.

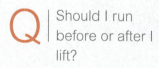

The cause of DOMS, although still not entirely understood, appears to be related to the **microtears** (tiny tears in muscle fibers) and injuries suffered within the muscle cell during new or intensive activity. The process starts with damage to the cell membrane, which is followed by a cascade of inflammatory responses, buildup of waste products, stimulated nerve endings, and the sensation of pain. During DOMS, you experience swelling, stiffness, and loss of strength that lasts 24–72 hours. Recovery from microtears is critical because when the fibers rebuild, they are a little stronger than they were before, thanks to the overload principle, making for increased muscle mass, strength, and endurance. So don't be fooled into believing that lifting every day is twice as good as lifting every other day. If you think this way, you'll find yourself quickly tiring and making little if any gain in your muscle fitness. Stick with the 48-hour rule at minimum, but don't wait too long between resistance workouts, as you don't want to miss the benefits of regular exercise.

Q | Should I run before or after I lift?

You should do whatever works best for you. If you are a recreational exerciser, it is not likely to make any difference. If you are a competitive athlete on your college team, then you should do what your coach suggests. Most of us do what is most comfortable and convenient. Some people find it difficult to run after doing muscle training on their legs, but others are not bothered and feel fine. There are many articles in muscle magazines about which order of exercise burns more fat or improves performance more, but in truth there is little if any difference, because you will have done the same amount of work at the end of the day. If you have a routine that you like,

delayed-onset muscle soreness (DOMS) Muscle soreness experienced 12–36 hours after increased exertion. The exact cause of DOMS is unknown, but it may be related to microtears in muscle cells. The discomfort usually subsides within 24 hours.

microtears Tiny tears in muscle fibers that are believed to be at least partly responsible for DOMS.

stick with it. If you are just starting, try different training schedules until you find what works best for you.

Making Progress

Q | What parts of my workout should I track?

Whether you are new to muscle-fitness training or an experienced lifter, you should consider tracking your progress on a regular basis. Options for tracking include writing in a notebook, creating a daily log to fill in, using an electronic spreadsheet, and signing up for a Web site that will store your data for you. The more information you track (sets, reps, resistance, recovery time, frequency of exercise, and so on), the more effective you will be at goal setting—and goal revising—as well as marking improvement and identifying problems.

You can modify the sample log in Figure 5-6 to track whatever factors are most relevant to your goals. An online workout tracker is available in your course materials; you can also download other sample logs to use from the same Web site.

Q | When can I increase the weight I'm lifting?

If you have been tracking your progress, you will have a good sense of when it is time to increase the resistance. Once you can perform all your sets at the upper end of your desired repetition range (8–12) while still maintaining good technique, it is time for more resistance. For example, when the individual whose program is shown in Figure 5-6 can complete 12–13 bench presses with good form, then it is time to add resistance. Generally, resistance increases of 5–10 percent are best—that would be about 5–10 pounds in the bench press example. Any more than that can lead to injury, and any less won't provide the overload stimulus needed to get stronger. When you are new to muscle-fitness training, 5–10

percent won't seem like much of an increase, but eventually it will become quite challenging to attempt an increase of that amount. You can't increase resistance indefinitely; once you reach your strength goal, you can maintain your strength gains by continuing to train at the same intensity.

Q | I didn't work out at all during spring break, and then I was busy with finals. How should I start back?

Restarting a muscle-fitness program need not be tricky. If the layoff has been less than about 3 weeks, you probably haven't lost much strength. In this case, you might want to reduce your FITT by about 10 percent at first, to ease back into your program. For example, reduce the resistance from 110 pounds to 100 pounds; drop the number of reps from 10 to 9, and do 1 less set than you previously did. You may even want to increase the rest period the first week back. These steps will help minimize DOMS, give your nervous system a reminder, and get you back to your pre–spring-break level within a week or two.

If you have had a longer layoff, drop your FITT by about 25 percent to ease the transition back to regular training. Reduce your resistance from 100 pounds to 75 pounds, do only 1 set, and if you are noticeably sore, take an extra day of rest between workouts. After a long layoff, you will require more time to get back to your previous fitness level, so be patient, keep track of your progress, and stick with it as best you can.

Q | How long do I need to keep lifting?

The longer you perform muscle-resistance training, the longer you will reap the benefits of fit muscles. Long-term benefits of muscle training include reduced risk of diabetes, musculoskeletal injury, and osteoporosis; improved control of blood pressure and body weight; and higher self-esteem. These advantages are surely enough motivation for anyone to start—and to continue—muscle training. Even among the elderly, those who have never performed resistance exercise show dramatic improvement in muscle strength and balance shortly after initiating a resistance-training program.[22] Although older adults typically use much less resistance than individuals 35 years younger, they experience significant positive changes in muscle fitness that make their daily activities easier and more enjoyable.

Exercise	Set 1 Weight	Set 1 Reps	Set 2 Weight	Set 2 Reps	Set 3 Weight	Set 3 Reps	Rest (time between sets)
Bench press	110 lbs.	11	110 lbs.	9			2 min.
Lat pull down	45 lbs.	10	45 lbs.	9			2 min.
Crunches	n/a	25	n/a	25	n/a	30	n/a
Side bridges	n/a	20 sec.	n/a	20 sec.	n/a	20 sec.	n/a
Dumbbell squats	5 lb. dumbbells	14	5 lb. dumbbells	11			2 min.

Figure 5-6 Sample muscle-fitness training log.

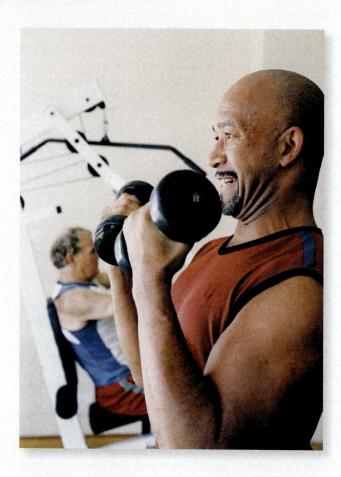

The push-up not only involves more muscles, but also is much more accessible and a lot less expensive—the exerciser just needs floor space.

Q | I keep hearing about functional training. Does that mean what I've been doing isn't functional? The same goes for core training—what's that?

Core training and **functional training** are nothing new, but there has been a recent increase in awareness of their value in overall fitness and sport performance.

The body's core muscles—the abdominals, obliques, and erectors—are the foundation for almost all types of movement, and they form the essential muscular connection between the upper and lower body. Located around the torso, the core muscles stabilize the spine to provide a solid foundation for movement, so "core stability training" is vital for improving fitness and reducing the risk of injury. To generate a powerful movement, it is necessary to first contract the core, which provides a solid base in the spine, pelvis, and shoulders. Training the core can also help improve posture and prevent injury. Although traditional core training includes crunches, a well-rounded program focused on core stability may focus on planks, side bridges, and hip extensions. Examples and instructions for popular core exercises appear at the end of this chapter. The biggest benefit of core training may be its ability to develop functional fitness.

Functional fitness is training the body in movement patterns that are needed in daily activity, ranging from sports to just getting around. Many people train with a focus on isolating specific joints or muscle groups (think biceps curl). Functional training is more concerned with movement patterns and therefore integrates multiple muscle groups rather than isolating them. Movements that incorporate squatting, lunging, pushing, and pulling develop stability, balance, and factors other than just strength; they require that all muscles be used in a coordinated, functional pattern. When you throw a baseball, kick a soccer ball, or jump high, your muscles are not working in isolation; they are working together to produce the specific movement pattern needed to complete the task. This is the heart of functional training.

The most basic functional-strength exercises are those that require the ability to control your body weight. Exercises such as body-weight squats, lunges, push-ups, and pull-ups are foundation functional exercises. As your functional strength develops, you can try more difficult exercises and progressions. Examples and instructions for popular functional exercises appear at the end of this chapter. Give the basic functional exercises a try—they are more challenging than most people think.

Q | I get bored with the same old workout and lose my motivation. Any ideas?

The short answer: For much-needed variety, try new exercises frequently or vary the number of sets, repetitions, and resistance in your usual workout.

Boredom can occur with any type of exercise program, and minimizing boredom can go a long way toward keeping your motivation high. Muscle-fitness training programs tend to be repetitious (do 2 sets, 10 reps, three times a week), so changing your routine frequently can stave off boredom. There is considerable interest today in functional muscle training, which relies primarily on body weight for resistance, in stark contrast to the more traditional programs using free weights or machines. Varying your routine between traditional training and functional training, as often as weekly, may reduce boredom.

Further, frequent changes in your routine will likely increase the number of muscles you are using, vary the way you are using them, and help you reach your goals more effectively. As an example, consider the difference between the bench press and the push-up. Both are primarily chest exercises (pectoralis major), yet compare the muscles involved in each:

- *Bench press:* pectoralis major, triceps, deltoid
- *Push-ups:* pectoralis major, triceps, deltoid, abdominals, erector spinae

core training Training that focuses on the muscles of the abdominal region and lower back. By stabilizing the spine, it can improve posture and decrease risk of falls.

functional training Training that mimics real-life movement patterns and integrates multiple muscle groups.

Q Do I need special equipment for core training and functional training?

No. Core training and functional training aren't limited to weight rooms or wellness center. All you need is your body weight and some floor space. We have seen that your body weight is a simple yet effective source of resistance that allows you to work out in the comfort and privacy of your own room.

Do you think body-weight squats are too easy for you? Then don't rest at the top; instead pause for 2 seconds at the bottom. This pause will eliminate the recoil effect typical of many gym lifts. Pausing at the bottom means that you must recruit more muscles to move your body instead of letting momentum help you along. You will definitely know which muscles are working! Squats, lunges, and push-ups can all be done in this manner.

Rubber bands and tubing can also take the place of free weights or machines when you work out away from the gym. You are limited only by your imagination in creating exercises to utilize the resistance that bands and tubing provide, ranging from simple curling exercises for the arms to more complex movements of the shoulder joint. Be aware that exercises utilizing tubing may be challenging at first, but the body will quickly adapt. To apply the overload principle and other tenets of progressive-resistance exercise, you will need to find ways to make the tubing and bands more challenging over time. For example, try thicker or shorter elastic bands or more sets and reps.

Stability balls are another common, commercially available piece of home exercise equipment often used for core exercises such as crunches, side crunches, and back extensions. However, with the addition of a pair of dumbbells, the stability ball can take the place of an exercise bench, and movements such as bench press or shoulder press can be done while sitting on the ball, increasing the demands on the core musculature.

Q Can I do Pilates for muscle-fitness training?

Yes, Pilates can build muscle fitness and provide other wellness benefits as well, including increased flexibility, improved body composition and body awareness, and reduced stress.[23] Pilates is named for its creator, German-born gymnast and boxer Joseph Pilates. It's a physical-movement program focused on developing strength and endurance (especially in the core), flexibility, posture, functional spinal alignment, and balance through whole body movements. A Pilates workout involves a small number of repetitions of exercises done with precise form—with careful attention to breathing patterns, coordinated and flowing movement, and body

alignment. Some Pilates exercises are done on the floor (mat work), and others involve specialized equipment such as the Reformer, an apparatus with cables, pulleys, and a sliding-board seat to provide resistance.

You can try Pilates at home for just a little money, using a floor workout based on an instructional book or a DVD. However, you may learn better by starting with a class or personal session led by an experienced instructor. Pilates is effective and, for most people, a safe activity choice. If you are looking for something other than traditional strength training to build muscle fitness—or if you are seeking to change your routine—Pilates may be an excellent choice. For more information about Pilates or to locate a certified instructor, visit the Web site of the Pilates Method Alliance (www.pilatesmethodalliance.org).

Avoiding Drugs and Supplements

Some people who want to add significant strength or size to their body resort to supplements, drugs, or steroids, many of which either are illegal or have no scientific evidence of effectiveness. Although these substances may be tempting, especially if you are highly competitive, the downside can be severe. Monetary fines, jail time, illness, disease, and death are all possible outcomes of use and abuse of illegal drugs. Supplements that are sold over the counter may be legal, but most have no scientific proof of effectiveness and rely on slick marketing. Ultimately, eating a healthy diet (see Chapters 8 and 9) and following a well-planned exercise program will help you achieve your goals and leave you with a much better sense of accomplishment than if you had you "supplemented" your progress—and risked your health in the process.

Q Creatine is a natural substance, so it's safe to take, right?

CREATINE. Although scientists have thoroughly studied the acute effects of creatine, the long-term impact of years of its use remains unclear. What exactly is creatine?

A substance typically found in fast-twitch muscle fibers, creatine is one of the basic muscle-energy stores. During exercise, creatine is thought to be an immediate energy source for explosive activities like sprinting and jumping. Creatine is created in the body, usually from the consumption of red meat, and is therefore readily available for most people. The balance of "creatine-in" through eating, and "creatine-out" through the urine, is in perfect harmony for healthy people. Some believe, however, that ingesting additional creatine may allow for greater explosive strength and power. Unfortunately, though, taking in extra creatine triggers an internal balance mechanism that causes the body to reduce its own creatine synthesis. Human muscle has a capacity of about 150 millimoles of creatine per kilogram of muscle, and once this level is reached, synthesis slows to maintain that level.

Why bother supplementing creatine in the first place? Well, if your creatine stores are low, supplementation does appear to improve performance in certain explosive activities.[24] The consensus is that creatine supplementation can increase the amount of work done by about 10 percent in the first few seconds of a maximal trial, such as a 1-RM strength trial. However, this gain isn't of practical benefit for most people.

People who choose to use creatine supplements should do so with caution. A better choice may be to improve their diet to increase the amount of quality protein they ingest, while not sacrificing other important nutrients.

DOLLAR STRETCHER
Financial Wellness Tip

Don't waste money on expensive protein supplements or other compounds advertised as muscle builders. A healthy diet with adequate protein is all you need. Try drinking low-fat or nonfat chocolate milk after your workouts and consuming more skim milk, beans, and skinless chicken breast to increase your protein intake inexpensively.

Q If steroids are so bad, why are athletes always using them?

STEROIDS. Money is usually the reason why athletes use steroids. Steroids can and do help athletes get stronger and perform better and longer—and enhanced performance typically means more and better paydays.[25] This temptation is too great for some professional athletes, regardless of the physical, emotional, and financial hardships steroid use brings. The desire to outperform others has trickled down to high schools, where some student athletes use steroids to improve their performance and therefore their chances of landing a college scholarship.

The sport of bodybuilding has long been known for rampant steroid use, to the point that today there is a worldwide bodybuilding competition for "clean" competitors. The idea is that those who are not "clean" can keep harming themselves all they want. Unfortunately, however, no evidence exists to support claims that steroid use causes biological or emotional harm. Most telling might be that steroids are banned by the majority of professional sport organizations due to their performance-enhancing effects, and the concern for human safety is still very much a question.

How do steroids work? All **anabolic steroids** are derived from testosterone. Steroids help to increase muscle size and strength by boosting protein synthesis. However, taking too much of a steroid also increases production of the by-product estradiol, which triggers a feedback mechanism that minimizes the steroid's potency. Anabolic steroids have been shown to increase weight gain, fat-free mass, and muscle fiber area if they are coupled with an aggressive strength-training program of the kind that is typical for highly trained individuals. Importantly, however: For anyone who is committed to muscle-fitness training, the combination of hard work, healthful eating, and plenty of rest is the only effective, safe, and legal way to achieve personal strength goals. There is no way around it: Steroid use is illegal, immoral, unethical, and extremely dangerous.

With respect to the safety issue, most side effects of steroids are undesirable, permanent, and serious. The additional load on the liver can lead to liver failure. Increased levels of natural testosterone act negatively on the pituitary gland, decreasing sperm production and levels of testosterone and luteinizing hormone. There is also a noticeable increase in risk for cardiovascular disease, because steroids decrease circulating HDL ("good") cholesterol and increase LDL ("bad") cholesterol. In addition, steroid use is linked to emotional problems, including irritability, increased aggressiveness, nervous tension, and frequent mood swings. Women using steroids experience hoarseness of voice, excessive hair growth (especially on the face), an enlarged clitoris, and decreased breast size. Men using steroids experience decreasing sperm count, shrinking testicles, and frequent mood swings and irritability. When the legal implications of steroid use are added to these negative physical effects, it makes sense to just say no.

Substances such as steroids, human growth hormone, insulin, and diuretics are all used to increase size and heighten performance. Regrettably,

anabolic steroids
Synthetic steroids designed to increase muscle mass. Anabolic steroids, although quite effective in increasing muscle size and strength, have many undesirable side effects, including severe mood swings, decreased libido, decreased testicle size, decreased sperm production, and increased male sexual traits in women.

Mind Stretcher
Critical Thinking Exercise

What do you think about the use of drugs and supplements to improve sports performance? Would you use a banned drug if you knew you could get away with it? What would you say about the ethics of drug use? What about the potential health risks? How would you distinguish between the performance benefit provided by using drugs and the performance benefit provided by inheriting an above-average muscle mass?

Steroids and related compounds increase muscle-fiber size and fat-free mass. But their use for performance enhancement is illegal, and they have many dangerous side effects, including liver damage, unhealthy cholesterol levels, increased cardiovascular disease risk, and hormonal and behavioral changes.

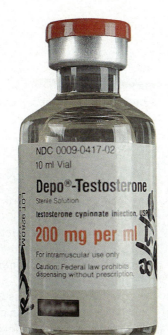

the use of performance-enhancing drugs is a not-so-secret problem within professional sports. Steroid scandals have shaken virtually every major sport, a sad reminder of how far some athletes will go to enhance their performance. These athletes are taking giant risks not only with their honor and credibility but also with their health.

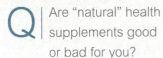

Q Are protein shakes really worth it?

PROTEIN. If you like their taste and can afford them, protein shakes pose little risk. On the other hand, if you eat a healthy diet and do regular moderate exercise, you probably won't get any benefit from them. Recommended daily protein intake for the average adult is 0.36 grams per pound of body weight. Therefore, a 140-pound woman needs about 50 grams of protein a day to meet her basic needs.

Moderate muscle-fitness training does not increase protein needs. Vigorous strength training or competing at a high level of sport (such as college scholarship athletes) may necessitate an increase in daily protein, but there is no need to exceed 1.0 gram per pound of body weight. Further, it is better to get protein from whole sources, especially those low in saturated fat, than to use supplements. Supplements tend to be more expensive than food sources, and their efficacy is not proven.

So, how about protein shakes? Shakes might be useful for the high-level athlete needing a lot of protein, since it is easier to drink shakes than to eat an equivalent amount of other protein. However, shakes can be expensive and can come with unwanted added ingredients. Skim milk might be one of the best and most cost-effective sources of supplemental protein.

And what about the value and safety of other protein supplements, beyond shakes? A high-protein energy bar goes for anywhere from $1.50 to $3.00 at most stores. That's two bars for the same price as ten PBJ sandwiches. At the same nutritional retailer, you can buy a popular brand of protein powder for $60.00 (yes, 60!), but it yields over 80 servings, for a per-serving price around 75 cents. That isn't a bad value, but a close look at the label reveals that the main ingredients are soybeans and milk, and there is frequent mention of "naturally occurring" ingredients. It would seem better, then, to consume "natural" foods since they are the source of these protein supplements. See the box on "Supplement Smarts: What's Really Safe?" for more on what is considered safe to use.

In short, if you are new to muscle-fitness training, you should strive to eat well, have a good exercise plan, and get plenty of rest. Leave the supplements to someone who has lots of money to waste.

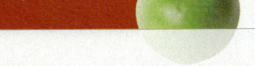

Wellness Strategies

Supplement Smarts: What's Really Safe?

Q Are "natural" health supplements good or bad for you?

When it comes to nutritional supplements, "natural" is not necessarily safe. In fact, most supplements have no governmental oversight, so consumers must be highly diligent in looking into what they are buying. Many supplements can be used safely by most people, but some herbs may cause cancer, some vitamins can be toxic at high doses, and some supplements can cause injury when mixed with medications. Sources of sound information to help you sort through the hype include:

National Center for Complementary and Alternative Medicine
http://nccam.nih.gov

National Institutes of Health Office of Dietary Supplements
http://dietary-supplements.info.nih.gov

Federal Trade Commission: Test Your Supplement Savvy
http://www.ftc.gov/bcp/edu/pubs/consumer/health/hea09.shtm

Summary

Muscle fitness is critical for a long and healthy life. If your muscles are not fit, many mundane tasks can be challenging—and will become especially difficult as you grow older. During your college years, good muscle fitness allows you to perform all types of tasks with more vigor and enjoyment than if your muscles were not fit. Increasing muscle fitness does not have to take lots of time or be done in a specialized facility. This chapter discusses plans for dorm-room workouts using nothing more than body weight, as well as strategies for more extensive workouts for those with the time, access to equipment, and desire. The key to muscle fitness is to do something, and do it regularly. Although it is possible to maintain your muscle fitness for up to 6 weeks with very little time and effort, it is much healthier to put in enough effort to ensure that your muscles are regularly stressed according to the overload principle. Muscle-fitness training a few days a week, coupled with regular cardiovascular exercise and a healthy diet, will keep you strong, healthy, and happy for many years to come.

More to Explore

American College of Sports Medicine
http://www.acsm.org
American Council on Exercise: Fit Facts
http://www.acefitness.org/fitfacts
National Strength and Conditioning Association
http://www.nsca-lift.org
Strongwomen.com: Fitness Programs
http://www.strongwomen.com/fitness.htm
University of Michigan: Muscles in Action
http://www.med.umich.edu/lrc/Hypermuscle/Hyper.html

Sample Resistance-Training Programs

▶ **WATCH IN CONNECT**   All the exercises in the Basic Program and Body-Weight Circuit, along with many others, are described in the following section and have corresponding video clips available online.

Program 1: Basic Muscle-Fitness Program (Using Machines or Free Weights)

UPPER BODY	LOWER BODY	CORE
Biceps curl (biceps, brachioradialis, brachialis)	Leg press (quadriceps, gluteals)	Curl-up (abdominals, hip flexors)
Triceps extension (triceps)	Leg curl (hamstrings)	Side bridge (abdominals, quadratus lumborum)
Bench press (pectoralis major, triceps, deltoid)	Heel raise (gastrocnemius, soleus)	Prone (forward) plank (anterior and posterior trunk and pelvis)
Lat pulldown (latissimus dorsi, pectoralis major, biceps)		
Shoulder press (triceps, deltoids, pectoralis major)		

Program 2: Upper- and Lower-Body Split Routine

Upper- and lower-body split routines alternate between upper-body exercises on one day and lower-body exercises on another. There are many ways to structure a split routine; in the sample program shown here, days 3 and 6 are rest days, and then the 6-day sequence repeats.

DAY 1	DAY 2	DAY 4	DAY 5
Barbell bench press	Front squat	Barbell shoulder press	Step-up
Triceps push-down	Dumbbell lunge	Dip	Deadlift
Dumbbell row	Heel raise	Lat pull-down	Back extension
Barbell biceps curl	Stability-ball curl-up	Dumbbell biceps curl	Cable woodchopper
	Side bridge		Prone (forward) plank

Program 3: Muscle-Group Split Routine

Muscle-group split routines divide workouts by muscle groups; individual muscle groups are typically rested for several days between training sessions. In the example shown here, day 4 is a rest day, and then the 4-day sequence repeats.

DAY 1: CHEST, SHOULDERS, TRICEPS	DAY 2: LOWER BODY	DAY 3: BACK, BICEPS
Incline bench press	Back squat	Bent-over row
Dumbbell fly	Lunge	Chin-up
Machine shoulder press	Deadlift	Shrug
Lateral raise	Leg curl	EZ bar biceps curl
Triceps extension	Heel raise	Reverse curl
	Curl-up	
	Reverse crunch	

Program 4: Body-Weight Circuit

This program includes exercises that exclusively use body weight for resistance.

Push-up	Body-weight squat
Pull-up	Curl-up
Prone (forward) bridge	Body-weight lunge
Chair dip	Quadruped hip extension (bird dog)
Inverted row	Body-weight step-up
Side bridge	

Strength-Training Exercises

▶ **WATCH IN CONNECT**   For each major muscle group of the body, several exercise options are presented using different types of equipment (or no equipment). Choose one or more exercises for each muscle group to put together a complete strength-training program that fits your needs. Exercises are organized by the key muscle group they develop, but many exercises work additional muscles; refer to the "Muscles developed" list in each exercise. For best results, pay close attention to the description of correct technique and the training tips. Always use proper body alignment and don't bounce or swing weights. You can make many exercises more challenging by pausing for 1–2 seconds at the bottom of each repetition.

MUSCLE GROUP **Chest**

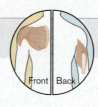

Front | Back

▶ **WATCH ONLINE**

Barbell Bench Press

Muscles developed: Pectoralis major, triceps brachii, deltoids

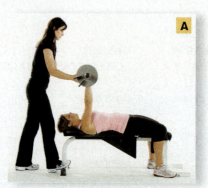

A

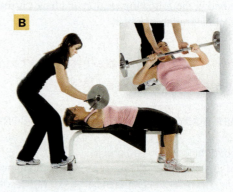

B

Instructions

A. Lie on your back on a bench with your feet flat on the floor. Adjust the bench so that your back is straight and not arched; if your feet don't reach the floor comfortably, place them on the bench with your knees bent. Grasp the bar with your palms upward and hands about shoulder-width apart. Start with the bar over the middle of your chest or slightly above it. Fully extend your arms, but don't forcefully lock your elbows.

B. Lower the bar slowly to your chest; then press it in a straight line back to the starting position. Each full repetition should take 2–4 seconds.

Training tips

- If the weight is resting on a rack, move it carefully with the help of spotters. If you have one spotter, he or she should stand behind you; if you have two spotters, they should stand at the ends of the bar.

- During the exercise, don't arch your back or bounce the bar off your chest.

Machine Chest Press

Muscles developed: Pectoralis major, triceps, deltoids

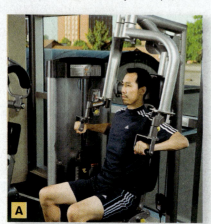

A

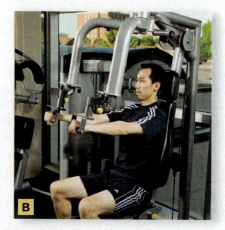

B

Instructions

A. Depending on the type of machine, sit or lie on the seat or bench with your feet flat on the floor or the foot support. Your back and hips should be against the machine pads, and the tops of the handles should be aligned with your armpits. Grasp the handles with your palms facing away from you.

B. Push the bars until your arms are fully extended, but don't forcefully lock your elbows. Return to the starting position. Each full repetition should take 2–4 seconds.

Training tips

- During the exercise, don't arch your back or bounce at the end of the movement.

- If the starting position of the bar is adjustable, set it so that your wrists can remain straight throughout the exercise.

Push-Up and Modified Push-Up
Muscles developed: Pectoralis major, triceps, deltoids

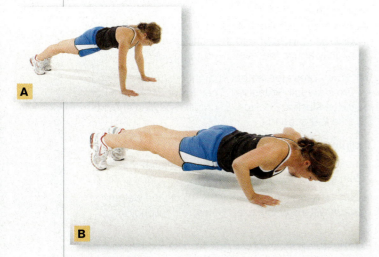

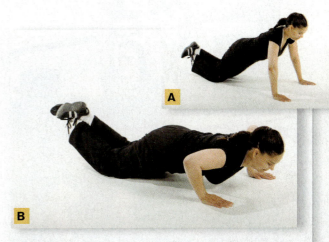

Instructions
A. For push-ups, start with your body in the upright position, supported by your hands and the balls of your feet. For modified push-ups, support your weight with your hands and knees; bend your knees about 90 degrees and keep your ankles together or crossed. Your back should be straight and your neck neutral. Your hands should be about 2–3 inches wider than shoulder-width apart, and your fingers should point forward.

B. Lower your chest to the floor so that your elbows are bent about 90 degrees. Then return to the starting position by fully straightening your arms. Each push-up should take 2–4 seconds.

Training tips
- Use the modified technique if you cannot do more than 8 push-ups; once you can do more than 20–25 modified push-ups, switch to the standard push-up technique.
- Keep your body straight throughout the exercise; don't let your back arch or your hips rise up or sag.
- To ensure that you lower yourself far enough during each repetition, touch your chest on a soft object on the floor, such as a pair of rolled-up socks, a tennis ball, or a friend's fist.
- Push-ups can be made more challenging by raising the level of your feet with a small bench or an exercise ball.

MUSCLE GROUP Shoulders

Front | Back

Barbell Shoulder Press
Muscles developed: Anterior deltoid, lateral deltoid, triceps brachii

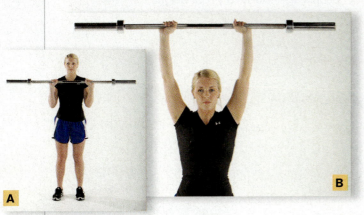

Instructions
A. Stand with your feet about shoulder-width apart. Grasp the bar with your palms facing away from you; the bar should be at the top of the chest.

B. Slowly press the bar straight overhead until your arms are fully extended. Then lower the weight back to the starting position in a controlled manner. Each full repetition should take 2–4 seconds.

Training tip
- Keep your back straight throughout this exercise; don't arch.

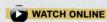
▶ **WATCH ONLINE**

Machine Shoulder Press

Muscles developed: Anterior deltoid, lateral deltoid, triceps brachii

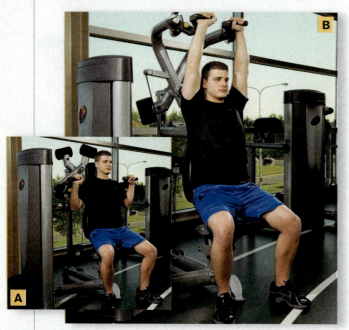

Instructions

A. Adjust the seat so that your feet are flat on the ground or foot bar and the handles or bars are slightly above the level of your shoulders.

B. Slowly press the weight straight overhead until your arms are fully extended. Then lower the weight back to the starting position. Each full repetition should take 2–4 seconds.

Training tips

- Lower the weight in a controlled fashion rather than letting it fall with gravity.
- Not lowering the weight all the way to the weight stack will make this exercise more challenging.

Dumbbell Lateral Raises

Muscles developed: Anterior deltoid, lateral deltoid, trapezius

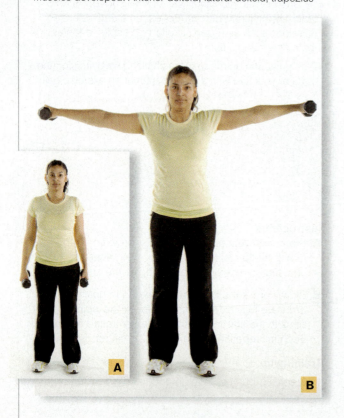

Instructions

A. Stand with feet about shoulder-width apart, holding a dumbbell in each hand by your side.

B. With your palms facing in and wrists held straight, slowly raise the weights out to the sides until your elbows are level with your shoulders. Return to the starting position slowly and in a controlled fashion.

Training tips

- Keep your back straight and your shoulders down throughout this exercise.
- This exercise can be quite challenging, so most people start with a very light weight.

MUSCLE GROUP **Back**

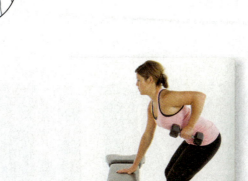

Dumbbell Row

Muscles developed: Posterior deltoid, latissimus dorsi, biceps brachii

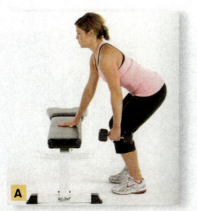

Instructions

A. Stand in front of a bench, grasping a dumbbell in one hand with your feet about shoulder-width apart. With your abdominals tight and your back straight, bend your knees and lean forward at the hips until your support hand is on the bench. The hand with the dumbbell should be directly below your shoulder.

B. Pull the dumbbell up to the side until it makes contact with your ribs or until your upper arm is just beyond horizontal. Lower the weight until your arm is extended and your shoulder is stretched forward. Repeat on the opposite side.

Training tips

- Try to hold your torso in a horizontal plane while pulling the weight upward. Adjust supporting knee and/or arm slightly forward or back as needed.

- The exercise can also be done with one knee and hand on the bench for support. Position the foot of your other leg slightly back and to the side.

Lat Pull-Down

Muscles developed: Posterior deltoid, latissimus dorsi

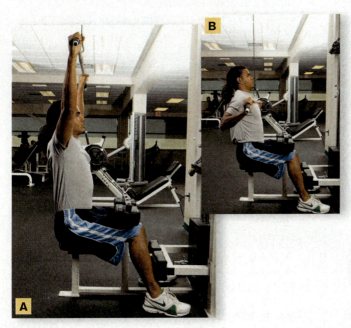

Instructions

A. Grasp the cable bar with a grip slightly wider than your shoulders, palms facing away. Sit with your thighs under the supports and your feet flat on the floor.

B. Pull down on the cable bar until it reaches your upper chest. Move your shoulder blades together and your elbows down. Return the weight to the starting position in a controlled fashion, until your arms and shoulders are extended.

Training tips

- Do not hold too wide a grip; otherwise, your range of motion will be compromised.

- Avoid swinging your body or leaning back to use your weight to pull the bar down; instead, focus on using the muscles of your arms and back to move the weight.

▶ WATCH ONLINE

Chin-Up (Pull-Up)

Muscles developed: Latissimus dorsi, biceps brachii, brachialis

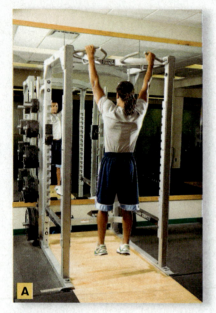
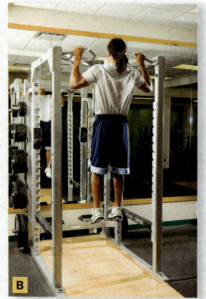
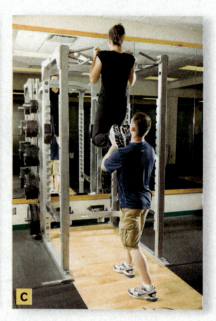

Instructions

A. Using a stable overhead bar, grasp the bar with your palms facing away from you. Ideally, your feet will still be on the ground.

B. Using your arm strength, pull yourself upward until your chin is over the top of the bar, then lower yourself back to the starting position. Don't let your feet rest on the floor until you are completely finished with the movement. Each full repetition should take 2–4 seconds.

Training tips

- Keep your body in a fairly straight position, and don't swing.
- If you can't complete a pull-up, assistance can be provided by a spotter (**C**) or by a weight-lifting band (a rubber-band-like device that supports some of your body weight during the pull-up).
- This exercise can be modified by doing it from a supine position—the "Australian" chin-up, in which you begin lying on your back with a stable bar an arm's length above you.

MUSCLE GROUP Biceps

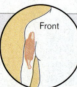

Front

Barbell Biceps Curl

Muscles developed: Biceps brachii, brachialis

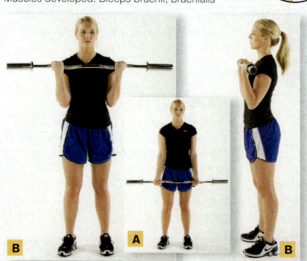

Instructions The exercise can be done with a straight barbell or a curl bar; the curl bar may place less stress on your wrists.

A. Stand with feet about shoulder-width apart, grasping the bar with your palms facing away from you and your hands about shoulder-width apart.

B. Slowly raise the weight until the bar is slightly below the level of your collarbone. Then without pausing, lower the weight back to the starting position. Each full repetition should take 2–4 seconds.

Training tips

- Keep your back straight throughout the exercise; don't let your back arch or your arms to swing through the motion.
- This exercise can also be performed with dumbbells.

Machine Biceps Curl

Muscles developed: Biceps brachii, brachialis

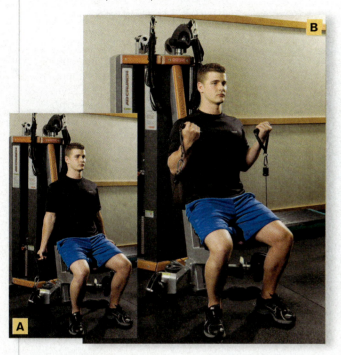

Instructions

A. Adjust the seat so that your feet rest on the ground or foot bar and your back is straight. Grasp the handles or hand grips with your palms facing up.

B. Keep your body still as you bend your elbows until the handles or hand grips are close to your collarbone. Return to the starting position. Each full repetition should take 2–4 seconds.

Training tip

- Keep your back straight throughout the exercise; don't let your back arch or move back during the exercise.

MUSCLE GROUP **Triceps**

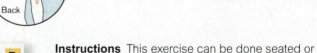

Back

Dumbbell Triceps Extension

Muscles developed: Triceps brachii

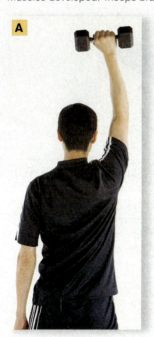
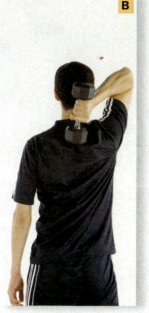

Instructions This exercise can be done seated or standing.

A. Holding one dumbbell, fully extend your arm overhead, palm facing forward.

B. Slowly lower the weight behind your head, keeping your elbow straight up and rotating your palm toward your body, until your arm is fully bent. Slowly raise the weight back to the starting position.

Training tips

- Keep your back straight throughout this exercise.
- Your elbow and upper arm should remain straight up throughout this exercise.

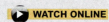
WATCH ONLINE

Machine Triceps Push-Down
Muscles developed: Triceps brachii

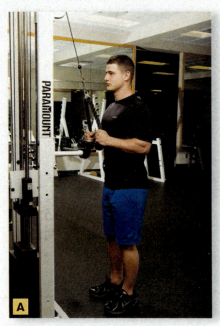

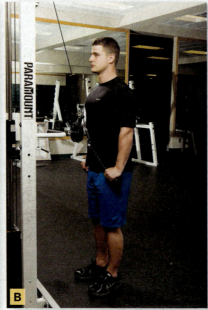

Instructions This exercise requires a lat pull-down machine.

A. Stand facing the machine with your feet about shoulder-width apart. Grasp the bar with your palms facing down. Your elbows should be at your sides, bent 90 or more degrees.

B. Keeping your elbows at your side, slowly push the weight down until your arms are almost straight. Then slowly raise the bar back to the starting position.

Training tip

- Keep your back straight throughout this exercise.

Chair Triceps Dip
Muscles developed: Triceps brachii

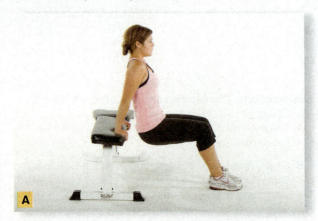

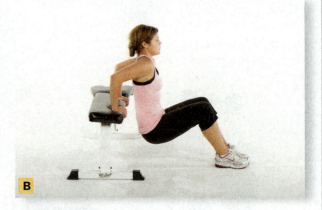

Instructions This exercise requires a stable chair or bench.

A. Start by sitting on the front edge of the chair, with your hands palm-down beside your hips. Use your hands to push your body up (your feet should remain on the floor), and move your hips forward away from the chair.

B. Lower your body in front of the chair by bending your elbows to about a 90-degree angle; then push back up with your arms to the starting position.

Training tips

- Keep your back straight and your elbows close to your body throughout the exercise.

- To make the exercise easier, move your feet closer to the chair. To make the exercise more challenging, move your feet farther from the chair, elevate them on a small bench, or place them on an exercise ball.

MUSCLE GROUP Quadriceps

Front

Note: Many of the exercises in this group also develop the gluteal muscles and the hamstrings.

Body-Weight Squat

Muscles developed: Quadriceps, hamstrings, gluteals, erector spinae

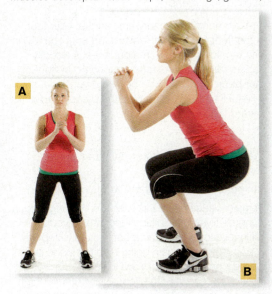

Instructions

A. Stand with your feet just wider than your shoulders and your toes pointed slightly out. For balance, your hands should be together and out in front of you at about shoulder height, with elbows bent.

B. Squat down until your thighs are parallel with the floor; then raise yourself back to the starting position. As you squat, push your hips back and keep your back neutral or slightly arched; don't round your lower back. Each repetition should take 2–5 seconds.

Training tips

- Don't lean forward as you squat down; keep your feet flat on the floor, chest up, and head forward.
- Think of squatting as sitting back on a toilet seat.
- Advanced users can do one-legged squats, which are the same as previously described with one leg held up and forward. This exercise can also be done standing on one leg on a slightly elevated, stable surface, while the other leg hangs over the edge.

Barbell Back Squat

Muscles developed: Quadriceps, hamstrings, gluteals, erector spinae

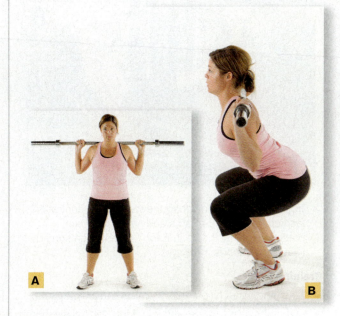

Instructions

A. Stand with your feet just wider than your shoulders and your toes pointing slightly out. The bar should rest on your upper back; grasp it slightly wider than shoulder-width, with your palms facing forward.

B. Squat down until your thighs are parallel with the floor; then raise yourself back to the starting position. As you squat, push your hips back and keep your back neutral or slightly arched; don't round your lower back. Each repetition should take 2–5 seconds.

Training tips

- Keep your head forward, chest up, and feet flat on floor.
- Unless you are using a specialized squat rack, you will need spotters. If you have one spotter, he or she should stand behind you; if you have two spotters, they should stand at the ends of the bar.
- Your knees should point the same direction as your feet throughout the movement.
- Maintain a natural curve (arch) in your back throughout the entire movement.

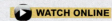 **WATCH ONLINE**

Dumbbell Lunge

Muscles developed: Quadriceps, gluteus maximus, adductors

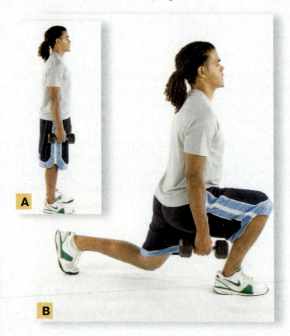

Instructions

A. Stand with your feet about shoulder-width apart. Hold a small dumbbell in each hand.

B. Take a larger-than-normal step forward, and let your foot land fully on the floor. Bend your forward leg until your thigh is parallel with the floor; make sure your knee is directly above your ankle rather than extending forward in front of your foot. Your back leg should be bent and your heel off the ground. Return to the starting position by pushing off with your forward leg.

Training tips

- Keep your back straight, maintaining its natural curves through the entire movement.

- Beginners can perform lunges without weights to start.

- There are two major variations of this exercise: walking lunges and reverse lunges. To do the walking lunge, once you are in the lunge position, instead of pushing back, simply step forward with the opposing leg, again going in to the lunge position. For a reverse lunge, step backward instead of forward, lowering your back knee toward the floor until your front thigh is parallel with the floor. Push back up to start, and repeat.

Machine Leg Press

Muscles developed: Quadriceps, gluteus maximus, hamstrings

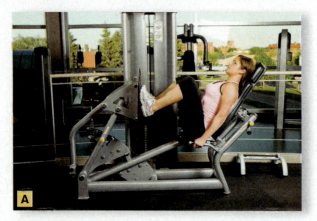

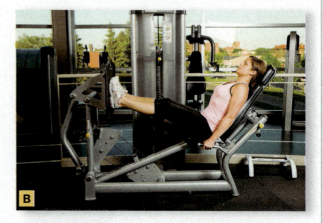

Instructions

A. Sit or lie on the seat or bench of the machine; adjust it so that your head, back, and buttocks are against the pads and your hands can grasp the handles. Your feet should be about shoulder-width apart, and your knees comfortably bent and in line with your feet.

B. With your feet flat on the footplate, push to straighten your legs; move through the full range of motion, but don't forcefully lock your knees. Return to the starting position by slowly lowering the weight in a controlled fashion. Keep your head steady and your back pressed against the seat. Each full repetition should take 4–5 seconds.

Training tips

- If the starting position feels cramped, adjust the seat.

- Keep your knees in line with your feet; don't allow them to bow inward or outward.

Machine Leg Extension

Muscles developed: Quadriceps

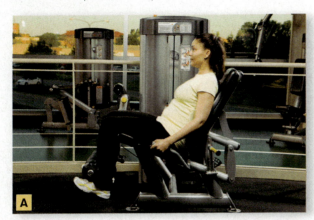

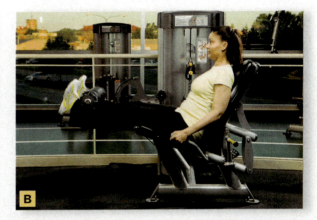

Instructions

A. Sit with your hips and back against the pads. Adjust the seat so that the pads rest comfortably on the top of your shins.

B. Keep your body still as you extend your knees until they are almost but not quite straight. Keep your head steady and your back pressed against the seat. Each full repetition should take 2–4 seconds.

Training tips

- If you feel any knee pain, don't perform this exercise.
- Tightening your abdominal muscles may help you keep your back from arching.

Step-Up

Muscles developed: Quadriceps, gluteus maximus

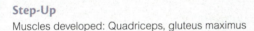

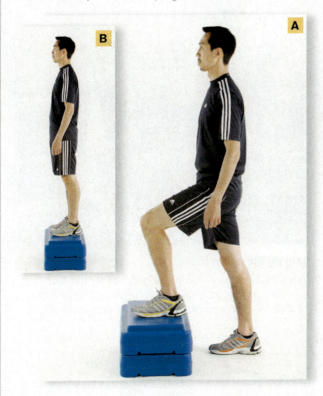

Instructions This exercise requires a stable step or low bench, between 12 and 18 inches high.

A. Start by standing about 2 feet from the bench, with your feet shoulder-width apart, as if you were about to walk up some stairs. Place one foot forward fully onto the step.

B. Step up. Once your forward leg is fully extended, slowly lower back down to the start position. This exercise can be done one leg at a time or alternating lead legs.

Training tips

- Maintain the natural curve (slight arch) in your back through the entire movement.
- This exercise can be made more challenging by holding a dumbbell in each hand or wearing a weighted vest.

MUSCLE GROUP **Hamstrings**

▶ **WATCH ONLINE**

Stability-Ball Leg Curl
Muscles developed: Hamstrings, gluteals, erector spinae

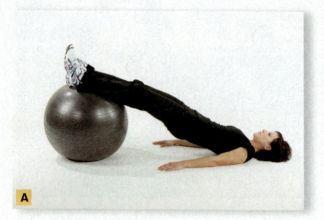

A

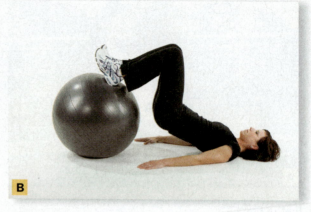

B

Instructions

A. Lie on your back on the ground with your feet up on an exercise ball (at least 15 inches high). Raise your hips so that your back is straight or slightly arched. Keep your arms extended on the floor beside you. You should be able to roll the ball with your feet.

B. Keeping your hips straight, roll the ball toward you until your knees are bent at a 90-degree angle.

Training tips

- Don't do the exercise if it causes low-back pain.
- Keep your hips straight throughout the movement. Bend only your knees and not your hips.
- This exercise can be made more challenging by using a larger ball. It can also be done with a chair or bench in place of the ball, slowly raising your hips up and down.

Machine Leg Curl
Muscles developed: Hamstrings

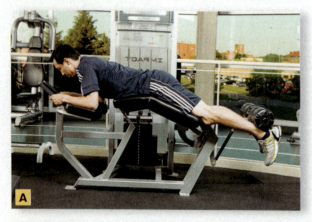

A

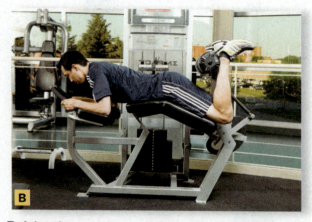

B

Instructions

A. Lie on the front of your body, with hips and forearms aligned with the appropriate pads. The leg pad should rest comfortably against your lower calves. Grasp the hand grips loosely.

B. Keep your body still as you flex your knees until they are bent at a 90-degree angle. Return to the starting position. Keep your head steady and your back straight. Each full repetition should take 2–4 seconds.

Training tip

- Use caution when doing this exercise for the first time. Use a light weight until you are comfortable with the movement, and increase the weight very gradually.

MUSCLE GROUP Core

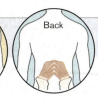

Front   Back

Prone (Forward) Plank

Muscles developed: Obliques, rectus abdominis, deltoids, erector spinae

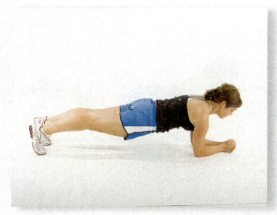

Instructions Lie face down on the floor with arms bent at your sides so your elbows and forearms are on the ground. Lift your body so that only your forearms and the balls of your feet are touching the ground and supporting your weight. Your body should be in a straight line from head to toe. Your head should be relaxed as you face the floor. Hold this position for 10 seconds, or longer as you get stronger.

Training tips

- Keep your body straight throughout the exercise; don't let your lower back arch or sag.

- You can make this exercise easier by spreading your feet wider.

- You can make this exercise more challenging by lifting one arm straight out to the side for 10–15 seconds or one leg off the ground for 10–15 seconds.

Side Bridge

Muscles developed: Obliques, transverse abdominis

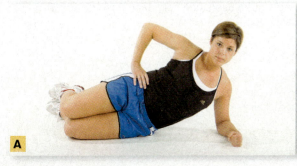

A

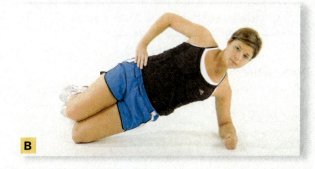

B

Instructions Side bridges can be done in several different positions

A. Lie on the floor on your side, with your knees bent. Your top arm can lie along your side, or you can place your hand on your hip.

B. Lift your hips so that your weight is supported by your forearm and knee. Hold this position for at least 10 seconds, slowly building up to 30 seconds. As you gain strength, you can make the exercise more difficult by supporting your weight with your forearm and your feet (**C**).

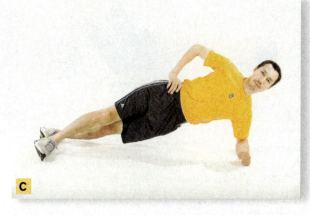

C

Training tips

- Keep your body firm and straight throughout this exercise.

- This exercise can be made more challenging by pointing your top arm straight up.

- An advanced variation involves "rolling" from a side bridge to a forward-plank position with forearms perpendicular to the body and then to a side bridge facing the other direction.

▶ **WATCH ONLINE**

Quadruped Hip Extension (Bird Dog)

Muscles developed: Erector spinae, rectus abdominis, gluteus maximus

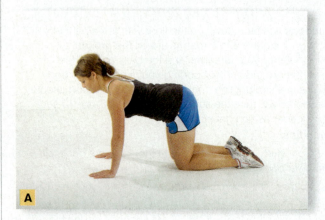

A

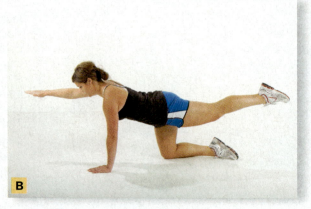

B

Instructions

A. Start on the floor, supporting your weight with your hands and knees. Your knees should be below your hips, and your hands should be below your shoulders and slightly wider.

B. Slowly extend one arm and the opposite leg, keeping your back straight. Hold this position for 5–10 seconds. Repeat on the other side.

Training tips

- Use a pad under your hands and knees for more comfort.
- Beginners can start by lifting an arm alone, then lowering it, and then lifting a leg alone.
- Advanced users can hold each pose for 10–15 seconds.

Back (Glute) Bridge

Muscles developed: Erector spinae, gluteals, hamstrings

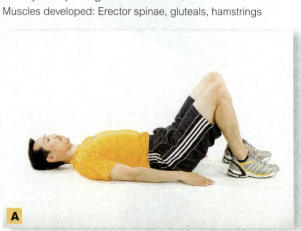

A

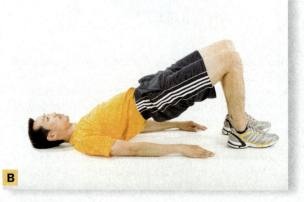

B

Instructions

A. Lie on your back with your arms extended along your sides, legs bent, and feet flat on the floor.

B. Tuck your pelvis under and tighten your gluteal muscles. Raise your hips so that your weight is supported by your head, shoulders, and feet. Hold this position for at least 10 seconds, and slowly build up to 30 seconds.

Training tips

- Keep your back straight throughout this exercise.
- This exercise can be made more difficult by lifting one leg so that the foot is pointing out, in line with the support leg.
- If you feel any pain in your back, don't perform this exercise.

Curl-Up

Muscles developed: Rectus abdominis

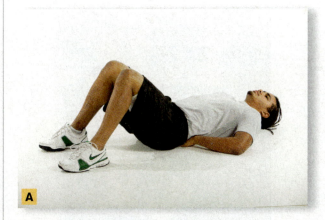

A

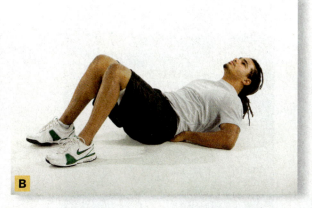

B

Instructions

A. Lie on the floor with your legs bent and your feet flat on the floor. Place your hands under the small of your back; maintain the natural curve of your lower back throughout this exercise.

B. Slowly lift your shoulder blades off the ground, keeping your nose pointed straight upward. Then slowly lower yourself back to the floor.

Training tips

- You can reduce the strain on your back by keeping one leg straight and one leg bent.

- Do not try to lift your entire back off the floor, just your shoulder blades.

- This exercise can be made more challenging with the use of an exercise ball. "Sit" on the ball and slowly lower your back until it is fully extended, and then return to the starting position. Your feet should be firmly on the ground.

MUSCLE GROUP **Calf/Soleus**

Back

Barbell Standing Heel-Raise

Muscles developed: Gastrocnemius, soleus

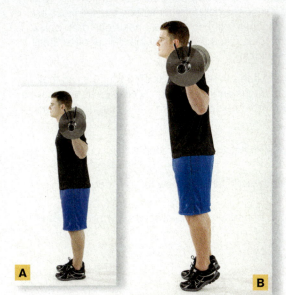

A

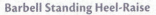

B

Instructions

A. Stand with your feet about shoulder-width apart and your toes pointing forward. Grasp the barbell with palms facing forward and rest it comfortably on your upper back.

B. Press down with your toes as you lift your heels. Then slowly lower your heels back to the floor. Don't let your ankles roll in or out during the exercise. Each full repetition should take 2–4 seconds.

Training tips

- Keep your back straight or slightly arched throughout the movement.

- Look forward and keep your neck in a neutral position.

- Don't bounce at the end of the range of motion.

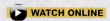 **WATCH ONLINE**

Machine Seated Heel-Raise

Muscles developed: Gastrocnemius, soleus

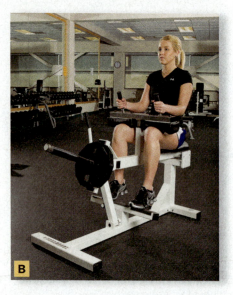

Instructions

A. Sit with the balls of your feet on the platform, your knees bent at 90 degrees, and the pads on top of your lower thighs; your toes should point forward.

B. Press down with your toes as you lift your heels. Then slowly lower your heels back to the starting position. Don't let your ankles roll in or out during the exercise, and keep your back straight. Each full repetition should take 2–4 seconds.

Training tip

- Don't bounce at the end of the range of motion.

Dumbbell Seated Heel-Raise

Muscles developed: Gastrocnemius, soleus

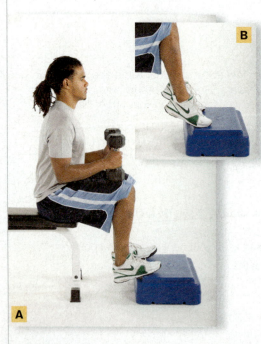

Instructions

A. Sit down on a chair or a bench, with your feet comfortably resting on the ground. Place the balls of your feet on a small block or a low step (2–4 inches high) so that your heels can drop below the level of your toes. Place a dumbbell, barbell, or other small weight on your thighs.

B. Starting with your heels lowered, press onto your toes so that the front of your thighs and knees slightly elevate, as your calves contract. Lower your heels back down to the starting position.

Training tips

- Keep your back straight or slightly arched throughout the exercise movement.
- The chair or bench height should allow for a 90-degree angle at the knee.
- This exercise can be made more challenging by using a heavier weight.

COMPLETE IN connect

NAME	DATE	SECTION

This lab includes tests for assessing muscular strength of the upper and lower body. The traditional test for strength is a one-repetition maximum (1-RM) test, which measures the greatest resistance that can be moved through one full range of motion with good form. The 1-RM test is the most accurate assessment, but it is not appropriate for people with little or no strength-training experience. For them, there are formulas, although somewhat less accurate, that can convert a multiple-repetitions result to an estimated 1-RM value; in this type of test, you perform multiple repetitions of an exercise just as you would during a strength-training workout. Choose tests that are appropriate for you. Scores and ratings are based on your age, sex, and body weight:

Age: [ ] Sex (male/female): [ ] Body weight: [ ] lb

Upper-Body Strength: Bench Press

Equipment

- Bench-press machine OR a flat bench, barbell, weight plates, collars, and at least one spotter
- Weight scale (for measuring body weight)

Preparation

Perform a general warm-up; then warm up for the bench press by performing several repetitions using a light weight. If you are using free weights, practice the exercise with your spotter(s).

Instructions

Follow the instructions for the bench-press technique given on p. 168. Keep your feet flat on the floor or bench, and don't arch your back. Push the weight up until your arms are fully extended. Don't hold your breath or bounce the weight on your chest.

For the 1-RM test: Start with a weight that is less than the amount you think you can lift (50%–70% of your estimated 1-RM). Lift that amount of resistance one time with good form. Increase the weight with each attempt, resting 3–5 minutes between attempts. If you lifted the weight easily, add 20 or more pounds; if you are close to your 1-RM, add a smaller amount of resistance (about 5 pounds). Your goal is to reach your 1-RM in 4–5 attempts. Your 1-RM is the final weight you lifted with good form.

Bench press 1-RM: [ ] lb

For estimating 1-RM from multiple repetitions: Choose a weight that is an amount you think you can lift about 10 times. Using correct form, perform as many repetitions as you can. Estimate your 1-RM for the bench press with the following formula:

$$\text{Bench press 1-RM} = \frac{\text{resistance} \boxed{} \text{lb}}{1.0278 - (0.0278 \times \text{repetitions} \boxed{})} = \boxed{} \text{lb}$$

Results

Divide your 1-RM score by your body weight:

1-RM [____] lb ÷ body weight [____] lb = [____] bench-press weight ratio

Find the rating for your bench-press weight ratio in the following table: [____]

BENCH-PRESS WEIGHT-RATIO RATINGS*

Males

AGE (YEARS)	SUPERIOR	EXCELLENT	GOOD	FAIR	POOR
20	>1.76	1.34−1.375	1.19−29	1.06−1.18	<1.01
20−29	>1.63	1.32−1.48	1.14−1.26	0.99−1.10	<0.96
30−39	>1.35	1.12−1.24	0.98−1.08	0.88−0.96	<0.86
40−49	>1.20	1.00−1.10	0.88−0.96	0.80−0.86	<0.78
50−59	>1.05	0.90−0.97	0.79−0.87	0.71−0.77	<0.70
60+	>0.94	0.82−0.89	0.72−0.79	0.66−0.70	<0.65

Females

AGE (YEARS)	SUPERIOR	EXCELLENT	GOOD	FAIR	POOR
<20	>0.88	0.77−0.83	0.65−0.76	0.58−0.64	<0.57
20−29	>1.01	0.80−0.90	0.70−0.77	0.59−0.68	<0.58
30−39	>0.82	0.70−0.76	0.60−0.65	0.53−0.58	<0.52
40−49	>0.77	0.62−0.71	0.54−0.60	0.50−0.53	<0.48
50−59	>0.68	0.55−0.61	0.48−0.53	0.44−0.47	<0.43
60+	>0.72	0.54−0.64	0.47−0.53	0.43−0.46	<0.41

*In terms of percentiles, *well above average* = over the 80th percentile; *above average* = between 60th and 80th percentiles; *average* = between 40th and 60th percentiles; *below average* = between 20th and 40th percentiles; and *well below average* = below the 20th percentile.

Source: Cooper Institute for Aerobics Research. (2009). *Physical fitness assessment and norms for adults and law enforcement.* Dallas, TX: Cooper Institute.

Lower-Body Strength: Leg Press

Equipment

- Leg-press machine
- Weight scale (for measuring body weight)

Preparation

Perform a general warm-up; then warm up for the leg press by performing several repetitions using a light weight.

Instructions

Follow the instructions for the leg-press technique given on p. 176. Keep your feet flat on the footplate about shoulder-width apart. Push the weight up until your legs are fully extended, but don't forcefully lock your knees. Don't hold your breath.

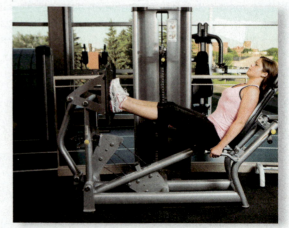

For the 1-RM test: Start with a weight that is less than the amount you think you can press (50%–70% of your estimated 1-RM). Press that amount of resistance one time with good form. Increase the weight with each attempt, resting 3–5 minutes between attempts. If you lifted the weight easily, add 25 or more pounds; if you are close to your 1-RM, add a smaller amount of resistance. Your goal is to reach your 1-RM in 4–5 attempts. Your 1-RM is the final weight you pressed with good form.

Leg press 1-RM: ☐ lb

For estimating 1-RM from multiple repetitions: Choose a weight that is an amount you think you can press about 10 times. Using correct form, perform as many repetitions as you can. Estimate your 1-RM for the leg press with the following formula:

$$\text{Leg press 1-RM} = \frac{\text{resistance } \boxed{} \text{ lb}}{1.0278 - (0.0278 \times \text{repetitions } \boxed{})} = \boxed{} \text{ lb}$$

Results

Divide your 1-RM score by your body weight:

1-RM ☐ lb ÷ body weight ☐ lb = ☐ bench-press weight ratio

Find the rating for your leg-press weight ratio in the following table: ☐

LEG-PRESS WEIGHT-RATIO RATINGS*

Males

AGE (YEARS)	WELL ABOVE AVERAGE	ABOVE AVERAGE	AVERAGE	BELOW AVERAGE	WELL ABOVE AVERAGE
20–29	>2.12	1.97–2.12	1.83–1.96	1.63–1.82	<1.63
30–39	>1.92	1.77–1.92	1.65–1.76	1.52–1.65	<1.52
40–49	>1.81	1.68–1.81	1.57–1.67	1.44–1.56	<1.44
50–59	>1.70	1.58–1.70	1.46–1.57	1.32–1.45	<1.32
60 +	>1.61	1.49–1.61	1.38–1.48	1.25–1.37	<1.25

Females

AGE (YEARS)	WELL ABOVE AVERAGE	ABOVE AVERAGE	AVERAGE	BELOW AVERAGE	WELL ABOVE AVERAGE
20–29	>1.67	1.50–1.67	1.37–1.49	1.22–1.36	4<1.22
30–39	>1.46	1.33–1.46	1.21–1.32	1.09–1.20	<1.09
40–49	>1.36	1.23–1.36	1.13–1.22	1.02–1.12	<1.02
50–59	>1.24	1.10–1.24	0.99–1.09	0.88–0.98	<0.88
60 +	>1.17	1.04–1.17	0.93–1.03	0.85–0.92	<0.85

*In terms of percentiles, *well above average* = over the 80th percentile; *above average* = between 60th and 80th percentiles; *average* = between 40th and 60th percentiles; *below average* = between 20th and 40th percentiles; and *well below average* = below the 20th percentile.

Source: Cooper Institute for Aerobics Research. (1994). *Physical fitness assessment and norms*. Dallas, TX: Cooper Institute.

Summary of Results

Fill in the scores and ratings for the tests you performed

TEST	ACTUAL 1-RM	ESTIMATED 1-RM	RATING OF RATIO
Bench press			
Leg press			

Reflecting on Your Results

Are you surprised by your test results and ratings? Did your results match what you thought about your own muscle fitness?

Planning Your Next Steps

Muscle strength is typically a function of training. If your scores were lower than you expected, then it may be time to start or change your muscle-fitness routine. If you scored well, then strive to maintain your current level of fitness, or add some new or more advanced exercises or training techniques to boost your results. Set realistic goals for improvement and create a plan to achieve them. Then repeat these tests in several weeks and note any improvements.

Describe your goals and the specific steps you will take to improve your muscular strength. If needed, refer to Lab Activity 5-3 on program planning.

What effect, if any, did your plan have on your muscular strength?

Source: Conversion formula for multiple reps to 1-RM from Brzycki, M. (1993). Strength testing: Predicting a one-rep max from reps to fatigue. *JOPERD 64:* 88–90.

COMPLETE IN connect

NAME	DATE	SECTION

Muscle endurance can be assessed by performing multiple repetitions of push-ups and curl-ups.

Upper-Body Endurance: Push-Up/Modified Push-Up

Most people can perform push-ups, and they require little training. For this test, the ratings are based on males performing standard push-ups and females performing modified push-ups.

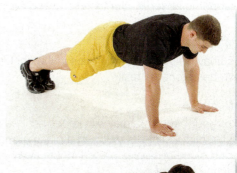

Equipment

- A mat or similar firm, padded surface

Preparation

If you haven't performed push-ups or modified push-ups in the past, practice to familiarize yourself with the movement. Do a general warm-up before the test.

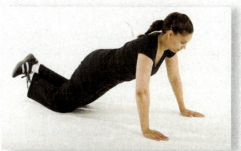

Instructions

The push-up test starts with hands shoulder-width apart, arms extended straight out under the shoulders, back and legs in a straight line, and toes curled under. For the modified push-up's starting position, the weight is supported by the knees and hands; the hands should be slightly ahead of the shoulders so that the hands are in the proper position for the downward motion.

For both versions of the test, the objective is to lower your body in a straight line, keeping your back straight, until your chin touches the mat. Your stomach should not touch the mat at any time. Once your chin touches the mat, you push back up to the start position, or until your arms are straight again. Continue for as many repetitions as possible until (1) no more push-ups can be completed, (2) your technique is no longer appropriate (back and/or legs not straight), or (3) there is a pause in the cadence.

Results

Your score is the number of push-ups or modified push-ups completed with good form. You can use the following chart to compare your push-up score to others of your age and sex.

Number of push-ups or modified push-ups ☐ Rating ☐

PUSH-UP/MODIFIED PUSH-UP RATINGS BY AGE AND SEX

	Age and Sex											
	15–19		20–29		30–39		40–49		50–59		60–69	
RATING	M	F	M	F	M	F	M	F	M	F	M	F
Excellent	≥39	≥33	≥36	≥30	≥30	≥27	≥25	≥24	≥21	≥21	≥18	≥17
Very good	29–38	25–32	29–35	21–29	22–29	20–26	17–24	15–23	13–20	11–20	11–17	12–16
Good	23–28	18–24	22–28	15–20	17–21	13–19	13–16	11–14	10–12	7–10	8–10	5–11
Fair	18–22	12–17	17–21	10–14	12–16	8–12	10–12	5–10	7–9	2–6	5–7	2–4
Needs improvement	≤17	≤11	≤16	≤9	≤11	≤7	≤9	≤4	≤6	≤1	≤4	≤1

Source: Canadian Society for Exercise Physiology. (2003). *The Canadian physical activity, fitness & lifestyle approach: CSEP-Health & Fitness Program's health-related appraisal and counseling strategy* (3rd ed.). Reprinted with permission from the Canadian Society for Exercise Physiology.

Abdominal Endurance: Curl-Up
Curl-ups measure strength and endurance of the abdominal muscles

Equipment
- A mat or similar firm, padded surface
- Metronome or other way to keep time (the cadence for the test is 50 beats per minute)
- Two strips of tape about 8–10 inches (20–25 cm) in length; these should be placed 4 inches (10 cm) apart
- Partner to observe your technique and count the number of curl-ups you complete

Preparation
If you haven't performed curl-ups in the past, practice to familiarize yourself with the movement. Do a general warm-up before the test.

Instructions
Lie on your back on a mat with knees bent 90 degrees. Place your arms at your sides, palms facing down, with the middle fingers touching a piece of masking tape. A second piece of tape is placed 10 cm away. Keep your shoes on during the test.

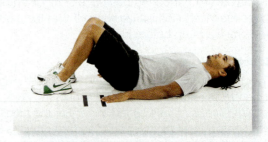

    Set the metronome to a pace of 50 beats per minute. Do slow, controlled curl-ups as you lift your shoulder blades off the mat in time with the metronome. You will curl up on one beat and lower down on the next beat, for a rate of 25 curl-ups per minute. As you curl up, slide your fingers forward until they reach the second piece of tape. Your trunk should make a 30-degree angle with the mat at the top of the curl-up. Your low back should be flattened before curling up. The test continues for 1 minute. Complete as many curl-ups as possible in time with the metronome without pausing or using poor technique. The maximum number is 25 curl-ups completed during the 1-minute test time. Make sure that the fingertips start behind the first line of tape and reach the second line of tape during each curl-up.

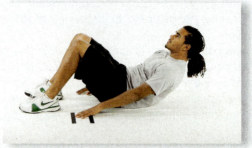

Results
One repetition is counted each time the shoulder blades touch the floor. After determining the total number of curl-ups, you can use the following chart to determine your abdominal endurance compared to others of the same age and gender.

Number of curl-ups ☐   Rating ☐

CURL-UP RATINGS BY AGE AND GENDER

| | Age and Gender | | | | | | | | | | | |
| | 15–19 | | 20–29 | | 30–39 | | 40–49 | | 50–59 | | 60–69 | |
RATING	M	F	M	F	M	F	M	F	M	F	M	F
Excellent	25	25	25	25	25	25	25	25	25	25	25	25
Very good	23–24	22–24	21–24	18–24	18–24	19–24	18–24	19–24	17–24	19–24	16–24	17–24
Good	21–22	17–21	16–20	14–17	15–17	10–18	13–17	11–18	11–16	10–18	11–15	8–16
Fair	16–20	12–16	11–15	5–13	11–14	6–9	6–12	4–10	8–10	6–9	6–10	3–7
Needs improvement	≤15	≤11	≤10	≤4	≤10	≤5	≤5	≤3	≤7	≤5	≤5	≤2

Source: Canadian Society for Exercise Physiology. (2003). *The Canadian physical activity, fitness & lifestyle approach: CSEP-Health & Fitness Program's health-related appraisal and counseling strategy* (3rd ed.). Reprinted with permission from the Canadian Society for Exercise Physiology.

Reflecting on Your Results

Are you surprised by your test results and ratings? Did your results match what you thought about your own muscle fitness?

Planning Your Next Steps

Muscle fitness is typically a function of training. If your scores were lower than you expected, then it may be time to start or change your muscle fitness routine. If you scored well, then strive to maintain your current level of fitness, or add some new or more advanced exercises or training techniques to boost your results. Set realistic goals for improvement and create a plan to achieve them. Then repeat these tests in several weeks and note any improvements.

Describe your goals and the specific steps you will take to improve your muscular fitness. If needed, refer to Lab Activity 5-3 on program planning.

What effect, if any, did your plan have on your muscular fitness?

LAB ACTIVITY 5-3 Creating a Program for Building and Maintaining Muscle Fitness

COMPLETE IN connect

NAME	DATE	SECTION

Equipment

None required; you may want to develop and track your program using a paper notebook, digital spreadsheet, smartphone application, or online program.

Preparation: None

Instructions

1. Set SMART goals: Set goals for your muscle-fitness program. Your goal could be something about training—number of workouts per week—or it could be based on one of the tests in Lab Activities 5-1 and 5-2.

Current status	Goal	Target date	Notes (rewards, special considerations)

2. Apply the FITT principle: Create a program that meets the recommended criteria for success and fits your schedule and preferences. Fill in the following exercises for your starting program:

- *Frequency:* 2–3 days per week, with muscle groups rested at least 48 hours between workouts
- *Intensity:* A resistance that allows 8–12 repetitions of each exercise to be performed to fatigue with good technique; usually 60%–80% of 1-RM
- *Time:* 2–4 sets of 8–12 repetitions of each exercise
- *Type:* Perform exercises to train each major muscle group

Muscle group	Exercise	Starting		
		Resistance	Sets	Reps
Chest				
Shoulders				
Back				
Core				
Quadriceps				
Hamstrings				
Lower legs				
Arms: Biceps				
Arms: Triceps				
Additional exercises:				

Results

Track your progress with a log like the one on the next page or one you create for yourself. Make as many copies as you need.

STRENGTH-TRAINING LOG

	Date: ________								Date: ________								Date: ________							
	Set 1		Set 2		Set 3		Set 4		Set 1		Set 2		Set 3		Set 4		Set 1		Set 2		Set 3		Set 4	
Exercise	Wt	Reps	Wt	Reps	Wt	Reps	Wt	Reps	Wt	Reps	Wt	Reps	Wt	Reps	Wt	Reps	Wt	Reps	Wt	Reps	Wt	Reps	Wt	Reps

	Date: ________								Date: ________								Date: ________							
	Set 1		Set 2		Set 3		Set 4		Set 1		Set 2		Set 3		Set 4		Set 1		Set 2		Set 3		Set 4	
Exercise	Wt	Reps	Wt	Reps	Wt	Reps	Wt	Reps	Wt	Reps	Wt	Reps	Wt	Reps	Wt	Reps	Wt	Reps	Wt	Reps	Wt	Reps	Wt	Reps

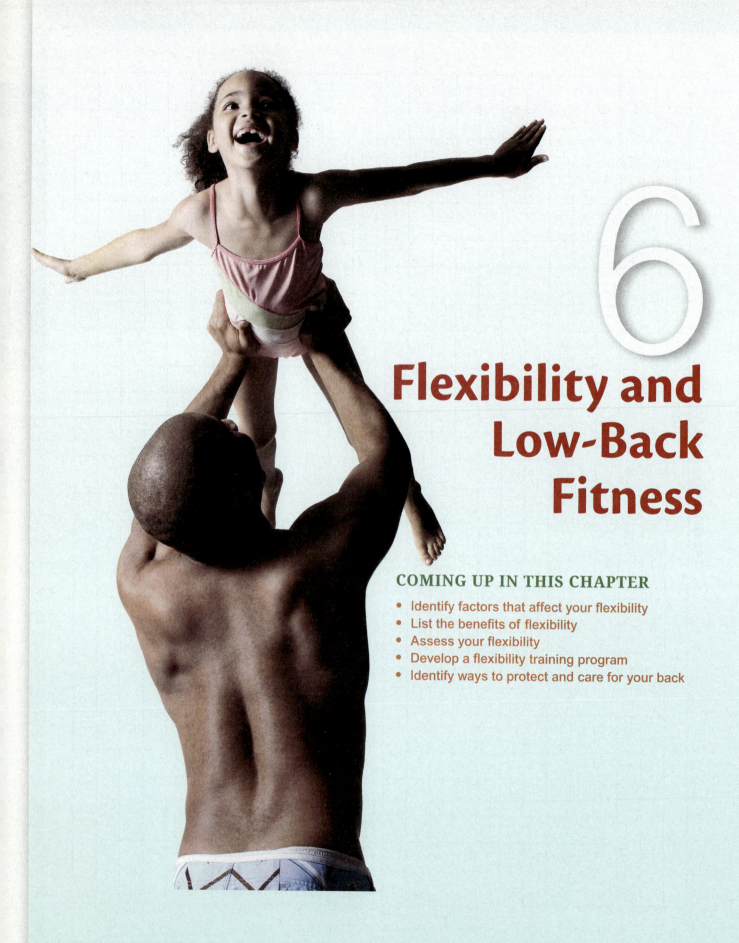

6

Flexibility and Low-Back Fitness

COMING UP IN THIS CHAPTER

- Identify factors that affect your flexibility
- List the benefits of flexibility
- Assess your flexibility
- Develop a flexibility training program
- Identify ways to protect and care for your back

How does flexibility affect wellness? The physical dimension of wellness is the most directly affected. An adequate range of motion in your joints lets you perform daily tasks easily and efficiently, and, over time, it helps prevent stiffness, soreness, and falls and their associated injuries. In addition to maintaining good flexibility, stretching exercises promote relaxation and reduce stress.

Low-back pain is often a result of poor flexibility, muscle fitness, and posture. Like any other physical health problem, it can have a negative impact on the other wellness dimensions. Pain and the inability to engage in normal activities with ease can lead to stress and depression, undermining emotional well-being. These in turn can affect your intellectual wellness by reducing your ability to think clearly. Your social wellness may be affected if you withdraw from others due to depression or physical limitations. On a larger scale, social as well as environmental wellness may be harmed by the high costs associated with chronic low-back pain, a common cause of missed workdays and reduced productivity. Any of these erosions of the other dimensions of wellness may affect your spiritual wellness. Fortunately, the converse is true also. A sufficient amount of physical flexibility boosts your overall physical functioning and enhances all the dimensions of your life.

Flexibility, our topic in this chapter, is a key component of health-related fitness, but despite the recent popularity of activities like Pilates and yoga, flexibility is often neglected. You can easily find information about aerobic or strength-training activities, but you'll rarely see an article about flexibility or hear from friends about their stretching routine. This is unfortunate because, just like the other components of fitness, flexibility affects all the dimensions of wellness and your day-to-day living.

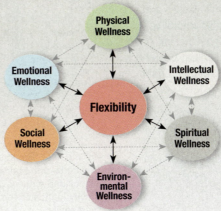

Factors Affecting Flexibility

Q | Why are some people more flexible than others?

As discussed in Chapter 3, **flexibility** is the ability of a joint to move through its full range of motion. You don't need an extremely high level of flexibility for good fitness and wellness. The goal of flexibility training is to be able to move a joint through its normal range of motion without experiencing pain or being limited in the performance of activities of daily living. Both too little and too much flexibility can be detrimental.

flexibility The ability of a joint to move through its full range of motion.

Flexibility is highly variable from person to person and joint to joint. A number of factors contribute to your level of flexibility—some of these are under your control, but others cannot be affected by training.

Joint Structure

Q | Why are some of my joints more flexible than others?

Some of your joints are designed to have a greater range of motion than others; in addition, your flexibility varies from joint to joint due to other factors.

A joint is a place where two or more bones meet. The structure of a joint plays a role in its range of motion. Some joints are designed to move very little, such as the ones

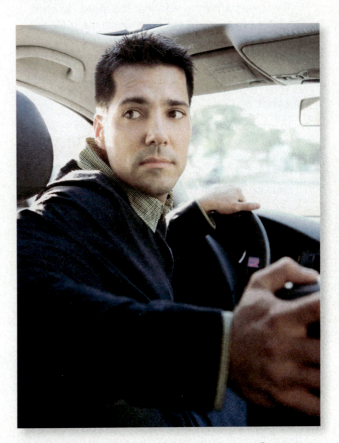

An extremely high level of flexibility isn't necessary for most people. Your goal should be a range of motion in your joints that allows you to perform daily activities easily and without pain.

Behavior-Change Challenge
Getting Back to a Healthy Back

At the start of school, you hurt your back helping a friend move a reclining chair up three flights of stairs. For a few weeks now, you've been experiencing moderate low-back pain. You've missed some classes and work. The pain has also kept you from intramural volleyball and your workouts, so you are getting out of shape—and have gained some weight. What behavior changes do you need to make in order to regain your fitness and your back health?

Meet Elena

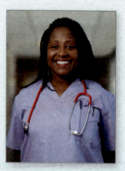

Elena, a nursing student, began having back pain after lifting a heavy piece of equipment without using the proper technique. At the advice of a doctor at her campus health center, she started a physical therapy program in which she did back-strengthening and stretching exercises at least twice a week. She also made it a point to sit and stand straight and avoided further heavy lifting. In addition, she dieted to shed the extra weight she'd put on while studying for her difficult exams last year. For continued maintenance, she is taking yoga classes. Gradually, Elena has gotten back to her pain-free self.

How might you benefit from Elena's experience? Consider:

- To what campus and community resources might you turn for professional advice and for therapy if it's needed?
- How can you modify your habits and daily tasks to avoid injuring your back again?

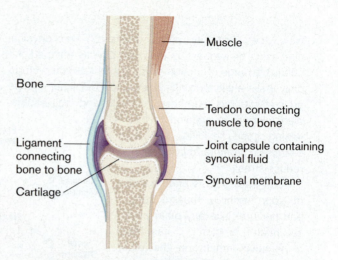

Figure 6-1 Basic structure of a joint. Inside the joint capsule, the ends of the bones are covered by cartilage that absorbs shock and reduces friction; the synovial fluid inside the joint cavity lubricates the tissues and helps the joint move smoothly and easily.

- Muscles connected to tendons around the joint contract and move the bones.

Problems with any of these components, including injury, inflammation, or stiffness, can limit a joint's range of motion.

The shape of the cartilage-covered surfaces and the way in which bones come together determine how—and how much—a joint can move. For example, elbow joints function somewhat like a hinge and primarily bend up and down in one direction. The hips and shoulders are ball-and-socket joints, in which the rounded end of one bone fits into a cup-shaped depression in the other bone. This type of joint allows for the widest range of motion, but it is less stable and has a greater risk of injury than other more stable types of joints.

Because each joint has a different structure, your relative flexibility varies from joint to joint, reflecting the principle of specificity (see Chapter 3). For example, you may have normal range of motion in your hips but limited mobility in your shoulders. For this reason, no single test can measure overall flexibility.

Connective Tissues and Nervous System Action

Q | How can I be more flexible? | You become more flexible by increasing the range of motion in a joint. The precise mechanisms are still being studied, but it is thought

cartilage A type of stiff but flexible tissue in various areas of the body, including joints, the ears and nose, and parts of the rib cage; it is not as hard as bone but stiffer than muscle.

joint capsule A sac or envelope enclosing a synovial joint, with an inner layer (the synovial membrane), which secretes synovial fluid, and a fibrous outer layer.

synovial fluid Fluid that lubricates and nourishes the tissues in the cavity of a synovial joint.

ligament Fibrous tissue that connects bone to bone.

where the bones of your skull come together. Others, like those in your spine, allow small movements. Joints such as those in your hips, shoulders, and limbs are called *synovial joints* and move much more freely. Figure 6-1 illustrates the main components of synovial joints:

- **Cartilage** covers and cushions the ends of the bones that meet in the joint, reducing friction as the joint moves and serving as a shock absorber.
- A fibrous **joint capsule** surrounds the joint; the inner layer of the capsule, known as the *synovial membrane,* surrounds the joint cavity and secretes **synovial fluid,** which lubricates and nourishes the tissues inside the cavity.
- **Ligaments** inside and around the joint connect the bones and provide stability.

that increases in range of motion occur through changes in the **connective tissues**—fibrous matter that provides support and structure—in muscles, tendons, and ligaments.[1] (Muscle fibers themselves aren't connective tissue, but they are held together in bundles by sheaths of connective tissues.) All the connective tissues affect your flexibility, but the tissues in your tendons and muscles probably play the largest role.

Both the length of tissues and their tolerance of stretching may affect flexibility.[2] **Collagen** is the key component of tendons, ligaments, and the connective tissue within muscle. It typically has a wavy structure when relaxed, but when stretched, the fibers first straighten and align and then may elongate as additional stretching force is applied. The overlapping fibers in muscle tissue shift to decrease the amount of overlap, also allowing tissues to elongate. Because connective tissues have elastic properties, they snap back to almost their resting length. Over time, however, the elasticity and resting length of some tissues may increase as they are repeatedly stretched, and these increases expand the joint's range of motion.

Tolerance of stretching has an important role in increasing flexibility.[3] When you hold a stretch for a period of time and then repeat the stretch, you will begin to feel less pain when you apply the same force of stretch. Although the exact mechanism isn't entirely clear, this increase in stretch tolerance increases range of motion. Changes in the activities of sensors and nerves in and around the joint and its associated muscles and tendons may reduce the pain felt during the stretch and allow for greater flexibility.[4]

Injury and Disease

Q | I recently recovered from a knee injury and don't have the same movement. Will I get it back?

Probably. Immobilization of bones and joints by casts or braces can lead to a loss in range of motion, but this is usually temporary. Loss of flexibility from the injury itself depends on the type and extent of your injury. In many cases, flexibility and strength exercises will help you maintain as much of your normal movement and strength as possible as you recover.

Some injuries can have longer-term effects on flexibility. For example, the condition known as *frozen shoulder,* in which the joint capsule thickens and contracts, causing pain and stiffness, can take 6 months to 2 years to resolve. Frozen shoulder affects about 10 percent of the general population and 30 percent of people with diabetes at some time in their lives.[5]

Osteoarthritis, which occurs when the cartilage inside a joint breaks down, is a common disease that affects flexibility. More than 20 million Americans have osteoarthritis; risk factors include obesity, age, injury, and overuse. Loss of range of motion in people with arthritis is associated

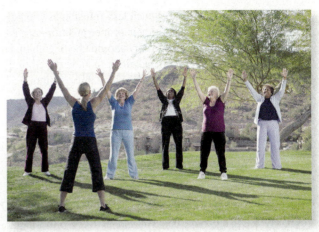

Although aging and osteoarthritis decrease range of motion, exercises to maintain flexibility can reduce pain and disability and prevent injuries.

with increased disability.[6] Treatment for osteoarthritis often includes strengthening and stretching exercises to help stabilize joints and improve range of motion and overall physical functioning.

Genetics

Q | Do double-jointed people have a higher flexibility level than others?

Some people are more flexible than others, and genetics is one reason for individual differences—for being a little or a lot more flexible than average.[7] Some people have extreme levels of flexibility: **Hypermobility** in a joint, or what some refer to as double-jointedness, runs in families and is thought to have a genetic basis. The prefix *hyper-* means "over" or "beyond." So people who are hypermobile are too flexible; their joints move beyond the normal range of motion. Specific examples of hypermobility include being able to bend your thumb to your forearm, bend your little finger backward to a 90-degree angle, bend forward with your knees straight and place your hands flat on the floor, and hyperextend your knees or elbows 10 degrees beyond their natural, straight position.

For some people, hypermobility causes no problems. However, hypermobile joints are less stable and can be more prone to injury and arthritis.[8] Muscles have to work harder to stabilize a hypermobile joint during activity, potentially causing muscle fatigue and reduced performance. Showing off hypermobile joints may have been a way to amuse your friends when

connective tissue A type of fibrous tissue in many body organs and systems, often providing support and structure; it may be soft and flexible or hard and rigid. Cartilage and bone are both types of connective tissue.

collagen Key protein in bone, cartilage, ligaments, tendons, skin, and connective tissue.

osteoarthritis Inflammation of the joint, usually involving damage to the cartilage-covered surfaces in the joint.

hypermobility Excessive range of motion in a joint, making it less stable and more susceptible to injury.

you were young, but it can be much less amusing as you age if your joints do not return to their proper position as easily. People with joint hypermobility should check with their health care provider; recommendations include developing and maintaining strong muscles to help stabilize joints.

Sex

Q Are women more flexible than men?

Although there is a broad range of flexibility within each sex, in general, yes, females are more flexible than males. Women's greater flexibility is primarily due to anatomical and hormonal differences. Larger muscles are less flexible and can block free movement at a joint, and men tend to have larger muscles than women. Women's wider hips contribute to their greater flexibility in the pelvic region and lower body. (Women have a wider pelvis to allow for childbirth.) Researchers have found that hormone levels also affect flexibility: Women have greater range of motion during certain points in the menstrual cycle.[9] Also, hormones released during pregnancy substantially relax women's joints to prepare the body, especially the pelvis, for delivery.

Use and Age

Q Why are people less flexible as they get older?

As with other areas of fitness, the "use it or lose it" adage is true. When considering flexibility, it's difficult to separate the effects of disuse from the effects of aging because the two often go together.

Once you have passed puberty, the only way to maintain your flexibility is through activity that utilizes the full range of motion of your joints. In your teens and twenties, you are likely to participate in recreational or competitive activities that do so. As you age, however, you will probably be less likely to include these activities in your regular routine. The problems that result from this decrease in activity are sometimes compounded by occupations or daily routines that require long hours of sitting or poor postural positions. In addition, the direct effects of aging and wear and tear over time—resulting in degeneration of collagen fibers and joint structures—adversely affect joints' flexibility.[10] Also, weight gain often comes with aging, and body-fat deposits can impair flexibility by physically blocking a joint from moving through its full range of motion.

Without regular full-range-of-motion activities, tissues may shorten and tighten. In most instances, activities designed to improve flexibility are necessary to prevent significant declines in flexibility. The human tendency to become less flexible with aging is primarily a result of inactivity rather than of the aging process itself. Studies have shown that unless people have an injury-related trauma or disease, a regular routine of flexibility exercises can

Fast Facts

Stretch and Bend

Ever wonder if you could be an acrobat or a contortionist? In getting at that question, consider that most contortionists have an unusually high degree of natural flexibility, enhanced through significant training. Most excel at one particular skill—such as front-bending, back-bending, over-splitting, or squeezing into a small container—depending on which way their spine is most flexible. Contortionists generally do not dislocate their joints when they flex or extend them very far. Studies have shown that despite their high degree of flexibility, contortionists can develop joint problems, including fractures.

- Do you know someone who is hypermobile? What makes that person so?
- How might this characteristic increase risk for injury?

Source: Peoples, R. R., Perkins, T. G., Powell, J. W., Hanson, E. H., Snyder, T. H., Mueller, T. L., & Orrison, W. W. (2008). Whole-spine dynamic magnetic resonance study of contortionists: Anatomy and pathology. *Journal of Neurosurgery: Spine, 8*(6), 501–509.

preserve sufficient flexibility throughout the life span—range of motion may decrease, but it will remain at a level that allows safe and effective movement. Studies also indicate that people of any age can benefit from beginning an appropriate flexibility-exercise routine.[11]

Benefits of Flexibility

Like the other components of health-related fitness, flexibility is needed so that you can perform your daily functions easily and efficiently and reduce your likelihood of injury. Other benefits of flexibility and stretching exercises are improved posture and reduced stress.

Improved Performance

Q Will flexibility help me play basketball better?

Possibly. As we considered in earlier chapters, performing stretching exercises right before an activity, such as basketball, that requires a high degree of muscle power can harm performance in the short term because stretching can temporarily decrease peak muscle force.[12] On the other hand, for gymnastics, diving, and other sports in which joints move through extreme ranges of motion, stretching exercises beforehand may improve performance.

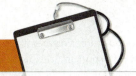

Research Brief

Stretch for Strength Gains

Are you new to strength training? If so, research indicates that you may become stronger faster if you also do regular stretching.

In a study of college students who were novice lifters, researchers paired students who had comparable starting strength. They assigned one student from each pair to a strength-training group and the other student to a strength-training-plus-stretching group. All the students did three sets of strength-training exercises 3 days a week; the stretching group also stretched twice a week for 30 minutes. After 8 weeks of progressive strength-training with knee-flexion, knee-extension, and leg-press exercises, the two groups were compared. Both groups significantly improved, but the strength-training-plus-stretching group had significantly greater gains in strength (see table, left bottom).

Analyze and Apply

- What does this study mean for your potential gains in strength if you're just starting a strength-training program?
- What do you think contributed to the additional gains in the strength-training-plus-stretching group?

Source: Kokkonen, J., Nelson, A. G., Tarawhiti, T., Buckingham, P., & Winchester, J. B. (2010). Early-phase resistance training strength gains in novice lifters are enhanced by doing static stretching. *Journal of Strength and Conditioning Research, 24*(2), 502–506.

	Increase in 1-RM	
	Strength-training group	Strength-training-plus-stretching group
Knee flexion	12%	16%
Knee extension	14%	27%
Leg press	9%	31%

Over time, flexibility training has the potential to improve performance in these sports and other skilled activities. Most athletes develop an optimal range of motion required for their particular sport as a result of regular participation in it. An optimal level of flexibility will afford you greater efficiency in the movements required for your sport—in your case, basketball.

Different sports require different amounts of flexibility for optimal performance. For example, gymnasts, ice skaters, and divers need greater flexibility than runners, but runners need enough flexibility in their legs and hips to achieve good running mechanics.[13] However, as we have seen, too much flexibility can hurt performance: Hypermobility can increase the risk of injury and reduce speed, strength, and power needed for a sport.

Although you may think first of sports when you hear the word *performance,* flexibility is also important for the performance of routine daily activities. You need flexibility to climb stairs, put on your shoes, back up your car, take clothes out of the dryer, feed your pets, lift your backpack or your kids, put away the groceries, and hang pictures. Unfortunately, many of us don't think of performance in these terms until we have trouble with some of these activities. Maintaining a normal range of motion in your joints through flexibility training will allow you to go about your day-to-day tasks with ease and efficiency. For non-athletes, a stretching program, done over time, can improve exercise performance and measures of muscle strength.[14] See the box "Stretch for Strength Gains" for more information.

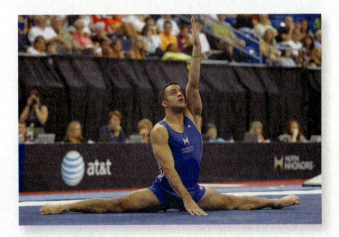

Only a few sports and activities—such as gymnastics, diving, dancing, and ice skating—require an extremely high level of flexibility for optimal performance.

Reduced Risk of Injury

 Does stretching prevent injuries?   It depends. The relationship between stretching, flexibility, and injury is somewhat controversial.[15] The answer to this question will depend on whether you're considering stretching's immediate effects on sport-injury risk or its longer-term effects on all types of injuries.

For many years, it was believed that stretching as part of a warm-up before an exercise session or competition would reduce muscle soreness and the risk of injury. Some more recent studies have not supported this idea, finding no reduction in sport injuries associated with stretching. Findings differ, however, depending on the type and intensity of the activity, the type of stretching, and other factors. When stretching is done as part of a warm-up, it can be difficult to distinguish the effects of stretching from the effects of the warm-up; warm-ups have been shown to reduce sport-injury risk. More research is needed, especially about different activities and stretching techniques. It may be that for each sport, a different combination of warm-up, stretches, and other pre-exercise activities will enhance performance and reduce injury risk.

What about the effects of stretching for non-athletes? Research findings have been mixed, but evidence suggests that routine stretching may reduce the rate of certain types of muscle and tendon injuries as well as some types of soreness from physical activity.[16] Stretching can also be a key component of rehabilitation of injuries—to return joints to a normal and healthy range of motion.[17]

Flexibility, along with muscular fitness, is also important for good posture, which in turn helps reduce joint strain and may decrease risk of certain types of injuries. Abnormal posture can strain ligaments and muscles and contribute to musculoskeletal problems, including low-back pain. For example, if the muscles and tendons in the front of your thighs and hips are tight, your back may be pulled into a more arched position than is normal. We will examine posture in greater detail later in this chapter.

Finally, maintaining flexibility in joints is critical as you age. If you don't stretch, your joints will stiffen—and having less than the normal range of motion in a joint increases your risk of injury. Loss of flexibility in the hips and ankles, for example, increases the risk of falls. Regular stretching will improve your flexibility and walking mechanics and reduce the risk of falls and associated injuries.[18]

Other Benefits of Flexibility and Stretching Exercises

Q | I feel better when I stretch after a workout. Does stretching help me relax?

Stretching exercises do have benefits beyond maintaining joint range of motion. As you have experienced, stretching can reduce muscle tension, blood pressure, and breathing rate—all indicative of a more relaxed physical state.[19] After stretching, people also report improved mood, reduced stress, and subjective feelings of relaxation. You can also use stretching to treat exercise-associated muscle cramps—painful muscle contractions that occur during or just after exercise.[20] If you get muscle cramps with exercise, try rest and stretching. (See the box "Flexible Body, Flexible Arteries?" for more on the benefits of stretching.)

Assessing Your Flexibility

Flexibility is assessed in several ways; there is no single test to assess flexibility because it is not a single general characteristic of the body. Rather, it is very specific to each joint.[21] Remember that more flexibility isn't necessarily better; your goal should be a normal range of motion in all your major joints.

Q | How is flexibility rated?

The most common test for flexibility is the sit-and-reach test, which primarily reflects the range of motion of the hamstrings. Lab Activity 6-1 includes instructions and norms for the

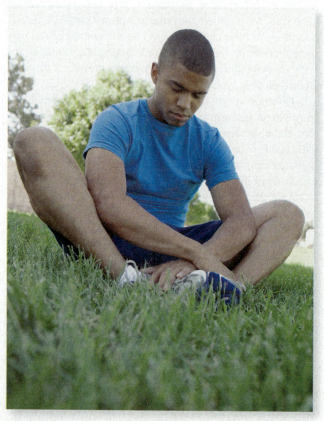

Stretching exercises can relieve stress by reducing muscle tension, blood pressure, and breathing rate.

Research Brief

Flexible Body, Flexible Arteries?

Healthy arteries are elastic, meaning they can expand to accommodate increased blood volume and then snap back to their original size. Stiff arteries are a risk factor for high blood pressure, heart disease, and death. Arteries become stiffer as we age, and physical activity has been shown to delay the process. But how does flexibility affect the arteries?

Researchers recently looked for an association between body flexibility and arterial flexibility in a group of healthy adults ranging in age from 20 to 83. They measured body flexibility using the sit-and-reach test, and they measured blood pressure and blood flow. For participants age 40 and older, there was a strong association between trunk flexibility and arterial stiffening: The more flexible people had more elastic arteries; they also had lower blood pressure, another sign of a healthy cardiorespiratory system. The findings were independent of cardiorespiratory fitness and muscular strength.

The researchers considered several possibilities in trying to explain the link between body flexibility and arterial flexibility. Arteries are made of many of the same types of tissues as muscles and tendons and so may be affected by some of the same factors, including stretching. In addition, stretching exercises cause short-term activation of the nervous system, which may reduce nervous-system activity at rest. (This is similar to the relationship of aerobic exercise and blood pressure—the short-term effect of exercise is to raise blood pressure, but in the long term, exercise reduces resting blood pressure.) Lower resting nervous-system activity may reduce both arterial stiffness and blood pressure.

More research is needed to determine the underlying mechanisms, but in the meantime, this study provides more evidence that a lifetime of stretching exercises will help you maintain good flexibility—in more ways than one.

Analyze and Apply

- What might be the connection between muscular flexibility and arterial flexibility?
- What other "hidden" benefits might be gained from increased flexibility?

Source: Yamamoto, K., Kawano, H., Gando, Y., and others. (2009). Poor trunk flexibility is associated with arterial stiffening. *American Journal of Physiology—Heart and Circulatory Physiology, 297,* H1314–H1318.

sit-and-reach test. For other joints, range of motion is measured with other tests. Lab Activity 6-1 includes assessments for shoulder, hamstring, and hip-flexor range of motion. There are no precise flexibility measures associated with peak performance or wellness, but averages can provide points of reference to help you determine if any of your joints have a range of motion that is significantly below normal.

The most important preparation for flexibility assessments is to warm up beforehand; you can stretch farther and more safely after a warm-up. Before you complete the flexibility tests in the lab activities, see Table 6-1 for factors that can affect your scores. You'll also want to take several of these factors into account when you plan and carry out your regular stretching program.

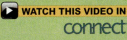

MYTH or FACT?

Static stretching before activities like sprinting or jumping decreases performance.

▶ **WATCH THIS VIDEO IN** connect

See page 476 to find out.

Q | How flexible should I be?

Unless you participate in a sport or an activity that requires significant flexibility, a good goal for a flexibility program is to achieve and maintain a normal range of motion in all your major joints. How did you score on the flexibility assessments in the lab activities? If you are significantly less flexible in one joint than the others, you might want to give special attention to it in your stretching program—but you should continue to stretch all your joints regularly. If you don't currently do any flexibility training, then a good goal is to start now.

Putting Together a Flexibility Program

As with any other component of fitness, flexibility must be purposely addressed. Exercises specifically designed to build and maintain flexibility should be a regular part of your routine. Although you may not feel that you need flexibility exercises at this point in your life, incorporating them into your routine will help you to maintain your flexibility. To reduce your likelihood of injuries later, develop good habits now. To put together a safe and effective program, consider the types of training and then apply the FITT formula.

Flexibility Training Techniques

Though you have already read that stretching is a type of exercise that affects your flexibility, you may not be aware of the different types of stretching you can use

TABLE 6-1 FACTORS THAT AFFECT FLEXIBILITY TESTS

FACTOR	CONSIDER THIS
TIME OF DAY	Most people are more flexible in the afternoon.
TEMPERATURE OF THE ROOM AND YOUR MUSCLES	Most people can stretch farther in a warm room and after they've completed a warm-up consisting of 5–10 minutes of light aerobic activity.
YOUR CLOTHING	Nonrestrictive clothing allows for easier stretching.
SORENESS OR INJURIES	Because soreness or an injury can limit flexibility, try to delay testing until you are pain-free. Always take care not to aggravate an existing problem.
YOUR LEVEL OF COMPETITIVENESS	Will you be in a group setting for testing? Do you have a competitive nature or a high pain tolerance that might cause you to push yourself too far?
YOUR ABILITY TO RELAX	You are likely to feel tense during testing if the situation is new to you. Try to relax and follow the specific guidelines for each test.
HUMAN ERROR	Will your testers know how to administer the tests? You may not have a choice, but keep this factor in mind when evaluating your scores.

Q What is the best way to stretch? What are the different kinds of stretches, and what are the benefits of each?

to increase or maintain flexibility. Stretching techniques include static stretching, ballistic stretching, dynamic stretching, and proprioceptive neuromuscular facilitation (PNF).

STATIC STRETCHING. In **static stretching,** you stretch each muscle group using a slow, steady stretch with a hold at the end of the range of motion. You relax the muscle being stretched as it lengthens. Because you hold the stretch for a while and then repeat it, you can usually stretch a little farther as your tissues adjust to the stretch.

Static stretching may be performed either actively or passively. In **active stretching,** you take an *active* role by contracting the muscles opposite those being stretched; the force for the stretch comes from your own muscle contraction. In **passive stretching,** you allow an outside force, rather than the contraction of a muscle group, to assist in the stretching. The external force for a passive stretch can be provided by another person, an object, gravity, or another body part. For example, to stretch your calves actively, you could sit on the ground with your legs out in front of you and contract the muscles in your shins to pull your toes back. To stretch the same muscle group passively, you could perform the exercise in the same seated position, but with a partner providing the force to gently move your toes back rather than using your own muscles. You could also do a passive stretch of the calf in a standing position by using the floor for resistance to move your toes closer to your shins without contracting the opposing muscle group (Figure 6-2). Static

stretching is a widely recommended technique because it is safe and easy to learn, may be performed without a partner or special equipment, and can be done fairly quickly.

BALLISTIC STRETCHING. In **ballistic stretching,** you use quick jerky or bouncing movements to stretch your joints and move them to the ends of their typical range of motion—and beyond it. Ballistic stretching uses the momentum of body movement to produce the force required to lengthen the muscles and other tissues; the endpoint of the stretch is not held. This type of stretching is effective for increasing flexibility, but because it is less controlled than other types of stretching, there is greater potential for overstretching, soreness, and injury. Ballistic stretching is generally not recommended for most people, but athletes in certain sports use it, especially if the activity involves ballistic movements such as throwing, kicking, running, and batting.

DYNAMIC STRETCHING. Like ballistic stretching, **dynamic stretching** involves movement. However, dynamic stretching uses controlled movement through the active range of motion for a joint rather than bouncing movement at the endpoints of the range of motion. For example, a lunge position

static stretching
A stretching technique that involves a slow, steady stretch with a hold at the end of the range of motion.

active stretching
A stretching technique in which the force for the stretch comes from a contraction of the muscles opposite those being stretched.

passive stretching
A stretching technique in which the force for a stretch comes from an object, a partner, or another body part.

ballistic stretching
A stretching technique that involves quick jerks or bounces to move joints to the ends of their range of motion; momentum provides the force for this stretch.

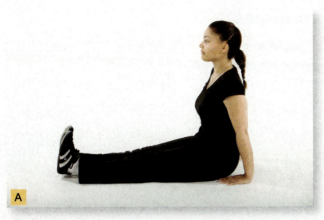

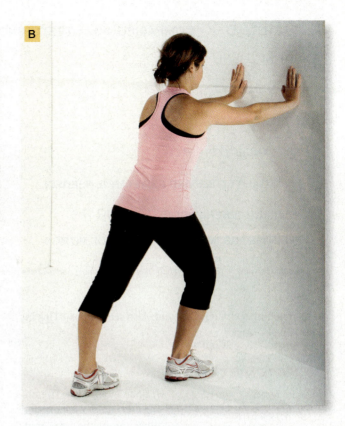

Figure 6-2 Active versus passive stretching. A. In an active stretch, the force for the stretch is provided by contraction of the opposing muscle group. B. In a passive stretch, the force comes from an outside source—another person, an object, gravity, or another body part—rather than from one's own muscle contraction.

stretches the hamstrings and the front of the hip. In a static stretch, you would slowly and gently move into the lunge position and hold it. In a ballistic stretch, you would repeatedly bounce in the lunge position at the end of the range of motion. In a dynamic stretch, you would do a series of lunges, moving through the full range of motion of a lunge in a controlled manner. For many dynamic stretches, completing the movement safely and with good form requires muscular strength and endurance.

Dynamic stretching has been found to be particularly useful as a prelude to other activities. For example, some athletes like to use this type of stretching in conjunction with a warm-up before an event because it elevates body and muscle temperature and may help prepare the body for optimum performance.[22]

PROPRIOCEPTIVE NEUROMUSCULAR FACILITATION. **Proprioceptive neuromuscular facilitation (PNF)** is group of techniques originally developed for rehabilitation; it has become a popular form of stretching in recent years. PNF techniques are designed to affect both connective tissues and nerves in order to increase flexibility; they typically combine muscle contraction and stretching. Some PNF stretches require a partner or another source of resistance. Here are two basic PNF techniques applied to a hamstring stretch:

- *Contract-relax:* After an initial stretch, you contract the muscle being stretched isometrically (6 seconds) against resistance. Then relax and stretch again. You should be able to stretch farther during the second and subsequent stretches. An example is an assisted stretch of the hamstring, in which a partner aids in a static hamstring stretch by pushing the extended leg gently toward your torso and provides resistance for the isometric contraction by stabilizing, or pushing against, your leg as you try to push it toward your partner (see Figure 6-3).

- *Contract-relax-opposite contract:* You perform a contract-relax stretch as just described, but during the second stretch, you assist the stretch by actively contracting the opposing muscle group. For example, during the second static hamstring stretch, you contract the muscles on the front of your leg (quadriceps) and hip to extend the stretch. This additional contraction is thought to elicit a reaction and a stretching of the target muscle group.

Although they are an effective means of increasing flexibility, PNF techniques are not often used for regular stretching routines because they require more time and often the use of partner. Like other stretching techniques, it isn't entirely clear why PNF stretching works—whether through changes to tissue length or changes to stretch tolerance, or both—but it does increase flexibility.[23]

Table 6-2 compares the three stretching techniques. Among the techniques described here, static stretching is the most widely recommended for general fitness. For this reason, the discussion in the next section about applying the FITT formula—as well as the sample exercises at the end of the chapter—are based on static stretching techniques. If you are an athlete involved in specialized activities or high-performance events, talk to your coach or trainer about the

dynamic stretching
A stretching technique that involves controlled movement through the active range of motion of a joint.

proprioceptive neuromuscular facilitation (PNF)
A group of stretching techniques that combine stretching and muscle contraction; the most common PNF techniques combine passive stretching and isometric contraction.

TABLE 6-2   COMPARISON OF STRETCHING TECHNIQUES

FACTOR	SLOW STATIC	BALLISTIC	PNF
RISK OF INJURY	Low	High	Medium
DEGREE OF PAIN	Low	Medium	High
RESISTANCE TO STRETCH	Low	High	Medium
PRACTICALITY (TIME AND ASSISTANCE NEEDED)	Excellent	Good	Poor
EFFICIENCY (ENERGY CONSUMPTION)	Excellent	Poor	Poor
EFFECTIVE FOR INCREASING RANGE OF MOTION	Good	Good	Excellent

Source: Heyward, V. (2010). *Advanced fitness assessment and exercise prescription* (6th ed.). Champaign, IL: Human Kinetics.

best stretching techniques for you. Also see the box "Tips for Safe Yoga Practice."

Applying the FITT Formula

Q | Can stretching hurt my muscles?

If done incorrectly, stretching can cause soreness and other problems. As with other components of fitness, the best way to avoid injury is to plan your exercise routine carefully. Applying the FITT formula (<u>f</u>requency, <u>i</u>ntensity, <u>t</u>ime, and <u>t</u>ype) to your flexibility training can help you come up with a sensible plan.

Q | How often should I stretch?

FREQUENCY. Most experts agree that you should perform stretching exercises at a minimum of two or three times per week.[24] Stretching every day isn't harmful and won't hurt the development of flexibility. As with all types of exercise, start with a

relatively low frequency if you are a beginner. Then work your way up to as many days per week as your comfort and schedule allow. You can incorporate stretching into training sessions for cardiorespiratory or muscular fitness; you don't have to schedule separate stretching workouts.

Q | How do I determine the right amount of stretch?

INTENSITY. Because flexibility is specific to each joint, you will have a different threshold and target zone for each exercise. You can't quantify these concepts as you can in other areas; you have to use your own abilities and perceptions to determine the appropriate levels of stretching.

As you perform each movement, stretch to the point where you feel *slight tension* or *mild tightness* but not discomfort or pain. This point of slight tension is your threshold. Once you reach the threshold, move slowly and carefully just *slightly* beyond it into your target zone. If you need to quantify this effort in your mind, imagine your threshold to be 75 percent of your maximum and your desired target zone to be 85 percent (or slightly above the threshold) of your maximum.

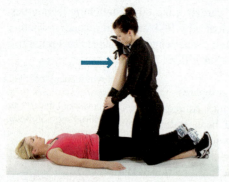

Figure 6-3 **Contract-relax PNF stretch of the hamstring.** After a passive static stretch of the hamstring, you push against a partner for a 6-second isometric contraction of the hamstring and then you do another passive static stretch. You could also use a towel or strap around your foot or ankle to provide resistance for the isometric stretch and force for the passive stretch.

Q | How long should I stretch?

TIME. The total time for your flexibility training depends on the type of stretches you do. A workout based on

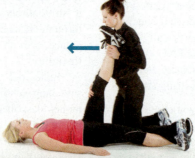

Wellness Strategies

Tips for Safe Yoga Practice

Q | Is yoga a way to do flexibility training?

Yoga is an effective way to build flexibility as well as to improve muscle fitness, balance, and coordination and to reduce stress. Keep these tips in mind when thinking about starting a yoga program:

- Although you can learn yoga at home from a book or DVD, learn with an instructor if you are a beginner. As with any new information or activity related to your well-being, do your research. Look for a yoga instructor who is highly trained—one who recognizes the variety of ability levels in a class and can adjust activities appropriately.
- Ask about the physical demands of the type of yoga in which you are interested, as well as the training and experience of the yoga teacher you are considering.
- Ask the instructor about any concerns you have—for example, whether a class is aimed at your goal (such as increased flexibility) and what you should bring to class (a mat or towel, for instance).
- If you have a medical condition, consult with your health-care provider before starting yoga. Yoga is generally safe, but people with certain medical conditions should not use some yoga practices. For example, people with disk or inflammatory disease of the spine, extremely high or low blood pressure, glaucoma, fragile arteries, a risk of blood clots, ear problems,

or severe osteoporosis should avoid some inverted poses.

- Although yoga during pregnancy is safe if practiced under expert guidance, after about the twentieth week of pregnancy, pregnant women should avoid poses that involve lying flat on the back.
- Always warm up to prepare your body for activity.
- Don't push yourself beyond the limits of your strength or flexibility to perform a specific pose. Don't force your body into a position that is difficult for you. Listen to your body and use common sense and self-awareness.
- Review the guidelines in this chapter regarding the intensity of stretches (see the section "Intensity"). Ask the instructor about alternative poses or methods. Your instructor should provide modifications appropriate for people at different levels of flexibility and yoga experience.

Sources: Adapted from National Center for Complementary and Alternative Medicine. (2008). *Yoga for health: An introduction* (http://nccam.nih.gov/health/yoga/introduction.htm). Crews, L. (2006, February). Injury prevention: Yoga. *IDEA Fitness Journal* (http://www.ideafit.com/fitness-library/injury-prevention-yoga).

---

static stretches will typically require the shortest amount of time. The American College of Sports Medicine (ACSM) recommends that for static stretches, each stretch be performed four or more times and held for 15–60 seconds each time.[25] Because you should do stretches for all major joints (muscle/tendon groups), the minimum time for a complete flexibility training cycle is about 10–15 minutes. A longer time would be required for a larger number of stretches or for different training techniques. If you haven't been stretching recently, you might start out with a small number of repetitions and short "holds" and then work your way up as your body adjusts to the training.

Q | Is stretching considered physical activity?

Yes, stretching is physical activity. However, time spent stretching doesn't count toward total daily or weekly aerobic or muscle-fitness time if you are measuring your activity time against the Department of Health and Human Services physical activity guidelines.[26]

Q | What are the best stretches?

TYPE. Your program should include a stretch for each major muscle/tendon group or joint: neck, shoulders, upper and lower back, pelvis, hips, and legs. As described in Table 6-3, one of the principles for flexibility training is the principle of specificity. The sample exercises on pp. 214–220 include choices for each, and Lab Activity 6-2 can guide you in setting up a flexibility program that fits your needs. You may want to do additional exercises for joints or areas where tests show that your range of motion is below average. The exercises at the end of this chapter are not the only choices for flexibility training; if you'd like to try dynamic or PNF stretches, check with your instructor or a trainer at a fitness facility. See the box "Flexibility Program Planning: FITT."

Q | Are there any stretches that are unsafe?

Yes. Certain stretches can place too much strain on your joints. Avoid stretches involving full bends of the knee, significant arching or rounding of the lower back, and

Wellness Strategies

Flexibility Program Planning: FITT

Q | How do I determine what the right amount of stretching is and what is safe to do solo?

The ACSM recommends the following basic program:

- **Frequency:** 2–3 days per week or more.
- **Intensity:** Stretch to the point of slight tension or mild tightness.

- **Time:** Hold the stretch for 15–60 seconds, and do four or more repetitions of each stretch.
- **Type:** Perform a stretch for each major muscle/tendon group or joint: neck, shoulders, upper and lower back, pelvis, hips, and legs.

And remember: Always warm up before you stretch.

TABLE 6-3 FLEXIBILITY AND TRAINING PRINCIPLES

WARM-UP AND COOL-DOWN	Warm muscles stretch farther. If you have not already warmed up, begin with a few minutes of light aerobic activity. Because most flexibility training isn't done at a heart-rate-raising intensity, cool-down is not as critical as with some other types of exercise. If you tend to push yourself too hard or go too quickly through your stretches, playing soothing music can help you maintain a slower pace. You can also follow your routine with a few deep-breathing exercises to help your body relax further.
SPECIFICITY	Choose exercises that will allow you to work specifically on each major muscle/tendon group. If you tested below average in a specific area, you may want to add additional exercises for it.
PROGRESSIVE OVERLOAD	Progressive overload happens naturally during static stretching exercises. You may be stretching farther (overloading) before you even realize it. Don't focus on stretching farther; instead, concentrate on the point of slight tension. If you're motivated by fitness-test results, you can repeat the assessment procedures after several weeks of training to see changes in your flexibility.
REVERSIBILITY	Although loss of flexibility is rarely as noticeable when you are young as are decreases in other fitness components, don't forget the factors discussed at the beginning of the chapter. Age and use play a big role in maintaining or increasing your flexibility.

pressure on the neck, especially when bent. Some widely known stretches aren't the best choices; see Figure 6-4 for alternatives.

Low-Back Fitness

Q | Why did my mother always nag me to sit up straight? Other than making me look a little better, what difference does it make?

Your mother was right to stress the importance of good posture. Poor posture gives the appearance of low self-esteem and apathy, and it can also have negative effects on your health. To see why, you must first understand the structure and function of your spine, as well as body mechanics.

Structure and Function of the Spine

The *spinal cord* is a long, thin bundle of nerves, fluid, and support cells that extends from the brain down the back. The spinal cord is enclosed in the bony *spinal column,* also called the backbone or spine (Figure 6-5). A healthy spine appears straight if you look at it from the back, but it has natural curves when viewed from the side. The human spine is made up of five sections of 33 individual bones called **vertebrae:**

- The cervical, or neck, section of the spine has seven vertebrae.
- The thoracic, or upper back, section has twelve vertebrae.
- The lumbar, or lower back, section has five vertebrae.
- The sacrum is formed by five fused vertebrae.
- The coccyx or tailbone is formed by four fused vertebrae.

Ligaments and muscles surround the spine to provide support and to aid movement.

Though they vary slightly in size and structure, the vertebrae in the top three sections of the spine have a similar design and characteristics; the vertebrae in the lower two sections are smaller and shaped differently. The vertebrae in the upper three sections

vertebra One of the 33 ring-like bones that make up the spine; together, they provide structural support, help protect the spinal cord, and aid in movement.

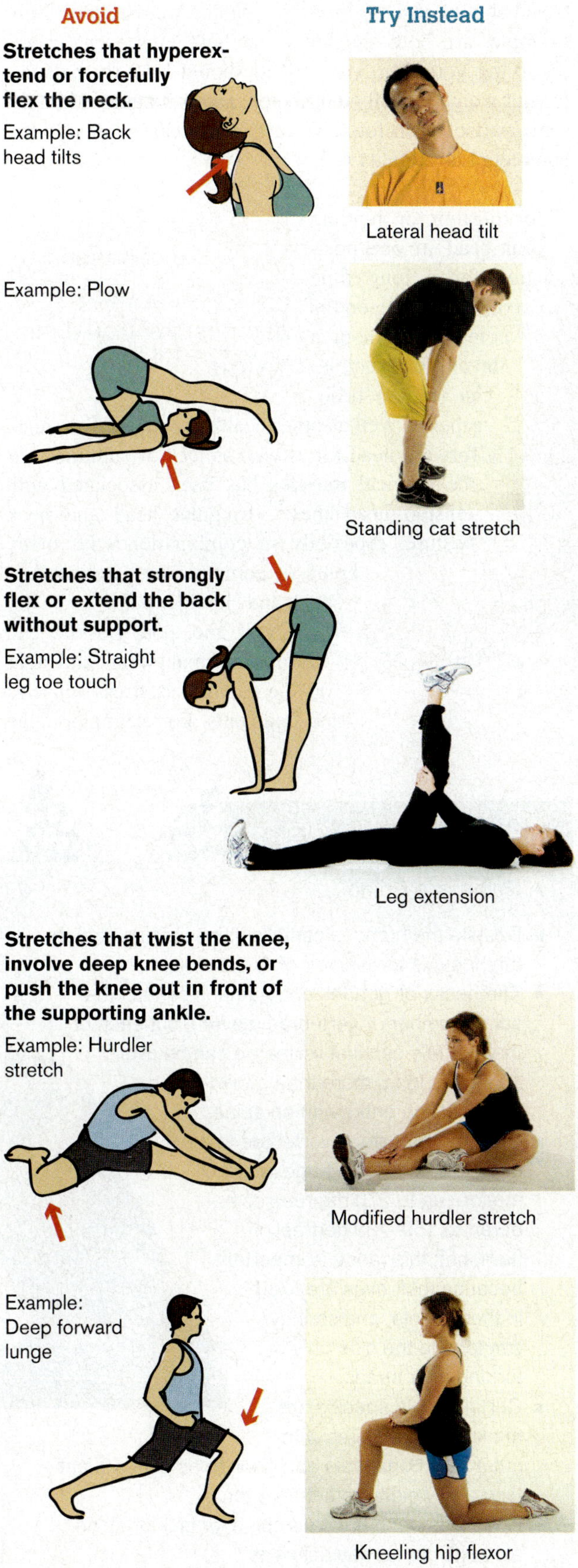

Avoid

Stretches that hyperextend or forcefully flex the neck.

Example: Back head tilts

Example: Plow

Stretches that strongly flex or extend the back without support.

Example: Straight leg toe touch

Stretches that twist the knee, involve deep knee bends, or push the knee out in front of the supporting ankle.

Example: Hurdler stretch

Example: Deep forward lunge

Try Instead

Lateral head tilt

Standing cat stretch

Leg extension

Modified hurdler stretch

Kneeling hip flexor

Figure 6-4 Types of stretches to avoid—and safer alternatives.

of the spinal column have a large, flat, cylindrical body that allows them to stack on top of one another. Between the vertebra are **intervertebral disks,** flat, elastic, gel-filled disks that act as shock absorbers and permit spinal column movement (see Figure 6-6). Protruding from the back of the body of the vertebrae is a horseshoe-shaped piece of bone with projections called *processes.* Like the body of the vertebra, this section of bone and its processes are sized and shaped differently in different locations in the spine. The special shapes of the processes form small synovial joints—the rounded end of a process on one vertebra fits into a matching hollow in a process on the neighboring vertebra. These joints both provide stability and allow for movement. The shapes of the vertebrae and processes create protected passageways for the spinal cord and for nerves that branch off the spinal cord and extend through the body.

The spinal column has many important functions, most of which you can probably guess from its structure:

- Provides structural support for the body
- Allows the upper body to bend and twist
- Protects the spinal cord and the roots of nerves
- Serves as an attachment site for muscles, tendons, and ligaments
- Supports and distributes much of the body's weight
- Absorbs impact and helps maintain balance

A healthy spine is essential for living an active life.

Understanding Body Mechanics and Good Posture

Q What does body mechanics mean?

Simply put, **body mechanics** is the application of basic mechanical principles to the human body. As a system made up primarily of levers, your body is designed to function optimally—that is, to perform activities in the most safe, efficient, and energy-conserving manner. Unfortunately, our habits and lifestyles tend to encourage poor mechanics more often than proper mechanics. Closely related to body mechanics is **posture,** or the position of body parts in relation to one another.

Q I think I have pretty good posture. Is there a way to tell?

Good posture is essential for optimal body function; good posture means that the body is properly aligned. To assess the condition of your posture, have a friend observe you from the side and from behind. From the side, your friend should look at your ear, shoulder, elbow, hip, knee, and mid-foot. Are these points in a straight line? From the back, your

intervertebral disk Fibrous, gel-filled disk between vertebrae that acts as a shock absorber and allows the spine to move.

body mechanics Application of basic mechanical principles to the human body.

posture Position of body parts in relation to each other.

friend should observe the same points. Are they level? For example, are both shoulders and both hips even? When observing your feet, your friend should look for balance. Is your weight equally distributed, and is it balanced on the same part of each foot? To further evaluate your posture, complete Lab Activity 6-3.

Poor posture or holding your head in one position for a long time (while working on the computer without a break, for example) can lead to head-aches as well as other health problems. Too much forward head tilt as well as lack of endurance of the cervical muscles has been associated with tension headaches.[27] Irregular head and neck posture, especially in combination with many hours of computer use, is linked to neck and shoulder pain.[28]

Q I've been told my headaches are probably caused by bad posture. Could this be true?

Over time, poor posture can cause abnormal wear and tear on the joints and stress muscles and ligaments. For example, if the

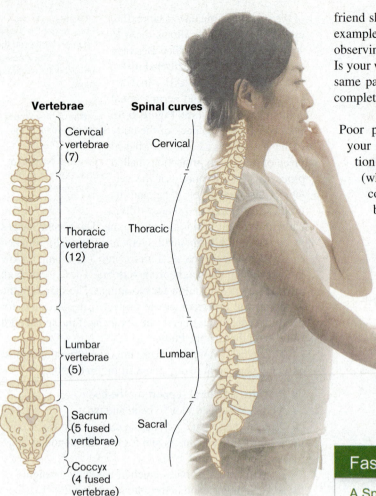

Figure 6-5 **The spine.** The spinal column is made up of five sections with a total of 33 individual bones called vertebrae. The spine is straight when viewed from the back but has natural curves when viewed from the side.

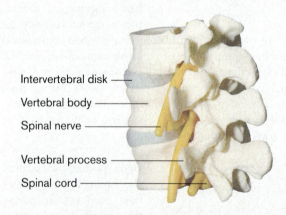

Figure 6-6 **Vertebrae and intervertebral disks.** The vertebrae are separated by flat, elastic, gel-filled disks. The processes that extend from the body of the vertebrae form small synovial joints, and the shapes of the vertebrae and processes create passageways for spinal nerves.

Fast Facts

A Spine Is a Spine . . .

- Despite the hump, a camel's spine is fairly straight; the hump is a reservoir of fatty tissue.
- The necks of giraffes and humans contain the same number of vertebrae (seven), but each of the giraffe's cervical vertebrae can be over 10 inches long, more than a third of the length of the entire human spine.
- Owls have fourteen vertebrae in their neck, giving them a huge range of motion (up to 270 degrees compared to 150–180 degrees in humans); this range is important because their eyes are fixed in the sockets, and so they can look to the side only by turning their heads.
- Certain squid species are the largest creatures without a backbone; they can grow to be over 40 feet long and weigh more than a ton.
- How does each animal's spine, or lack of spine, aid in its day-to-day activities?
- How does the structure of the human spine help to accommodate your day-to-day activities?

Research Brief

Heavy Backpack, Heavy Price

You know how tiring it can be to haul your books and supplies all over campus. But chances are, if your backpack is very heavy, you may be getting more than just tired—you may also be injuring yourself. Recent studies have investigated the high toll heavy backpacks can take on the body. An easily recognizable sign of an overweight backpack is discomfort that typically increases as the weight goes up. What else happens with increased backpack weight?

According to those recent studies, there's likely to be an increase in abdominal muscle activity and neck curvature, a decrease in mid- and lower-back curvature and pelvic tilt, and a possible decline in lung and breathing capacities. Furthermore, the longer you carry the backpack, the longer it takes for the body to reposition itself in its normal posture. Continued and/or prolonged use of heavy backpacks can increase the likelihood of injury. What may be even more surprising is that a heavy backpack can slow your walking speed and alter your perception of the environment, increasing your chances of being a casualty of a pedestrian-related accident. Research results indicate that participants with heavier packs walked more slowly, missed safe opportunities for crossing streets, left less time to spare when crossing, and experienced more frequent hits or close calls with a vehicle.

Many of the study samples were small, and more research is needed, but these results speak to the need to lighten your backpack load. Most studies agree that carrying 10 percent of a person's body weight is a reasonable backpack goal.

Analyze and Apply
- What impressed or surprised you most about the results of these studies?

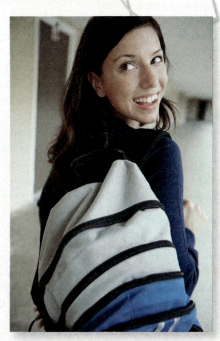

- How can you apply lessons from this research to your daily habits—in particular, to the weight you carry around in your backpack and/or in other carrying equipment?

Sources: Chow, D., and others. (2011). Carry-over effects of backpack carriage on trunk posture and repositioning ability. *International Journal of Industrial Ergonomics 41*(5), 530–535.

Dominelli, P., and others. (2011). Effect of carrying a weighted backpack on lung mechanics during treadmill walking in healthy men. *Medicine & Science in Sports & Exercise, 43*(5), 631.

Schwebel D., and others. (2009). The influence of carrying a backpack on college student pedestrian safety. *Accident Analysis and Prevention, 41*(2), 352–356.

Yusuf, S., and others.(2008). The effect of backpack heaviness on trunk–lower extremity muscle activities and trunk posture. *Gait & Posture, 28*(2), 297–302.

spine is misaligned, there may be pressure on the spinal nerves, resulting in pain. If the neck is tilted or the shoulders are hunched over, muscles become fatigued and weak, leading to muscle and joint pain and increasing the risk of injury. (See the box "Heavy Backpack, Heavy Price" for a good example.) Proper posture, on the other hand, can help prevent fatigue because the body can move with good body mechanics.

Poor posture has many causes. Postural problems can result from hereditary or congenital conditions, disease, or injuries that are beyond our control. The majority of postural problems, however, are within our control. Ill-fitting clothing, inappropriate furniture, and excessive sitting and standing in place can lead to poor posture, as can fatigue, excess weight, weak muscles, and emotional issues such as low self-esteem. There are many actions you can take to improve your posture and avoid the problems associated with poor posture. See the box "Adjustable Tables and Chairs for Better Posture and More" for an interesting example of the effects of posture improvement.

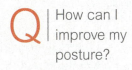

Q | How can I improve my posture?

One of the most important things you can do is to think about your posture. Become aware of your posture, and

Research Brief

Adjustable Tables and Chairs for Better Posture and More

Do you ever get tired of just sitting at a desk? In Finland, a group of 30 high school students were subjects for research to compare the effects of adjustable tables and chairs on posture, pain and tension levels, and learning success. Half the students were a control group, and the other half received tables and chairs that were personally adjusted for their size and shape.

At the onset of the study, students who used the new adjustable tables and chairs reported immediate reduction in lower-back and neck tension. Additional improvements were observed at the end of the 2-year research period, including better posture while sitting and standing, less frequent headaches, and a continued decrease in tension in the lower back and neck—as well as significantly better grades.

Analyze and Apply

- What does this study show about the influence of posture on various aspects of wellness?
- In what specific ways can you benefit from the researchers' findings?

Source: Koskelo, R., Vuorikari, K., & Hänninen, O. (2007). Sitting and standing postures are corrected by adjustable furniture with lowered muscle tension in high-school students. *Ergonomics, 50*(10), 1643–1656.

correct it when you notice that you are slouching or arching your back. Increasing your muscular endurance and flexibility can also improve your posture. See the box "Keys to Good Posture" for further tips.

The cause of poor posture for most of us is the muscles surrounding the spine rather than the spine itself. The muscles of the neck, trunk, and legs work together to support proper alignment and posture. These muscles must have both sufficient strength and flexibility to provide proper alignment during our many movements.

Good posture is not just about standing straight or sitting straight. That's only one kind of posture, and it's typically referred to as *static posture. Dynamic posture* is the alignment of your body when in motion. As with static posture, the proper dynamic posture involves using the stance and movements that are most mechanically efficient and least stressful on your body. See the box "Maintaining Good Posture and Body Mechanics" for specific strategies. Later in the chapter, you'll learn more tips for improving posture and body mechanics while using a computer.

Wellness Strategies

Keys to Good Posture

Q | What are some basics and tips for proper posture?

Important factors for correct posture include:

- Good muscle flexibility
- Normal motion in the joints
- Strong postural muscles
- A balance of the muscles on both sides of the spine
- Awareness of differences between one's posture and proper posture, leading to conscious correction

Practicing good posture isn't difficult. Try the wall test. With your heels about 4 inches from the wall, stand so that the back of your

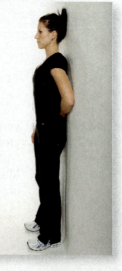

head, your shoulder blades, and your buttocks lightly touch the wall. You should be able to slide one hand into the curve of your lower back with your palm against the wall. Arch your back a little if you need more room to slide your hand behind you. If you need to decrease the arch to bring your posture into alignment, try tightening your abdominal muscles. Maintain this posture as you step away from the wall.

Sources: Adapted from MayoClinic.com. (2009). *Prevent back pain with good posture* (http://www.mayoclinic.com/health/back-pain/LB00002_D &slide=4). Cleveland Clinic. (2009). *Posture for a healthy back* (http://my.clevelandclinic.org/healthy_living/Back_health/hic_Posture_for_a_Healthy_Back.aspx).

Wellness Strategies

Maintaining Good Posture and Body Mechanics

Q | What steps can I take to improve my posture?

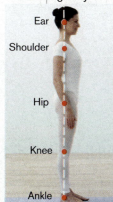

Vertical gravity line

Ear

Shoulder

Hip

Knee

Ankle

Standing

- Hold your head up with your neck straight and your chin neutral, making sure your earlobes are in line with the middle of your shoulders.
- Keep your shoulder blades back and chest forward; tuck your stomach in.
- Keep your pelvis straight (not tilted forward or backward) and maintain the natural curves in your upper and lower back without excessive rounding or arching.
- Provide support for the arches in your feet. Wear low-heeled shoes.
- If possible, adjust the height of your work table to a comfortable level to avoid bending.
- When standing for an extended period, elevate one foot by resting it on a stool or box; change feet every 5–15 minutes.

Walking

- Maintain your good standing posture when walking.
- Keep your head up and eyes looking 10–20 feet ahead.
- Keep your arms bent, and swing your arms from the shoulder.
- With each step, strike with your heel first and then roll through the step from heel to toe, followed with a push-off from the toe.
- Make sure your stride is longer in back of your body than in front.

Sitting

- Sit up with your back straight, shoulders back, and buttocks touching the back of your chair.
- Distribute your body weight evenly on both hips. Don't cross your legs, and keep your feet flat on the floor.
- Bend your knees at a right angle, keeping them even with or slightly lower than your hips. Use a foot rest (such as your backpack) if necessary.
- Avoid sitting for a long time whenever possible.
- It's OK to assume other sitting positions for short periods, but spend most of your sitting time as described above to minimize spinal stress.

Driving

- As when you are at your desk, sit up with your back straight, shoulders back, buttocks touching the back of your seat, and body weight distributed evenly across both hips.
- Position the seat close enough to the steering wheel to support your back and to allow your knees to bend at least slightly and your feet to reach the pedals.
- Position your knees at the same level as your hips, or higher.
- Use a back support (a lumbar roll) at the curve of your back if your seat does not support your back adequately.
- Maintain a forward facing position, with both hands on the wheel. Avoid leaning to the side on the armrests.

Lifting

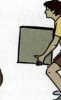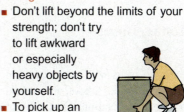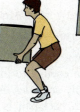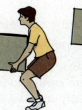

- Don't lift beyond the limits of your strength; don't try to lift awkward or especially heavy objects by yourself.
- To pick up an object that is lower than waist level, establish firm footing and use a wide stance. Stand close to the object to be lifted. Keep your back straight and bend at your knees and hips. Do not bend forward at the waist with your knees straight. Tighten your stomach muscles and lift the object using your leg muscles. Straighten your knees in a steady motion. Don't jerk the object up to your body. Stand completely upright without twisting. Always move your feet forward when lifting. Use the reverse action to place the object down, focusing on bending the legs, not the waist.
- To lift an object from a table, slide it to the edge of the table so that you can hold it close to your body. Bend your knees so that you are close to the object. Use your legs to lift the object and come to a standing position.
- Carry items close to your body.

Carrying a backpack or computer bag

- If possible, use packs on wheels, which are the best solution for reducing back strain. If a wheeled pack is impractical, choose a lightweight pack that doesn't add a lot of weight to your load. It should have two wide, padded shoulder straps and a padded back; a waist belt; and multiple compartments to help distribute the weight evenly.
- If you must use a tote or similar bag, choose one with a long shoulder strap. Slip it over your head onto the opposite shoulder (across the body like a seat belt) to distribute the weight more evenly.
- Maintain good walking and standing posture while carrying your load.

(continued)

(*continued*)

Sleeping

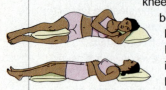

- Sleep in a position that allows you to maintain the natural curve in your back. If you sleep on your side, bend your knees slightly and try placing a pillow between your knees; don't pull your knees too far up toward your chest. If you sleep on your back, try placing a pillow under your knees or a lumbar roll under your lower back. Avoid sleeping on your stomach, especially if your mattress sags in the middle.
- Regardless of your sleeping position, place your pillow under your head (not your shoulders) and opt for a thickness that allows your neck to be at a neutral angle.
- Avoid using too soft a mattress and box spring. For back pain, a medium-firm mattress is recommended.

See Lab Activity 6-3 for more information on evaluating your posture.

Sources: Adapted from Cleveland Clinic. (2008). *Posture for a healthy back* (http://my.clevelandclinic.org/healthy_living/Back_health/hic_Posture_for_a_Healthy_Back.aspx). Maurer, E., & Spinasanta, S. (2010). *A head's up on posture: Don't be a slouch!* (http://www.spineuniverse.com/displayarticle.php/article1290.html). Kovacs, F. M., Abraira, V., Peña, A., and others. (2003). Effect of firmness of mattress on chronic non-specific low-back pain: Randomised, double-blind, controlled, multicentre trial. *Lancet, 362*(9396), 1599–1604.

Prevention and Management of Low-Back Pain

At some point in life, nearly all of us will have back pain severe enough to interfere with work, school, recreation, or daily activities. According to the National Institutes of Health, back pain is the most common cause of job-related disability and second only to headaches as a neurological problem; Americans spend at least $50 billion each year on low-back pain.[29] Back pain can occur at any time during adulthood, with pain varying from mild to severe and from short to long term.

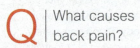 **Q** | What causes back pain?

CAUSES OF BACK PAIN. There are many potential causes of back pain. Because the lower back bears the majority of the body's weight, it is the most frequent site of pain or injury. The lower back provides the core from which the body generates power and mobility along with the strength to stand, walk, and lift, all while allowing for turning, twisting, and bending movements. Proper low-back function is critical for almost all activities of daily living. Without efficient low-back function, people begin to experience pain, discomfort, and restriction of typical activities. If left untreated for too long, disability can occur.

Pain may come from muscle strains, spasms, or soreness or from the compression of nerves. Short-term (acute) back pain lasts from a few days to a few weeks; it may be the result of trauma, overuse, or an underlying condition such as arthritis. Acute back pain often resolves with time and self-help measures, although it can return if the underlying causes, such as weak core muscles and poor posture, are not addressed. If pain persists for 3 months or more, it is considered chronic back pain, which can be difficult to treat successfully.

Triggers for back pain include lifting or moving something too heavy, overstretching while lifting, and doing more physical activity than usual—for example, being sedentary during the week and then engaging in heavy yard work or high-intensity recreational activities during the weekend. Back pain can also develop slowly over time, from frequent but less intense stresses—for example, sitting every day for long periods with poor posture. Whether you develop back pain from your activities depends on other factors, including some you can't control (such as age and heredity) and many that you can.

Degeneration of the intervertebral disks is a relatively normal part of the aging process and is a contributor to back problems. As people age, the disks begin to wear away, lose water content, and shrink; in some cases, a disk may collapse completely and no longer provide a cushion between the vertebrae. In other cases, a disk may bulge out from between vertebrae and put pressure on one of the spinal nerves, causing pain. Compression of a sciatic nerve, a large nerve that extends from the lower back down the leg, can lead to severe and debilitating leg or foot pain known as *sciatica*. Importantly, however, not everyone with back pain has a bulging disk, and not everyone with a bulging disk has back pain. Other risk factors for back pain include heredity and a family or personal history of a degenerative disease such as arthritis or osteoporosis.

Many other important risk factors for back pain are controllable, including the following:

- Poor physical fitness—especially limited muscular strength, endurance, and flexibility in and around the core
- Poor posture, especially as a result of sitting for long periods
- Overweight, especially excess weight around the middle
- A job that involves frequent heavy lifting, twisting, or bending or activities that vibrate the spine (such as operating machinery or driving a truck)
- Smoking—past or current[30]
- Stress and fatigue

The link between smoking and back pain may seem surprising, but smoking can damage arteries and restrict the flow of blood and nutrients to the disks and joints in the back; it also increases the risk of osteoporosis and slows healing from injuries.

Q What helps prevent back pain? Are there special exercises?

PREVENTION OF BACK PAIN. If you look at the list of risk factors for low-back pain in the previous section, you'll probably think of many steps you can take to reduce your risk. Being physically active and building strength and flexibility in the back and core muscles helps prevent overweight and aids in the maintenance of good posture and good body mechanics. Eating a moderate diet will help you maintain a healthy weight and get enough calcium and vitamin D to keep your bones strong (see Chapter 8). In addition, don't smoke, and manage stress effectively. See pp. 219–220 in this chapter for descriptions of specific exercises designed to help prevent and manage low-back pain.

Follow the suggestions in the box "Maintaining Good Posture and Body Mechanics" for appropriate posture and biomechanics while sitting, standing, walking, and lifting. If you spend many hours every day on a computer, pay special attention to your posture and the placement of your computer equipment (Figure 6-7):

- Position the monitor directly in front of you, about an arm's length away, with the top of the monitor tilted back about 10–20 degrees. The top of the viewing screen should be at or slightly below eye level when you sit up straight.
- Sit in the position suggested earlier in the chapter, with your back against the backrest and the backrest (or a lumbar pad) adjusted to fit the curve of your lower back. Your feet should be flat on the floor or on a footrest, your thighs parallel to the floor, and your knees at about the same level as your hips.
- Place the keyboard at about elbow level so that you can hold your forearms and wrists relatively straight and parallel to the floor.
- Take a break every 30 minutes. Stand up and walk around. Stretch your neck, shrug your shoulders, and place your hands gently behind your head and pull your shoulders back. Hold your arms straight out in front of you and stretch your wrists by pulling your hands backward and then pressing them down; alternate between making a fist and extending your fingers.

Laptops are designed for short-term mobile use and usually require you to hold your neck, arm,

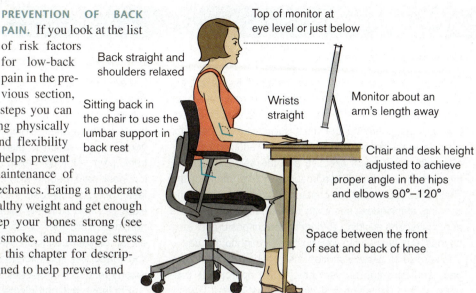

Back straight and shoulders relaxed

Top of monitor at eye level or just below

Sitting back in the chair to use the lumbar support in back rest

Wrists straight

Monitor about an arm's length away

Chair and desk height adjusted to achieve proper angle in the hips and elbows 90°–120°

Space between the front of seat and back of knee

Feet flat on the floor or on foot rest

Figure 6-7 Recommended sitting posture and computer placement.

and wrist at stressful angles. Pay particular attention to your posture when you use a laptop. Whenever possible, dock your laptop at a desktop computer station or hook it up to a separate monitor, keyboard, and/or mouse. If you aren't already keyboard literate, set that as a goal: Looking down at the laptop keyboard while you type puts a lot of stress on your neck.

Q If you have back problems, what can you do to help them improve?

MANAGEMENT OF BACK PAIN. Most cases of back pain improve within a short time. Typically, a few days of rest along with a safe dose of acetaminophen or a nonsteroidal anti-inflammatory drug such as ibuprofen can help to manage discomfort. Hot or cold packs (or both) can reduce muscle spasms, pain, and swelling. Stronger medications, such as muscle relaxants and prescription painkillers, should be reserved for severe pain and be used only under a doctor's supervision. Prolonged bed rest (more than 2 or 3 days) is no longer recommended for managing low-back pain. Gradually getting back to your usual activities—provided they are appropriate—will help prevent stiffness and weakness that can worsen back problems over time. Once your pain eases, address any underlying risk factors, such as poor posture and faulty body mechanics. Making careful note

DOLLAR STRETCHER
Financial Wellness Tip

If the chairs you typically sit in don't have adjustable lumbar support, create your own inexpensive version. Roll up a small towel or shirt and place it to maintain the natural curve of your lower back. Try this at home, work, and school and in your car.

Living *Well* with . . .

Low-Back Pain

Although medication and injections can decrease pain in the short term, they don't address the root causes or help prevent or reduce the severity of future episodes of low-back pain. Among the most successful methods for minimizing the risk of low-back pain or reducing its reoccurrence are physical exercise and the establishment of proper body mechanics. Approaches include many of the strategies described in this chapter, including safe lifting and carrying techniques, adequate lumbar support on seats and chairs, and avoiding stationary upright posture for long periods. Pay attention to your posture throughout the day.

Exercise to restore motion and strength to the lower back and core can be very helpful. An appropriate program should center on activities to boost overall fitness, including aerobic activities such as walking, swimming, and so on; resistance training with machines, free weights, bands, or body resistance; and whole-body flexibility. Some of the most effective low-back exercises strengthen the core. Three core exercises that help low-back pain are the following (see instructions on pp. 219–220):

- Side bridge
- Modified curl-up
- Quadruped hip extension (bird dog)

Performing these core exercises along with aerobic, resistance, and flexibility exercises to promote overall fitness will go a long way toward maintaining good back health. In addition, regular exercise helps maintain a healthy body weight, which is also important for reducing low-back pain. Although exercise won't absolutely prevent low-back pain, people who exercise regularly suffer much less from low-back pain throughout their lifetime. If some exercises and activities cause you pain, check with your health care provider for advice on which are safe and beneficial for your condition. Avoid any exercise that strains your back; see the exercises at the end of this chapter recommended for low-back health.

For those with chronic back pain, relaxation techniques to reduce stress can also help. The causes of back pain are usually physical, but emotional stress influences the severity and duration of the pain.

Sources: McGill, S. (2007). *Low back disorders: Evidenced-based prevention and rehabilitation.* Champaign, IL: Human Kinetics. American Academy of Orthopaedic Surgeons. (2009). *Low back pain* (http://orthoinfo.aaos.org/topic.cfm?topic=A00311). National Institute of Arthritis and Musculoskeletal and Skin Diseases. (2010). *Handout on health: Back pain* (http://www.niams.nih.gov/health_info/back_pain/default.asp).

of, and addressing, the types of activities that cause or lead to pain and can be particularly helpful in preventing recurring problems.

If your pain is severe or accompanied by other symptoms—weakness, numbness, or tingling; fever; trouble urinating; or unexpected weight loss—see a physician. Back pain is usually diagnosed through a physical exam, a history of your symptoms, and possibly a diagnostic test such as a standard X-ray or a magnetic resonance imaging (MRI). It is not unusual for the cause of back pain to remain undetermined. In addition to the self-help measures described above, a doctor may prescribe stronger medications or recommend a treatment such as electrical stimulation, physical therapy, spinal manipulation, or acupuncture.[31] A physician can inject a local anesthetic or steroids (to reduce pain and inflammation) or both, but such injections are usually a last resort after more conservative treatments have failed to provide relief. Most people with back pain do not need surgery.

Chronic low-back pain is difficult to treat and may recur. See the box "Living Well with . . . Low-Back Pain" for more information on treatment and management. Whatever your level of pain, it's important that you take an active role in your treatment and recovery.

Summary

Flexibility—the ability of joints to move through their full range of motion—is an often overlooked component of health-related fitness, ignored until later in life when problems develop. Your level of flexibility in a particular joint is affected by the structure of the joint, genetics, age, biological sex, history of injuries and disease, and whether you engage in some form of stretching exercises. Benefits of flexibility include fewer of certain types of injuries and less muscle soreness as well as maintenance of the ability to perform daily activities with ease. By initiating a regular stretching program now, utilizing FITT principles, you may be able to avoid many problems in the future. Stretching exercises also promote relaxation.

Flexibility, along with muscle strength and endurance, will reduce the risk of low-back pain. Good posture, accompanied by a program of regular exercise, helps prevent and manage many types of low-back problems. Flexibility training and improvement of posture through small changes in your day-to-day routine can make a big difference in the long run.

More to Explore

American Academy of Orthopaedic Surgeons: Your Orthopaedic Connection
    http://orthoinfo.aaos.org
Cornell University Ergonomics Web
    http://ergo.human.cornell.edu
Mayo Clinic
Slideshow: How to Stretch Your Major Muscle Groups
    http://www.mayoclinic.com/health/stretching/SM00043
Slideshow: Prevent Back Pain with Good Posture
    http://www.mayoclinic.com/health/back-pain/LB00002_D
Slideshow: Core Exercises
    http://www.mayoclinic.com/health/core-strength/SM00047
MedlinePlus: Back Pain
    http://www.nlm.nih.gov/medlineplus/backpain.html
Spine Universe
    http://www.spineuniverse.com

FLEXIBILITY EXERCISES

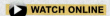 **WATCH ONLINE**

Head Tilt and Turn

Muscles stretched: Splenius muscles, sternocleidomastoid, medial layer of erector spinae

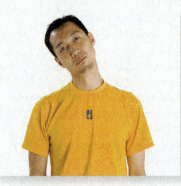 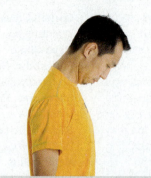 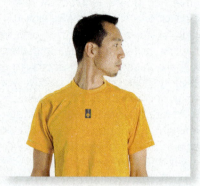

Instructions

Head tilts: Stand or sit comfortably. Begin by leaning your head to one side, moving your ear toward your shoulder. Keep your shoulders relaxed. Hold the stretch. Then gently roll your neck so that your chin moves forward and downward toward your chest. Hold. Then continue the movement until your other ear and shoulder are aligned. Hold. Repeat in the opposite direction.

Head turns: Keeping your shoulders relaxed, turn your head to the right and hold the stretch. Repeat on the left side.

Training tip

■ Keep your shoulders relaxed and in a neutral position. Don't perform full neck circles, and take care not to extend your neck back

Triceps Stretch

Muscles stretched: Triceps brachii

Instructions

In a sitting or standing position, raise one arm directly overhead, bending the arm at the elbow to reach toward your back, in the middle of your shoulders. With the opposite arm, reach across the back of your head and grasp the elbow of the first arm. Gently push up and back on your elbow and hold the stretch. Repeat on the other side.

Training tip

■ Keep your neck straight, and hold the stretched arm directly beside your head.

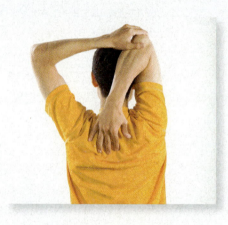

Across-the-Body Shoulder Stretch

Muscles stretched: Deltoid

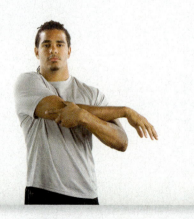

Instructions

Keep your back straight and your torso forward as you cross your right arm in front of your body and grab your elbow or back of the upper arm with your left hand. Gently pull your right arm toward your body. Hold the stretch. Repeat on the other side.

Training tip

■ Keep your shoulders relaxed and down. Look forward and keep your neck neutral.

Wall Stretch for Chest

Muscles stretched: Pectoralis major, pectoralis minor, subscapularis

Instructions

Stand in front of a wall and extend one arm out against the wall, palm facing away from you. Turn away from the wall until you feel a stretch in your chest and upper arm. Hold the stretch. Repeat on the other side.

Training tip

- Keep your arm parallel to the floor.

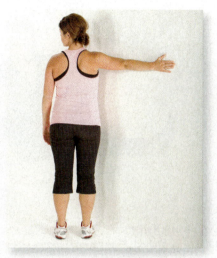

Standing Cat Stretch

Muscles stretched: Deltoid, latissimus dorsi, teres major, erector spinae

Instructions

Stand with your feet about shoulder-width apart. Bend forward, and place your hands on your knees or lower thighs. Keep your head stationary as you round your back. Hold the stretch and then straighten your back to return to the starting position. Repeat.

Training tip

- Don't bend your neck excessively; this is a stretch of the upper back and not the neck.

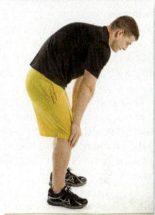

Overhead Reach and Lateral Stretch

Muscles stretched: Latissimus dorsi, internal and external obliques, erector spinae

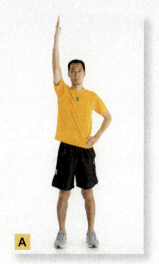
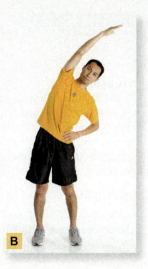

Instructions

Stand comfortably, with your feet about shoulder-width apart and knees slightly bent.

A. With one hand on your hip, reach straight up with the other arm. Hold the stretch. Repeat on the other side.

B. If you can perform this exercise comfortably, try a more advanced lateral stretch. From the same position, bend sideways from the waist as you support your trunk with your opposite hand on your hip or thigh for support. Keep your pelvis tucked in. Hold the stretch, and then repeat on the other side.

Training tips

- Keep the movement directly to the side—don't lean forward or backward.
- Bend at the waist, keeping the lower body stable.

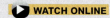

Hip and Trunk Rotation

Muscles stretched: Internal and external obliques, piriformis, erector spinae, gluteal muscles

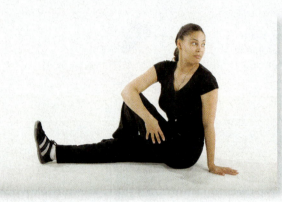

Instructions

Sit comfortably on the floor with your right leg straight out in front of you. Bend your left knee and cross it over your right leg, placing your left ankle against the outside of your right knee. Place your left hand on the floor next to your left hip. Rotate your trunk to the left, using your right elbow to aid in the stretch by placing it on the outside of your left knee. Hold the stretch. Repeat on the other side.

Training tip

- Turn with your trunk, not your neck. Don't let your lower back round excessively

Lying Trunk Twist

Muscles stretched: External and internal obliques

Instructions

Lie on your left side with your left leg straight, right knee bent, right lower leg resting on the ground, and left arm extending out on the floor perpendicular to your body. Leading with your right shoulder, twist your trunk to the right as you push down with your right knee. If needed, you can use your left hand to gently hold your right leg in place. The goal is to get both your shoulders and your upper body flat on the floor while keeping your right knee on the ground. Hold the stretch. Repeat on the other side.

Training tip

- Move your neck in line with your torso; look toward the ceiling rather than over one shoulder.

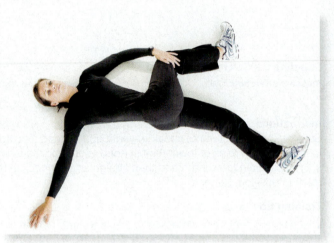

Modified Hurdler's Stretch

Muscles stretched: Hamstrings, erector spinae, gastrocnemius

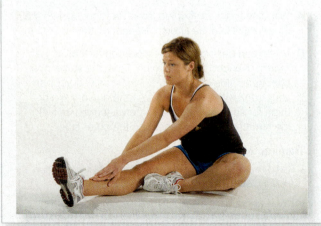

Instructions

Sit on the floor with your right leg extended and the sole of the left foot pressed against the inner right thigh or knee. Keeping your back straight, lean forward at the hips and reach toward your right foot. Hold the stretch. Repeat on the other side. If you are very flexible, grab the toes of the extended leg.

Training tips

- Don't round your shoulders or flex your upper back; keep your back straight.
- Keep your extended leg straight and don't roll your leg out.

Knee-to-Chest and Leg Extension Stretch

Muscles stretched: Hamstrings, gluteus maximus, erector spinae

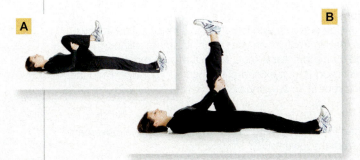

Instructions

Lie on your back with your knees extended.

A. Bend your right leg and grasp it behind your knee, at the back of your thigh. Keeping your left leg flat on the ground, pull your right leg toward your chest. Hold the stretch.

B. Then extend your right leg toward the ceiling; your hands can rest at the back of the thigh. Hold the stretch. Repeat on the other side.

Training tip

- Take care not to flex your neck or arch your back. Keep the straight leg flat on the ground throughout the stretch.

Gluteal Stretch

Muscles stretched: Gluteus maximus

Instructions

Lie on your back with your knees bent and feet flat on the floor. Place your right ankle just above your left knee, with your hip turned out. Reach through with both hands to get a hold of the back of your left knee. (Your right arm will reach through between your legs, your left arm will be outside your left leg.) Gently pull your left knee toward your chest. Your head and torso should be resting on the floor. Hold the stretch. Repeat on the other side.

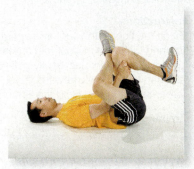

Training tip

- Don't force the movement or arch or strain your back. For an easier variation, place your right foot on your left knee and gently pull your right knee toward your chest with your hands.

Standing Quad Stretch

Muscles stretched: Quadriceps

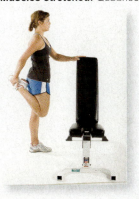

Instructions

Stand comfortably. Begin the stretch by bending one knee, raising your foot to the rear. Grasp the raised ankle with the same hand and pull gently toward your buttocks. Rest the opposite hand on the back of a chair or other support to help maintain your balance. Hold the stretch. Repeat on the other side.

Training tips

- Take care not to arch your back or lean forward.
- Keep your knees together and don't let the bent knee move out to the side. If you feel pain in your knee, stop the stretch.

Kneeling Hip-flexor Stretch

Muscles stretched: Quadriceps, iliopsoas, sartorius, tensor fasciae latae

Instructions

Start in a half kneeling position, with your left knee and your right foot on the ground. Your right knee should be directly above your right ankle. Rest both hands on your right knee. Keeping your abdominals and gluteals tight, shift your entire body forward until you feel a stretch at the front of the hip and in the upper thigh. Your right knee should not extend out in front of your right foot. Hold the stretch, and repeat on the other side.

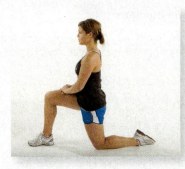

Training tip

- Don't let your lower back arch. Tuck your pelvis under and tighten your abdominals if you feel your back start to arch.

▶ **WATCH ONLINE**

Standing Side Lunge Stretch
Muscles stretched: Hip adductors

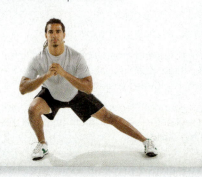

Instructions
Stand in a wide straddle with legs turned slightly out. With your hands clasped in front (or on your thighs for more balance), lunge to the side by bending one knee. Keep the knee directly over the ankle and don't let it extend out in front of your foot. Hold the stretch and repeat on the other side.

Training tip
- Don't lean forward or to the side with your torso; the movement comes from the lower body.

Groin Stretch (Butterfly)
Muscles stretched: Hip adductors

Instructions
Sit on the floor with your torso upright. Bend your knees and rotate your thighs out to bring the soles of your feet together in front of you. Place your hands around your feet or ankles and gently pull your feet toward your body. Keeping your back straight, lean slightly forward. If you can, gently push your knees down with your forearms or elbows. Hold the stretch.

Training tips
- Be sure to use slow, smooth motions and go only to the point of a comfortable stretch.
- Keep your back straight and don't round your shoulders or upper back.

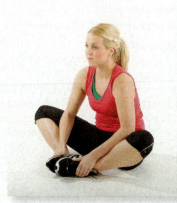

Calf, Soleus, and Shin Stretch
Muscles stretched: Gastrocnemius, soleus, tibialis anterior

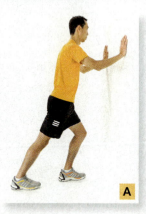
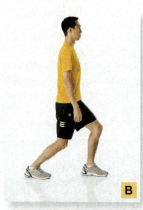
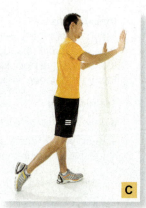

Instructions

A. Stand facing a wall with your toes about 12 inches from the wall. Lean forward and place both hands on the wall. Step back with your right leg about 2 feet as you bend your left leg. Extend your right leg and keep your foot flat on the floor. If you don't feel a stretch in the right calf, bend your elbows slightly and move your hips and torso toward the wall until you feel a stretch. Hold the stretch.

B. Pull your right foot in, bend your right knee, and shift your weight as you remove your hands from the wall. Support your weight with your right leg. Hold the stretch.

C. Straighten your legs, shift your weight forward onto your left leg, and rest your hands lightly on the wall. Place the top of your right foot on the ground; try to point your toenails toward the floor. Push down gently to stretch the front of your shin. Repeat on the other side.

Training tip
- Push only to the point of a comfortable stretch.
- Keep your toes pointed forward throughout parts A and B.

EXERCISES FOR THE LOWER BACK

Cat and Camel

Purpose: Reduces joint friction and resistance to movement

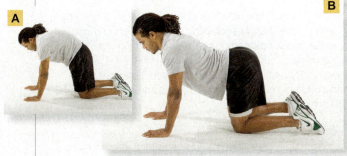

Instructions

A. Kneel on your hands and knees, with your hands directly below your shoulders and your knees directly below your hips. Begin by pushing up your back, pulling in your abdomen, dropping your head slightly, and tucking your pelvis down and under.

B. Next, slowly lower your back, shift your pelvis up, and lift your chin slightly until your back is flexed. Stop if you feel any pain. Complete 5–10 gentle cycles of flexion and extension, taking care not to push the maximum range in either direction.

Training tips

- This is a movement and not a stretch—move gently through the entire range of motion and don't press at the ends of the range of motion.
- Keep your hands and hips facing directly forward for both positions.

Modified Curl-up

Purpose: Builds endurance in the rectus abdominis

Instructions

A. Lie on your back with one leg straight and the other knee bent. Place both hands under your lumbar spine to help keep your spine neutral during the exercise. Your elbows should touch the floor.

B. To perform the curl, raise your head and upper shoulders off the floor. Alternate the bent leg midway through your repetitions.

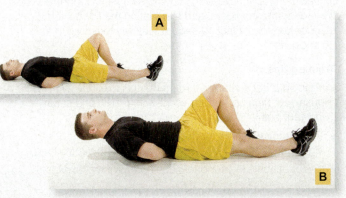

Training tips

- Don't curl up with your head; the movement should come from your thoracic region.
- You can make the exercise more challenging by raising your elbows off the floor.

Side Bridge

Purpose: Builds endurance in the quadratus lumborum, abdominal obliques

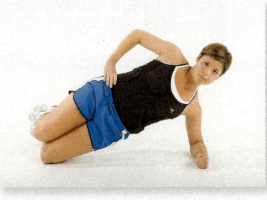

Instructions

Start by lying on the floor on your side, with your knees bent. Your top arm can lie along your side or across your chest, or you can place your hand on your hip. Lift your hips so that your weight is supported by your forearm and knees. Hold this position for 7–8 seconds. Return to the starting position. Repeat. As you gain strength, you can make the exercise more difficult by supporting your weight with your forearm and your feet.

Training tips

- Keep your body firm and straight throughout this exercise.
- This exercise can be made more challenging by pointing your top arm straight up.

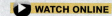

Quadruped Hip Extension (Bird Dog)

Purpose: Builds endurance in the erector spinae, multifidus spinae, and rectus abdominis

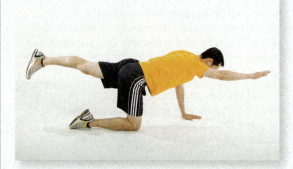

Instructions

Start on the floor on your hands and knees. Knees should be below the hips and hands should be below the shoulders and slightly wider. Slowly extend one arm and the opposite leg, keeping your back straight. Hold this position for 7–8 seconds, then lower your hand and knee and "sweep" the floor with them before raising them for the next repetition. Alternate to the opposite arm and leg.

Training tips

- Use a pad under your hands and knees for more comfort.
- Beginners can start by lifting an arm alone, then lowering it, and then lifting a leg alone.

Back (Glute) Bridge

Purpose: Builds strength and endurance in the gluteus maximus, erector spinae, hamstrings

Instructions

Start by lying on your back with your arms extended along your side. Tuck your pelvis under and tighten your gluteal muscles. Raise your hips so that your weight is supported by your head, shoulders, and feet (flat on the floor). Hold this position for at least 10 seconds, slowly building up to 30 seconds.

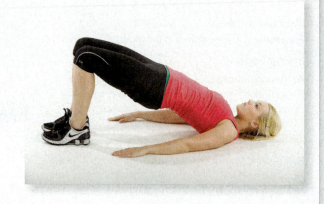

Training tips

- Keep your back straight throughout this exercise. Don't push your hips up, forcing your back to arch and straining your neck.
- This exercise can be made more difficult by lifting one leg so the foot is pointing out, in line with the support leg.
- If you feel pain in your back, don't perform this exercise.

Wall Sit (Squat)

Purpose: Builds endurance of the quadriceps, hamstrings, gluteus maximus, and rectus abdominis

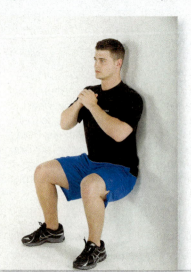

Instructions

Stand in front of a wall and lean against it with your back. Walk your feet out and then bend your knees and slide down the wall until you are in a squat position. Imagine you are sitting in a chair; focus on using the muscles in your thighs, buttocks, and abdomen. Begin by holding the position for 10–15 seconds and work your way up to a 1-minute hold.

Training tip

- Make sure that your knees don't extend out in front of your toes; stop if you feel any pain in your knees.

COMPLETE IN connect

NAME	DATE	SECTION

Complete one or more of the tests for flexibility described in this lab activity and then answer the questions in the "Reflecting on Your Results" section at the end.

- Sit-and-reach test (flexibility of the lower back and hamstrings)
- Shoulder flexibility test
- Hip range of motion and hamstring flexibility test
- Hip-flexor flexibility test (Thomas Test)

Sit-and-Reach Test

Equipment

- Sit-and-reach box with the footline set at 26 centimeters (cm). You can also create your own measuring device from a firm box or pieces of wood and a metric ruler. The ruler should be set so that the 26-cm mark is aligned with the end of the box or board. (If you can reach past your feet, your score will be higher than 26 cm; if you can't reach as far as your feet, your score will be below 26 cm.)
- Partner to check measurement

Preparation

Warm up for 5–10 minutes, using low-intensity aerobic activity. Stretch your hamstrings and lower back.

Instructions

Remove your shoes and sit with your feet flat against the sit-and-reach box. As described, your feet should be at the 26-cm mark of the metric ruler or measuring device. The inner edges of your feet should be within 2 cm of the ruler or scale. With your hands parallel and in contact with the measuring portion of the sit-and-reach box or the ruler, slowly reach forward as far as possible. Your fingertips can be overlapped, but do not lead with one hand. Your knees should be extended but not pressed down. Don't hold your breath; to aid in your performance on the test, exhale and drop your head between your arms as you reach forward. Hold the position of farthest reach for about 2 seconds. Your partner should note this measurement. Repeat the test.

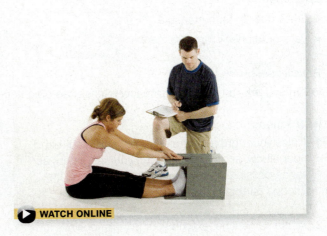

▶ **WATCH ONLINE**

Results

Your score is the most distant point (in centimeters) you reached with your fingertips. Find the rating that corresponds to your score. (Note: If the sit-and-reach box has a different footline or zero point, adjust the score accordingly. For example, if the footline of your box is 23 cm, you would add 3 cm to your score.)

Trial 1: [   ] cm   Trial 2: [   ] cm   Best trial: [   ] cm   Rating (from table): [   ]

RATINGS FOR THE SIT-AND-REACH TEST (IN CENTIMETERS)*

	Age (years)					
	15–19	20–29	30–39	40–49	50–59	60–69
MEN						
Excellent	≥39	≥40	≥38	≥35	≥35	≥33
Very good	34–38	34–39	33–37	29–34	28–34	25–32
Good	29–33	30–33	28–32	24–28	24–27	20–24
Fair	24–28	25–29	23–27	18–23	16–23	15–19
Needs improvement	≤23	≤24	≤22	≤17	≤15	≤14
WOMEN						
Excellent	≥43	≥41	≥41	≥38	≥39	≥35
Very good	38–42	37–40	36–40	34–37	33–38	31–34
Good	34–37	33–36	32–35	30–33	30–32	27–30
Fair	29–33	28–32	27–31	25–29	25–29	23–26
Needs improvement	≤28	≤27	≤26	≤24	≤24	≤22

*Footline of box set at 26 cm.

Source: Canadian Society for Exercise Physiology. (2003). *The Canadian physical activity, fitness and lifestyle approach: CSEP health and fitness program's health-related appraisal and counselling strategy* (3rd ed.). Ottawa, ON: CSEP.

Shoulder Flexibility Test

Equipment

- Small ruler or tape measure
- Partner to check measurement

Preparation

Warm up for 5–10 minutes, using low-intensity aerobic activity. Stretch your shoulders.

Instructions

1. Raise your right arm straight over your head, bend your elbow, and reach between your shoulders as far as possible, palm against your back (see the Triceps Stretch in this chapter).

2. At the same time, extend your left arm down toward the ground, bend at the elbow and reach up behind your back, trying to touch or overlap the fingers of both hands.

3. Your partner should measure the distance of finger overlap or the distance between your fingers to the nearest quarter inch. If your fingers overlap, the score is a positive number. If your fingers fail to meet, the score is a negative number.

4. Repeat with the left arm up and right arm down.

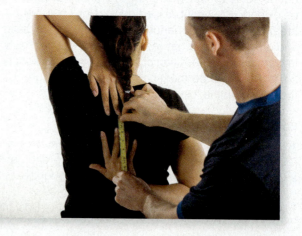

Results

Your score is the average of the two measurements: The distance between your fingertips (negative number) or the distance of overlap of your fingers (positive number). Find your rating in the table.

Right elbow up: [ ] in.

Left elbow up: [ ] in.

Average of two measurements: [ ] in.

Rating: [ ]

LAB ACTIVITY 6-1

RATINGS FOR SHOULDER FLEXIBILITY TEST

RATING	AVERAGE OF TWO SIDES IN INCHES
Excellent	≥5
Above average	2 to 4.75
Average	0 to 1.75
Below average	−1 to −0.25
Poor	<1

Source: Nieman, D. (2003). *Exercise testing and prescription: A health-related approach* (5th ed., pp. 185, 197). New York: McGraw-Hill.

Hip Range of Motion and Hamstring Flexibility Test

Equipment

- Partner to check range of motion
- Goniometer or other joint measurement tool (optional)

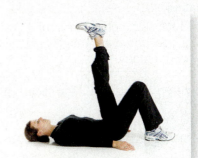

Preparation

Warm up for 5–10 minutes, using low-intensity aerobic activity. Stretch your hamstrings and lower back.

Instructions

Lie on your back with your arms at your sides. Bend one knee and place your foot flat on the floor. Keeping your other leg straight, raise it. Compare the range of motion in the raised straight leg relative to a 90-degree position perpendicular to the floor. If a partner and a measuring instrument such as a goniometer are available, you can obtain a more precise measurement of the joint angle. Repeat the test on the other leg.

Results

Average flexibility for this test is about 90 degrees. If you cannot raise your leg so that it is at least perpendicular to the floor, then your hamstring flexibility is below average. Note for each leg whether hamstring flexibility is below average, average, or above average:

Right leg: [ ]   Left leg: [ ]

If you used a goniometer for joint angle measurement, record the results here:

Right leg: [ ] degrees   Left leg: [ ] degrees

Hip-Flexor Flexibility Test (Thomas Test)

Equipment

- Partner to check range of motion
- Training table or bench (optional)

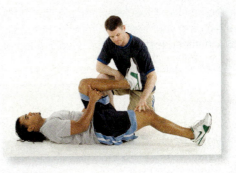

Preparation

Warm up for 5–10 minutes, using low-intensity aerobic activity. Stretch your hip flexors, quadriceps, and hamstrings.

Instructions

If you are performing the test on the floor: Lie on your back and bring both knees to your chest. Grab your right leg behind the knee and hold your knee at your chest. Let your left leg straighten and lower it toward the floor or mat by relaxing your hip. Have your partner note whether the straight leg is flat on the floor or the knee and lower thigh are "floating" above the floor. Repeat the test on the other leg.

If you are performing the test on a training table or bench:
Sit so that your tailbone is at the edge of the table. Lie back on the table, pulling your knees to your chest. Grab your right leg behind the knee and hold it to your chest. Gently lower your left leg beyond the edge of the table or bench. The table or bench should be tall enough that your leg can hang freely. Your lower back should maintain its natural curve throughout the movement by touching the table or bench at all times. Have your partner note the angle of your thigh on the extended leg. If your leg is lifted above the level of the table, this indicates poor hip-flexor flexibility; if your leg extends below the level of the table, this indicates good hip-flexor flexibility. Repeat the test with the other leg.

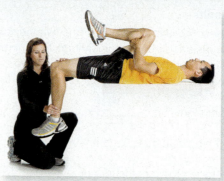

Rating

For each side, note the position of the test leg. If your leg does not lower all the way—if your knee and lower thigh float above the ground or come off the table—then your hip flexors are tight and their range of motion is below average.

Right leg: ☐ (flat / floating)   Rating: ☐ (OK / below average)

Left leg: ☐ (flat / floating)   Rating: ☐ (OK / below average)

Reflecting on Your Results

Record the results of the tests you completed.

	SCORE	RATING
Sit-and-reach test		
Shoulder flexibility test		
Hip range of motion and hamstring flexibility test	Right: Left:	Right: Left:
Hip-flexor flexibility test	Right: Left:	Right: Left:

Are you surprised by your ratings? Did your results match what you thought about your level of flexibility?

Planning Your Next Steps

If the results of the tests indicate that the flexibility in some of your joints is below average, consider starting or expanding your flexibility training. Set realistic goals for improvement and create a plan to achieve them. Then repeat these tests in several weeks and note any improvements.

Describe the specific steps you will take to improve your flexibility:

What effect, if any, did your plan have on your flexibility?

LAB ACTIVITY 6-2 Creating a Program for Flexibility

COMPLETE IN connect

NAME	DATE	SECTION

Equipment

None required, but you may want to develop and track your program in a paper notebook, digital spreadsheet, smartphone application, or online program.

Preparation: None

Instructions

1. **Set SMART goals** (specific, measurable, achievable, realistic, time-bound): The goals for your flexibility program can be about training—such as number of stretching workouts per week—or they can be based on one of the flexibility tests you completed in Lab Activity 6-1.

Current status	Goal	Target date	Notes (rewards, special considerations)

2. **Apply the FITT principle:** Create a program that meets the recommended criteria for success and fits your schedule and preferences.

- *Frequency:* 2–3 days per week or more
- *Intensity:* Stretch to the point of slight tension or mild tightness.
- *Time:* Hold the stretch for 15–60 seconds, and do four or more repetitions of each stretch.
- *Type:* Perform a stretch for each major muscle/tendon group or joint: neck, shoulders, upper and lower back, pelvis, hips, and legs. Fill in the exercises for your starting program below.

EXERCISE	MUSCLE/TENDON GROUP OR JOINT STRETCHED

Results

Track your progress with a log like the one below or one you create for yourself.

FLEXIBILITY TRAINING LOG

DATE	DURATION/TIME	WORKOUT (IF DIFFERENT FROM STARTING PROGRAM)	NOTES (E.G., CHANGES IN FLEXIBILITY, HOW STRETCHING PROGRAM MAKES YOU FEEL)

Reflecting on Your Results and Planning Your Next Steps

Have you been sticking with your program plan for flexibility training? How have you responded to the program? Has your flexibility increased? How does your stretching routine make you feel? Do you plan to change your program going forward? If so, describe the changes. How do you plan to stick with your program going forward?

LAB ACTIVITY 6-3

COMPLETE IN *connect*

NAME	DATE	SECTION

Standing Posture

Equipment: Partner

Preparation

None. The assessment is easier to complete if you wear clothing that allows your posture and body lines to be easily seen. Remove your shoes.

Instructions

Have a partner compare your *typical* standing posture to the illustrations and key points listed below. Your partner should describe any differences between your posture and the recommended posture.

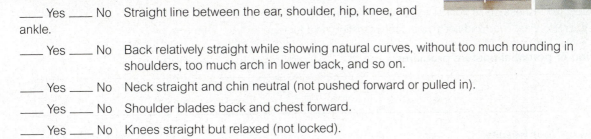

From the side:

____ Yes ____ No   Straight line between the ear, shoulder, hip, knee, and ankle.

____ Yes ____ No   Back relatively straight while showing natural curves, without too much rounding in shoulders, too much arch in lower back, and so on.

____ Yes ____ No   Neck straight and chin neutral (not pushed forward or pulled in).

____ Yes ____ No   Shoulder blades back and chest forward.

____ Yes ____ No   Knees straight but relaxed (not locked).

From the back:

____ Yes ____ No   Ears level.

____ Yes ____ No   Shoulders level.

____ Yes ____ No   Hips level.

____ Yes ____ No   Feet parallel, with weight evenly balanced on both feet; ankles tilted neither inward nor outward.

Description of potential posture problems:

Desk/Computer Posture

Equipment

- Partner
- Computer and desk/chair where you typically use your computer

Preparation

None. The assessment is easier to complete if you wear clothing that allows your posture and body angles to be easily seen.

Instructions

Have a partner compare your *typical* sitting posture when you use your computer to the illustration below. Your partner should note and describe any problems.

____ Yes ____ No   Eyes level or just above top of monitor.

____ Yes ____ No   Eyes about arm's length away from monitor.

____ Yes ____ No   Elbows bent and close to body, angle of 90–120 degrees.

____ Yes ____ No   Wrists straight (not angled upward, downward or to either side).

____ Yes ____ No   Upper back relatively straight while showing natural curves, without rounding of the shoulders.

____ Yes ____ No   Shoulders down and relaxed, directly over hips (not lifted or pulled forward).

____ Yes ____ No   Lower back relatively straight while showing natural curves, without too much arch or rounding.

____ Yes ____ No   Sitting all the way back in the chair, with a backrest supporting lower back.

____ Yes ____ No   Hips bent to achieve angle of 90–120 degrees.

____ Yes ____ No   Knees out in front of the edge of the chair.

____ Yes ____ No   Feet even and flat on the floor or resting on a footrest.

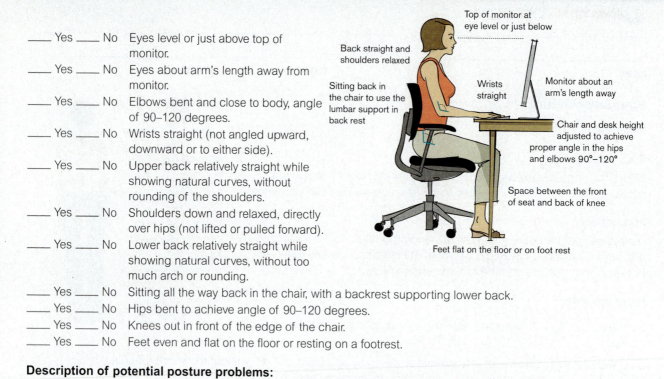

Description of potential posture problems:

[ ]

Reflecting on Your Results

How did you do? How close or far is your typical posture from the recommendations? Do you ever think about your posture or have problems that might be attributed to your posture (such as a sore neck or back)?

[ ]

Planning Your Next Steps

Practice using correct posture. First, for standing posture, practice realigning your body to match the recommendations; you can use the checklist in the lab and also try the wall test on p. 208. If you need to pull your shoulders back and open your chest, try the following: With your arms hanging loosely in front, place your palms toward your body and point your thumbs inward at each other. Then rotate your arms (at the shoulder joint) so your thumbs are pointing outward. After you try correct standing posture a few times, describe what you did to achieve it and how it feels. What can you use as a reminder to periodically check and correct your posture until the recommended posture becomes habit?

[ ]

For your desk/computer posture, determine what steps are needed to improve your posture so that it matches the guidelines. You may need to adjust your chair and desk in addition to your body positions. List and describe the changes needed in your work area and include a plan for each. (If you make significant changes to your work area, you may need to reevaluate your desk/computer posture.) Next, list and describe the changes needed in your posture. What specific steps can you take to work on improving your desk/computer posture?

[ ]

■ COMPLETE IN connect

NAME	DATE	SECTION

Side-Bridge Endurance Test

Equipment

- Floor mat
- Stopwatch, watch, or clock with a second hand
- Partner

Preparation

Warm up for 5–10 minutes, using low-intensity aerobic activity. If you haven't performed side bridges before, practice.

Instructions

Lie on your side with your legs extended. Place your top foot slightly in front of your lower foot for support. Lift your hips off the mat so that your weight is supported by your forearm and your feet. Your body should form a straight line. Keep your neck neutral and don't hold your breath. Hold the position as long as possible. Your score will be the total time you maintain the position with good form. A partner can monitor the time and watch your form. Rest for several minutes and then repeat the test on the other side.

Results

Your score is the total number of seconds you held the side bridge position.

Right side: [　　　] seconds   Left side: [　　　] seconds

Reflecting on Your Results

The table at right shows mean endurance times for both men and women. Compare your scores with the means shown in the table.

Check the appropriate line for your score.

Right side bridge: Above mean [　　]   At mean [　　]
　　　　　　　　　　Below mean [　　]

Left side bridge: Above mean [　　]   At mean [　　]
　　　　　　　　　Below mean [　　]

Average Endurance Times (in seconds)

TEST	MEN	WOMEN
Right side bridge	95	75
Left side bridge	99	78

Source: McGill, S. M. (2003). *Low back disorders: Evidence-based prevention and rehabilitation*. Champaign, IL: Human Kinetics.

Are you surprised by your ratings? Did your results match what you thought about your own level of muscle endurance and low-back health?

[　　　　　　　　　　　　　　　　　　　　　　　　　　]

Planning Your Next Steps

If the results of the lab indicate your low-back muscle endurance is below average, consider incorporating some specific exercises to build endurance in the muscles that help support back health. Set realistic goals for improvement and create a plan to achieve them. Then repeat these tests in several weeks and note improvements.

Describe the specific steps you will take to improve your muscle endurance for low-back health:

_____

What effect, if any, did your plan have on your muscle endurance?

_____

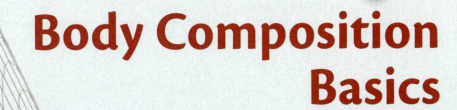

7

Body Composition Basics

COMING UP IN THIS CHAPTER

- Understand the basic composition of your body
- Identify factors that influence your body composition
- Examine the relationship between body composition and health
- Assess your body composition
- Identify strategies for making changes in your body composition

How does body composition relate to your overall wellness? The impact on your physical wellness is fairly clear, especially if you have significantly too much or too little body fat. Either situation can cause serious health problems and severely limit your daily activities. Body composition also affects other wellness dimensions. Your perceptions of your body weight and shape influence your emotional, spiritual, and social wellness. Do you experience positive or negative emotions when you think about your body? Does your body image affect your decisions about recreational or social activities? Are you missing out on anything because of your body image?

The planning and critical thinking skills of intellectual wellness can help you make good decisions about lifestyle choices that affect your body composition. These skills can also

help you evaluate media messages that may hurt your body image and emotional wellness. Your environment, too, plays a large role in determining your body composition; it can provide opportunities for healthy food choices and physical activity, or it can limit your ability to make healthy changes. In turn, you can positively influence your environment—for example, by campaigning for streets that are safe for walking and bicycling, for grocery stores and restaurants with healthful food, and for a positive focus on healthy body image.

This chapter presents basic information about body composition. You'll learn about the body's makeup and its influence on your health; factors affecting your body composition; methods of assessing it; and steps for altering your body composition.

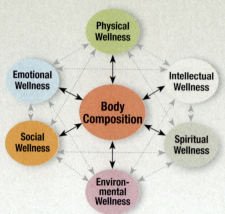

Basics of Body Composition

There are different ways to think about the makeup of the body—its joints, muscle groups, limbs, organs, and more. Let's define body composition and begin to examine how the proportion of muscle, fat, and other body tissues affects your short- and long-term health and well-being.

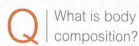 **What is body composition?**

Body composition refers to the makeup of the body. It is typically defined as the relative proportions of different types of body tissues:

- Muscle
- Bone
- Fat
- Other vital tissues

For adults of all ages, the proportion of body weight that is fat—**percent body fat**—is the measure most often used to define and evaluate body composition. For example, an individual who weighs 150 pounds and who is estimated to have 30 pounds of fat would have percent body fat of 20 percent. As we'll consider later in the chapter, too much or too little body fat has adverse effects on health, so percent body fat is an important consideration and body composition is a major health-related component of physical fitness. Percent body fat is one of the ways—but not the only way—of defining underweight, overweight, and obesity. Among older adults, the density and weight of bone tissue are also

important measures of health since loss of bone mass (known as *osteoporosis*) with aging can lead to fractures.

Q **Is there such a thing as good body fat?**

Yes. Your body needs fat in order to function—and body fat is much more than just a reservoir of energy. You can think of body fat in two categories: essential fat and storage fat.

Essential fat is the fat found in the central nervous system, in bone marrow, and in various organs. Fat is a key component of cell membranes and of the sheath that surrounds nerve fibers in the brain and enables the transmission of messages. Fat is necessary for normal physiological functioning—to maintain life and for reproductive functioning. Women typically have more essential fat than men due to hormonal and reproductive demands; essential fat is about 8–12 percent of women's body weight and about 3–5 percent of men's body weight (Figure 7-1). Women have more fat tissue in the breasts and pelvic area. Both women and men need a certain amount of fat for healthy hormone production.

Storage fat, also called *adipose tissue,* can be further divided into two

body composition Relative proportions of muscle, fat, bone, and other vital tissues; often expressed in terms of fat and fat-free body mass.

percent body fat The proportion (percentage) of total body weight that is fat; the measure most often used to evaluate body composition.

essential fat Fat necessary for normal body functioning; found in nerves, cell membranes, bone marrow, the central nervous system, and other organs.

Behavior-Change Challenge
Targeting Body Fat

You recently got the opportunity to have your percent body fat measured with skinfold method, using state-of-the-art spring-loaded calipers. Cool, you thought. But your mood deflated when the test revealed that your percent body fat is on the high end of the "recommended" range for your age and sex. Bummer! You know from a friend, though, that there are programs for changing body composition and that many people have success with them. You resolve to make one of these regimens your friend. At the same time, you want to set realistic goals. Where should you begin?

Meet Oscar

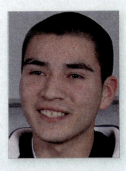

Oscar, a community college student, has been accepted to a 4-year school in the architectural program. He is physically active and currently has a percent body fat in the healthy range, but he is concerned about his family history of diabetes and what will happen when he goes away to college and is no longer eating at home. Oscar has set a specific goal for lowering his percent body fat. View the video to learn more about Oscar, his behavior-change goals and plan, and his achievements over the initial weeks of his program. As you watch, consider:

- How realistic are Oscar's goals and his starting program plan? How would his approach work for you?
- Does Oscar have enough motivation and environmental support for his program? What are likely to be his biggest challenges?
- What will be your greatest obstacles as you begin a program to revamp your body composition? What can you learn from Oscar's experience that will help you in your behavior-change efforts?

VIDEO CASE STUDY   WATCH THIS VIDEO IN connect

subcategories. The first type is found deep within the abdominal cavity surrounding internal organs. This fat is known as *internal storage fat* or **visceral fat,** and it provides a cushiony protection for organs such as the kidneys and intestines. The other type, known as **subcutaneous fat,** is storage fat found just beneath the skin; this is the fat you can see and pinch with your fingers (Figure 7-2). Subcutaneous fat helps to insulate the body and regulate temperature. It can be found in many parts of the body, but the largest deposits are typically in the abdomen, hips,

buttocks, and thighs. You need a certain amount of each type of storage fat, but too much, especially visceral fat, has negative health effects.

As indicated by its name, storage fat is a site for the storage of energy. As described in Chapter 4, the body can used stored fat as fuel to produce ATP for energy. Fat tissue also serves other functions: It releases many different kinds of molecules and hormones that affect appetite, blood pressure, immune system function, insulin and glucose levels, and various other body systems and processes.[1]

Q My friends and I look about the same, but most of them weigh around 15 pounds less than I do. How is that possible?

Body weight and body size are obviously related, but they don't tell the entire story. Different types of tissue vary in density, so two people who are the same size can have different weights and different body compositions. Muscle is denser than fat, so a pound of muscle takes up less space—about 18 percent less—than a pound of fat. Fat is even less dense than water, which means that it floats, whereas muscle is denser than water; this difference is the reason underwater weighing is sometimes used to estimate body composition (see p. 249). If an exercise program causes you to gain muscle mass and lose body fat, your weight on a scale may not change, but you are likely to notice your clothes getting looser because your new muscle takes up less space than the fat you lost.

If two people are about the same size, the heavier one likely has more muscle and less fat. Similarly, two people of the same weight can look very different and have different body compositions. Consider two people who both weigh 150 pounds. One might have 20 percent body fat, and the other 40 percent body fat. These two people would look significantly different from each other and would have very different health risks associated with their body composition.

Q What is metabolism?

Metabolism is all the processes that occur in your body to maintain its functioning. These processes require energy (calories), which you take in as food. The amount of energy your body requires depends on three criteria:

- *Resting metabolic rate (RMR):* The energy required to maintain essential body processes at rest,

storage fat Fat stored under the skin (subcutaneous fat) and surrounding internal organs (visceral fat); provides insulation, protects organs, serves as an energy store, and releases hormones and other chemical messengers.

visceral fat Storage fat found around and between organs in the abdominal cavity.

subcutaneous fat Storage fat found just under the skin.

metabolism All the processes within the body required to maintain its functioning.

resting metabolic rate (RMR) The energy required to maintain essential body processes at rest, including breathing, blood circulation, and temperature regulation.

Body composition (percent)

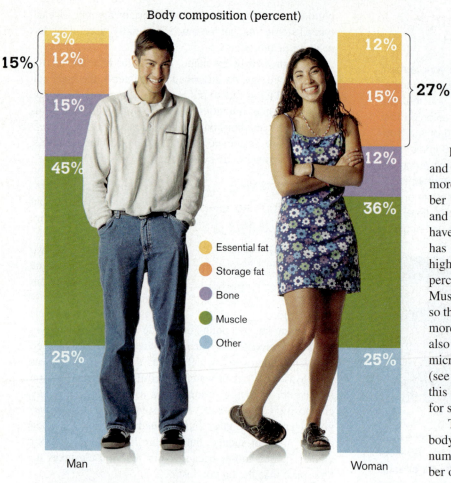

Man

Woman

Figure 7-1 **Body composition of young adults (ages 20–24).** The values here are not goals or averages; they only provide a basis for comparison. Note the larger percentage of essential fat for women compared to men.

Source: Behnke, A. R., & Wilmore, J. H. (1974). *Evaluation and regulation of body build and composition* (p. 123). Englewood Cliffs, NJ: Prentice Hall.

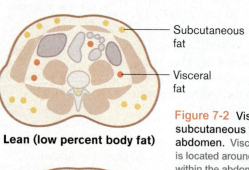

Subcutaneous fat

Visceral fat

Lean (low percent body fat)

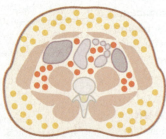

Excess body fat

Figure 7-2 **Visceral and subcutaneous fat in the abdomen.** Visceral fat is located around organs within the abdominal cavity, whereas subcutaneous fat is located just beneath the skin. Excess body fat of any kind carries health risks, but excess visceral fat is particularly unhealthy.

Source: Adapted from Stehno-Bittel, L. (2008). Intricacies of fat. *Physical Therapy: Diabetes Special Issue, 88*(11), 1265–1278.

including respiration, circulation, and temperature regulation

■ *Dietary thermogenesis:* The energy required for digesting and processing the foods you eat

■ *Physical activity:* The energy required for the tasks of daily living as well as formal exercise sessions

People with a higher resting metabolic rate and higher level of physical activity require more calories. Your RMR depends on a number of factors, including genetics, body size, and body composition. Larger people generally have a higher RMR simply because their body has more tissue to maintain. People with a higher proportion of muscle tissue and a lower percent body fat also have a higher RMR: Muscle is more metabolically active than fat, so the more pounds of muscle in your body, the more calories you require. Resistance training also increases RMR; research suggests that the microtears in muscle tissue caused by training (see Chapter 5) require energy to repair, and this tissue-remodeling process increases RMR for several days following a workout.[2]

The connection between metabolism and body composition is *energy balance*—the number of calories you take in versus the number of calories your body burns. See p. 252 for more information.

Q How do we get fat, literally? What causes the body to retain fat, and where does it go?

The body produces and stores fat when more energy is consumed than is used to maintain body functions and fuel activities, including regular daily tasks plus exercise. Stored body fat is an adaptation that protects humans from starvation when food is scarce or infrequent—something that is rare in contemporary life in many parts of the world. Stored body fat can also be used as a source of energy when energy demands increase, as they do, for example, during times of significant body growth or during pregnancy.

Mind Stretcher
Critical Thinking Exercise

How do you feel about your own body weight, size, and shape? Do you have strong feelings about what an ideal male or female body should look like? How do you think you developed these ideals? Are they realistic?

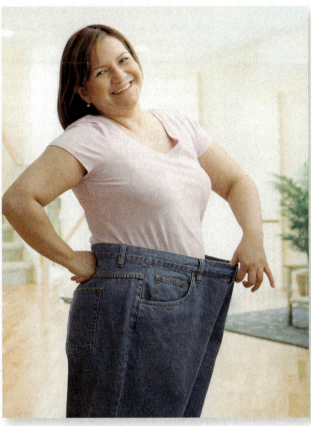

Muscle is denser than fat, so a pound of muscle takes up less space than a pound of fat. If you lose a pound of fat and add a pound of muscle, your body weight won't change but your body size will.

Calories from any source, whether fat, protein, carbohydrate, or alcohol, can cause increases in body fat if consumed in excess. You'll learn more about this delicate balance of energy later in the chapter. For now, consider that 3,500 calories is the equivalent of a pound of body weight, so if you consume 3,500 calories more than your body uses, you will gain a pound. Over the course of a year, consuming just 150 extra calories a day—the number of calories in one can of beer or regular soda—can add up to 15 pounds.

Most fat is stored in fat deposits, which are about 80 percent fat and 20 percent support cells, immune cells, and blood vessels. Droplets of fat are stored in specialized fat cells in these deposits. The number of fat cells stays fairly constant throughout adulthood. If you gain weight as fat, these fat cells enlarge, storing more

fat. If you lose body fat, your fat cells shrink. Some evidence suggests that significant fat gain may also increase the number of fat cells.[3]

It is possible to gain weight as muscle rather than fat, but it requires a careful program of increased energy intake combined with resistance training. See Chapter 9 for specific strategies for healthy weight gain.

overweight Body weight above the recommended range for good health.

obesity A serious degree of overweight characterized by an excessive amount of body fat.

Q | Do *overweight* and *obese* mean the same thing?

Although there are several ways to assess and define overweight and obesity, obesity is considered a more extreme and serious condition than overweight. **Overweight** generally means a body weight above a recommended range, based on large-scale population surveys or studies. **Obesity** is a higher degree of overweight, characterized by excessive body fat; obesity may also be defined by body weight or a related measure. In addition to body weight and percent body fat, height and waist circumference may be considered in evaluating the health risks associated with a particular body weight or shape. See the section "Assessing Body Composition" later in this chapter for more about specific fat percentage ranges as well as other means of defining overweight and obesity.

Q | Have Americans gotten fatter?

On average, yes. Twenty years ago, the average weight for American men and women in their twenties was about 15 pounds less than the average weight for adults in their twenties today. Furthermore, 50 years of tracking body mass index, a measure related to body weight and body composition (see pp. 246–247), shows that the prevalence of obesity among Americans has increased significantly, particularly in the 1980s (Figure 7-3).

DOLLAR STRETCHER
Financial Wellness Tip

Don't waste money on gadgets or supplements promising fat loss. There's no way to burn calories effortlessly or to reduce body fat in a specific spot. Physical activity is free, and consuming fewer calories can also save you money. Visit the Web site of the Federal Trade Commission for additional tips: http://www.ftc.gov/bcp/menus/consumer/health.shtm.

Factors Affecting Body Composition

Q | Do shorter people have a higher body-fat percentage?

Shorter people don't necessarily have a higher percentage of body fat. Your body composition depends on a combination of factors, and although height may be related to some of them,

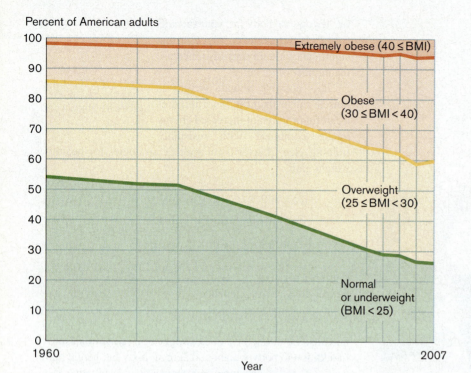

Percent of American adults

Figure 7-3 Prevalence of overweight, obesity, and extreme obesity among U.S. adults.

Source: Ogden, C. L., & Carroll, M. D. (2010). Prevalence of overweight, obesity, and extreme obesity among American adults, June 2010. *National Center for Health Statistics Health E-Stat* (http://www.cdc.gov/nchs/data/hestat/obesity_adult_07_08/obesity_adult_07_08.htm).

it doesn't directly predict the amount of fat within your body. Like height, some of the factors that determine body composition are beyond your control. But there are other influences on body composition that you can do something about.

Genetics

Q Is my body composition going to be similar to that of my parents? Is body composition based at all on genetics?

Genes do influence body size, amount and distribution of body fat, resting metabolic rate, response to exercise and overeating, and other factors related to energy balance. Depending on the factor, the contribution of heredity will be between 25 and 75 percent.[4] However, it can be difficult to separate the effects of genetic inheritance from environmental influences such as the eating and activity habits that you "inherit" from the family you grow up in.

Scientists have identified hundreds of genes that appear to have an effect on levels of body fat. For example, the *INSIG2* gene controls insulin and slows the synthesis of cholesterol and fatty acids, but about 10 percent of people

carry a gene variation that makes them less able to inhibit this synthesis and more likely to build up excess body fat.[5] The *fat-mass-and-obesity-related (FTO) gene*—dubbed the "fatso" gene—is associated with increased size and body fat. Researchers found that people with one copy (from one parent) of a particular variant in the FTO gene are likely to be fatter than those with no copies, and people with two copies (from both parents) are likely to be fatter than those with one copy.[6] About one in six adults carries two copies of the FTO gene variant. Other genes influence where fat is most likely to be stored—in the abdomen or hips, for example, or as visceral fat versus subcutaneous fat.

Genes do not tell the full story, however. Body composition is a complex trait, influenced by numerous environmental factors as well as many genes. Some genes that influence body composition come into play only under conditions of excess energy intake or inactivity. For example, researchers have found that for people who are physically active, having a variant of the FTO gene that predisposes them to obesity has no effect;[7] see the box "Beating the 'Fatso' Gene."

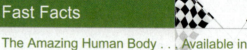

Fast Facts

The Amazing Human Body . . . Available in All Shapes and Sizes

Height

Average American man:	5 ft, 9 in.	Average American woman:	5 ft, 4 in.
Tallest man:	8 ft, 11 in.	Tallest woman:	8 ft, 2 in.
Shortest man:	21.5 in.	Shortest woman:	24 in.

Weight

Average American man:	195 lb	Average American woman:	165 lb
Heaviest man:	1,400 lb	Heaviest woman:	1,200 lb

Sources: Guinness World Records (http://www.guinness-worldrecords.com/); CDC National Center for Health Statistics (http://www.cdc.gov/nchs/).

- What is your first thought when you see someone who is especially thin or heavy? Short or tall?
- Is it fair and accurate to associate particular personality traits with different body types? How do you think people develop these ideas?

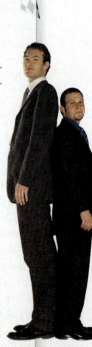

Research Brief

Beating the "Fatso" Gene

Researchers have identified many genes linked to excess body fat and unhealthy body-fat distribution. But do these genes alone explain the rapid rise in the number of Americans who are obese? It seems unlikely that our genes have changed dramatically in the past 20–30 years. What can researchers tell us about the relationship between genes and other factors?

One recent study looked at the effect of variations of the FTO gene, which is clearly associated with obesity. Researchers tested adults to identify which variants of FTO they carried and then compared their body mass index values (body mass index is a method of classifying and evaluating body weight). They also had the study participants wear a device called an *accelerometer* for a week to track their physical activity.

The researchers found that the FTO gene has a significant effect on whether people are overweight—but only people who are not physically active. Among the study participants who were physically active, body fatness was about the same regardless of the version of the gene they carried. Physical activity overcomes the effects of the obesity-promoting variations of the FTO gene.

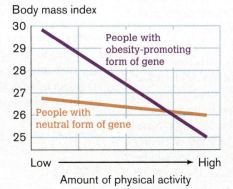

Body fatness versus physical activity for two variations of the FTO gene.

The results of this study highlight the interaction between genes and environment. Humans have long carried genes that can potentially promote obesity, but these genes came into play only in recent centuries, when a sedentary lifestyle and an abundance of food became possible for many people. It may seem unfair that some of us are born with genes that predispose us to gain body fat and others are not, but the results of this research are good news! A genetic predisposition for obesity is rarely destiny, because we do have some control over our genes through the food and activity choices we make.

Analyze and Apply

- What can those of us with obesity-promoting genes do to help prevent unhealthy fat gain?
- If you had such genes, what specific changes would you make to address this problem?

Sources: Rampersaud, E., Mitchell, B. D., Pollin, T. I., and others. (2008). Physical activity and the association of common FTO gene variants with body mass index and obesity. *Archives of Internal Medicine, 168*(16), 1791–1797.
Vimaleswaran, K., Li, S., Zhao, J., Luan, J., Bingham, S., Khaw, K., Ekelund, U., Wareham, N., & Loos, R. (2009). Physical activity attenuates the body mass index–increasing influence of genetic variation in the FTO gene. *American Journal of Clinical Nutrition, 90*(2), 425–428.

Q Why is it so hard for skinny guys to gain muscle mass?

As described in Chapter 5, people are born with different numbers of muscle cells and a different proportion of muscle-cell types. Some people are also less likely to gain body weight of any kind—fat or muscle—because their resting metabolic rates are high and their bodies simply aren't designed for weight or muscle gain. Although "skinny guys" can certainly build muscle, they won't be able to radically change their body type. See Chapter 5 for more about muscle tissue and strength training and Chapter 9 for weight-gain strategies.

The same is true for all general body types: We can't change our genetic structure or, in most cases, radically alter our body shape. But we don't all have to be shaped the same in order to have healthy bodies.

Biological Sex

Q I know men and women's bodies are different, but when my boyfriend and I eat together, it seems as if I am more susceptible to weight gain than he is. Why?

It's hard to compare any two people, even when they are similar in age or genetic makeup, because so many factors contribute to each person's body composition. As described in the earlier section "Basics of Body Composition," if your boyfriend is larger, weighs more, and has more muscle mass than you do, then he can eat more than you without gaining weight because his resting metabolic rate is likely to be higher. Even if a given man and woman are the same weight, the man will likely have a higher metabolic rate than the woman due to differences in their proportion of muscle and fat, with women having a higher proportion of essential body fat. But other sex differences are related to body composition as well, and these differences change with age.

On average, male babies are heavier at birth and in the first few months of life than female babies. However, male and female babies often have a similar amount of fat mass. This means girl babies typically are proportionally fatter than boy babies (a higher percent of their total weight is fat). Between ages 1 and 6, both boys and girls tend to lose body fat. After that point, girls' fat levels typically increase, while boys' lean mass increases. As boys and girls move into puberty and adolescence, the differences become even greater, with girls gaining fat mass but very little lean mass, and boys gaining lean mass but very little fat. By early adulthood, although males and females are often similar in weight-height ratios, males tend to have less body fat (Figure 7-4). Female reproductive maturity and childbirth can further contribute to the disparities in body-fat mass.[8]

In midlife, both men and women tend to begin to lose muscle mass, and this change leaves a higher proportion of fat mass. For men, this process typically begins in their fifties. For women, it often starts in their forties and is frequently accompanied by increases in fat mass.[9] These declines typically continue for both males and females as they grow older, though by the time they hit their seventies and eighties, both men and women may begin to lose total mass.[10]

Q | Why do men gain fat in their belly, and women in their hips?

Although there is a great deal of individual variation, on average, men are more likely to store excess fat in the abdomen, and women are more likely to store it in the hips and thighs (Figure 7-5).

- *Android,* or apple-shaped, fat distribution is more common in men and postmenopausal women.
- *Gynoid,* or pear-shaped, fat distribution is more common in premenopausal women.

The difference is due at least in part to the effects of estrogen in premenopausal women. After menopause, women's estrogen levels drop, and their body shape tends to change to an apple form. As we'll see later in the chapter, the apple-shaped pattern of fat distribution is associated with more health risks than the pear-shaped pattern of fat distribution. People with an apple shape tend to have a higher proportion of unhealthy visceral fat. You'll have a chance to evaluate your own shape in Lab Activity 7-1.

Age

Q | Does body composition always get worse as we get older?

It's hard to separate the effects of age from use, because we tend to become less active as we age. With each decade they don't strength train, adults lose about 4–6 pounds of muscle mass, and their resting metabolic rate also declines.[11] If calorie intake is not decreased, the energy that had been used to maintain the lost muscle tissue will be stored as fat, thereby increasing percent body fat. Studies have found that older adults usually have a higher percent body fat than younger adults.[12] Excess body fat in young adults is a serious concern because we typically gain fat and lose muscle as we age; an unhealthy amount of body fat in young adulthood makes achieving and maintaining a healthy body composition over time more challenging. Fortunately, physical activity, especially resistance training, can maintain muscle mass as we age; strength training can help build muscle and reduce fat at any age.

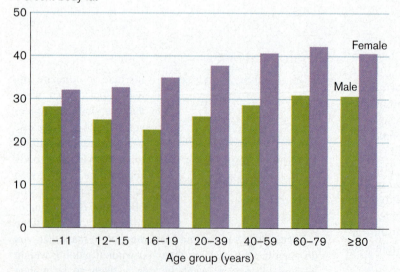

Percent body fat

Figure 7-4 Average percent body fat by age and sex.
Source: U.S. Department of Health and Human Services. (2009). Mean percentage body fat by age group and sex—National Health and Nutrition Examination Survey, United States, 1999–2004. *MMWR Weekly, 57*(552), 1383 (http://www.cdc.gov/mmwr/preview/mmwrhtml/mm5751a4.htm).

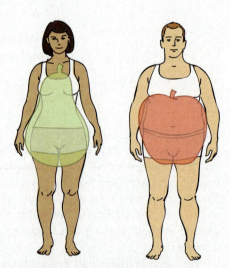

Figure 7-5 Body-fat distribution. Are you an apple or a pear? A pear shape is healthier because it typically means less visceral fat.

Ethnicity

Q | Do different ethnic groups have different body compositions?

Research tells us the body-composition patterns related to sex and age are true across all ethnic groups.[13] However, ethnic differences have been found in average height, weight, and body composition. The extent of the differences can be affected by lifestyle and environmental factors related to culture and ethnicity. More research is needed, especially on how these differences may affect the health and fitness risks and benefits associated with different body compositions. Table 7-1 shows the findings from one study involving detailed body scans of nearly 2,000 adults. General trends don't apply to every individual in an ethnic group, but findings from this and other research may be relevant when you assess your body composition:

- At a given body weight, Asian Americans and Latinos have a higher percent body fat and a higher percent of abdominal fat than whites and African Americans.

- At a given body weight, African Americans have a lower percent body fat and lower percent of abdominal fat than other ethnic groups, indicating greater relative bone density and muscle mass.

These trends reinforce that each of us is different and there is no single body size or body composition that is best or even possible for everyone.

Lifestyle and Environment

Q | Some of my cousins are really fat, but my brothers and I are skinny. Why aren't we more alike since we have many of the same genes?

Genetics is one factor in body composition, but there are other influences as well, including age and sex. Different lifestyles and environments may also play a role in your different body compositions, including these four factors:

- *Energy intake:* The amount of energy you take in as food obviously affects body composition. If you

TABLE 7-1 COMPARISON OF AVERAGE HEIGHT, WEIGHT, BODY MASS INDEX, AND TOTAL AND ABDOMINAL FAT AMONG ADULTS FROM FOUR ETHNIC GROUPS*

	WHITE	AFRICAN AMERICAN	LATINO	ASIAN AMERICAN
MEN				
HEIGHT	69 in.	69 in.	67 in.	67 in.
WEIGHT	176 lb	177 lb	173 lb	152 lb
BODY MASS INDEX**	25.7	26.0	27.1	23.6
ABDOMINAL FAT	9.3 lb	7.9 lb	9.1 lb	9.9 lb
PERCENT BODY FAT	20.4%	18.6%	20.9%	22.5%
WOMEN				
HEIGHT	64 in.	64 in.	61 in.	62 in.
WEIGHT	156 lb	174 lb	150 lb	120 lb
BODY MASS INDEX**	27.0	29.2	28.4	22.2
ABDOMINAL FAT	12.7 lb	12.2 lb	12.7 lb	13.3 lb
PERCENT BODY FAT	35.6%	35.3%	37.4%	36.8%

*Based on measurement and dual-energy X-ray absorptiometry of 604 men and 1,192 women ages 18–96 years.
**Body mass index, described on pp. 246–247, is a measure of relative body weight.

Source: Adapted from Wu, CH, Heshka, S., Wang, J., Pierson, R. N., Heymsfield, S. B., Laferrère, B., Wang, Z., Albu, J. B., Pi-Sunyer, X., & Gallagher, D. (2007). Truncal fat in relation to total body fat: Influences of age, sex, ethnicity and fatness. *International Journal of Obesity, 31(9),* 1384–1391.

consume more calories than you burn, you will gain weight and possibly fat. If you consume fewer calories than you burn, you will lose weight and possibly fat. Whether you gain or lose weight as muscle or fat depends on factors such as your genes and activity level.

- *Physical activity:* The amount of energy you burn during daily activity and purposeful exercise also obviously affects energy balance and body composition.
- *Sleep:* Consistent short sleep duration is associated with increased overall body fat and increased abdominal body fat. Lack of sleep may interfere with the regulation of appetite, causing people to eat more, and with the balance of glucose and insulin, possibly increasing diabetes risk.[14]
- *Stress:* Excess psychological stress is linked to increased energy intake, weight gain, and excess abdominal fat.[15] During the stress response, the liver produces more glucose to provide energy. If you don't use all the extra glucose, your body reabsorbs it. But if you are frequently or chronically stressed, the extra blood sugar can contribute to glucose intolerance, insulin resistance, and type 2 diabetes. Excess insulin in the blood also encourages the body to store fat.

The good news about lifestyle factors affecting body composition is that you can control or at least influence many of them. However, some environmental factors linked to your body composition, such as the socioeconomic status of the household where you grew up and your parents' educational attainment, may be beyond your control. The characteristics of your neighborhood can also influence your body composition. Is it walkable, so that you have many easy opportunities for daily physical activity? Are there healthy grocery options? How many fast-food restaurants are there? Living in a neighborhood with limited opportunities for physical activity and poor access to healthy foods is a risk factor for unhealthy body composition.[16] These neighborhood characteristics are most often associated with socioeconomically disadvantaged populations and ethnic minorities.

Finally, it's important to remember that overall body size isn't necessarily an indicator of a higher percent of body fat. Just because your cousins are larger doesn't mean they are automatically fatter. You would have to assess their body composition in order to determine their degree of fatness or overfatness.

Body Composition and Wellness

Q | Why is it important to know how much fat is in your body? What can one statistic like percent body fat tell you about health?

Body composition is just one component of health-related fitness. However, as with the other components, there is a desired range for easy performance of daily activities and long-term health maintenance. Maintaining an appropriate level of body fat is vital to a healthy, longer life.

Your body composition can tell you a lot, but as will be described in the section "Assessing Body Composition," you will need to consider more than just a single number (percent body fat). A certain amount of fat is healthy and necessary, but too much or too little fat can harm your health. As the next two sections discuss, an extremely high or low percent body fat can significantly compromise your quality of life and reduce your life expectancy.

Problems Associated with Excess Body Fat

Q | My dad is really big (I don't like to say "fat") and I worry about him. What are his greatest health risks?

The main problem for people who are overweight and have a high percent body fat is the increased risk for a number of deadly chronic diseases, leading to reduced life expectancy.

- *Cardiovascular disease:* Obesity is linked to high blood pressure, unhealthy blood fat levels, and heightened risk of developing and dying from cardiovascular disease.
- *Type 2 diabetes:* Excess body fat is the main risk factor for type 2 diabetes, and rates of diabetes among Americans have increased along with the rates of overweight and obesity.
- *Cancer:* Excess body fat drives up the risk for cancer of the breast, prostate, colon, pancreas, esophagus, endometrium (part of the uterus), kidney, and other sites. One recent report estimated that obesity causes 100,000 cases of cancer in the United States each year.[17]

MYTH or **FACT?**

It's healthier to be 25 pounds overweight and physically active than to be at an optimal weight and sedentary.

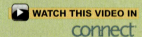 **WATCH THIS VIDEO IN** connect

See page 476 to find out.

Other health problems associated with overweight and obesity include joint problems such as osteoarthritis, sleep apnea, asthma and other respiratory problems, gallbladder and liver diseases, and reproductive problems.

As we have seen, the risk for some health problems is greater if the excess fat is in the abdomen instead of the hips. Visceral fat is closely linked to unhealthy cholesterol levels, problems with insulin regulation, and increased blood pressure. Researchers are still investigating the mechanisms by which visceral fat harms health. One idea relates to its proximity to the liver; substances released by visceral-fat stores may influence the liver's production of cholesterol in unhealthy ways.

So although subcutaneous fat may be what most people have in mind when they think about losing excess body fat, visceral fat can do more damage to your health. Removal of subcutaneous fat through liposuction doesn't improve

Research Brief

Screen Time and Waistlines

Many studies conducted over the past few decades have demonstrated an increase in the average number of hours of television people watch each day. Studies have also shown a connection between hours of television and obesity, especially in children. What about for adults?

Researchers recently looked at the number of reported hours of screen time (television and computer) among nearly 100,000 adults to determine if there was a relationship among screen time, physical activity, obesity, and other factors. They found that the risk of obesity rose for

Relative risk of obesity

Screen time and relative risk of obesity.

Average daily hours of screen time: <2, 2–3, 4–5, 6–7, ≥8

both men and women with increasing amounts of screen time, no matter what their physical activity level was. Adults who averaged 6 or more hours of screen time per day had almost double the rate of obesity risk of adults who averaged less than 2 hours of daily screen time.

Analyze and Apply

- What does this research mean with respect to achieving or maintaining a healthy body composition?
- What policy should parents take regarding their children's TV viewing and computer time? Why?

Source: Banks, E., Jorm, L., Rogers, K., Clements, M., & Bauman, A. (2010). Screen time, obesity, ageing, and disability. *Public Health Nutrition*, 34–43.

---

metabolic measures such as insulin sensitivity, whereas weight loss through diet and exercise does. Losing body fat through changes in diet and physical activity reduces the amount of dangerous visceral fat in the body.[18]

In addition to shortening life expectancy, obesity can also reduce years of healthy life. Obese people spend a greater portion of their life with disabilities that interfere with day-to-day living. Obesity has many serious consequences, but obesity can be reversed. It is never too late to start making changes that can lead to a longer and healthier life.

Q Can you be sort of overweight or overfat and healthy at the same time?

Maybe. The health consequences of a moderate degree of excess body fat and weight are controversial and the subject of ongoing research. The following factors can make a difference:

- *Age and weight history:* Overweight in someone young is of extra concern because unless a healthy weight is established, the person's body will be exposed to the effects of overweight for a longer period. Also, people usually gain weight and fat as they age, so someone who is moderately overweight as a young adult is at increased risk of becoming dangerously obese in later life. Has your weight remained stable, or has it gone up as you've gotten older?

Fast Facts

As Waistlines Grow, Life Expectancy Shrinks

Overweight and obesity are associated with reduced life expectancy. The number of years lost increases if the individual is also a smoker. The table shows the reduced life expectancy, by biological sex, for overweight nonsmokers and for obese nonsmokers and smokers relative to the life expectancy of normal-weight nonsmokers.

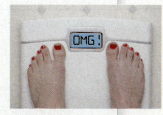

Group	Change in Years of Life Expectancy Relative to Normal-Weight Nonsmoker
Overweight	
Female nonsmoker	−3.3 years
Male nonsmoker	−3.1 years
Obese	
Female nonsmoker	−7.1 years
Female smoker	−13.3 years
Male nonsmoker	−5.8 years
Male smoker	−13.7 years

Source: Peeters, A., Barendregt, J. J., Willekens, F., Mackenbach, J. P., Al Mamun, A., & Bonneaux, L. (2003). Obesity in adulthood and its consequences for life expectancy: A life-table analysis. *Annals of Internal Medicine, 138*(1), 24–32.

- *Body-fat distribution:* Health risks from body fat are greater if the excess fat is stored in the abdomen rather than in the hips and thighs.
- *Other health risk factors:* Someone who is overweight and who has, for example, high blood pressure and elevated glucose levels is at greater risk for health problems than someone who is overweight but doesn't have additional risk factors.
- *Lifestyle:* Even if it doesn't significantly lower a person's weight, regular exercise can improve body composition and reduce some of the risks associated with overweight, including high blood pressure and unhealthy cholesterol levels. (See the box "Screen Time and Waistlines" for some insight into a common problem associated with lack of physical activity.)

Once gained, excess fat is difficult to shed. If you have a slightly or moderately elevated percent body fat, strive to adopt a healthy diet and physical activity habits that will help prevent weight and fat gain and reduce other risk factors.[19] One of the biggest concerns about a small degree of overweight is that it won't stay small.

Problems Associated with Too Little Body Fat

Q What is the lowest body-fat percentage you can have and still maintain a healthy lifestyle? Is it even possible for a woman to have absolutely no body fat?

It's not possible for a woman (or a man) to have zero body fat, and no one should want to. As noted earlier, a certain amount of fat is essential for the body to function properly and to sustain life. Underweight people with low body fat are often malnourished. As a result they may have fluid imbalances, vitamin and mineral deficiencies, and kidney problems. They are more likely as well to lose bone mass and develop osteoporosis. Women may also experience reproductive disorders. Appropriate body fat ranges are presented in the section "Assessing Body Composition."

Q If I exercise a lot and my period stops, is that a good thing or a bad thing?

Usually that is a bad thing. Some women develop a condition known as the **female athlete triad.** It is most common in those participating in sports that emphasize leanness, such as gymnastics, diving, ice skating, and cross-country running, but it can occur in any sport or with any form of regular

---

strenuous exercise.[20] The disorder is called a triad because it has three components, each of which can occur on a continuum between optimal/healthy and unhealthy (Figure 7-6):

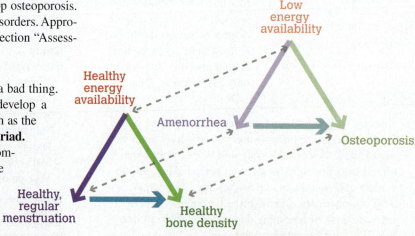

Figure 7-6 **The female athlete triad.**

■ *Energy availability:* A healthy level of available energy supports physical activity, bone health, and menstruation. Insufficient energy intake leads to loss of bone density and menstrual disorders. Low energy availability is usually the result of insufficient calorie intake or increased energy expenditure through exercise without increasing calorie intake. The triad can be caused by disordered eating patterns or full-blown eating disorders.

■ *Menstruation:* Healthy energy availability supports hormonal function and regular menstruation. Low energy availability leads to menstrual disorders and eventually to *amenorrhea* (absence of menstruation for more than 90 days), which can reduce bone density. Amenorrhea and other types of menstrual dysfunction are associated with a state of estrogen deficiency similar to that in menopause. Menstrual irregularities and low bone mass increase the risk of stress fractures.

■ *Bone health:* Low energy availability reduces bone density in two ways—by suppressing hormones that promote bone formation and by causing amenorrhea. The loss of bone density may not be fully reversible even if the issues underlying the triad are addressed.

If you experience any of the signs of developing the triad, you should consult a medical professional and be assessed for all the components. Many athletes can continue with their regular training and deal with triad-related health problems with adequate nutrition and energy intake.

Body Composition and Athletic Performance

Q | I'm a runner. Will decreasing my body fat help make me faster?

That's a difficult question because many factors beyond body composition determine your running speed. Other factors being equal though, a decreased level of body fat (that is still in the healthy range) might improve your performance and reduce your susceptibility to performance-related injuries.[21]

Most athletes rely on two things for good performance: the ability to sustain both aerobic and anaerobic power and the ability to overcome resistance, or what is often referred to as "drag." This presents a dilemma for athletes who associate overcoming drag with eating less and losing weight, which they may think equates to losing body fat. However, most of them also know they need to eat more in order to increase energy and sustain their activity.

With the intention of losing weight and decreasing fat, some athletes fall into a bad cycle of eating too little, burning a lot of calories through activity, losing lean muscle mass (and thus increasing percent body fat), decreasing performance, eating even less, and so on. This spiral can sometimes lead to eating disorders that pose serious risks to health (see Chapter 9) as well as to the female athlete triad in women.

Decreased body fat can improve performance in some athletes, but only if it's still at a healthy level. Athletes must consume enough calories to fuel their efforts and maintain lean body mass and a healthy level of body fat. Too little energy intake and body fat harm both health and athletic performance.

There is no ideal percent body fat for each sport. However, your coach, trainer, or doctor can help you find an appropriate range for your sport.

Body Composition, Body Image, and Emotional Wellness

"I'm too fat." "I'm too skinny." "I'd be happy if I were taller / shorter / had bigger muscles / longer legs. . . ." Do any of these statements sound familiar? Many of us have difficulty accepting our body, and this dissatisfaction can hurt our self-esteem and emotional wellness.

Q | What exactly is body image?

Body image is your own mental picture of your body and how you feel about it. It is subjective, so what you "see" in the mirror may not be the same as what others see. Your body image may be realistic or unrealistic, just like your goals for your body shape or size. Many of us have internalized cultural ideals of appearance that are far removed from what is possible, or even healthy, for us to achieve.

A negative body image can cause stress, anxiety, and depression; in some cases, it can lead to disordered patterns of eating and other negative health habits (see

female athlete triad A condition in active females that develops because excess exercise or insufficient energy intake or both results in insufficient available energy; characterized by amenorrhea and loss of bone density.

body image An individual's subjective mental representation of his or her own body

Mind Stretcher
Critical Thinking Exercise

Think about your work, recreational, home, and school activities. How could a body-fat percentage that is too low or too high negatively impact your daily activities? What about your closest friends and family members: Is body composition affecting their lives either positively or negatively?

Chapter 9 for more on eating disorders). A positive body image supports emotional wellness and healthy attitudes, behaviors, and self-esteem.

Many of us have small or moderate body-image issues, but a few people develop an extremely negative and unrealistic body image. **Body dysmorphic disorder (BDD)** is characterized by extreme preoccupation with an imagined defect in appearance. The focus might be on a particular feature, such as the skin or nose, or on body shape in general. People with BDD typically isolate themselves from others out of fear of being judged for their "defect," and they have very low self-esteem. They may engage in compulsive behaviors such as mirror checking, use cosmetics or clothing to camouflage the imaged defect, and seek multiple plastic surgeries. Although more common in women, BDD can also affect men. A form of BDD more common in men is **muscle dysmorphia,** or becoming obsessed with the idea of not being big or muscular enough. People with muscle dysmorphia may spend all of their time at the gym while ignoring other parts of their life; they use exercise compulsively to feel better about themselves and may also take supplements or even steroids in an effort to fix the perceived problem. BDD is different from eating disorders, but like them, it is considered a psychological disorder that requires professional treatment.

body dysmorphic disorder (BDD)
A psychological disorder characterized by extreme preoccupation with an imagined defect in appearance.

muscle dysmorphia
A form of BDD more common in males, characterized by preoccupation with perceived lack of muscularity.

Q Where does body image come from?

Two key sources of body image (and self-esteem) are family and the media. Parents who criticize their children and the way they look create a negative self-image and lower their kids' self-esteem. These family influences are often subtle and are frequently dismissed ("It's no big deal; my mom says that about everyone"), but over time they have a cumulative harmful effect on body image and self-esteem. Peers and teachers can also influence attitudes about body image through their comments and the ways they treat people of different body shapes and sizes.

The media are a major influence on body image. The pressure to look a certain way, whether one is male or female, is everywhere. All forms of media contain messages about how we should look, and they imply that if we don't conform, something is wrong. These daily messages have a powerful impact, especially on young people already predisposed toward a negative body image. Here are some sobering statistics:

- In surveys, the biggest wish of girls ages 10–14 is to lose weight.
- For adolescent girls, the media tend to be the main source of information about women's health issues; the majority of middle school girls read at least one fashion magazine regularly.
- Women's magazines have more than ten times more advertisements and articles promoting weight loss than men's magazines.

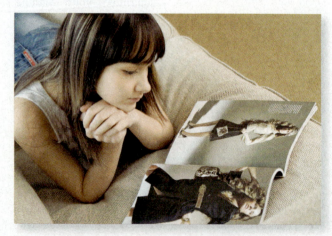

Body image is our subjective mental picture of how our body looks and how we feel about it. A negative body image can cause stress and impair emotional wellness.

- A study of over 4,000 network television commercials revealed that 1 of every 3.8 commercials sends some sort of "attractiveness message," telling viewers what is or is not attractive; the average adolescent sees over 5,260 "attractiveness messages" per year.[22]

Barbie dolls are a classic example of body-image distortion promoted by the media. We all know that Barbie and Ken's body proportions are absurdly unreal, yet they continue to be regarded as having ideal, albeit unattainable, bodies. Similarly, male action figures have grown increasing large and muscular over the years and now have a degree of muscularity not found even in bodybuilders. Another example is fashion models and the winners of the Miss America pageant, who have gotten significantly thinner since the 1920s and many of whom now would be classified as underweight (Figure 7-7). The growing gap between actual and idealized body type can contribute to a negative body image.

Q So we're supposed to worry about how we look for health reasons but not worry about how we look. How does that work?

For body composition and body image, what's important is what is healthy for you. Assess your body composition according to health criteria (see the next section), and avoid comparing yourself to unachievable cultural and media ideals. Instead of trying to change your appearance, which isn't always easy, change the way you think about your body. Recognize that regardless of its size and shape, your body is a gift to you. Treat it as such and you will begin to appreciate the marvel your body is. See the box "Accepting Your Body" for ideas to improve your body image.

Figure 7-7 **Average young women versus fashion models and Miss America (1920s–2000s).** In the 1920s, the idealized body type represented by Miss America and fashion models was very close to the typical body type of young women. Over the course of the twentieth century, however, the gap widened between real and idealized young women.

Sources: Byrd-Bredbenner, C., Murray, J., & Schlussel, Y. R. (2005). Temporal changes in anthropometric measurements of idealized females and young women in general. *Women & Health, 41*(2), 13–30. National Center for Health Statistics. (2008). Anthropometric reference data for children and adults. *National Health Statistics Reports, 10.*

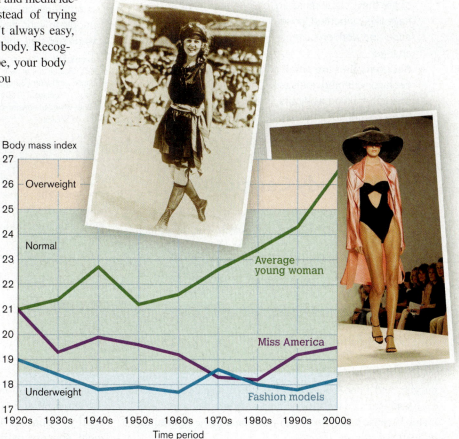

Wellness Strategies

Accepting Your Body

Q | How can I improve my self-image?

To avoid body-image problems and raise your self-esteem, concentrate on good physical and emotional health and engage in some body acceptance.

- **Focus on the positives.** Think about your body's unique beauty and functionality. Remember, too, that body composition, weight, and shape are just one aspect of wellness. Your self-esteem and self-image should be based on all the things you think and do.
- **Focus on health and healthy habits.** Evaluate your body composition based on health criteria. Engage in healthy eating and physical activity habits, and feel good about yourself for making positive wellness choices. For many people, regular exercise can provide feelings of competency and mastery that boost self-esteem and body image, even if it doesn't change their weight or shape.
- **Realistically evaluate which aspects of your body you can change.** If you're like everyone else, you have things you can't change and need to accept, such as your height and your shoe size. Do most of your family members have narrow shoulders or broad hips or are they "small-muscled" or "big-boned?" If so, you have likely inherited those characteristics. Acknowledge and work on accepting the things you can't change.
- **Set goals that are small and attainable.** Focus on behavior-oriented goals, such as engaging in regular strength-training workouts, rather than on unrealistic goals related to specific aspects of your body.

- **Avoid negative self-talk about your body.** Don't compare yourself to others or to media ideals. Remember that the models you see in the media typically have atypical body types enhanced by expensive cosmetics and clothing as well as photographic touch-ups. Emphasize the good things you do and the positive aspects of your life.
- **Recognize advertisements from the fitness and beauty industries as what they are.** These promotions are attempts to make you dissatisfied with yourself and your life so that you will buy certain products. Be a media-literate consumer.
- **Just as you don't judge yourself by appearance, don't judge others.** Body size and shape are only external characteristics. Judge the people in your life based on what they say and do, not on how they look.

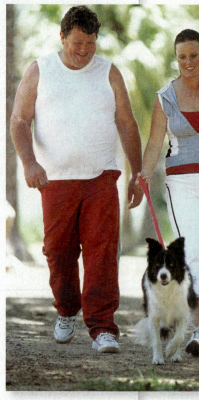

Sources: Wood-Barcalow, N. L, Tylka, T. L., & Augustus-Horvath, C. L. (2010). "But I like my body": Positive body image characteristics and a holistic model for young-adult women. *Body Image, 7*(2), 106–116. Vocks, S., Hechler, T., Rohrig, S., & Legenbauer, T. (2009). Effects of a physical exercise session on state body image. *Psychological Health, 24*(6), 713–728.

Assessing Body Composition

Q | What's my ideal weight?

That's a tough question to answer. We have seen that body weight and even percent body fat don't provide a full picture of how your body composition might affect your health and wellness. A healthy body composition for you also depends on other health risk factors, including fat distribution, blood pressure, and your exercise habits.

Percent body fat is a better indicator of health status than overall body weight—a scale can't distinguish between fat, muscle, and bone—but it is difficult to measure. In fact, even sophisticated tests for percent body fat yield mere estimates because exact body composition can be determined only after death.

This section will review techniques for evaluating body weight, percent body fat, and body-fat distribution. Lab Activity 7-1 walks you through the steps of calculating and evaluating your own BMI, percent body fat, and body-fat distribution.

Body Mass Index: An Indirect Measure of Body Fat

Q | How do I determine my BMI?

Body mass index (BMI) is one of the most common techniques for assessing body fatness, and it is useful if you don't have access to equipment for estimating percent body

body mass index (BMI) An indirect measure of body fatness calculated by dividing body weight (in kilograms) by the square of height (in meters); for non-athletic populations, BMI correlates closely with more precise measures of body composition.

Wellness Strategies

Calculating Body Mass Index

Q | How do I calculate my BMI?

Visit the book's Web site for an online BMI calculator. To compute by hand, use the formulas below or in Lab Activity 7-1. Measure your height with shoes off and your weight with minimal clothing. To measure waist

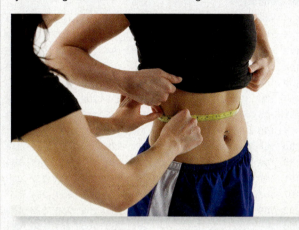

circumference, place a measuring tape flat against your skin, above the iliac crest (hipbone) at the narrowest point of your waist; keep the tape horizontal as you measure. Look up your BMI and waist circumference in Table 7-2.

If you know your body weight in kilograms and your height in meters:

Formula	Example	
$\dfrac{\text{Weight (kg)}}{(\text{Height [m]})^2}$	$\dfrac{70 \text{ kg}}{(1.7 \text{ m})^2}$	$= 24.2 \text{ kg/m}^2$

If you only know your body weight in pounds and your height in inches:

Formula	Example	
$\dfrac{\text{Weight (lb.)}}{(\text{Height [in.]})^2} \times 703$	$\dfrac{165 \text{ lb.}}{(68 \text{ in.})^2} \times 703$	$= 25.1 \text{ kg/m}^2$

Note: 1 pound = 0.4536 kilograms; 1 inch = 0.0254 meters; in the second formula, the multiplier 703 converts the units to kg/m^2.

fat. Many research studies have compared BMI against the risk of developing health problems, so BMI can provide guidance in determining if your weight places you at risk. Although, like the old insurance company tables, BMI is based on height and weight, it is a more accurate indicator.

BMI is calculated by dividing your weight (in kilograms) by the square of your height (in meters); see the box "Calculating Body Mass Index" or refer to Figure 7-8. Because BMI doesn't distinguish between weight from fat and weight from lean tissue, measurement of waist circumference is used to help classify the health risks associated with different BMI values. Again, excess fat in the abdomen is linked to greater health risks than fat stored in other places.

Q | Is BMI relevant and accurate for both athletes and people who are out of shape?

Not entirely, no. BMI is only an indirect measure of body composition. BMI is most accurate for non-athletes and people who don't do a lot of strength training; for them, BMI measures have been highly correlated with more precise measures of body fat. However, athletes and people with an above-average amount of muscle mass are likely to have a BMI in the overweight range when they actually have a healthy body composition. If you are athletic or heavily muscled, one of the methods of estimating percent

body fat is probably a more accurate assessment for you. Look as well at waist circumference and some of the other measures of body-fat distribution described in the next section.

BMI may also be less accurate for older adults, who tend to have more fat mass and less muscle mass than younger people of the same weight. Older adults may be classified in the normal BMI range when they actually have excess body fat. In addition, there has been a significant amount of debate about whether there should be different cutoffs for people in different ethnic groups. As mentioned earlier in the chapter, Asian Americans tend to have a higher percent body fat and African Americans a lower percent body fat at a given weight. For Asian Americans, researchers have proposed lower BMI cutoff points for the classification of overweight and obesity; however, there is no universally agreed upon standard.[23]

Despite its limitations, BMI can be relatively accurate for the average adult. Although it's not the most accurate way to estimate body composition, it is a good place to start if you don't have access to more direct methods of assessment.

Methods for Estimating Percent Body Fat

Q | How can you determine body-fat percentages?

There are a number of different ways to estimate percent body fat. Some methods require expensive

Figure 7-8 Body mass index. Find your height in the left column and then your weight in the appropriate row. Your BMI will be in the top row of the table above your weight. For example, if you are 5' 7" and weigh 160 pounds, your BMI is 25.

Source: Ratings from the National Heart, Lung, and Blood Institute. (1998). *Clinical guidelines on the identification, evaluation, and treatment of overweight and obesity in adults.* Bethesda, MD: National Institutes of Health.

BMI	17	18	19	20	21	22	23	24	25	26	27	28	29	30	31	32	33	34	35	36	37	38	39	40
Height (inches)													Body weight (pounds)											
58	81	86	91	96	101	105	110	115	120	124	129	134	139	144	148	153	158	162	168	172	177	182	187	192
59	84	89	94	99	104	109	114	119	124	129	134	139	144	149	154	159	163	168	173	178	183	188	193	198
60	87	92	97	102	108	113	118	123	128	133	138	143	149	154	159	164	168	174	179	184	190	195	200	205
61	90	95	101	106	111	117	122	127	132	138	143	148	154	159	164	169	174	180	185	191	196	201	207	212
62	93	98	104	109	115	120	126	131	137	142	148	153	159	164	170	175	180	186	191	197	202	208	213	219
63	96	102	107	113	119	124	130	136	141	147	153	158	164	169	175	181	186	191	198	203	209	215	220	226
64	99	105	111	117	122	128	134	140	146	152	157	163	169	175	181	186	192	197	204	210	215	222	227	233
65	102	108	114	120	126	132	138	144	150	156	162	168	174	180	186	192	198	204	210	216	222	229	235	241
66	105	112	118	124	130	136	143	149	155	161	167	174	180	186	192	198	204	210	217	223	229	236	242	248
67	109	115	121	128	134	141	147	153	160	166	173	179	185	192	198	205	211	217	224	230	236	243	249	256
68	112	118	125	132	138	145	151	158	165	171	178	184	191	197	204	211	216	223	230	237	244	250	257	263
69	115	122	129	136	142	149	156	163	169	176	183	190	197	203	210	217	224	230	237	244	251	258	264	271
70	119	126	133	139	146	153	160	167	174	181	188	195	202	209	216	223	230	237	244	251	258	265	272	279
71	122	129	136	143	151	158	165	172	179	187	194	201	208	215	222	230	237	244	251	258	265	273	280	287
72	125	133	140	148	155	162	170	177	184	192	199	207	214	221	229	236	243	251	258	266	273	280	288	295
73	129	137	144	152	159	167	174	182	190	197	205	212	220	228	235	243	250	258	265	273	281	288	296	303
74	132	140	148	155	164	171	179	187	195	203	210	218	226	234	242	249	257	265	273	281	288	296	304	312
75	136	144	152	160	168	176	184	192	200	208	216	224	232	240	248	256	264	272	280	288	296	304	312	320
76	140	148	156	164	173	181	189	197	206	214	222	230	238	247	255	263	271	280	288	296	304	312	321	329

Category ranges:
- <18.5 Underweight
- 18.5–24.9 Normal
- 25–29.9 Overweight
- 30–34.9 Obesity (class I)
- 35–39.9 Obesity (class II)
- >40 Extremely obese

TABLE 7-2 BODY MASS INDEX (BMI) CLASSIFICATION AND DISEASE RISK*

	BMI (KG/M^2)	DISEASE RISK RELATIVE TO NORMAL WEIGHT AND WAIST CIRCUMFERENCE*	
		MEN: WAIST ≤40 IN. (102 CM) WOMEN: WAIST ≤35 IN. (88 CM)	MEN: WAIST >40 IN. (102 CM) WOMEN: WAIST >35 IN. (88 CM)
UNDERWEIGHT	<18.5		
NORMAL	18.5–24.9		
OVERWEIGHT	25.0–29.9	Increased	High
OBESITY (CLASS I)	30.0–34.9	High	Very high
OBESITY (CLASS II)	35.0–39.9	Very high	Very high
EXTREME OBESITY (CLASS III)	≥ 40.0	Extremely high	Extremely high

*Disease risk for type 2 diabetes, hypertension, and cardiovascular disease; increased waist circumference can be a marker for increased risk even in persons of normal weight.

Source: National Heart, Lung, and Blood Institute. (1998). *Clinical guidelines on the identification, evaluation, and treatment of overweight and obesity in adults.* Bethesda, MD: National Institutes of Health.

medical equipment, but others can be done in a gym or classroom. Check with your instructor or your campus or community health center to find out what methods are available to you.

Table 7-3 gives an overview of common methods for estimating percent body fat, along with information about each method's accuracy. The margin of error refers to how close the estimate is likely to be to your actual percent body fat; if you have 20 percent body fat, then a method with a 2.5 percent margin of error may yield a result between 17.5 percent and 22.5 percent body fat.

For the best results, follow your test provider's instructions about what type of clothing you should wear and whether you should refrain from eating, drinking, or exercising for any period before the test. If you repeat the assessment method in the future to compare results, replicate the conditions as closely as possible—for example, the same time of day—for more accurate results.

TABLE 7-3 PERCENT-BODY-FAT ASSESSMENT METHODS

METHOD	MARGIN OF ERROR	DESCRIPTION
SKINFOLD MEASUREMENTS	±3.5%	Folds of skin and subcutaneous fat at specific body locations are measured with an instrument called a *caliper*. These measurements are used in equations that link the thickness of skinfolds to percent-body-fat calculations made from more precise assessment methods. The accuracy of skinfold calculations depends on the skill of the person taking the measurements as well as the caliper's quality. Spring-loaded metal calipers with parallel surfaces are generally best.
UNDERWATER (HYDRO-STATIC) WEIGHING	±2.5%	The person is weighed under typical conditions and then submerged and weighed under water. Percentages of body fat and fat-free weight are calculated from the results. This method is based on the differing densities of fat and muscle. A person with a greater proportion of body fat will weigh relatively less under water.
BIOELECTRICAL IMPEDANCE ANALYSIS (BIA)	±3.5–5.0%	The person stands on or holds a specialized scale, or electrodes are attached to the skin, or both. A small electrical current is sent through the body, and the body's resistance (*impedance*) to the current is recorded. The signal is impeded most in fatty areas because there is less water in body fat. The amount of resistance relates to the amount of water in the body, and the measurement is used in calculations that estimate percent body fat.
AIR DISPLACEMENT PLETHYSMOGRAPHY	±2.2–3.7%	The person sits in a small sealed chamber; the best-known is the BodPod. Sensors measure the amount of air the person displaces, and percent body fat is calculated from the results. The BodPod is expensive and not widely available.
DUAL X-RAY ABSORPTIOMETRY (DXA)	±1.8%	A specialized medical scanner aims two X-ray beams with differing energy levels at the person. DXA scans were initially developed to measure bone density, but the results can also be used to estimate body-fat content. DXA has a small margin of error and is non-invasive; however, the scanners are not widely available outside medical settings or for routine use.

Source: Margin of error data from American College of Sports Medicine. (2009). *ACSM's resource manual for guidelines for exercise testing and prescription* (6th ed.). Baltimore, MD: Lippincott Williams & Wilkins.

Women

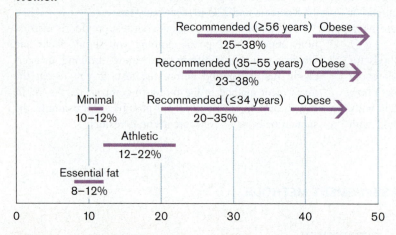

Men

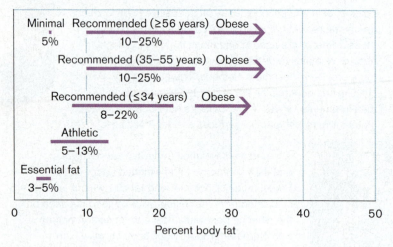

Figure 7-9 **Percent-body-fat standards for men and women.**
Source: American College of Sports Medicine. (2009). *ACSM's resource manual for guidelines for exercise testing and prescription* (6th ed.). Baltimore, MD: Lippincott Williams & Wilkins.

Q | What's the right percent body fat for me?

There are no universally accepted standards for percent body fat for either health or athletic performance. Figure 7-9 shows the standards published by the American College of Sports Medicine. The appropriate, right, or ideal level of body fat for you depends on your age, sex, current body composition and health status, and, to some extent, your goals. For example, women have and need more fat than men, and the level of fat typically increases with age. Therefore, an appropriate, healthy level of fat for a 20-year-old-man is not the same as that for a 45-year-old woman, which is not the same as what is appropriate and healthy for a 60-year-old woman.

If you are an athlete whose performance may be affected by body fat, you may choose to work to maintain a lower level of fat than the average person. Of course, you should always maintain a sufficient level of energy and nutrient intake to support performance and good long-term health.

Methods for Assessing Body-Fat Distribution

Q | Does body shape make any difference when assessing weight and percent body fat?

Yes, it does. Recall that fat in the abdomen poses a greater health risk than fat stored in other areas. DXA scans can estimate the amount of fat in the abdomen, but other, simpler methods provide information about whether your body-fat distribution is healthy.[24] Instructions for each of these methods appear in Lab Activity 7-1.

- *Waist circumference:* Measuring your waist can provide an estimate of body fat distribution. Women with waist measurements over 35 inches and men with waist measurements over 40 inches are at higher risk for health problems. See Lab Activity 7-1 for a detailed set of waist circumference standards.
- *Waist-to-hip ratio:* Comparing your waist measurement and your hip measurement is another means of assessing abdominal obesity. Divide your waist measurement by your hip measurement; your waist should be measured at its narrowest point and your hips at the widest point. Women with waist-to-hip ratios over 0.71 and men with waist-to-hip ratios over 0.83 are at higher risk for health problems. See Lab Activity 7-1 for a detailed set of standards for waist-to-hip ratio.
- *Waist-to-height ratio:* A third way to judge abdominal obesity is to compare your waist measurement to your height (both measured in either inches or centimeters). A healthy ratio is less than 0.5, meaning that your waist is no larger than half your height.[25] Waist-to-height ratio reflects your overall body shape.

These three tests provide some estimate of the risks associated with abdominal fat. However, they cannot distinguish between subcutaneous and visceral fat. Tests based on waist circumference may not identify people who have little subcutaneous fat in their abdomen but an unhealthy amount of visceral fat. In most cases, though, people with significant visceral fat have enough combined subcutaneous and visceral abdominal fat that the tests described in this section—waist circumference, waist-to-hip ratio, and waist-to-height ratio—will identify them as at risk.

Making Changes in Body Composition

Achieving and maintaining a healthy body composition are huge challenges in our society given that most people have sedentary jobs and are surrounded by technological conveniences and tempting, high-calorie foods. (See the box "You Are What You Drink" to examine a common "high-calorie" problem among college students.) But you can take control, set goals, and develop strategies that will work for you. Your eating choices and activity patterns are the two main factors determining body composition that are under your control. You've learned a lot about exercise and physical activity in Chapters 3–6; healthy foods and dietary patterns are described in detail in Chapters 8 and 9. This section introduces the energy balance equation (Figure 7-10).

Setting Appropriate Goals

Q What's a good goal for body weight and body fat?

Before setting a goal, review the results of your assessment tests and any related health-risk factors. Do the assessments indicate that your body composition is a potential risk factor? If so, choose a goal based on BMI, percent body fat, or body-fat distribution. If you are close to the healthy range for body composition, you might want to set a goal based on lifestyle, such as increasing daily physical activity or starting a strength-training program. Exercise can improve measures of health even if it doesn't significantly change your body composition or body weight. Exercise is also extremely helpful for preventing future increases in body fat and weight.

Apply the SMART criteria to your goal. Remember that your goal needs to be realistic and achievable. Genetics limits your capacity to change, whether your goal is to lose body fat or gain muscle, and any goal you set should be consistent with overall good physical and emotional wellness. BMI and percent body fat can guide you in setting a goal, but consider your individual health and lifestyle factors as well. Set a goal that you will be able to maintain over the long term.

If you are significantly overweight or overfat, or if you have a risk factor such as high blood pressure or diabetes, consult a physician in order to set an appropriate body-composition goal. For obese individuals, even modest fat loss, especially if combined with increased exercise, is likely to bring significant health improvements. It is better to maintain a modest amount of fat loss than to lose much more and then quickly gain it all back.

To track progress toward your goal, you can periodically weigh yourself, even though weight isn't a precise measure of your body composition. If you are shedding pounds at a slow rate while maintaining an exercise program, it is likely that you are losing body fat. For some people, checking their weight provides motivation to keep their behavior-change program on track; for others, checking their weight is stressful and decreases motivation. Pick a monitoring strategy that works best for you.

You can repeat percent-body-fat tests periodically as well. However, don't get hung up on any particular measure, whether body weight, BMI, or body fat. None is

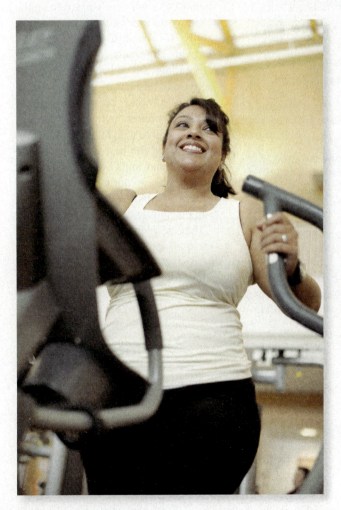

For people with excess body fat, even a small amount of weight loss can significantly improve health, especially if exercise is part of the plan.

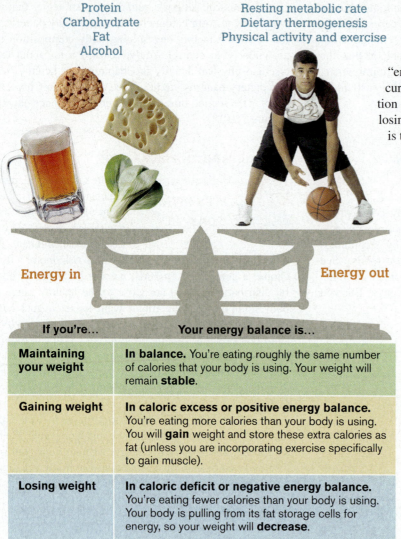

Protein
Carbohydrate
Fat
Alcohol

Resting metabolic rate
Dietary thermogenesis
Physical activity and exercise

Energy in   **Energy out**

If you're...	Your energy balance is...
Maintaining your weight	**In balance.** You're eating roughly the same number of calories that your body is using. Your weight will remain **stable.**
Gaining weight	**In caloric excess or positive energy balance.** You're eating more calories than your body is using. You will **gain** weight and store these extra calories as fat (unless you are incorporating exercise specifically to gain muscle).
Losing weight	**In caloric deficit or negative energy balance.** You're eating fewer calories than your body is using. Your body is pulling from its fat storage cells for energy, so your weight will **decrease.**

Figure 7-10 Energy balance.
Source: Adapted from Centers for Disease Control and Prevention. (2009). *Balancing calories* (http://www.cdc.gov/healthyweight/calories/index.html).

precise, and none tells the whole story about your particular body composition. Also consider how you feel—your energy level, the fit of your clothes, and your success in sticking with the lifestyle strategies you planned for improving your body composition.

Focusing on Energy Balance

Q What's the best way to lose body fat?

There's no one best way to lose body fat, and it's important to look at both sides of the *energy balance equation* (Figure 7-10). You can choose strategies that affect both the "energy in" side of the balance (calories consumed) as well as

the "energy out" side. (See the box "Snack Packing for Your Body . . . Your Brain . . . and Your Bank Balance" for a good way to positively impact your "energy in" side of the scale.) If your weight is currently stable, then the two sides of the equation are balanced. If you're currently gaining or losing weight, or would like to, then the balance is tipped in one direction or the other.

Q Why do I lose weight but not body fat?

Weight loss doesn't automatically equal fat loss. Any weight decrease can be in the form of fat, water, or muscle, and if you lose weight as muscle, your body composition will not improve. Losing more muscle than fat is most likely if you focus only on the "energy in" side of the balance, especially if you lose weight quickly through large cuts in energy intake. Depending on other factors, your body may respond by slowing resting metabolism and preserving its fat stores—definitely not your goal. Dieting can lead to weight loss, but dieting alone is not the best way to decrease body fat and improve body composition. Exercise during a weight-loss program helps preserve muscle so that the weight lost is in the form of fat.

The best programs for fat loss include increased exercise and modest reductions in energy intake. Chapters 8 and 9 provide more information about healthy food choices, including recommended strategies for adjusting your diet to lose or gain weight safely.

Q What's the best kind of exercise to lose body fat?

Just as the intake side of the balance scale shouldn't be tackled alone, neither should the energy-output side. On the "energy out" side of the scale, body composition is best improved by a combination of activity types. Aerobic activities are essential for burning calories and fat. Research tells us that high-intensity exercise works best for improving body composition, and as we get progressively better at aerobic exercise, we begin to burn body fat better and more efficiently.[26] However, as described in Chapter 4, moderate-intensity exercise may be easier for

Research Brief

You Are What You Drink

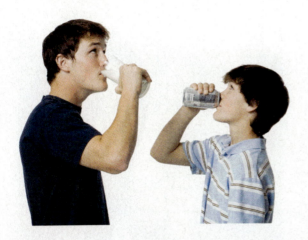

In a recent study researchers followed 47 overweight subjects to examine the effects of the consumption of different types of beverages. Subjects were randomly assigned to one of four groups: sugar-sweetened soft drinks (SSSD), semi-skim milk (which has half the cream removed), water, or no-calorie soft drinks. Participants were instructed to drink 1 liter of the designated beverage daily for 6 months while changing none of their other habits.

Results indicated interesting differences in the groups:

- A higher relative amount of VAT (visceral adipose tissue) was found in the SSSD group: 31 percent higher than the milk group, 24 percent higher than the water group, and 23 percent higher than the diet cola group.

- Lean mass did not differ significantly but did show slight increases among the participants in the milk group.
- Triglycerides increased 32 percent and cholesterol increased 11 percent in the SSSD group. No significant differences were noted in the other groups.
- Both systolic and diastolic blood pressure decreased significantly in the milk group and slightly in the diet cola group.
- No significant differences in glucose levels were noted for any group.
- Slight changes in bone mass were found, with an increase for the milk group and decreases for the other groups.

Analyze and Apply

- Do you drink any of the beverages that were used in the study? If so, what are the positives and negatives of your preferred drinks?
- If you drink SSSDs but are not ready to give them up, how could you at least cut back?
- What effect could one of these changes or some other change have on your fat levels, blood pressure, or other dimensions of health?

Source: Maersk, M., Belza, A., Stødkilde-Jørgensen, H., Ringgaard, S., Chabanova, E., Thomsen, H., Pedersen, S., Astrup, A., & Richelsen, B. (2012). Sucrose-sweetened beverages increase fat storage in the liver, muscle, and visceral fat depot: A 6-mo randomized intervention study. *American Journal of Clinical Nutrition, 95*(2), 283–289.

---

people to maintain over the long term. The best endurance activities are those you stick with, regardless of intensity. In addition, you'll definitely want to incorporate resistance training into your program. It increases muscle mass, thereby improving body composition directly, and it also helps to increase metabolism and utilize the body's fat more efficiently.

If the thought of engaging in multiple types of exercise or intense exercise in order to address body composition seems overwhelming, keep in mind that these types of exercise also increase your cardiorespiratory and muscular fitness. So, you will get multiple gains for your efforts. Also bear in mind that intensity is specific to you. You don't have to be an athlete or highly trained in order to exercise at an intense level. The key is to participate in activities that are safe and appropriate for your needs—and that you can stick with throughout your life.

Q | How much exercise do I need to do to maintain my weight range over time? The answer to this question is different for each person due to genetic variations and other factors. The U.S. Department of Health & Human Services provides the following estimates for the amount of exercise needed for weight management.[27]

- *To prevent weight gain:* Engage in a minimum of 150 minutes per week of moderate-intensity aerobic exercise or 75 minutes of high-intensity exercise. Some people may need to engage in more exercise in order to prevent increases in weight and fat over time.
- *To lose a modest amount of weight or to maintain weight loss:* The general advice might be "more is better," but further research is needed to determine

Wellness Strategies

Snack Packing for Your Body . . . Your Brain . . . and Your Bank Balance

Q What are some snacks that are low calorie, healthy, and handy?

Your body needs to refuel every few hours, but hectic class schedules, along with work and home responsibilities, don't always allow time for regular sit-down meals. Taking a little extra time in the morning or at the beginning of the week to pack a few healthy take-along snacks will pay off. Healthy, regular snacks not only give you energy and needed nutrients but also help to control total calorie, fat, and sugar intake; regulate blood glucose levels; and fend off hunger and fatigue. As well, studies have shown that well-timed snacks can improve cognitive abilities, including memory, attention span, reading speed, reasoning skills, and math skills. Finally, having readily available snacks helps you avoid the convenient temptation of vending machines and drive-through windows and thus can save you money.

When meals are more than 4 hours apart, satisfy yourself with a snack from your pack. Try small whole-grain bagels, fruits, raw vegetables, whole-wheat crackers with peanut butter or low-fat cheese, nuts and seeds, low-fat granola, flavored rice cakes, pretzels, bran muffins, string cheese, tuna, plain popcorn, or low-fat or nonfat yogurt. (Remember, though, that some snacks can be deceiving, so be sure to check the sodium, fat, and sugar content.) And don't forget water. You can carry a refillable bottle to limit the extra weight in your pack.

Some of your choices will be limited by the season or your location. Always err on the side of food safety. With creativity you may be surprised to discover what travels well. Also, remember to choose snacks that fit your

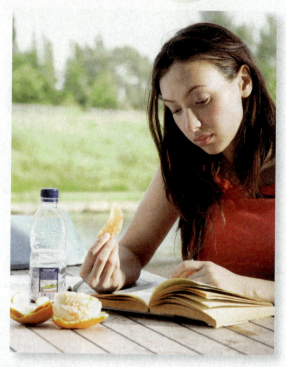

schedule—both prep time and eating time. You won't continue to make the effort if the packing becomes cumbersome or the snacks aren't enjoyable.

Sources: AARP. (2007). *Healthy snacking* (http://www-static-w2-md .aarp.org/health/healthyliving/articles/snacking.html). Mayo Clinic. (2010). *Snacks: How they fit into your weight loss plan* (http://www. mayoclinic.com/health/healthy-diet/HQ01396). Family Education. (n.d.). *Stocking up on smart snacks* (http://life.familyeducation.com/snacks/ nutrition-and-diet/48798.html). Women Fitness. (n.d.). *Top 10 healthiest snacks: You can just keep on eating* (http://www.womenfitness.net/top10_ healthiest_snacks.htm).

---

exactly how much. Based on current evidence, about 50 minutes a day of moderate-intensity exercise or 25 minutes a day of high-intensity exercise will help you shed a modest amount of weight and keep it off.

- *To lose a more significant amount of weight:* To drop more than 5 percent of body weight, engage in more than 300 minutes of moderate-intensity exercise or 150 minutes of high-intensity exercise per week.

In studies of people who lost a significant amount of weight and maintained the loss over the long term, physical activity levels averaged about 60 minutes per day.[28]

See Chapters 3–6 for more information on creating a fitness program that is right for you. Be sure to include strength training, because although it doesn't burn many calories directly, it helps maintain your muscle mass, and your body's

response to strength training (repair of muscle microtears) raises your resting metabolic rate for several days after your workouts. If you want to increase your "energy out" by a specific number of calories, refer to Table 7-4 for approximate calorie costs of some common activities.

Q Why can't I just focus on improving one part of my body, such as getting rid of unwanted fat in one area?

It is impossible to target one area for fat burning (so-called spot reduction). You can strengthen the muscles in a particular area of your body through exercise, but such workouts will not reduce fat from that specific area. When you exercise, fat is burned from the body generally; the exact areas where the body will

TABLE 7-4 APPROXIMATE CALORIE COSTS OF SELECTED PHYSICAL ACTIVITIES

ACTIVITY	CALORIES PER POUND PER MINUTE*	ACTIVITY	CALORIES PER POUND PER MINUTE*
Sitting in class or at computer	0.014	Cycling, moderate	0.060
Child care (dressing, bathing)	0.023	Cycling, vigorous	0.076
Vacuuming or heavy cleaning	0.026	Swimming laps, moderate effort	0.053
Shoveling snow	0.045	Basketball, game (moderate/vigorous)	0.060
Walking, brisk (3.5 mph)	0.029	Roller blading, vigorous	0.091
Walking, very brisk (4.5 mph)	0.048	Tennis, singles	0.060
Jogging, moderate (5 mph, 12 min/mile)	0.060	Frisbee, ultimate (vigorous effort)	0.060
Jogging (7.5 mph, 8 min/mile)	0.095	Weight lifting	0.045
Cycling, light effort	0.045	Circuit training	0.060

*To determine the approximate number of calories burned, multiply the value in the right column by your total body weight and the number of minutes you engage in the activity. For example, if you weigh 150 pounds and walk briskly for 30 minutes, you will burn about $0.29 \times 150 \times 30 = 130$ calories. The values given here are estimates; due to metabolic differences, some people will burn more or fewer calories than indicated by this table.

Source: Adapted from Centers for Disease Control and Prevention, National Center for Chronic Disease Prevention and Health Promotion. (1999). *General physical activities defined by level of intensity* (www.cdc.gov/nccdphp/dnpa/physical/pdf/PA_Intensity_table_2_1.pdf); a complete listing of MET values for many different physical activities can be found in *The Compendium for Physical Activities* at http://sites.google.com/site/compendiumofphysicalactivities/home

mobilize fat for fuel depend on a number of factors, including genetics. Many people find this reality frustrating, but it is true. Thankfully, however, research has shown that exercise will reduce dangerous visceral fat.

Don't focus too much of your attention on aspects of your body that you can't change. Strive to make healthy changes in your body composition, and accept that healthy bodies come in many shapes and sizes.

Summary

Body composition includes the relative amounts of muscle, fat, bone, and other tissues that make up the body. It is typically assessed in terms of the percent of total body weight that is fat. A number of factors contribute to body composition, including genetic heritage, biological sex, age, ethnicity, lifestyle, and environment. A certain percentage of body fat is necessary and healthy, but high fat levels can contribute to functional problems as well as deadly chronic diseases. Too little body fat is also dangerous and can affect athletic performance, bone density, and hormonal balance. Along with a healthy body composition, people should strive to develop a positive and realistic body image.

Body mass index (BMI) is a common method of indirectly measuring body fat and classifying the health risks associated with body weight, but it is not accurate for all body types. There are several methods of estimating percent body fat, including skinfold measurement, underwater weighing, and bioelectrical impedance analysis.

A program to change body composition should include realistic goals and attention to both sides of the energy balance equation—"energy in" as food and "energy out" as physical activity. Both aerobic exercise and resistance training contribute to positive changes in body composition.

More to Explore

Centers for Disease Control and Prevention: Assessing Your Weight
http://www.cdc.gov/healthyweight/assessing/index.html

MedlinePlus: Obesity
http://www.nlm.nih.gov/medlineplus/obesity.html

Department of Nutrition and Food Science, University of Vermont: Methods of Body-composition Analysis Tutorials
http://nutrition.uvm.edu/bodycomp

National Heart, Lung and Blood Institute: What Are Overweight and Obesity?
http://www.nhlbi.nih.gov/health/dci/Diseases/obe/obe_whatare.html

The Surgeon General's Vision for a Healthy and Fit Nation
http://www.ncbi.nlm.nih.gov/books/NBK44660/

womenshealth.gov: Body Image
http://www.womenshealth.gov/bodyimage/

⬛ **COMPLETE IN** connect

NAME	DATE	SECTION

This lab includes several tests for measuring and evaluating factors related to body composition:

- Body mass index, with waist circumference
- Percent body fat using skinfold measurement
- Body-fat distribution, using waist circumference, waist-to-hip ratio, waist-to-height ratio

Standards for evaluating percent body fat are also included in the lab activity, and these can be applied to any method of measuring percent body fat that you complete.

Calculating and Evaluating Body Mass Index

Equipment

- Weight scale
- Tape measure or other means of measuring height and waist circumference
- Partner (optional)

Preparation: None

Instructions

Measure and record your height, weight, and waist circumference. Don't forget to note the unit of measurement. Measure your waist at the smallest point. For best results, have a partner measure your waist while standing at your side; be sure to keep the measuring tape flat against your skin and parallel to the ground. Measure your height with shoes off and your weight with minimal clothing.

Height: [ ] in./m   Weight: [ ] lb/kg   Waist circumference: [ ] in./cm

Calculate your BMI using the following formulas. You need to complete steps 1 and 2, which convert the units of measurement, only if your height was measured in inches or your weight in pounds.

1. **Convert your body weight to kilograms by dividing your weight in pounds by 2.2.**

   Body weight [ ] lb ÷ 2.2 lb/kg = body weight [ ] kg

2. **Convert your height measurement to meters by multiplying your height in inches by 0.0254.**

   Height [ ] in. × 0.0254 in./m = height [ ] m

3. **Square your height measurement (in meters, from step 2).**

   Height [ ] m × height [ ] m = height [ ] m^2

4. **BMI equals body weight in kilograms (from step 1) divided by height in meters squared (from step 3).**

   BMI = body weight [ ] kg ÷ height squared [ ] m^2 = [ ] kg/m^2

Results

Refer to the table for a rating of your BMI. Use your waist circumference to further classify your level of risk. Record the results here and on the final page of this lab.

BMI classification: [   ]   Disease risk from waist circumference (if any): [   ]

BODY MASS INDEX (BMI) CLASSIFICATION AND DISEASE RISK

	BMI (KG/M^2)	Disease risk relative to normal weight and waist circumference	
		MEN: WAIST ≤ 40 IN. (102 CM) WOMEN: WAIST ≤ 35 IN. (88 CM)	MEN: WAIST > 40 IN. (102 CM) WOMEN: WAIST > 35 IN. (88 CM)
Underweight	<18.5		
Normal	18.5–24.9		
Overweight	25.0–29.9	Increased	High
Obesity (Class I)	30.0–34.9	High	Very high
Obesity (Class II)	35.0–39.9	Very high	Very high
Extreme obesity (Class III)	≥40.0	Extremely high	Extremely high

Source: National Heart, Lung, and Blood Institute. (1998). *Clinical guidelines on the identification, evaluation, and treatment of overweight and obesity in adults.* Bethesda, MD: National Institutes of Health.

Calculating Percent Body Fat: Skinfold Measurements

Equipment

- Skinfold calipers
- Partner to take measurements (Note: results are most accurate if the person measuring the skinfolds is experienced)
- Water-soluble marking pen (optional)
- Tape measure (optional)

Preparation

- Wear clothing that allows easy access to the skinfold sites being measured. The skinfold sites for males are chest, abdomen, and thigh; for females, triceps, suprailiac, and thigh.
- If needed, the person taking measurements should practice. Grasp the skin with the thumb and forefinger about 3 inches apart; the pinched skinfold should contain two layers of skin with just fat in between. If it feels like there may be any muscle tissue in the skinfold, the person being measured should contract the muscle to allow the measurer to more easily distinguish muscle from skin and fat.

Instructions

1. ***Locate the correct sites for measurement.*** The subject should stand, with all measurements taken from the right side of his or her body. The person taking the skinfold measurements may want to mark the correct sites with a water-soluble pen before taking any measurements.
   - *Chest.* Pinch a diagonal fold halfway between the nipple and the shoulder crease.
   - *Abdomen.* Pinch a vertical fold about 2 cm to the right of the navel.
   - *Thigh.* Pinch a vertical fold midway between the top of the kneecap and the inguinal crease (hip).
   - *Triceps.* Pinch a vertical skinfold on the back of the right arm midway between the shoulder and elbow. The arm should be held freely at the side of the body.
   - *Suprailiac.* Pinch a fold at the top front of the right hipbone. The skinfold will be slightly diagonal in line with the natural angle of the top of the hipbone.

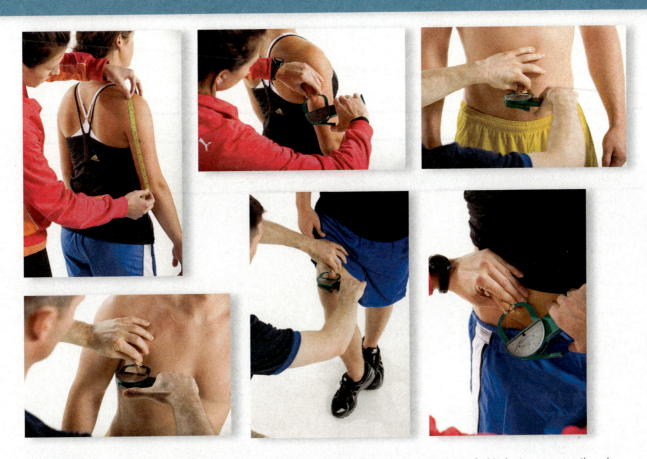

2. ***Measure the appropriate skinfolds and record the values.*** Raise and hold a fold of skin between your thumb and forefinger. Make sure that you are not including any muscular tissue. Be careful not to pinch too hard. Place the calipers directly on the skin surface at a right angle to the fold, and measure the skinfold about 1 cm away from your fingers. Wait 1–2 seconds before reading the caliper. Take readings to the nearest half millimeter. Don't let go of the skinfold until you've removed the caliper from the skin. Take at least two measurements at each site, and retest if the measurements are not within 1–2 mm. Allow the skin to regain its normal position and appearance before repinching a fold. Make a note of the final measurements for each site.

Results

To determine percent body fat, average the measurements for each site and then add the three average measurements together for a sum of the three skinfolds. Then refer to the appropriate table on pp. 260–261 and the figure on p. 262 to determine your estimated percent body fat and rating. Record the result below and in the chart at the end of the lab.

	TRIAL 1	TRIAL 2	AVERAGE OF TWO TRIALS
MEN			
Chest	mm	mm	mm
Abdomen	mm	mm	mm
Thigh	mm	mm	mm
Sum of three skinfolds			**mm**
WOMEN			
Triceps	mm	mm	mm
Suprailiac	mm	mm	mm
Thigh	mm	mm	mm
Sum of three skinfolds			**mm**

Percent body fat (from table): [   ]%   Rating of percent body fat (from figure): [   ]

PERCENT BODY-FAT ESTIMATE FOR MEN: SUM OF CHEST, ABDOMEN, AND THIGH SKINFOLDS

SUM OF SKINFOLDS (MM)	AGE								
	UNDER 22	23–27	28–32	33–37	38–42	43–47	48–52	53–57	OVER 57
8–10	1.3	1.8	2.3	2.9	3.4	3.9	4.5	5.0	5.5
11–13	2.2	2.8	3.3	3.9	4.4	4.9	5.5	6.0	6.5
14–16	3.2	3.8	4.3	4.8	5.4	5.9	6.4	7.0	7.5
17–19	4.2	4.7	5.3	5.8	6.3	6.9	7.4	8.0	8.5
20–22	5.1	5.7	6.2	6.8	7.3	7.9	8.4	8.9	9.5
23–25	6.1	6.6	7.2	7.7	8.3	8.8	9.4	9.9	10.5
26–28	7.0	7.6	8.1	8.7	9.2	9.8	10.3	10.9	11.4
29–31	8.0	8.5	9.1	9.6	10.2	10.7	11.3	11.8	12.4
32–34	8.9	9.4	10.0	10.5	11.1	11.6	12.2	12.8	13.3
35–37	9.8	10.4	10.9	11.5	12.0	12.6	13.1	13.7	14.3
38–40	10.7	11.3	11.8	12.4	12.9	13.5	14.1	14.6	15.2
41–43	11.6	12.2	12.7	13.3	13.8	14.4	15.0	15.5	16.1
44–46	12.5	13.1	13.6	14.2	14.7	15.3	15.9	16.4	17.0
47–49	13.4	13.9	14.5	15.1	15.6	16.2	16.8	17.3	17.9
50–52	14.3	14.8	15.4	15.9	16.5	17.1	17.6	18.2	18.8
53–55	15.1	15.7	16.2	16.8	17.4	17.9	18.5	19.1	19.7
56–58	16.0	16.5	17.1	17.7	18.2	18.8	19.4	20.0	20.5
59–61	16.9	17.4	17.9	18.5	19.1	19.7	20.2	20.8	21.4
62–64	17.6	18.2	18.8	19.4	19.9	20.5	21.1	21.7	22.2
65–67	18.5	19.0	19.6	20.2	20.8	21.3	21.9	22.5	23.1
68–70	19.3	19.9	20.4	21.0	21.6	22.2	22.7	23.3	23.9
71–73	20.1	20.7	21.2	21.8	22.4	23.0	23.6	24.1	24.7
74–76	20.9	21.5	22.0	22.6	23.2	23.8	24.4	25.0	25.5
77–79	21.7	22.2	22.8	23.4	24.0	24.6	25.2	25.8	26.3
80–82	22.4	23.0	23.6	24.2	24.8	25.4	25.9	26.5	27.1
83–85	23.2	23.8	24.4	25.0	25.5	26.1	26.7	27.3	27.9
86–88	24.0	24.5	25.1	25.7	26.3	26.9	27.5	28.1	28.7
89–91	24.7	25.3	25.9	26.5	27.1	27.6	28.2	28.8	29.4
92–94	25.4	26.0	26.6	27.2	27.8	28.4	29.0	29.6	30.2
95–97	26.1	26.7	27.3	27.9	28.5	29.1	29.7	30.3	30.9
98–100	26.9	27.4	28.0	28.6	29.2	29.8	30.4	31.0	31.6
101–103	27.5	28.1	28.7	29.3	29.9	30.5	31.1	31.7	32.3
104–106	28.2	28.8	29.4	30.0	30.6	31.2	31.8	32.4	33.0
107–109	28.9	29.5	30.1	30.7	31.3	31.9	32.5	33.1	33.7
110–112	29.6	30.2	30.8	31.4	32.0	32.6	33.2	33.8	34.4
113–115	30.2	30.8	31.4	32.0	32.6	33.2	33.8	34.5	35.1
116–118	30.9	31.5	32.1	32.7	33.3	33.9	34.5	35.1	35.7
119–121	31.5	32.1	32.7	33.3	33.9	34.5	35.1	35.7	36.4
122–124	32.1	32.7	33.3	33.9	34.5	35.1	35.8	36.4	37.0
125–127	32.7	33.3	33.9	34.5	35.1	35.8	36.4	37.0	37.6

PERCENT BODY-FAT ESTIMATE FOR WOMEN: SUM OF TRICEPS, SUPRAILIUM, AND THIGH SKINFOLDS

SUM OF SKINFOLDS (MM)	AGE								
	UNDER 22	23–27	28–32	33–37	38–42	43–47	48–52	53–57	OVER 57
23–25	9.7	9.9	10.2	10.4	10.7	10.9	11.2	11.4	11.7
26–28	11.0	11.2	11.5	11.7	12.0	12.3	12.5	12.7	13.0
29–31	12.3	12.5	12.8	13.0	13.3	13.5	13.8	14.0	14.3
32–34	13.6	13.8	14.0	14.3	14.5	14.8	15.0	15.3	15.5
35–37	14.8	15.0	15.3	15.5	15.8	16.0	16.3	16.5	16.8
38–40	16.0	16.3	16.5	16.7	17.0	17.2	17.5	17.7	18.0
41–43	17.2	17.4	17.7	17.9	18.2	18.4	18.7	18.9	19.2
44–46	18.3	18.6	18.8	19.1	19.3	19.6	19.8	20.1	20.3
47–49	19.5	19.7	20.0	20.2	20.5	20.7	21.0	21.2	21.5
50–52	20.6	20.8	21.1	21.3	21.6	21.8	22.1	22.3	22.6
53–55	21.7	21.9	22.1	22.4	22.6	22.9	23.1	23.4	23.6
56–58	22.7	23.0	23.2	23.4	23.7	23.9	24.2	24.4	24.7
59–61	23.7	24.0	24.2	24.5	24.7	25.0	25.2	25.5	25.7
62–64	24.7	25.0	25.2	25.5	25.7	26.0	26.7	26.4	26.7
65–67	25.7	25.9	26.2	26.4	26.7	26.9	27.2	27.4	27.7
68–70	26.6	26.9	27.1	27.4	27.6	27.9	28.1	28.4	28.6
71–73	27.5	27.8	28.0	28.3	28.5	28.8	29.0	29.3	29.5
74–76	28.4	28.7	28.9	29.2	29.4	29.7	29.9	30.2	30.4
77–79	29.3	29.5	29.8	30.0	30.3	30.5	30.8	31.0	31.3
80–82	30.1	30.4	30.6	30.9	31.1	31.4	31.6	31.9	32.1
83–85	30.9	31.2	31.4	31.7	31.9	32.2	32.4	32.7	32.9
86–88	31.7	32.0	32.2	32.5	32.7	32.9	33.2	33.4	33.7
89–91	32.5	32.7	33.0	33.2	33.5	33.7	33.9	34.2	34.4
92–94	33.2	33.4	33.7	33.9	34.2	34.4	34.7	34.9	35.2
95–97	33.9	34.1	34.4	34.6	34.9	35.1	35.4	35.6	35.9
98–100	34.6	34.8	35.1	35.3	35.5	35.8	36.0	36.3	36.5
101–103	35.3	35.4	35.7	35.9	36.2	36.4	36.7	36.9	37.2
104–106	35.8	36.1	36.3	36.6	36.8	37.1	37.3	37.5	37.8
107–109	36.4	36.7	36.9	37.1	37.4	37.6	37.9	38.1	38.4
110–112	37.0	37.2	37.5	37.7	38.0	38.2	38.5	38.7	38.9
113–115	37.5	37.8	38.0	38.2	38.5	38.7	39.0	39.2	39.5
116–118	38.0	38.3	38.5	38.8	39.0	39.3	39.5	39.7	40.0
119–121	38.5	38.7	39.0	39.2	39.5	39.7	40.0	40.2	40.5
122–124	39.0	39.2	39.4	39.7	39.9	40.2	40.4	40.7	40.9
125–127	39.4	39.6	39.9	40.1	40.4	40.6	40.9	41.1	41.4
128–130	39.8	40.0	40.3	40.5	40.8	41.0	41.3	41.5	41.8

Source: Jackson, A. S., & Pollock, M. L. (1985). Practical assessment of body composition. *The Physician and Sportsmedicine, 13*(5), 76–90, Tables 6 & 7.

PERCENT BODY FAT STANDARDS FOR MEN AND WOMEN

Women

Men

Source: American College of Sports Medicine. (2009). *ACSM's resource manual for guidelines for exercise testing and prescription* (6th ed.). Baltimore, MD: Lippincott Williams & Wilkins.

Percent Body Fat: Other Techniques

If you use a different method for estimating percent body fat, record the type of assessment and the result below and in the chart at the end of the lab activity. Find your body-composition rating on the table.

Method used: [_____]   Percent body fat: [_____] %

Rating of percent body fat (from figure): [_____]

Evaluating Body-fat Distribution

To evaluate your body-fat distribution, complete one or more of the assessments in this section:

- Waist circumference
- Waist-to-hip ratio
- Waist-to-height ratio

Equipment

- Tape measure or other means of measuring waist and hip circumferences and height
- Partner (optional)

Preparation: None

Instructions and Results

For ease of calculation, use the same units (inches or centimeters) for all measurements.

For waist circumference:

1. Measure your waist at the smallest point. For best results, have a partner measure your waist while standing at your side; be sure to keep the measuring tape flat against your skin and parallel to the ground. Record the measurement and the units:

Waist circumference: [_____] in./cm

2. Find your rating in the appropriate table. Record it here and in the chart at the end of the lab:

Waist circumference rating: ☐

For waist-to-hip ratio:

1. Measure your waist (see instructions just described). Waist circumference: ☐ in./cm

2. Measure your hips at the widest point. For best results, have a partner measure your hip circumference while standing at your side; keep the measuring tape flat against your skin and parallel to the ground.

Hip circumference: ☐ in./cm

3. Calculate your ratio by dividing your waist circumference by your hip circumference; make sure both measurements are in the same units:

Waist-to-hip ratio = waist circumference ☐ ÷ hip circumference ☐ = ☐

4. Find your rating in the appropriate table. Record it here and in the chart at the end of the lab:

Waist-to-hip ratio rating: ☐

For waist-to-height ratio:

1. Measure your waist (see instructions just described). Waist circumference: ☐ in./cm

2. Measure your height with shoes off and record the results:

Height: ☐ in./cm

3. Calculate your ratio by dividing your waist circumference by your height; make sure both measurements are in the same units:

Waist-to-height ratio = waist circumference ☐ ÷ height ☐ = ☐

4. If your ratio is 0.5 or less, record a rating of "OK"; if your ratio is above 0.5, record a rating of "increased risk":

Waist-to-height ratio rating: ☐

WAIST CIRCUMFERENCE AND HEALTH RISK

Waist circumference (inches, centimeters)

RISK CATEGORY	WOMEN	MEN
Very low	<27.5 in. (70 cm)	<31.5 in. (80 cm)
Low	27.5–35.0 in. (70–89 cm)	31.5–39.0 in. (80–99 cm)
High	35.5–43.0 in. (90–109 cm)	39.5–47.0 in. (100–120 cm)
Very high	>43.0 in. (109 cm)	>47.0 in. (120 cm)

Source: Adapted from Bray, G. A. (2004). Don't throw the baby out with the bath water. *American Journal of Clinical Nutrition, 79*(3), 347–349.

WAIST-TO-HIP RATIO AND HEALTH RISK

	AGE	RISK			
		LOW	MODERATE	HIGH	VERY HIGH
MEN	20–29	<0.83	0.83–0.88	0.89–0.94	>0.94
	30–39	<0.84	0.84–0.91	0.92–0.96	>0.96
	40–49	<0.88	0.88–0.95	0.96–1.00	>1.00
	50–59	<0.90	0.90–0.96	0.97–1.02	>1.02
	60–69	<0.91	0.91–0.98	0.99–1.03	>1.03
WOMEN	20–29	<0.71	0.71–0.77	0.78–0.82	>0.82
	30–39	<0.72	0.72–0.78	0.79–0.84	>0.84
	40–49	<0.73	0.73–0.79	0.80–0.87	>0.87
	50–59	<0.74	0.74–0.81	0.82–0.88	>0.88
	60–69	<0.76	0.76–0.83	0.84–0.90	>0.90

Source: Heyward, V. (2010). *Advanced fitness assessment and exercise prescription* (6th ed.; p. 222, table 8.8). Champaign, IL: Human Kinetics.

Summary of Results

Fill in the scores and ratings for the tests you performed.

	RESULT	RATING
BMI [WAIST CIRCUMFERENCE]	kg/m² in./cm	OK/increased risk
SKINFOLDS	% body fat	
OTHER METHOD: _____	% body fat	
WAIST CIRCUMFERENCE	in./cm	
WAIST-TO-HIP RATIO		
WAIST-TO-HEIGHT RATIO		OK / increased risk

Reflecting on Your Results

Are you surprised with your test results and ratings? Did your results match what you thought about your own body composition?

Planning Your Next Steps

Body composition is a function of your individual energy balance. If your body composition rates as healthy, then strive to maintain it. If the results of your assessment indicate that your body composition places you at elevated risk, then it may be time to make changes in your exercise or eating habits. Set realistic goals for improvement and create a plan to achieve them. As a first step here, describe the type of goal you'd like to set for body composition and the lifestyle parameters you plan to focus your efforts on. For assistance in setting a more precise goal, complete Lab Activity 7-2.

Lab Activity 7-2   Setting Body-Composition Goals

COMPLETE IN connect®

NAME	DATE	SECTION

If the results of the assessment tests in Lab Activity 7-1 indicate that your body composition is a health risk for you, then you can use this lab activity to set a goal for weight based on BMI or percent body fat. (As described in the chapter, if you lose weight slowly and incorporate exercise into your program, then your weight loss will likely be fat loss.) Alternatively, you might want to set a lifestyle goal, such as starting a strength-training program or increasing physical activity, instead of a specific body-composition goal.

Equipment

None required, although a calculator is helpful for doing the calculations. You'll also need the data and results from Lab Activity 7-1.

Height: [＿＿] in./cm/m   Weight: [＿＿] lb/kg

Current BMI: [＿＿] kg/m^2 Current percent body fat: [＿＿] %

Preparation: None

Instructions and Results

Body weight goal based on BMI:

Based on the BMI ratings and your current BMI, select a BMI goal:

Current BMI: [＿＿] kg/m2   Goal BMI [＿＿] kg/m2

To calculate a target body weight based on your BMI goal, use the following steps:

1. If needed, convert your height measurement to meters by multiplying your height in inches by 0.0254.

   Height [＿＿] in. × 0.0254 m/in. = height [＿＿] m

2. Square your height measurement (in meters, from step 1).

   Height [＿＿] m × height [＿＿] m = height [＿＿] m^2

3. Multiply your target BMI (from above) by the square of your height (from step 2) to get your body-weight goal (in kilograms).

   Body-weight goal = target BMI [＿＿] kg/m^2 × height squared [＿＿] m^2 = [＿＿] kg

4. If needed, convert your body-weight goal (in kilograms) to pounds by multiplying your weight in kilograms by 2.2.

   Body-weight goal = [＿＿] kg × 2.2 lb/kg = [＿＿] lb.

Body-weight goal based on estimated percent body fat:

Based on the percent-body-fat ratings and your current percent body fat, select a goal for percent body fat:

Current percent body fat: [＿＿] %   Goal percent body fat [＿＿] %

To calculate a target body weight based on your percent body fat goal, use the following steps. You can do the calculations for either pounds or kilograms as long as you are consistent.

1. Multiply your current weight by your percent body fat to obtain your current body-fat weight; express percent body fat as a decimal (20% would be 0.20).

   Current weight [＿＿＿] lb/kg × current percent body fat [0.＿＿＿] = current fat weight [＿＿＿] lb/kg

2. Subtract your current fat weight (from step 1) from your total weight to get your current fat-free weight.

   Current weight [＿＿＿] lb/kg – current fat weight [＿＿＿] lb/kg = current fat-free weight [＿＿＿] lb/kg

3. Subtract your target percent body fat (expressed as a decimal) from 1 to calculate your goal fat-free percent of body weight.

   1 – Goal percent body fat [0.＿＿＿] = Goal percent fat-free weight [0.＿＿＿]

4. Divide your current fat-free weight (from step 2) by your goal percent fat-free weight (from step 3).

   Body-weight goal = current fat-free weight [＿＿＿] lb/kg ÷ goal percent fat-free weight [0.＿＿＿]

   = [＿＿＿] lb/kg

Reflecting on Your Results and Planning Your Next Steps

BMI goal: [＿＿＿] kg/m² or percent-body-fat goal: [＿＿＿] %

Body-weight goal (calculated from BMI or percent body fat): [＿＿＿] lb/kg

Check your goal against the SMART criteria described in Chapter 2 (specific, measurable, achievable, realistic, and time-bound). Describe why you think this goal is a good one for you, or revise your goal to make it a better fit for your situation. Consider your current body composition and body type, heredity, health status, and personal preferences in setting your goal.

Based on what you've learned so far, list several specific strategies you could use to help achieve your body-composition goal; additional advice and strategies related to food choices are found in Chapters 8 and 9.

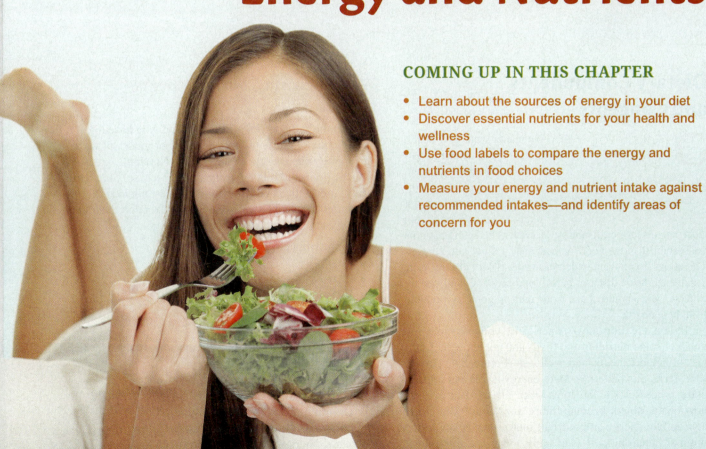

8

Nutrition Basics: Energy and Nutrients

Food provides the nutrients (nourishing components) and the energy you require to realize your wellness potential. In the short term, healthy eating is needed for optimal daily physical functioning; in the long term, it affects your risk for chronic diseases.

Following a healthy eating plan can give you confidence and satisfaction, boosting your self-esteem and emotional wellness. Having positive ways to deal with difficult emotions and spiritual challenges can also help keep you from using unhealthy food choices as a coping mechanism. Intellectual and social wellness also influence your eating habits. Are you thinking critically about your food choices? Can you stay committed to a dietary plan and personal nutrition goals? Can you avoid being overly influenced by the unhealthy food choices of those around you?

Finally, consider your environment. Be aware of whether the foods easily available to you include healthy choices. And pay attention to how your food

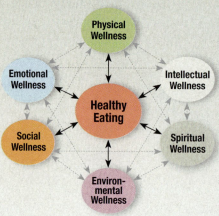

choices affect the environment. What resources were used to grow and ship the foods you eat? How much food packaging do you use and then discard? Your food choices can affect environmental wellness both locally and globally.

This is the first of two chapters on healthy eating. It describes the nutrients essential for being healthy and meeting your energy (calorie) needs. Chapter 9 examines how to combine foods into eating patterns that help prevent chronic diseases and maintain healthy weight; it also addresses the problems of overweight and obesity.

Americans today consume more calories than in the past, but many of us do not get all the nutrients we need. We are both overfed and undernourished.[1] Learning about nutrients—where they come from, what they do in the body, and how much of each you need—can help you put together a diet that is right for you.

Dietary Components and Concepts

Q I'm already healthy, so does it matter what I eat?

No matter what your health status, your dietary patterns are always important. If you are a typical-age college student, you are not likely to be suffering from a chronic disease or disability. However, the eating patterns you establish now, good or bad, may follow you forever. Therefore, if you want to decrease your risk of obesity, type 2 diabetes, heart disease, high blood pressure, and certain cancers, you should make your diet as good as possible from here on out.

If you are like most Americans, you consume too much of some nutrients and foods and not enough of others to support health and wellness (Figure 8-1). In the short term, this pattern reduces energy levels and impairs body processes; in the long term, all the health risks previously noted become more prevalent. Therefore, appropriate energy and nutrient intake *now* is key to the optimal functioning of your body, today and throughout your life.

Macronutrients, Micronutrients, and Energy

To reap the full benefits offered by food, you have to eat a healthy mix of nutrients from a variety of foods, all within an appropriate energy intake range. **Nutrients** are substances you must obtain from foods because your body can't produce them on its own—or at least not in sufficient quantities to maintain its structure and function. Nutrients are typically divided into six classes:

- Carbohydrates
- Fats
- Proteins
- Vitamins
- Minerals
- Water

Your body obtains nutrients through digestion, in which mechanical and chemical processes break down the foods you eat into small compounds (Figure 8-2). Food is chewed, mixed with digestive enzymes, and moved through the digestive tract. Nutrients are broken down into molecules that can be absorbed

nutrients Carbohydrates, fats, proteins, vitamins, minerals, and water—the compounds required for growth and survival that must be obtained from food.

Behavior-Change Challenge
Cleaning Up Your Diet

You don't have a weight problem, but you seriously want to improve your diet. Every day, you feast on junk food, even as you cringe with each new report you hear about its bad effects on body and mind. You're unsure how to get started on a healthier eating regimen, but your hectic schedule leaves you little time to figure out how to begin.

Meet Sharnita

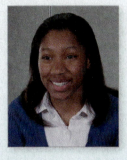

Sharnita is a fit 20-year-old who plays on her college basketball team. She doesn't have trouble with her weight, but she hates how eating fried food and fast food makes her feel. She wants to establish good eating habits now. Watch the video to learn more about Sharnita, her challenges, her behavior-change goals and plan, and her achievements over the course of her program. As you view the video, consider:

- Does Sharnita have enough motivation, environmental support, and specific strategies to succeed? What do you think her biggest challenges will be?
- What will be your key sources of support as you embark on a plan to improve your diet? What are the main obstacles you will face?
- What strategies that Sharnita adopted will help you in your own behavior-change efforts?

VIDEO CASE STUDY   WATCH THIS VIDEO IN connect

Intake as percent of goal or limit

Eat more of these:

Whole grains — 15
Vegetables — 59
Fruits — 42
Milk — 52
Oils — 61
Fiber — 40
Potassium — 56
Vitamin D — 42
Calcium — 75

Goal

Eat less of these:

Added sugars — 242
Solid fats — 281
Refined grains — 200
Sodium — 229
Saturated fat — 158

Limit

Figure 8-1 Dietary intake of selected nutrients and foods in comparison to recommended intake or limit. The bars show the intake of various nutrients and foods as a percentage of the recommended goal or limit. Clearly, Americans consume too much in the way of added sugars, sodium, unhealthy fats, and refined grains and too little fiber and certain micronutrients.

Source: Dietary Guidelines Advisory Committee. (2010). *Report of the Dietary Guidelines Advisory Committee on the dietary guidelines for Americans, 2010* (http://www.cnpp.usda.gov/DGAs2010-DGACReport .htm).

---

into the bloodstream and then circulated and used throughout the body.

Most foods contain a mix of nutrients. For example, whole milk has carbohydrate, fat, protein, calcium (a mineral), water, and other nutrients. However, some foods are especially good choices for specific nutrients. Along with carbohydrates and other nutrients, one large orange contains a full day's supply of vitamin C, and half a cup of cooked sweet potato has a full day's supply of vitamin A.[2] Your daily food choices must work together to provide all the nutrients and energy you need.

Q | Do we really need to eat from all the categories?

In an absolute sense, yes, because you are not likely to find any one food that contains everything you need. To simplify your food choices, think about the six classes just listed as two distinct groups: macronutrients and micronutrients (Table 8-1). **Macronutrients** are nutrients, such as carbohydrates, proteins, and fats, that provide calories and that you need to consume in fairly large amounts. Each macronutrient class liberates energy with a different level of efficiency, and the number of calories each provides also differs. As you'll learn later in this chapter, macronutrients provide more than just calories, and each

macronutrients
Nutrients such as carbohydrates, fats, and proteins that must be consumed in large amounts and that provide calories.

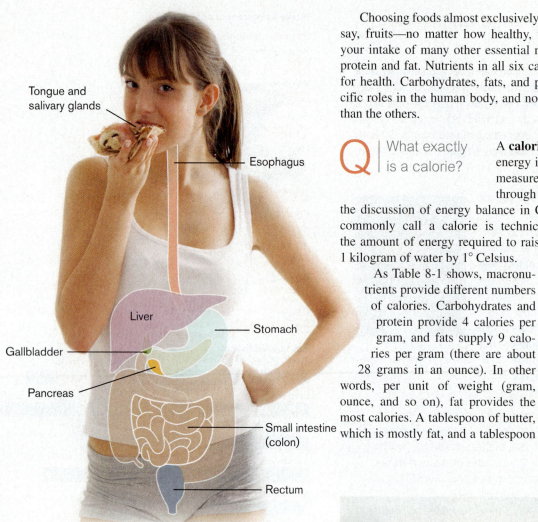

Tongue and
salivary glands

Esophagus

Liver

Stomach

Gallbladder

Pancreas

Small intestine
(colon)

Rectum

Figure 8-2 **The digestive system.** Food enters the body through the mouth, where it is partially digested by the process of chewing and by enzymes in our saliva. It then passes through the esophagus to the stomach, where it is dissolved by stomach acids. The next stop is the small intestine, where it is further broken down by enzymes and other chemicals released by the liver, gallbladder, pancreas, and small intestine lining. Undigested food is concentrated in the colon, collected in the rectum, and expelled via the anus.

affects your health in different ways. A balance of macronutrients is best for health. Water doesn't provide energy, but it is also needed daily in large amounts.

Micronutrients—nutrients in the form of vitamins and minerals—are needed in smaller amounts than macronutrients but are just as critical. Micronutrients occur naturally in food, and many processed foods (such as bread, cereal, orange juice, and milk) are fortified with micronutrients. Micronutrients do not supply calories, but they provide necessary compounds for the effective liberation of energy from the macronutrients; this energy is crucial for everyday activities. Micronutrients also help regulate many chemical reactions in the body that are critical for healthy functioning.

Choosing foods almost exclusively from one category—say, fruits—no matter how healthy, would severely limit your intake of many other essential nutrients, in this case protein and fat. Nutrients in all six categories are required for health. Carbohydrates, fats, and proteins all play specific roles in the human body, and none is more important than the others.

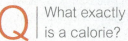

Q What exactly is a calorie?

A **calorie** is a measure of the energy in a food as well as a measure of the energy burned through physical activity (see the discussion of energy balance in Chapter 7). What we commonly call a calorie is technically a *kilocalorie*—the amount of energy required to raise the temperature of 1 kilogram of water by 1° Celsius.

As Table 8-1 shows, macronutrients provide different numbers of calories. Carbohydrates and protein provide 4 calories per gram, and fats supply 9 calories per gram (there are about 28 grams in an ounce). In other words, per unit of weight (gram, ounce, and so on), fat provides the most calories. A tablespoon of butter, which is mostly fat, and a tablespoon

micronutrients
Nutrients such as vitamins and minerals needed in small or trace amounts.

calorie A measure of the energy in food; usually refers to a kilocalorie, or the amount of energy required to raise the temperature of 1 kg of water by 1°C.

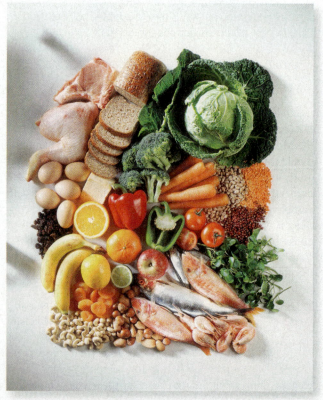

Choose a variety of foods daily to meet all your nutrient needs.

TABLE 8-1 ESSENTIAL NUTRIENTS

	NUTRIENT CLASS	ENERGY	MAJOR FUNCTIONS	MAJOR SOURCES
MACRONUTRIENTS	**CARBOHYDRATE**	4 cal/g	Energy for the body; nondigestible forms aid in elimination and help regulate glucose and cholesterol	Grains (breads, cereals), vegetables, fruits, milk products
	PROTEIN	4 cal/g	Growth and repair of bone and muscle; components of cells, blood, enzymes, and certain hormones; energy for the body	Meat, poultry, fish, milk products, eggs, legumes, nuts
	FAT	9 cal/g	Energy for the body; aid in absorption of certain vitamins; thermal insulation, cushioning of organs, and maintenance of cells	Meat, poultry, fish, milk products, eggs, nuts, seeds, some vegetables
MICRONUTRIENTS	**VITAMINS**	—	Regulation of body processes, including tissue growth and repair; liberation of energy; preservation of healthy cells, nerves, and immune function	Fruits, vegetables, grains
	MINERALS	—	Regulation of growth and development; liberation of energy	Many foods
	WATER	—	Digestion and absorption of food; lubrication, cushioning, and temperature control; medium for chemical reactions and transport of chemicals throughout the body	Water and other liquids,* fruits, vegetables

*Alcohol is a liquid that provides energy (7 cal/g) but is not an essential nutrient.

of sugar, all carbohydrate, weigh about the same, 11–12 grams; but the butter has more than twice the calories of the sugar.

Q | If I go out drinking a couple nights a week, does that mean I consume more calories?

If your food intake is the same on those nights as in a typical day, then yes, since alcohol has 7 calories per gram. These calories can add up fast. Some alcoholic beverages also contain carbohydrates, for instance, from juice; therefore their calorie total is higher. One standard 12-ounce beer has about 150 calories, while 1.5 ounces of hard liquor (the amount in a shot or a typical mixed drink) has about 100 calories. Multiply your total number of drinks by these values to get the approximate calorie intake of one of your evenings out.

Alcohol has other effects on health beyond its calorie contribution; see Chapter 13 for more information.

Energy and Nutrient Recommendations

Q | How many calories should I eat every day?

Depending on your sex, age, weight, and activity level, you need between 1,600 and 3,600 calories per day to maintain your current weight (Table 8-2). Lab Activity 8-1 will help you more precisely

Mind Stretcher
Critical Thinking Exercise

How do you feel after you eat or drink a healthy meal or snack? How do you feel after you consume foods and beverages you know are poor choices? Are your feelings physical, emotional, or both? How might you use your feelings to improve your eating habits?

TABLE 8-2 ESTIMATED CALORIE REQUIREMENTS FOR ADULTS, AGE 20 YEARS*

HEIGHT	ACTIVITY LEVEL**	CALORIES PER DAY	
		MEN	WOMEN
5 FT (60 IN.)	Sedentary	1,950–2,200	1,700–1,850
	Low active	2,150–2,400	1,900–2,100
	Active	2,400–2,700	2,150–2,300
	Very active	2,650–3,000	2,400–2,600
5 FT, 6 IN. (66 IN.)	Sedentary	2,200–2,500	1,900–2,100
	Low active	2,400–2,750	2,150–2,300
	Active	2,700–3,050	2,400–2,600
	Very active	3,000–3,410	2,700–2,950
6 FT (72 IN.)	Sedentary	2,450–2,800	2,150–2,350
	Low active	2,700–3,050	2,350–2,600
	Active	3,000–3,400	2,650–2,900
	Very active	3,350–3,850	3,000–3,300

* Values show the range for 20-year-olds with a body mass index (BMI) between 18.5 and 25.0. For each year above age 20, subtract 7 cal/day for women and 10 cal/day for men.

** Activity levels: *Sedentary* (activities of daily living); *low active* (activities of daily living plus the equivalent of 30 min/day of moderate activity); *active* (activities of daily living plus the equivalent of about 60–90 min/day of moderate activity); *very active* (activities of daily living plus the equivalent of about 150–240 min/day of moderate activity). Thirty minutes of vigorous activity is equivalent to about 60 min of moderate activity.

Source: National Academies, Institute of Medicine, Food and Nutrition Board. (2005). *Dietary reference intakes for energy, carbohydrate, fiber, fat, fatty acids, cholesterol, protein, and amino acids (macronutrients).* Washington, DC: National Academies Press.

determine the energy intake that is appropriate for you, as daily caloric needs vary greatly from person to person.

The **Dietary Reference Intakes (DRIs)** are a major tool for planning a healthy diet. Established by the Food and Nutrition Board of the National Academies, the DRIs are based on the best available research. The DRIs specify recommended intake levels of nutrients for Americans of all ages. For some nutrients, they also provide safe upper limits, and intakes above those levels could be harmful. Several different nutrient standards make up the DRIs, and you'll see those varying standards discussed throughout this chapter. The goal of the DRIs is to provide guidance on nutrient intake levels that will prevent deficiencies and help reduce the risk of chronic disease.

Q | Do I have to count calories every day?

Not necessarily, although close tracking of your diet can be helpful from time to time, especially if you're trying to make changes. A periodic self-check is a useful practice. Do you know how many calories you currently consume? How close are you to meeting the recommendations for individual nutrients? Lab Activity 8-2 will help you perform just such an analysis.

Keeping careful track of what you eat for several days can help give you a good picture of your current diet—and how you might improve it. Track your food intake on both weekdays and weekends, especially if your schedule and eating patterns vary, as is the case for most of us. You don't have to meet the recommended intakes for each nutrient every day, but your average intakes should be in line with the Dietary Reference Intakes.

Are you paying attention to what—and how much—you are eating on a daily basis? Relatively small deviations from recommended intakes add up. On average, Americans gain a

Dietary Reference Intakes (DRIs) A set of standards that includes recommended intakes of all essential nutrients, recommendations for balancing intakes of macronutrients, and upper safe limits for selected nutrients.

Fast Facts

Invisible Calories?

Researchers have found that most people significantly underestimate their energy intake in terms of both individual meals and daily totals. Underestimation by 15–25 percent is typical. The number is even higher for bigger meals: One study of college students found that for large fast-food meals, calorie estimations were nearly 40 percent below the actual energy content of the meal!

■ How many calories per day do you think you take in?
■ For a reality check, carefully track and measure all your food for a day or two (see ChooseMyPlate.gov/supertracker for tools such as the Food-A-Pedia resource in the SuperTracker). How do the results compare with your estimate of your daily calorie intake?

Source: Wansink, B., & Chandon, P. (2006). Meal size, not body size, explains errors in estimating the calorie content of meals. *Annals of Internal Medicine, 145*(5), 151.

pound a year between ages 20 and 60—a small change in one year but a big change over time.

Energy Density and Nutrient Density

Q What are the most filling foods with the fewest calories?

Your question relates to the important concept of **energy density,** or the amount of energy in a food per unit of weight. Foods with high energy density have a large number of calories, usually because they are high in fat and low in water and fiber. On the flip side, foods high in water and fiber have a low energy density, meaning they have a small number of calories by weight, so they can help fill you up without providing a lot of calories. For example, one small slice of cheese weighs about 1 ounce and has about 100 calories. For that same 100 calories, you could have:

■ Five small (5-inch) carrots
■ One large apple
■ Six apricots

If you want to fill up with fewer calories, try large portions of foods that are low in energy density. Many fruits, vegetables, and whole grains, if eaten without added sugars or fats, are low in energy density. The energy density of your overall diet should be relatively low, and it's best if the high-energy-density foods you consume are also rich in nutrients.

Q What are "super foods"?

"Super foods" is a good concept for thinking about foods that are **nutrient rich,** meaning naturally abundant in vitamins, minerals, and other beneficial food compounds but with relatively few calories. Nutrient-rich foods are the opposite of energy-dense foods. Nutrient-rich foods are the best way to ensure healthy nutrient intake while also maintaining a healthy level of energy intake. Good examples of nutrient-rich foods are vegetables, fruits, whole grains, fish, low-fat dairy products, and lean cuts of meat and poultry. Typically these are foods that are as close to their natural state as possible—that is, relatively unprocessed and without a lot of added sugars and/or fats.

A food can be nutrient rich and calorie dense, as in the case of nuts. Although such a food is good for you, you should not eat too much of it. You'll learn more about identifying nutrient-rich foods in the discussion of food labels on pp. 299–300 and in Chapter 9.

If you think of your daily calories in terms of a budget, you'll want to "spend" your calories wisely—get as much nutrient bang for your calorie buck as you can. Unfortunately, most adults choose many foods that are low in nutrient richness, often opting for energy-dense foods instead. For example, top sources of calories in the diets of young adults ages 19–30 include sodas and sports drinks, grain-based desserts (cakes, cookies, doughnuts, and the like), alcoholic beverages, and pizza.[3] These choices are high in calories and low in nutrients, especially fiber, vitamins, and minerals.

energy density
The amount of energy (calories) in a food per unit of weight.

nutrient rich Provides a substantial amount of vitamins, minerals, and other nutrients and relatively few calories.

DOLLAR STRETCHER
Financial Wellness Tip

Substitute no-cost water for some of your more expensive beverages. Analysis of the nutrient density and energy costs of foods reveals that most popular sweetened beverages are not a low-cost source of any nutrients. They are bad for your financial budget as well as your calorie budget. Track your weekly spending on beverages, including bottled water, and you might be surprised at the total amount.

Research Brief

Does Beverage Choice Make Kids Fat?

Over the past 30 years, the United States has seen a threefold rise in obesity rates for children. Increased consumption of sugary beverages is one of several factors cited in this spurt. These beverages also tend to displace the amount of milk children consume, thereby detracting from overall healthy eating. Initially, sweetened soda was was viewed as the main culprit, but today there is also concern over the potential role of 100-percent fruit juice and sweetened fruit drinks in the increased obesity observed among young children.

Researchers recently used nationally representative data from the National Health and Nutrition Examination Survey to investigate associations between types and amounts of beverages consumed and weight status in preschool-age children. Beverages were classified in broad categories, including cow's milk (with appropriate subtypes based on fat percentage); 100-percent fruit juice; fruit drinks (sweetened beverages that contain at least part juice); sweetened soft drinks; and diet drinks, including fruit drink, tea, or soda sweetened by a low-calorie additive. More than 1,100 children were then categorized by BMI as underweight (less than 5 percent), normal weight (60 percent), at risk for overweight (24 percent), or overweight (11 percent).

Most of the children (83 percent) drank milk daily. Also, 48 percent drank 100-percent fruit juice, 44 percent drank fruit drinks, and 39 percent drank soda. The children averaged about 27 ounces of fluid per day, which included 12 ounces of milk, 5 ounces of 100-percent fruit juice,

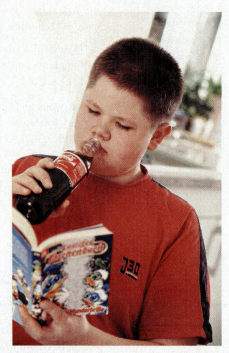

5 ounces of fruit drinks, 3 ounces of soda, and 2 ounces of other fluids. Interestingly, the weight status of the child had no association with the amount of total beverages—milk, 100-percent fruit juice, fruit drinks, or soda—consumed. However, daily total calorie intake rose with increased consumption of milk, 100-percent fruit juice, fruit drinks, and soda.

From this study, the researchers learned that (1) milk consumption was less than the recommended 16 ounces per day; (2) fewer than 10 percent of the children drank low-fat or skim milk, as recommended for children older than 2 years; and (3) drinking more beverages increased overall daily calorie intake. Although there is a clear beverage-to-calorie relationship, there is no apparent association with weight status. However, given the nature of biological maturation and the slowing of growth that comes with late adolescence, it seems reasonable to conclude that with a continuation of an increased beverage intake, body weight might creep up as a result of the increased calories entailed.

Analyze and Apply

- What are your beverage habits today? If you are overweight, how might the beverages you drink be contributing?
- What changes can you make to your beverage habits in the interest of good health and weight control?

Source: O'Connor, T. M., Yang, S. J., Nicklas, T. A. (2006). Beverage intake among preschool children and its effect on weight status. *Pediatrics 118*(4):e1010–8.

The American Diet and the Recommended Diet

The dietary recommendations in this chapter are based on the *Dietary Guidelines for Americans, 2010,* issued by the Departments of Agriculture and Health and Human Services every 5 years (http://health.gov/dietaryguidelines/). The guidelines incorporate the DRIs and reflect expert reviews of nutrition research. They provide authoritative advice about dietary habits that promote health and reduce risk for major chronic diseases.

There are two overarching recommendations in the 2010 *Dietary Guidelines:*

- Maintain calorie balance over time to achieve and sustain healthy weight.
- Focus on consuming nutrient-rich foods and beverages.

These two important pieces of advice are in evidence throughout this book, as they are the key to maintaining wellness. Also see the box "Recommendations for Macronutrients."

Wellness Strategies

Recommendations for Macronutrients

Q | How can I assess and improve my diet?

The Dietary Reference Intakes set several different types of standards for carbohydrates and the other macronutrients you can use.

Minimum Adequate Intake

	Women	Men
Carbohydrate	130 g	130 g
Protein*	46 g	56 g
Fat**		
Omega-6 fatty acid (linoleic acid)	12 g	17 g
Omega-3 fatty acid (alpha-linolenic acid)	1.1 g	1.6 g

* Protein requirements can be calculated more precisely by multiplying body weight (in pounds) by 0.36 g (see p. 282).
** See pp. 282–283 for more on specific types of fats.

Acceptable Macronutrient Distribution Ranges

	Percent of Total Daily Calories
Carbohydrate	45%–65%
Fat (total)	20%–35%
Protein	10%–35%

Additional Recommendations

Added sugars	No more than 25% of total daily calories*
Dietary fiber	14 g of dietary fiber per 1,000 cal consumed (about 25 g/day for women and 38 g/day for men)
Dietary cholesterol	As low as possible while consuming a nutritionally adequate diet
Saturated fats	As low as possible while consuming a nutritionally adequate diet
Trans fats	As low as possible while consuming a nutritionally adequate diet

*Added sugars should not displace other nutrients, and a much lower intake is appropriate for most people. The American Heart Association recommends limits of 150 cal (38 g, equivalent to 9 tsp) per day for men and 100 cal (25 g, equivalent to 6 tsp) per day for women.

Sources: National Academies, Institute of Medicine, Food and Nutrition Board. (2005). *Dietary Reference Intakes for energy, carbohydrate, fiber, fat, fatty acids, cholesterol, protein, and amino acids (macronutrients).* Washington, DC: National Academies Press. Johnson, R. K., and others. (2009). Dietary sugars intake and cardiovascular health: A scientific statement from the American Heart Association. *Circulation, 120,* 1011–1020.

Carbohydrates

Carbohydrates, one of the three classes of macronutrients, are typically the source of the largest proportion of calories in the diet, or our primary energy source. Most people consume plenty of carbohydrates daily because they are the main component of bread, pasta, cereal, grains, vegetables, fruit, and many other foods.

When carbohydrates are digested, they break down into **glucose,** which circulates in the blood as a readily available energy source for cells. Glucose that is not immediately used for energy can also be stored as **glycogen** in the liver and skeletal muscles. When energy is needed, glycogen can be converted back into glucose. However, there are limits to how much glucose can be stored as glycogen. Consumption of excess carbohydrate, as with any macronutrient, can lead to weight gain and increased body fat.

Simple and Complex Carbohydrates

Q | What is a meant by a "simple" and a "complex" carbohydrate?

Simple carbohydrates are one of two general categories of carbohydrates—simple and complex—based on chemical structure. Simple carbohydrates contain one or two units of sugar per molecule and usually have a sweet taste. Simple carbohydrates include glucose, sucrose, fructose, and lactose. These are different from *refined sugars,* which are sugars that undergo a process of refining and are commonly found in many baked and packaged goods.

Simple carbohydrates occur naturally in fruits, honey, sweet potatoes, milk products, and some cereal products. Simple carbohydrates are also often added to foods during processing and preparation and at the table. These **added sugars** provide calories but few other essential nutrients (thus they are energy dense), and high intake of added sugars is associated with unhealthy blood cholesterol levels, elevated blood pressure, poor vitamin and mineral intakes (Figure 8-3), and possibly weight gain.[4] Americans

carbohydrates
A category of essential nutrients that includes sugars, starches, and dietary fiber.

glucose A simple carbohydrate derived from plant sources that circulates in the blood and is used to produce energy; also called blood sugar.

glycogen A form of stored glucose; primarily found in skeletal muscle and the liver.

simple carbohydrates
Carbohydrates containing one or two units of sugar per molecule; occur naturally in fruits, milk, and other foods; commonly added to processed foods.

added sugars Simple carbohydrates added during processing and preparation of foods.

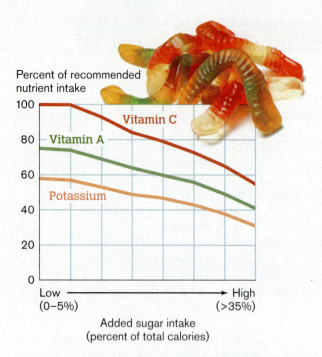

Figure 8-3 axis labels:
Percent of recommended nutrient intake

100
80
60
40
20
0

Vitamin C
Vitamin A
Potassium

Low
(0–5%)
High
(>35%)

Added sugar intake
(percent of total calories)

Figure 8-3 Added sugars and intake of selected nutrients. As added sugar consumption goes up (horizontal axis), intake of key vitamins and minerals goes down (vertical axis). **Source:** Data from Marriott, B., Olsho, L., Hadden, L., & Connor, P. (2010). Intake of added sugars and selected nutrients in the United States, National Health and Nutrition Examination Survey (NHANES) 2003–2006. *Critical Reviews in Food Science and Nutrition, 50,* 228–258.

currently consume far above the recommended amount of added sugars, with the top sources being regular soft drinks, candy, cakes, cookies, pies, fruit drinks, and milk- and grain-based desserts (such as ice cream and sweet rolls). One regular 12-ounce soft drink has about 40 grams, or 10 teaspoons, of added sugars and about 130 calories.

Complex carbohydrates, which include starches and fiber, contain longer molecular chains made up of many sugar units. Starches occur naturally in many foods, includ- ing grains (wheat, oats, rice, and barley), **legumes** (beans and peas, including pinto beans, kidney beans, and len- tils), and other vegetables. Most starches break down dur- ing digestion into simple sugars, which the body can then use. Some starches, however, such as those in legumes, are resistant to digestion and don't break down completely, so they can cause intestinal gas. Dietary fiber, discussed in more detail below, doesn't decompose during digestion and passes relatively intact into the large intestine.

Grains are edible seeds of certain types of grasses (Figure 8-4). In foods, they can be in the form of **whole grains**—grains that contain the entire seed (or kernel) of a plant—or refined grains—those with the seed removed through processing. In its natural state, a kernel of grain has three parts:

- *Bran:* An outer protective covering that is rich in fiber and contains several vitamins

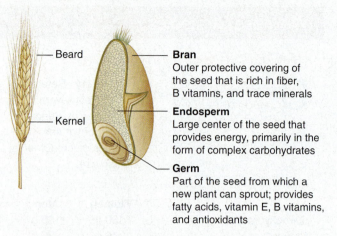

Figure 8-4 labels:
- Beard
- Kernel

Bran
Outer protective covering of the seed that is rich in fiber, B vitamins, and trace minerals

Endosperm
Large center of the seed that provides energy, primarily in the form of complex carbohydrates

Germ
Part of the seed from which a new plant can sprout; provides fatty acids, vitamin E, B vitamins, and antioxidants

Figure 8-4 Anatomy of a whole grain. Because whole grains include the bran, germ, and endosperm from the grain kernel, they are naturally higher in nutrients and dietary fiber than refined grains.

- *Germ:* The inner part of the seed from which a new plant can sprout; a concentrated source of certain vitamins
- *Endosperm:* The large center of the seed, containing complex carbohydrates

When whole grains are refined, they are stripped of their germ and bran, and only the starchy endosperm remains. The process converts whole grains to refined grains, pro- ducing foods like white flour and white rice; it also removes most of the nutrients. For this reason, whole grains are a richer source of nutrients than refined grains and are there- fore recommended.

Some studies have found that whole-grain intake pro- tects again cardiovascular disease, type 2 diabetes, certain types of cancer, and weight gain.[5] Most Americans do not consume adequate amounts of whole grains and thus miss out on the fiber, nutrients, and other beneficial com- pounds they contain. To improve the quality of your carbohydrate choices, choose whole grains over refined grains at least half the time. For good health, follow the practice "Make Half Your Grains Whole." In addition, select foods with naturally occurring sugars, and limit your consumption of added sugars. The box "Go for the Whole Grains—and Beware Added Sugars" will help you make good choices.

Q What is the glycemic index?

Glycemic index (GI) is a measure of how quickly carbohydrates you con- sume increase the level of glucose in your blood. When you consume sim- ple or complex carbohydrates, they

complex carbohydrates Carbohydrates such as starches and dietary fiber containing chains of many sugar units.

legumes Peas and beans, such as white, black, and pinto beans; soybeans; lentils; and chickpeas.

whole grain The entire grain kernel, including the bran, germ, and endosperm.

glycemic index (GI) A scale that quantifies the effect of a carbohydrate- containing food on the level of glucose in the blood.

Wellness Strategies

Go for the Whole Grains—and Beware Added Sugars

Q | What are good foods to choose if you want to eat carbohydrates like bread, crackers, pasta, and cereals?

A wise approach is to seek out the whole grains and shun added sugars. When you are shopping for packaged carbs, search the ingredient list for the items listed below. The higher the item in the package's ingredient list, the more of it in the product. Therefore, whole-grain ingredients listed first on a package indicate that they are the food's primary component. In addition, the Whole Grains Council has an international program that provides a stamp of approval for high whole-grain products, making it even easier to identify these foods.

Don't be fooled by healthy-sounding options like "wheat bread," "multigrain," and bread "made with whole wheat." These products are not necessarily whole-grain rich. Be a savvy consumer and read the ingredient list carefully.

In the case of sugars, total amounts are listed on food labels, but the label doesn't distinguish between naturally occurring versus added sugars.

However, be aware that if a food doesn't include fruit or milk products, then all its sugar likely comes from added sugars.

Choose foods with these whole grains high in the ingredient list:

Amaranth	Sorghum
Buckwheat	Triticale
Bulgur (cracked wheat)	Whole-grain barley
Brown rice	Whole-grain cornmeal
Millet	Whole rye
Oats and oatmeal	Whole wheat
Popcorn	Wild rice
Quinoa	

Limit foods with these added sugars in the ingredient list:

Brown sugar	Honey
Corn sweetener	Invert sugar
Corn syrup	Lactose
Dextrose	Maltose
Fructose	Malt syrup
Fruit juice concentrate	Molasses
Glucose	Raw sugar
High-fructose corn syrup	Sucrose
	Sugar

are converted into sugar (glucose) in your body. Simple carbohydrates are more quickly and readily converted into glucose than many types of complex carbohydrates are. The higher a food's glycemic index, the faster and higher blood sugar levels increase—and the faster the subsequent drop when the glucose is used up. *Glycemic load* is a related measure, which takes into account the amount of carbohydrate in a food or a meal. For example, carrots have a high glycemic index but a small amount of carbohydrate, or a low glycemic load, so they don't cause as big a rise in blood sugar as a food with a high GI and a large amount of carbohydrate.[6] However, not every food with a low GI value is a good choice—for example, premium full-fat ice cream has a low GI but is very high in calories and fat—and GI isn't listed on food labels or easily calculated. For these reasons, using GI to choose foods can be difficult and complex. However, you can use the following principles related to glycemic index to improve your food choices:

- Choose foods high in fiber, including whole grains, legumes, vegetables, and fruits.
- Choose fresh or raw foods rather than processed foods.
- Limit your intake of added sugars.

A food that causes a rapid rise in blood sugar gives you a fast energy boost but then quickly leaves you feeling hungry again. A food with a lower GI value gives you more of a feeling of satiety (fullness) and keeps you satisfied longer, even if it has the same number of calories as the higher GI food. The dilemma is that when you're hungry, you're looking for something to give you a quick boost, and simple carbohydrates—like candy or a sweet beverage—can do that really well. But then you're hungry again before too long, which can be the start of a poor eating cycle. The better strategy is to avoid becoming overly hungry so you're not tempted to eat foods high in added sugars.

Recommended Carbohydrate Intake

Q | How much carbohydrate should I eat daily? Is there an amount or a percentage?

The DRIs specify a minimum amount of carbohydrate that the body needs in order to function. It is a fairly small amount: 130 grams for adults, or about the amount in two baked potatoes. Most American should consume—and do consume—more. The

DRIs also include recommendations for carbohydrate intake as a percentage of total daily calories, a value that depends on the amount of protein and fat consumed.

The **Acceptable Macronutrient Distribution Ranges (AMDRs)** provide a range of healthy values for intake of all macronutrients. For carbohydrates, the range is 45–65 percent of total daily calories. If you're sedentary or have a low overall calorie intake, go with a value at the lower end of the range; if you're active, consume carbohydrates at the high end of the AMDR range.[7] The 2010 *Dietary Guidelines* put solid fats and added sugars (abbreviated as *SoFAS*) in the same category and recommend that no more than 5–15 percent of total daily calories come from SoFAS. Currently, Americans consume about 35 percent of their daily calories from SoFAS!

Lab Activity 8-2 will help you determine your current intake of carbohydrates, protein, and fats. If any are too high, you can then set goals for change.

Q Does eating carbs make me fat?

Almost any food or beverage can make you fat if you eat too much of it, from ice cream to alcohol and from pizza to pineapple. If you overeat, you can gain weight regardless of the foods. To change your body weight, you need to create an excess or a deficit of calories. If you eat more than you need, you will eventually gain weight, and if you eat less than you need, you will slowly lose weight. So, can carbohydrates make you fat? You bet. Can any food make you fat? Absolutely.

Simple carbohydrates can be tasty and easy to eat, so overeating them is common. And anytime you overeat, you risk gaining weight. Keep in mind, though, that good evidence exists for consuming plenty of complex carbohydrates, especially whole grains, as a means of reducing your risk of obesity and many other chronic diseases such as heart disease, diabetes, and certain cancers.[8] So don't avoid carbohydrates—just remember to "Make Half Your Grains Whole," or even more than half if you can.

Fiber

Q What's the deal with fiber? Isn't that like prune juice for old people?

Fiber is for old people—and also for young people who want to grow old gracefully. **Dietary fiber** is a nondigestible carbohydrate with tremendous health benefits; populations that eat fiber-rich diets tend to have very low rates of many chronic diseases.[9] Fiber protects against cardiovascular disease, obesity, and type 2 diabetes, and it also helps to lower blood pressure and to improve blood cholesterol and glucose levels. What's more, by adding fiber, or "bulk," to your diet, you will feel full faster and thus reduce your appetite.

Fiber promotes digestive health.[10] Dietary fiber reduces constipation, and certain types of fiber may alleviate the symptoms of irritable bowel syndrome in some people.[11] (Irritable bowel syndrome is a common disorder of intestinal functioning characterized by abdominal pain, cramping, bloating, constipation, and diarrhea.) Although research findings are mixed, some studies have suggested that dietary fiber may reduce the risk of colon cancer.[12]

The two types of dietary fiber are soluble fiber and insoluble fiber:

- **Soluble (viscous) fiber** soaks up water and turns into a gel during digestion. It slows the body's absorption of glucose, improves insulin sensitivity, and may delay the return of hunger after you eat. It also binds with cholesterol in the intestine for quick removal. Examples of foods that contain soluble fiber are peas,

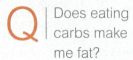

Fast Facts

I'll Take Some Sugar with My Sugar . . . and Fat and Alcohol

On average, American adults consume about 350 calories of added sugars per day. That adds up to the equivalent of 65 pounds of granulated sugar each year! On a daily basis, those 350 calories of added sugars contribute to excess energy intake (too many calories) and poor intake of other nutrients (too few nutrients).

The other sources of "empty" calories in the American diet are alcohol and solid fats such as butter and fats in fatty meats. Together, these three energy-dense, nutrient-poor food sources contribute between 700 and 1,000 calories per day to the average American diet, squeezing out healthier, more nutrient-rich foods.

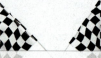

- What strategies can you use to meet your nutrient needs without consuming too many calories?
- What *specific* healthy foods that you currently enjoy will you focus on?

Source: National Cancer Institute, Risk Factor Monitoring and Methods Branch. (2010). Usual energy intake from solid fats, alcoholic beverages & added sugars (SoFAS). *Diet* (http://riskfactor.cancer.gov/diet/usualintakes/sofaas.html).

Acceptable Macronutrient Distribution Ranges (AMDRs) One of the standards that make up the Dietary Reference Intakes; recommended intake ranges for protein, fat, and carbohydrate as percentages of total daily calories.

dietary fiber Complex carbohydrates that cannot be broken down by the digestive system.

soluble (viscous) fiber Form of dietary fiber that soaks up water and turns into a gel during digestion; it may improve the body's insulin sensitivity and cholesterol levels.

soybeans, oats, plums, bananas, the pulp (fleshy parts) of apples and pears, broccoli, carrots, and sweet potatoes.

- **Insoluble fiber** binds water in the intestines, thereby making digested food bulkier and softer and speeding the transit of food through the digestive system. Elimination is easier and more complete. Examples of foods that contain insoluble fiber are whole grains, wheat bran, nuts and seeds, potatoes, the skin of apples and pears, flax, green beans, and cauliflower.

insoluble fiber Form of dietary fiber that binds water but does not dissolve; it adds bulk to the diet and improves elimination.

Consuming fiber, especially if you suddenly boost your intake, can temporarily increase intestinal gas and flatulence. However, given all the long-term benefits of dietary fiber, that's not a bad trade-off—and your body will adjust to the change.

Q | What is the best way to get fiber into your diet?

Dietary fiber is found naturally only in plant foods. Virtually all plant foods have some amount of fiber, and some have particularly high levels (Figure 8-5). Recommended fiber consumption is based on calorie intake—14 grams per 1,000 calories of

Grains, cereals, pasta, rice	Serving size	Fiber (grams)
Bran cereal	1/3 cup	9.1
Shredded wheat cereal	1 cup	5.6
Oat bran flakes cereal	1 cup	5.2
Rye (wafer) crackers	2	5.0
Whole wheat English muffin	1	4.4
Wheat bulgur, cooked	1/2 cup	4.1
Spaghetti, whole wheat	1/2 cup	3.1
Oat bran muffin, small	1	3.0
Barley, pearled, cooked	1/2 cup	3.0
Popcorn, air popped	1 1/2 cups	2.0
Oatmeal, plain, cooked	1/2 cup	2.0
Whole wheat bread	1 slice	1.9
Rye bread	1 slice	1.9
Brown rice	1/2 cup	1.8

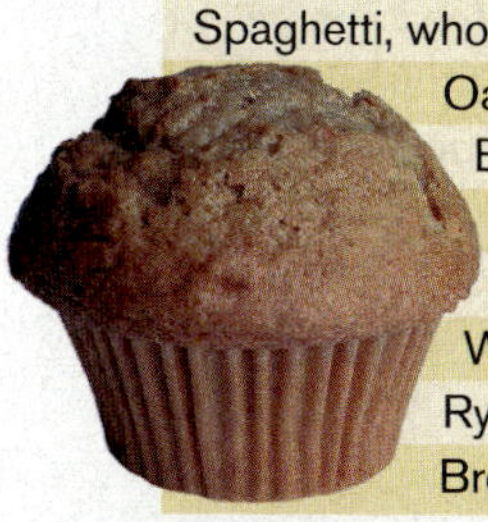

Fruits	Serving size	Fiber (grams)
Pear, medium	1	5.5
Avocado, cubed	1/2 cup	5.0
Apple, medium	1	4.4
Asian pear, small	1	4.4
Raspberries	1/2 cup	4.0
Blackberries	1/2 cup	3.8
Prunes, stewed	1/2 cup	3.8
Figs, dried	1/4 cup	3.7
Banana, medium	1	3.1
Orange, medium	1	3.1
Guava	1	3.0
Dates	1/4 cup	2.9
Apricots	3	2.1
Kiwifruit	1	2.1

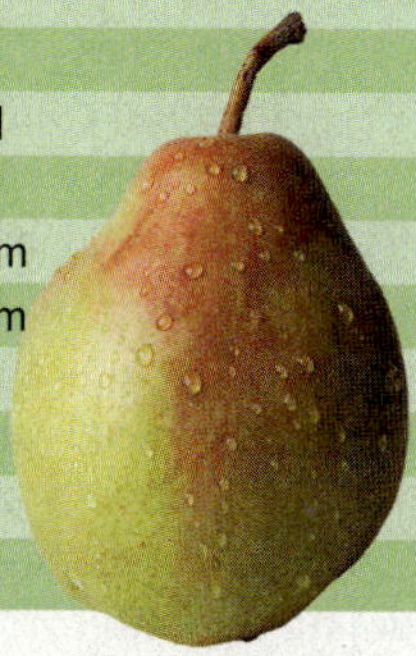

Legumes, nuts, seeds	Serving size	Fiber (grams)
Navy beans	1/2 cup	9.6
Split peas	1/2 cup	8.1
Lentils	1/2 cup	7.8
Pinto beans	1/2 cup	7.7
Black beans	1/2 cup	7.5
Kidney beans	1/2 cup	6.8
Lima beans	1/2 cup	6.6
White beans	1/2 cup	6.3
Chickpeas	1/2 cup	6.2
Soybeans (mature)	1/2 cup	5.2
Almonds	1 oz	3.5
Sunflower seed kernels, dry roasted	1 oz	3.1
Pistachio nuts	1 oz	2.9
Pecans	1 oz	2.7

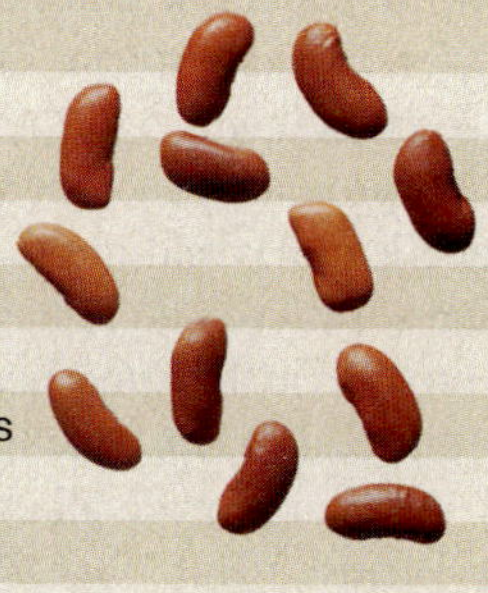

Vegetables	Serving size	Fiber (grams)
Artichoke hearts	1/2 cup	7.2
Green peas	1/2 cup	4.4
Sweet potato, medium, baked with skin	1	3.8
Potato, medium, baked with skin	1	3.8
Soybeans, green	1/2 cup	3.8
Pumpkin, canned	1/2 cup	3.6
Spinach, frozen, cooked	1/2 cup	3.5
Sauerkraut, canned	1/2 cup	3.4
Winter squash, cooked	1/2 cup	2.9
Tomato paste	1/4 cup	2.7
Collards, cooked	1/2 cup	2.7
Broccoli, cooked	1/2 cup	2.6
Okra, cooked	1/2 cup	2.6
Turnip greens, cooked	1/2 cup	2.5

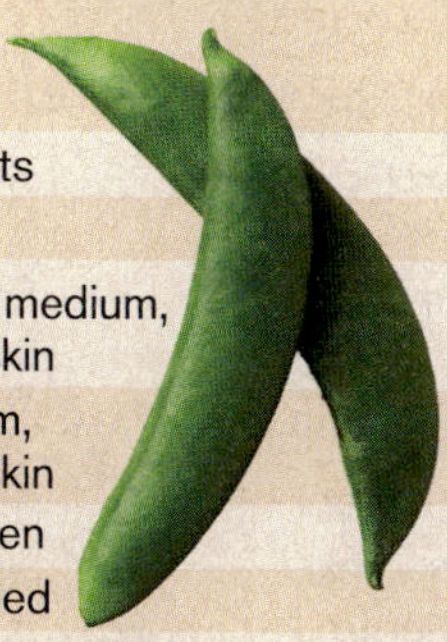

Note: All the food servings listed in this table have fewer than 200 calories.

Figure 8-5 Fiber content of selected high-fiber foods. Keep in mind that about 25 grams of fiber per day for women and about 38 grams per day for men are recommended.

Source: Data from U.S. Department of Agriculture, Agricultural Research Service, Nutrient Data Laboratory. (2009). *USDA national nutrient database for standard reference,* Release 22 (http://www.ars.usda.gov/ba/bhnrc/ndl).

daily diet. This works out to about 25 grams of fiber per day for women and 38 grams per day for men. On average, however, American adults consume only about 15 grams of fiber per day, at least half of which tends to come at breakfast.

You can increase your fiber intake by regularly consuming whole-grain products (ones with a whole grain first on the food ingredient list), whole fruits with the skin, legumes, and high-fiber breakfast cereals, which also make nutritious and delicious snacks. Many high-fiber foods are also rich in other nutrients and—if they're not prepared with lots of added fats—low in calories.

So, to get enough fiber, favor whole grains along with whole fruits and vegetables. That way, you'll likely meet the daily requirements for healthy carbohydrate intake.

Protein

Q | I don't eat meat. Protein is just for big muscles anyway, isn't it?

Protein is for everyone, regardless of muscle size. It's an essential macronutrient that is the major structural component of all your body cells. You need protein for the repair and growth of muscle and bone. Proteins and their components also function as enzymes and hormones and as carriers of important molecules throughout the body. Like carbohydrates, proteins provide about 4 calories per gram; however, the energy in protein is not liberated quite as easily, so protein is not considered a primary source of energy or fuel for the body.

Complete and Incomplete Proteins

Q | Is red meat the best kind of protein?

Red meat is an excellent source of protein, but there is more to the story. Protein is made up of molecules called **amino acids**—that is, amino acids are the building blocks of the body's protein molecules. There are twenty amino acids, eleven of which can be made by the body and nine of which cannot. *Essential amino acids* are the nine that cannot be made by the body and must be supplied in the diet. Your body can make the eleven *nonessential amino acids* if you consume enough essential amino acids and calories. You can easily obtain essential amino

acids if you eat a variety of protein-containing foods, including but not limited to red meat.

Complete proteins contain all the essential amino acids and are found in animal foods and soy: meat, fish, poultry, soybeans and soy products, eggs, and dairy products. (Some of the less widely available grains such as quinoa and amaranth are also complete proteins.) Foods that lack one or more of the essential amino acids are referred to as **incomplete proteins.** Except for soy, plant sources of protein—beans and other vegetables, nuts, seeds, and grains—are incomplete proteins. Meeting protein needs is easy when you include a variety of both types of proteins in your diet, but vegetarians can obtain adequate protein by combining different types of plant proteins.

When selecting animal proteins, consider the type and amount of fat and the total calories. Some food sources of animal protein are high in both unhealthy saturated fats and calories; you can choose healthier, more nutrient-rich alternatives. Table 8-3 shows the protein and saturated fat content of some popular protein sources, along with lower-fat alternatives. Fish and shellfish tend to be low in saturated fat, and the fat in many varieties of fish is a type that has been shown to improve heart health.

Plant sources of protein naturally contain little or no saturated fat, although fats may be added during processing. For plant proteins, your concern should be consuming a variety of sources. Different types of plant proteins are deficient in different amino acids, so combinations of these incomplete proteins create complete proteins. So-called *complementary protein pairs* include legumes and grains, legumes and nuts, and legumes and seeds. You don't have to consume complementary proteins in the same meal; a variety of plant foods eaten over the course of a day can provide all essential amino acids.[13] But it's easy to combine proteins in one meal: say, pinto beans and a tortilla, hummus with pita bread, vegetable chili with cornbread, salad with chickpeas and sunflower seeds, or split pea soup with rye crackers. Plant foods can be a source of protein for both vegetarians and non-vegetarians. In addition, they contain fiber and are lower in fat and calories than many animal protein sources—in many cases, they are also less expensive.

protein A category of essential macronutrient; a compound made of amino acids.

amino acids Molecules that are the building blocks of proteins; the 9 essential amino acids cannot be made by the body and must be obtained from food; the 11 nonessential amino acids can be made by the body.

complete proteins Dietary sources of protein that provide all the essential amino acids; found in animal foods and soy.

incomplete proteins Dietary sources of protein that are missing one or more essential amino acids; found in plant sources of protein.

DOLLAR STRETCHER
Financial Wellness Tip

Economize on protein by buying lean meat, poultry, and fish on sale. Also, keep in mind that although fattier cuts of meat may be cheaper, more goes to waste. For example, there are 29 cuts of lean beef, including eye of the round, sirloin tip, top round, and 95 percent lean ground beef. Another economizing tip is to choose less expensive protein sources often, including plant proteins and nonfat dairy products.

TABLE 8-3 PROTEIN, SATURATED FAT, AND ENERGY CONTENT OF SELECTED PROTEIN SOURCES

FOOD	PROTEIN (GRAMS)	SATURATED FAT (GRAMS)	CALORIES
Regular ground beef patty (30% fat)	21.6	6.2	232
Extra lean ground beef patty (5% fat)	22.4	2.5	145
Veggie burger or soyburger patty	11.0	1.0	124
Fried chicken breast (½) with skin	31.2	2.4	218
Roasted chicken breast (½) without skin	26.7	0.9	142
Salami, sliced (3 oz)	19.5	8.9	323
Roast beef, fat trimmed (3 oz)	21.9	3.4	177
Turkey breast, sliced (3 oz)	11.3	0.1	94
Regular cheddar cheese (1 oz)	7.1	6.0	114
Low-fat cheddar cheese (1 oz)	6.9	1.2	49
Whole milk (1 cup)	7.7	4.6	149
Low-fat (1%) milk (1 cup)	9.7	1.8	118
Nonfat milk (1 cup)	8.3	0.1	83
Yogurt, fruit, low-fat (8 oz)	9.9	1.6	232
Yogurt, plain, nonfat (8 oz)	14.0	0.3	137
Egg (1 large)	6.3	1.6	78
Salmon (3 oz)	18.8	2.1	175
Tuna, canned in water (3 oz)	20.1	0.7	109
Shrimp (3 oz)	17.8	0.2	84
Tofu (½ cup)	10.0	0.9	94
Soybeans (½ cup)	14.3	1.1	149
Lentils (½ cup)	8.9	0.1	113
Pinto beans (½ cup)	5.8	0.2	103
Kidney beans (½ cup)	6.7	0.1	108
Spaghetti (½ cup)	4.1	0.1	110
Whole-wheat bread (1 small slice)	3.6	0.2	69
Flour tortilla (8-in.)	3.8	0.9	144
Peanut butter (2 tbsp)	7.7	2.6	188
Sunflower seed kernels, roasted (1 oz)	5.5	1.5	165
Pumpkin seeds, roasted (1 oz)	5.3	1.0	126

Source: Data from U.S. Department of Agriculture, Agricultural Research Service, Nutrient Data Laboratory. (2009). *USDA national nutrient database for standard reference,* Release 22 (http://www.ars.usda.gov/ba/bhnrc/ndl).

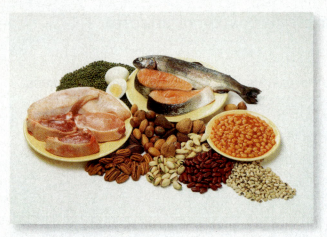

When selecting animal proteins, choose those that are low in unhealthy fats. For plant proteins, consume a variety of protein sources over the course of the day to obtain all essential amino acids.

So yes, red meat is a valuable source of complete protein, but eating a variety of proteins is healthier than sticking to any single protein source. If you shun red meat—and many people do for cultural, religious, ethical, or health reasons—you can meet your daily protein requirement with other lean complete proteins such as chicken, fish, or soy or with a combination of incomplete proteins such as beans, nuts, grains, and vegetables.

Recommended Protein Intake

Q | How much protein should I eat?

Healthy adults need to consume about 0.36 grams of protein per pound (0.8 grams per kilogram) of body weight, almost regardless of biological sex. Here are some examples:

- 36 grams of protein per day for a 100-pound adult
- 54 grams of protein per day for a 150-pound adult
- 72 grams of protein per day for a 200-pound adult

Lab Activity 8-1 will help you set a personal protein goal based on the Dietary Reference Intakes.

The AMDR for protein is 10–35 percent of total daily calories. If your diet is relatively low in calories, then the percent of total daily calories from protein may need to be at the higher end of the range in order to meet your daily requirement. For example, for a 200-pound person with a diet of 1,700 calories per day, 72 grams of protein would be 17 percent of total daily calories; with a diet of 3,000 calories per day, only 10 percent.

Some people need more protein. Infants, children, adolescents, and women who are pregnant or breastfeeding have higher protein requirements—up to 0.59 grams per pound of body weight for a breastfeeding woman, for example. The DRIs state that athletes do not need additional protein, but the American College of Sports Medicine recommends a somewhat higher protein intake for both endurance athletes (0.54–0.64 grams per pound) and resistance athletes (0.54–0.77 grams per pound) who are engaged in serious training.[14] Athletes typically consume high-calorie diets, so this higher protein intake can be achieved with food (supplements are not recommended) and remain within the AMDR for protein.

Diets very high in protein—above the AMDR—are generally not recommended. However, there is little evidence linking high protein diets with health problems.[15] Nor is there evidence that consuming high levels of protein from foods or supplements, or taking supplements of specific amino acids, will improve athletic performance. And with regard to weight loss, there is only mixed evidence that high-protein diets are better than other types of diets, so personal preferences and consultation with a health care provider may be the best guide. In the long term, it is the total energy content of the diet that matters for weight management, not the macronutrient distribution (see Chapter 9).

On average, Americans consume about 15 percent of total daily calories as protein, so most Americans take in adequate amounts.[16] More worrisome than total protein intake is the nutrient profile of the most common sources of protein in the U.S. diet—high in calories and solid fats.

Fats

Q | I know, I know— fats are bad and should always be avoided, right?

Not all fats are bad—and some are even essential. **Fats** are needed in sufficient quantities for cellular integrity, healthy reproduction, absorption of fat-soluble vitamins, support and cushioning of organs, and thermal insulation. As described earlier, fats also provide energy, lots of energy (9 calories per gram). Consuming healthy fats in limited amounts can actually benefit your health. Conversely, choosing the wrong fats can increase your risk of cardiovascular disease and type 2 diabetes, and consuming too much fat of either type can lead to weight gain, just as consuming too much protein or carbohydrate can.

Types of Fats

Fats in food are made up of different types of *fatty acids*. These fatty acids are found in the form of **triglycerides,** which contain three fatty-acid molecules and a glycerol molecule. Fatty acids are chains of carbon atoms with hydrogen atoms attached to some or all of the carbon atoms. Chemical differences—in the length of carbon chains, the types of bonds between the carbon atoms, and the number of hydrogen atoms attached

fats A category of essential macronutrient; an organic compound made up of fatty acids; lipid.

triglycerides Major form of fat found in foods and stored in the body, consists of three fatty-acid molecules and a glycerol molecule.

to the carbon chains—give rise to the differing effects of various types of fats on health. Most food fats contain a mix of different types of fatty acids.

Q | What's the difference between saturated and unsaturated fats?

The difference lies in their chemical structure and behavior in the body (Figure 8-6).

■ **Saturated fatty acids:** All the bonds between carbon atoms on the chain are single bonds, and every available bond from each carbon atom is attached to a hydrogen atom. In other words, the fatty-acid chain is "saturated" with hydrogen atoms. Saturated fats are generally solid at room temperature; think butter.

■ **Unsaturated fatty acids:** One or more of the available bonds on the carbon chain are not attached to a hydrogen atom, and neighboring carbon atoms form a double bond. Fatty acids with one double bond are called *monounsaturated,* and those with two or more double bonds are called *polyunsaturated.* Unsaturated fats are usually liquid at room temperature; think oils.

Food fats typically contain multiple types of fatty acids, and the predominant types determine the fat's characteristics. Butter is about two-thirds saturated fat and one-third unsaturated fat, so it is fairly solid at room temperature. Corn oil is about 85 percent unsaturated fatty acids, so it is liquid at room temperature. Generally speaking, saturated fats are found primarily in animal products, whereas unsaturated fats come from plant sources. There are exceptions: Fish contains polyunsaturated fatty acids, and certain plant oils (coconut and palm) are highly saturated.

Q | Why is saturated fat so bad?

When you consume saturated fats, they act on your liver to increase the amount of low-density lipoproteins (LDLs), or "bad" cholesterol, in your blood. High levels of LDLs increase

saturated fatty acid A fatty acid with a carbon chain full of hydrogen atoms; usually from animal sources and solid at room temperature.

unsaturated fatty acid A fatty acid with a carbon chain that includes one or more carbon-carbon double bonds; usually from plant sources and liquid at room temperature. Monounsaturated fatty acids have one carbon-carbon double bond, and polyunsaturated fatty acids have two or more double bonds.

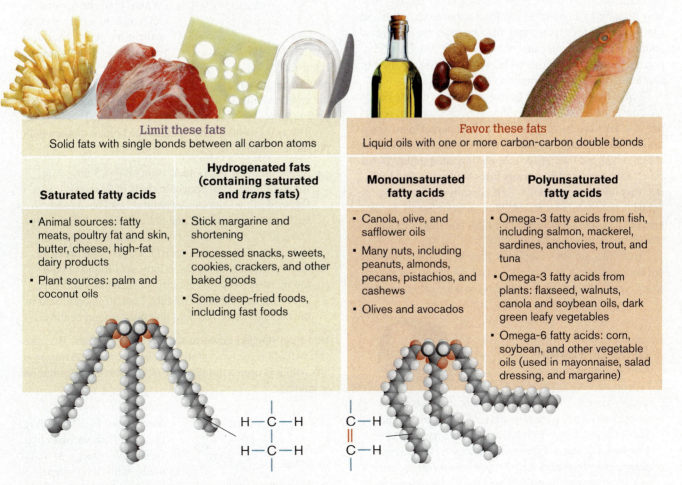

Limit these fats — Solid fats with single bonds between all carbon atoms

Favor these fats — Liquid oils with one or more carbon-carbon double bonds

Saturated fatty acids	Hydrogenated fats (containing saturated and *trans* fats)	Monounsaturated fatty acids	Polyunsaturated fatty acids
• Animal sources: fatty meats, poultry fat and skin, butter, cheese, high-fat dairy products • Plant sources: palm and coconut oils	• Stick margarine and shortening • Processed snacks, sweets, cookies, crackers, and other baked goods • Some deep-fried foods, including fast foods	• Canola, olive, and safflower oils • Many nuts, including peanuts, almonds, pecans, pistachios, and cashews • Olives and avocados	• Omega-3 fatty acids from fish, including salmon, mackerel, sardines, anchovies, trout, and tuna • Omega-3 fatty acids from plants: flaxseed, walnuts, canola and soybean oils, dark green leafy vegetables • Omega-6 fatty acids: corn, soybean, and other vegetable oils (used in mayonnaise, salad dressing, and margarine)

Figure 8-6 Types of fats. Although all food fats are in the form of triglycerides, fatty acids differ in their chemical properties and structure. These differences affect their behavior in the body and their long-term impact on health.

your risk for heart attack and stroke. Saturated fat is also associated with insulin resistance in cells, which increases your risk for type 2 diabetes. Your body can make all the saturated fats you require, so saturated fatty acids from the diet have no redeeming health value. Replacing some of the saturated fats you consume with unsaturated fats can reduce your risk for serious health problems.

Saturated fats occur naturally in many foods from animal sources, including fatty cuts of beef and pork; poultry with skin; and cream, butter, cheese, and other dairy products made from whole milk or reduced-fat (2 percent) milk. Many processed foods—fried and baked desserts and snack foods, for example—also contain high levels of saturated fat. Top sources of saturated fat in the U.S. diet include cheese, pizza, grain- and dairy-based desserts, sausage and other fatty meats, whole and reduced-fat milk, and mixed dishes containing beef and chicken.[17]

Q | What are trans fats, and why are they so bad?

Trans fats are produced during the process of **hydrogenation,** in which hydrogen atoms are added to polyunsaturated fatty acids, turning some of them into saturated fatty acids. Food manufacturers use this process because hydrogenated fats have a longer shelf life and can be reused for frying; they also improve the texture of some baked goods. Because they are solid or semisolid at room temperature, hydrogenated vegetable oils are used to create shortening, margarine, and spreadable fats.

Typically, only some of the carbon-carbon double bonds are converted to single bonds during hydrogenation, resulting in a "partially hydrogenated" oil. The partial hydrogenation of oils affects the remaining double bonds on the carbon chains, changing their shape to a configuration referred to as *trans*. Like saturated fats, **trans fatty acids** raise bad LDLs, but they also lower HDLs (high-density lipoproteins, or "good" cholesterol)—a double blow to heart health. Hydrogenated fats contain both saturated fats and trans fats and so should be limited in your diet.

Trans fats are found in foods fried in hydrogenated oils or shortening, such as french fries and doughnuts, as well as many types of baked goods, including cookies, cakes, pastries, pie crust, and biscuits. Stick margarines can be another source. Small amounts of trans fats also occur naturally in some meat and dairy products, but it's unclear if these naturally occurring trans fats are as bad for health as those that have been manufactured.

In response to the significant negative health effects of trans fats, the U.S. Department of Agriculture mandated that trans fat content be listed on food labels by 2006, and some U.S. cities began banning it in restaurant foods. Food manufacturers have started reducing or eliminating trans fat from their products, and it's possible that artificially produced trans fats will cease to be a part of our national diet. In the meantime, read food labels and use caution when you see the word *hydrogenated* in the ingredient list or trans fat indicated on the food label. When it comes to trans fat, the less you consume, the better. Ideally, the only trans fats in your diet should be those that occur naturally.

Q | What are omega fatty acids?

When you see *omega* in reference to a fat, it is an indication of the chemical structure of a polyunsaturated fat. In *omega-3 fatty acids,* the first carbon-carbon double bond starts with the third carbon from the end of the carbon chain; similarly, in *omega-6 fatty acids,* the first double bond is at the sixth carbon from the end.

The two essential fatty acids in the human diet are both polyunsaturated:

- *Alpha-linolenic acid (ALA)* is an omega-3 fatty acid found in fairly high concentrations in flaxseeds and flaxseed oil, walnuts and walnut oil, soybeans and soybean oil, canola oil, and fish and fish oil. The body converts ALA into other types of fats. The top food source of ALA in the American diet is salad dressing.
- *Linoleic acid* is an omega-6 fatty acid found in commonly used food oils, including safflower, sunflower, corn oils, and fish and fish oils. Lack of linoleic acid in the diet can cause hair loss and poor wound healing.

Don't get bogged down in the chemistry of fats. Because you will often see news stories about omega-3 and omega-6 fats, you just need a little background to put the information in context.

Q | I hate tuna but hear it has fats that are good for you. Is this true?

Yes, some fish, including tuna, are rich in particular types of omega-3 fatty acids with long names— eicosapentaenoic acid (EPA) and docosahexaenoic acid (DHA). These fats are considered heart-healthy because they reduce blood clots, decrease inflammation (which is a

hydrogenation A process that adds hydrogen atoms to polyunsaturated fats to produce a more solid and stable fat; hydrogenated fats include saturated fatty acids and standard and *trans* forms of unsaturated fatty acids.

trans fatty acid An unsaturated fatty acid with an atypical chemical shape that affects its functioning in the body; found naturally in small amounts in certain foods and produced during the process of hydrogenation.

Mind Stretcher
Critical Thinking Exercise

When you make your daily food choices, do you ever consider basic dietary guidelines and nutritional recommendations? Do you look at food labels and the other nutritional information provided in stores and restaurants? What criteria do you use in selecting foods? If you were a public health official, what strategies would you use to get people like yourself and your peers to put more emphasis on nutrition recommendations in making food choices?

precursor to heart disease), normalize heart rhythms, and lower the risk of developing or dying from high blood pressure, coronary heart disease, and stroke for some people. These omega-3 fatty acids are found not only in tuna but also in many other fish, including salmon, herring, sardines, trout, mackerel, and anchovies. The body can also synthesize these compounds from plant sources of alpha-linolenic acid, but the process is very inefficient and doesn't produce much EPA and DHA.

Because of the health benefits of these omega-3 fats, health authorities recommend that we eat several servings of fish per week. There are cautions, however, about consuming certain types of fish, which may be contaminated by mercury and other heavy metals (see Chapter 9 for more on food safety). If you don't like tuna, then try other fish and seafood—and try them prepared in different ways. If you dislike all fish and seafood, you can obtain some healthy omega-3 fats from plant sources such as flaxseed and walnut oils, although they yield only very small amounts of EPA and DHA.

Cholesterol

Q | Is there good and bad cholesterol in foods?

Not exactly, though we often refer to cholesterol as "good" or "bad" due to its effect on heart disease risk. **Dietary cholesterol** is a waxy substance in the cell membranes of animal tissues, so it is found only in animal products. The top sources of dietary cholesterol in the American diet are egg yolks, dairy products, and meats and meat products (beef, chicken, sausage, bacon, and so on). There is no dietary requirement for cholesterol because your body can manufacture all the cholesterol it needs.

Although a high intake of dietary cholesterol can raise blood cholesterol levels, the cholesterol ingested in foods is not considered as much of a culprit as are dietary saturated and trans fats. These two dietary fats promote cholesterol production by the liver, where most blood cholesterol is formed; only about a quarter or less of your body's cholesterol comes from the foods you eat. So, consuming dietary cholesterol in moderation is OK, and limiting saturated and trans fats is even better. Blood cholesterol circulates through your body in protein packages called *lipoproteins:*

dietary cholesterol
A waxy substance in the cell membranes of animal tissues; in humans, produced by the liver and consumed in animal products.

phytosterol A plant-based compound that competes with dietary cholesterol for absorption by the body, resulting in lower blood cholesterol levels.

- *Low-density lipoprotein (LDL)* carries cholesterol from the liver to the rest of the body. High levels of LDL can cause dangerous accumulation of cholesterol on the walls of blood vessels.
- *High-density lipoprotein (HDL)* carries cholesterol from the body back to the liver, where it can be eliminated.

Plant foods contain related cellular compounds called **phytosterols.** These compounds are similar in structure to cholesterol and they compete with dietary cholesterol for absorption during digestion. In effect, phytosterols reduce the amount of dietary cholesterol absorbed by the body—a real health benefit.[18] Phytosterols are found naturally in plant foods and are sometimes added as supplements in margarine spreads, salad dressings, and other foods. Phytosterol supplements may be recommended for some people with high blood cholesterol or heart disease.

Recommended Fat Intake

Q | How much fat is too much in my diet?

As you've seen, there are many recommendations related to your fat intake—for both type and amount (see the box "Tips for Meeting Dietary Fat and Cholesterol Recommendations"). Most Americans get plenty of fat in their diet and meet the requirement for essential fatty acids, which is equivalent to about 4 teaspoons of vegetable oil. The Acceptable Macronutrient Distribution Range for fat is 20–35 percent of total daily calories, with most

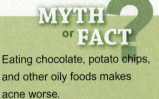

MYTH or FACT?

Eating chocolate, potato chips, and other oily foods makes acne worse.

▶ **WATCH THIS VIDEO IN** connect

See pages 476–477 to find out.

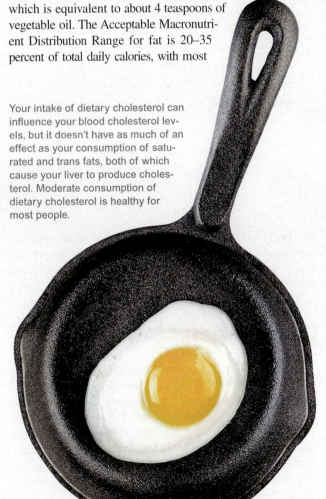

Your intake of dietary cholesterol can influence your blood cholesterol levels, but it doesn't have as much of an effect as your consumption of saturated and trans fats, both of which cause your liver to produce cholesterol. Moderate consumption of dietary cholesterol is healthy for most people.

Wellness Strategies

Tips for Meeting Dietary Fat and Cholesterol Recommendations

 Q What constitutes a proper fat intake?

When you complete Lab Activity 8-2, you'll find out where you stand in relation to most of the guidelines for fat and cholesterol intake. Then develop strategies for change that are right for you.

Targets

- Overall fat intake: 20%–35% of total daily calories
- Saturated fat: 10% or less of total daily calories (initial goal), working toward 7% or less of total daily calories
- Trans fat: Avoid artificially produced trans fats; the small amount of trans fats in the diet should be from natural sources
- Dietary cholesterol: 300 mg or less per day for healthy adults, 200 mg or less per day for people with or at high risk for cardiovascular disease or type 2 diabetes

General Strategies

- Read food labels and nutrition information available at restaurants to identify the type and amount of fat you consume; use the information to make better choices.
- Trim obvious fat from cuts of meats.
- Monitor and limit portion sizes of foods high in unhealthy fats and cholesterol.

Substitutions to Try

Instead of:	Try:
Regular cheese	Low-fat or fat-free cheese, or select a favorite cheese and cut your portion size in half
Full-fat ice cream and other desserts	Low-fat or fat-free ice cream, frozen yogurt, and dessert toppings
Pizza with cheese and meat toppings	Pizza with vegetable toppings; ask for half the usual amount of cheese
Sausage, bacon, salami, high-fat lunch meats	Canadian bacon, sliced turkey, other lower-fat lunch meats
Butter, stick margarine	Tub or squeeze margarine spreads, vegetable oils
Cream- or cheese-based salad dressings, sour cream	Vegetable-based salad dressings, low-fat or nonfat sour cream or plain yogurt
Pasta with cream sauce or alfredo sauce	Pasta with tomato or other vegetable-based sauce
Fried chicken or fish	Baked chicken (without skin) or fish
Ground beef, ribs, pork chops, prime grades of beef	Ground turkey, veggie burgers, extra-lean ground beef, sirloin steak, choice grades of beef
Biscuits, muffins, coffee cake, pastries	Fruit, yogurt, or small serving of a sweet treat
Fruit pie with crust	Baked fruit or fruit crisp (no pastry crust)

---

of that coming from unsaturated fats from plant and fish sources instead of saturated and trans fats from animal fats and hydrogenated oils. Replacing some of the saturated and trans fats in your diet with unsaturated fats is a great change to make for reducing your risk of chronic disease.

Water

 Q Why is drinking water important?

Water is a vital macronutrient. It is needed for the digestion and absorption of food; it is the main ingredient in blood; and it provides lubrication, cushioning, and temperature control throughout the body. Adult males are about 60 percent water by weight, and adult females about 55 percent.

To maintain a healthy water balance and sustain life, you must consume enough fluids to balance what you lose through urine, sweat, evaporation in the lungs, and bowel movements. There is no precise formula for determining what this amount is. So, you need to be attentive to your thirst, to environmental and weather conditions (drink more when it is hot or dry), and the simple need to consume water throughout any given day.

Sources of Water

Liquids, fruits, and vegetables are good food sources of water, though almost all foods contain some water.

 Q Can I drink juice or soda instead of water?

Juice, like all types of fluids you consume, can help you meet your daily water requirement. On average, fluids are the source of about 80 percent

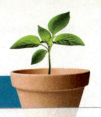

Living *Well* with . . .

Lactose Intolerance

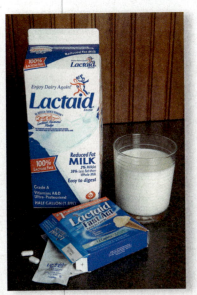

Lactose intolerance is the inability to digest significant amounts of lactose, the predominant sugar in milk. This condition may affect more than 30 million Americans. Its occurrence is lowest among European Americans and higher among African Americans, Latinos, Asian Americans, and Native Americans.

The problem stems from a shortage of the enzyme lactase, which is normally produced by cells lining the small intestine. Lactase breaks down milk sugar into simpler forms that can then be absorbed into the bloodstream. When there is not enough lactase to digest the amount of lactose consumed, the results, although not usually dangerous, may be distressing. Common symptoms include nausea, cramps, bloating, gas, and diarrhea, which can begin shortly after eating or drinking foods containing lactose.

The best treatment for lactose intolerance is prevention, which usually occurs through trial and error.

Many lactose-intolerant individuals can consume some lactose—the equivalent of 1 cup of milk—without developing symptoms and so can enjoy small servings of dairy products throughout the day. For those who react to very small amounts of lactose or have trouble limiting their intake of foods that contain it, nonprescription lactase enzymes can convert the lactose in milk to a more digestible form. Lactose-reduced milk and other dairy products are available at most supermarkets. These products contain all the nutrients found in regular dairy products.

If you are lactose intolerant, make sure your diet includes the recommended amount of calcium even if you don't consume dairy products. Nondairy foods high in calcium are green vegetables such as broccoli and kale and fish with soft, edible bones such as salmon and sardines. Recent research indicates that yogurt with active cultures may be a good source of calcium for many people with lactose intolerance, even though it is fairly high in lactose. Evidence shows that the bacterial cultures used to make yogurt produce some of the lactase enzyme required for proper digestion of lactose.

Sources: NIH Consensus Development Conference: Lactose Intolerance and Health. (2010, February). *Final panel statement* (http://consensus. nih.gov/2010/lactosestatement.htm). National Digestive Diseases Information Clearinghouse. (2009). *Lactose intolerance* (http://digestive.niddk .nih.gov/ddiseases/pubs/lactoseintolerance).

---

of daily water intake for most people, and the water in foods accounts for the remaining 20 percent. Many fruits and vegetables are very high in water content.

Water, however, is usually the best source for meeting the body's hydration needs. That said, many people consume other types of beverages daily. Milk is an important source of calcium, especially for children. Yet some people have trouble digesting milk; see the box "Living Well with . . . Lactose Intolerance." Orange juice is a favorite breakfast drink and contains lots of vitamin C and potassium, and calcium-fortified orange juice has as much calcium as milk. Fruit juice can be a good source of water if it fits in your overall nutrient and calorie needs. Although whole fruits are more nutrient rich than fruit juice, 100-percent fruit juices are healthier beverage choices than fruit drinks or punches (which often have little fruit and much added sugar) or other types of beverages high in calories and sugar.

Soda also counts as a source of water, though it often isn't the best choice. Regular soda is loaded with added sugars, has no vitamins or minerals, and contains phosphoric acid, which can speed the body's elimination of calcium.[19] Unfortunately, soda consumption in children and adolescents

has replaced milk consumption.[20] There is concern that over the long term, drinking soda instead of milk may result in lower bone mineral density,[21] thereby putting youths at greater risk for osteoporosis later in life. Drinking empty-calorie beverages such as regular sodas may also be linked with increased rates of overweight and obesity in children.

Regardless of your drink(s) of choice, bear in mind that most non-water drinks contain calories, of which water has none. So too much fruit juice or regular soda may be adding a lot of unnecessary and unwanted calories to your daily total.

Recommended Intake of Water

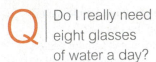

Q | Do I really need eight glasses of water a day?

Drinking eight glasses of water a day was long considered the norm. However, the *Dietary Guidelines for Americans, 2010,* reinforces that the combination of quenching thirst and practicing usual drinking patterns (especially fluid consumption with meals) is sufficient to maintain a normal level of hydration in most cases. Further, individual fluid needs

Research Brief

A Tax on Sweetness?

The rise in obesity among Americans has been associated with eating more meals away from home and drinking more sweetened beverages. Together, sodas, energy drinks, and sports drinks are now the leading source of calories for Americans ages 14 and over. These beverages contain added sugars but few if any other nutrients.

Some organizations and state and local governments have suggested a tax on caloric sweetened beverages. A recent study analyzed the effects of a hypothetical tax that would increase the price of caloric sweetened beverages by 20 percent. Researchers estimated that the tax would reduce the total calorie intake from the taxed beverages by 13 percent for adults and 11 percent for children. Assuming all else remained equal, the daily calorie reductions would translate into an average loss of 3.8 pounds over a year for adults and 4.5 pounds over a year for children.

Analyze and Apply

- If you consume these types of beverages, would such a tax reduce your intake? Why or why not?
- What do you think of the general strategy of taxing "empty" calories?

Source: Smith, T. A., Lin, B.-H., & Lee, J.-Y. (2010). *Taxing caloric sweetened beverages: Potential effects on beverage consumption, calorie intake, and obesity.* USDA Economic Research Service report no. ERR-100 (http://www.ers.usda.gov/Publications/err100/).

vary and depend on factors such as daily physical activity level and heat exposure.

How can you tell if you are drinking enough water? Do you rarely feel thirsty? Is your urine usually clear or slightly yellow? If so, then your fluid intake is probably sufficient. Healthy people who regularly participate in physical activity or are exposed to excess heat may need more purposeful drinking to maintain adequate hydration levels. See Chapter 3 for specific recommendations for fluid intake during exercise.

Fast Facts

Water of Life

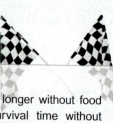

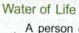

A person can survive much longer without food than without water. Survival time without water depends on the individual and the conditions. A baby or a child left in a hot car, an athlete exercising in hot weather, or a senior left alone without air conditioning during a heat wave might become dehydrated and overheated and die within a few hours. In less extreme conditions, an adult might live for 7–10 days without water—but he or she would be very ill. A person can live for more than a month without food, as long as he or she has water.

- Why do you think people generally live longer without food than water?
- If you unexpectedly found yourself without access to drinking water for more than a few hours, what strategies would you use to stay hydrated for as long as possible?

Source: Environmental Protection Agency. (2007). *Water trivia facts* (http://www.epa.gov/safewater/kids/water_trivia_facts.html).

Fast Facts

The Average American Drinker

Americans consume about 400 calories a day in beverages. Although the sources of the bulk of those calories differ between children (2–18 years) and adults (19 years and over), regular soda and sports/energy drinks take most of the top spots regardless of age. The table here shows, in descending order, the leading sources of beverage calories, respectively, for adults and children. How do you compare?

Most Common Adult Beverages:	Most Common Youth Beverages:
(Water is preferred)	(Water is preferred)
Regular soda	Milk
Energy and sports drinks	Regular soda
Alcohol	Energy and sports drinks
Milk	Fruit drinks
100% fruit juice	100% fruit juice
Fruit drinks	

Source: Dietary Guidelines For Americans, 2010. *http://www.cnpp.usda.gov/dietaryguidelines.htm*

- In terms of the amount of each type of beverage you consume, how do your beverage preferences stack up against those of the average adult?
- Why might it be "a good thing" to be different from the average American when it comes to beverage intake?

Vitamins and Minerals

Q | Are minerals different from vitamins?

Both **vitamins** and **minerals** are micronutrients, but vitamins are organic compounds and minerals are inorganic compounds, meaning that vitamins contain carbon and minerals don't. Humans need about fourteen different vitamins and seventeen different minerals.

Vitamins are divided into two groups: *water-soluble* (vitamin C and the B vitamins) and *fat-soluble* (vitamins A, D, E, and K). Water-soluble vitamins travel throughout the body in the bloodstream, and excess amounts are excreted in the urine, so these vitamins need to be regularly replaced. Fat-soluble vitamins are absorbed differently and can be stored in the liver and fatty tissues, so it is not as critical to consume them daily.

Minerals, also called elements, are divided into two groups: *major minerals* and *trace minerals.* The major minerals (at least 100 milligrams needed daily) include sodium, calcium, phosphorus, magnesium, potassium, and chloride. The trace minerals, or those needed in much smaller amounts, include copper, fluoride, iodine, iron,

vitamins Organic (carbon-containing) compounds needed in small quantities by the body for normal functioning.

minerals Inorganic compounds essential for normal metabolism, growth and development, and regulation of cell activity.

selenium, and zinc. Although the daily requirement for the trace minerals is much lower than for the major minerals, they are no less important.

Q | What do vitamins and minerals do?

First, vitamins don't provide energy, regardless of what you might read. However, adequate vitamin intake is necessary to regulate certain body functions and processes, including tissue growth and repair; releasing energy from nutrients; preserving healthy cells; and maintaining the nerves, skeletal tissue, red blood cells, and immune function. In addition, some vitamins are believed to help reduce the risk of chronic diseases; see the discussion of antioxidants on pp. 293–294. Minerals perform functions similar to those of vitamins, including the liberation of energy and the regulation of growth and development. To learn more about what specific vitamins and minerals do, see Tables 8-4 and 8-5.

If you consume significantly less than the recommended amount of a particular vitamin or mineral, symptoms of a deficiency disease can develop. For example, people who consume little or no vitamin C for a month or longer will develop scurvy, whose symptoms include weakness, bleeding gums, and tooth loss. Full-blown deficiency diseases are rare among Americans. However, many people do not consume recommended amounts of certain vitamins and minerals, and although the shortfalls may not be sufficient to cause

TABLE 8-4 VITAMINS: SOURCES, FUNCTIONS, AND RECOMMENDED INTAKES

VITAMIN	MAJOR FUNCTIONS	KEY FOOD SOURCES	RECOMMENDED DAILY INTAKE*
FAT-SOLUBLE VITAMINS			
VITAMIN A 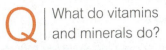	Maintenance of normal vision; immune system functioning; reproduction and fetal development; health of the skin and the surface linings of the nose, mouth, and digestive tract	Liver and other organ meats, oily fish, eggs, milk and other fortified dairy products, dark-colored fruits and leafy vegetables (e.g., tomatoes, red peppers, sweet potatoes, kale, carrots)	Males: 900 μg Females: 700 μg
VITAMIN D	Absorption of calcium and phosphorus for maintenance of healthy bones and teeth; support for healthy cellular metabolism	Fortified dairy products, orange juice, cereals; eggs, liver, oily fish (skin also produces vitamin D in response to sunlight exposure)	Males: 15 μg (600 IU) Females: 15 μg (600 IU)
VITAMIN E	An antioxidant that protects cells from damage by free radicals; may help prevent chronic disease	Vegetable oils, whole grains, nuts, seeds, leafy green vegetables	Males: 15 mg Females: 15 mg
VITAMIN K	Blood clotting, bone metabolism	Leafy green vegetables, brussels sprouts, cabbage, soy, asparagus, green beans, dried plums	Males: 120 μg Females: 90 μg

(continued)

TABLE 8-4 *(continued)*

VITAMIN	MAJOR FUNCTIONS	KEY FOOD SOURCES	RECOMMENDED DAILY INTAKE*
WATER-SOLUBLE VITAMINS			
BIOTIN	Synthesis of fats, glycogen, and amino acids	Egg yolk, legumes, nuts, cereals, yeast, liver; smaller amounts in fruits and meat; also synthesized by intestinal bacteria	Males: 30 µg Females: 30 µg
CHOLINE	Maintenance of cell membranes; precursor for acetylcholine, a neurotransmitter involved in muscle control, memory, and other functions	Milk, eggs, liver, pork, fish, soy milk, peanuts	Males: 550 mg Females: 425 mg
FOLATE	Metabolism of DNA, RNA, and amino acids; synthesis of new cells; prevents one form of anemia	Enriched grain products, green vegetables (spinach, broccoli, asparagus), orange juice, legumes, beets, whole grains, liver	Males: 400 µg Females: 400 µg
NIACIN	Energy metabolism	Meat, fish, poultry, enriched and whole-grain breads and cereals, leafy green vegetables, potatoes, peanuts	Males: 16 mg Females: 14 mg
PANTOTHENIC ACID	Energy metabolism; synthesis of fats, neurotransmitters, hormones, and hemoglobin	Chicken, beef, fish and shellfish, whole grains, legumes, egg yolk, oats, potatoes, tomatoes, broccoli	Males: 5 mg Females: 5 mg
RIBOFLAVIN (VITAMIN B$_2$)	Energy metabolism, many cellular processes	Wide variety of foods, including milk, meats, grains, and fortified cereals	Males: 1.3 mg Females: 1.1 mg
THIAMINE (VITAMIN B$_1$)	Metabolism of carbohydrates and protein	Enriched, fortified, and whole-grain foods; organ meats, leafy green vegetables, nuts, legumes	Males: 1.2 mg Females: 1.1 mg
VITAMIN B$_6$	Metabolism of amino acids and glycogen; support for cellular functioning and immune response	Meat, chicken, fish, liver and other organ meats, whole grains, nuts, legumes, fortified products	Males: 1.3 mg Females: 1.3 mg
VITAMIN B$_{12}$	Synthesis of amino acids, DNA, red blood cells; support for nervous system functioning	Fish and seafood, meat, poultry, fortified grain products, milk and yogurt	Males: 2.4 µg Females: 2.4 µg
VITAMIN C	Aids in iron absorption, promotion of healing, immune function, and protein metabolism; an antioxidant that protects cells from damage by free radicals	Most vegetables and fruit, especially citrus fruits, tomatoes, berries, potatoes, green vegetables	Males: 90 mg Females: 75 mg

*Recommended daily intakes for adults ages 19–30; for information on other age groups and life stages, including pregnancy, visit http://iom.edu/Activities/Nutrition/SummaryDRIs/DRI-Tables.aspx; to calculate your personal DRIs, go to the Interactive DRI website (http://fnic.nal.usda.gov/interactiveDRI).

Sources: Adapted from Food and Nutrition Board, National Academies. (2010). *Dietary Reference Intakes: Vitamins* (http://fnic.nal.usda.gov/nal_display/index.php?info_center=4&tax_level=3&tax_subject=256&topic_id=1342&level3_id=5140). Dietary Guidelines Advisory Committee. (2010). *Report of the Dietary Guidelines Advisory Committee on the dietary guidelines for Americans, 2010* (http://www.cnpp.usda.gov/DGAs2010-DGACReport.htm).

TABLE 8-5   SELECTED MINERALS: SOURCES, FUNCTIONS, AND RECOMMENDED INTAKES

MINERAL	MAJOR FUNCTIONS	KEY FOOD SOURCES	RECOMMENDED DAILY INTAKE*
CALCIUM	Formation of bones and teeth, control of blood clotting, muscle and nerve functioning	Milk and other dairy products, calcium-set tofu, fortified orange juice and bread, green leafy vegetables, broccoli, bones in fish	Males: 1,000 mg Females: 1,000 mg
FLUORIDE	Maintenance of tooth and bone structure; prevention of dental decay	Fluoridated water, tea, certain fish eaten with bones	Males: 4 mg Females: 3 mg
IODINE	Essential part of thyroid hormones, regulation of body metabolism	Iodized salt, seafood, processed foods	Males: 150 μg Females: 150 μg
IRON	Component of hemoglobin, myoglobin, and enzymes; regulation of cell growth and differentiation; prevention of anemia	Meat and poultry, fish and seafood, fortified grain products, legumes, dark-green vegetables, dried fruit, pumpkin seeds	Males: 8 mg Females: 18 mg
MAGNESIUM	Maintenance of normal muscle and nerve function; energy transfer; activation of many enzymes	Widespread in foods, especially nuts, seeds, whole grains, legumes, leafy green vegetables, soy milk, yogurt	Males: 400 mg Females: 310 mg
PHOSPHORUS	Maintenance of acid-base balance; bone growth and maintenance; energy storage and transfer in cells; synthesis of DNA and RNA	Widespread in foods, especially milk and other dairy products, fish, seeds, whole grains, meat, poultry	Males: 700 mg Females: 700 mg
POTASSIUM	Maintenance of body water balance and cellular function; assistance in muscle contraction; moderation of rise in blood pressure from excess sodium; decrease in bone turnover and recurrence of kidney stones	Fruits and vegetables, especially leafy greens, cantaloupe, bananas, orange juice, mushrooms, potatoes, tomato sauce, legumes, dairy products, nuts, fish, pork	Males: 4,700 mg Females: 4,700 mg
SELENIUM	Defense against oxidative stress from free radicals; regulation of thyroid hormone action	Seafood, meat, eggs, whole grains, nuts	Males: 55 μg Females: 55 μg
SODIUM	Maintenance of body water balance, acid-base balance, cellular function	Salt, soy sauce, and processed foods with added salt, especially lunch meats, canned soups and vegetables, salty snacks, processed cheese	Males: 1,500 mg Females: 1,500 mg
ZINC	Synthesis of amino acids, RNA, DNA; aids in wound healing and immune response; important for proper senses of taste and smell	Whole grains, meat, eggs, liver, seafood (especially oysters)	Males: 11 mg Females: 8 mg

Sources: Adapted from Food and Nutrition Board, National Academies. (2001). *Dietary reference intakes: Electrolytes and water* (http://fnic.nal.usda.gov/nal_display/index.php?info_center=4&tax_level=3&tax_subject=256&topic_id=1342&level3_id=5140). Dietary Guidelines Advisory Committee. (2010). *Report of the Dietary Guidelines Advisory Committee on the dietary guidelines for Americans, 2010* (http://www.cnpp.usda.gov/DGAs2010-DGACReport.htm).

a deficiency disease in the short term, there can be long-term effects. For example, below-recommended intakes of calcium and vitamin D can limit peak bone-mass development; in later life, this increases the risk of osteoporosis, fractures, and related disabilities.

Sources and Recommended Intakes of Vitamins and Minerals

Q | How much calcium and iron do I need?

Dietary Reference Intakes (DRIs) have been established for the essential vitamins and minerals—that is, they include standards for the amounts individuals should consume to prevent nutrient deficiencies and reduce the risk of chronic diseases. There are two sets of standards: **Recommended Dietary Allowances (RDAs)** and *Adequate Intakes (AIs)*. RDAs are set at intakes established to meet the needs of almost all individuals; but if there are insufficient data to set an RDA, then an AI value is set. The DRIs are reviewed and updated as new research is completed. Regardless of the type of standard (RDA or AI), the DRIs represent the best available information on healthy vitamin and mineral intakes.

The recommendations in Tables 8-4 and 8-5 are for young adults (ages 19–30). For information on other age groups and life stages, including pregnancy, visit the Web site for the Food and Nutrition Board (http://www.iom.edu/fnb). To calculate your personal DRIs, go to the Interactive DRI Web site (http://fnic.nal.usda.gov/interactiveDRI).

Recommended Dietary Allowance (RDA) A standard for dietary intake of a nutrient set at a level to meet the needs of almost all (97%–98%) individuals in the population in order to maintain good health.

Q | Is it really possible to get all the recommended vitamins each day?

Yes, most healthy adults can meet all their vitamin and mineral needs by eating nutrient-rich foods—without taking supplements and without exceeding moderate calorie intake. There are a few situations for which supplements or extra care might be required, including smoking, as noted in the box "Beta-Carotene and Smokers."

Vitamins and minerals are abundant in food, especially in whole grains, vegetables, fruits, legumes, lean meats, and nonfat dairy products. They are also added to some processed foods, including breakfast cereals. However, a diet high in empty calories from added sugars, solid fats, and alcohol and low in nutrient-rich foods *can* leave you short on some vitamins and minerals—another reason to choose nutrient-rich foods. If the dietary analysis you complete in Lab Activity 8-2 indicates you need to increase your intake of a particular vitamin or mineral, refer to Tables 8-4 and 8-5 for particularly good food sources.

A few vitamins are also produced by the body. Biotin (vitamin B_7) is produced by bacteria found naturally in your intestines. Vitamin D is produced by the skin in response to exposure to sunlight. See pp. 294–295 for more on vitamin D.

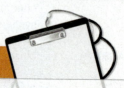

Research Brief

Beta-Carotene and Smokers

Beta-carotene is one of the carotenoids that the body can convert into vitamin A; it can also act as an antioxidant. After a number of studies found a lower lung cancer risk among people with higher blood levels of beta-carotene, several research trials tested whether high doses of beta-carotene supplements over an extended time would lower smokers' risk of lung cancer. The findings were surprising: The risk of developing and dying from lung cancer *went up* among the smokers taking beta-carotene compared with smokers not taking the supplement. The excess risk disappeared after the participants in the studies stopped using the supplements. Further review of the findings found that consumption of fruits and vegetables reduced the risk of lung cancer.

What are possible explanations for the findings? One may be the interaction of the effects of smoking on beta-carotene; it appears that cellular changes caused by smoking alter the actions of beta-carotene to produce more free radicals rather than reducing the number of

these cell-damaging compounds. Beta-carotene supplements have not been found to be harmful (or beneficial) in nonsmokers. In addition, there may be different effects from consuming supplements compared with ingesting beta-carotene in whole foods. Carrots and red peppers, for example, are rich in beta-carotene, but they also contain many other substances—and their benefits may be the result of a variety of phytochemicals working in combination.

Analyze and Apply

- What key conclusion emerges about smokers and the consumption of beta-carotene supplements?
- Why might there be a difference in outcomes between taking in beta-carotene through supplements versus through beta-carotene-rich whole foods given that they both contain beta-carotene?

Source: Druesne-Pecollo, N., and others. (2010). Beta-carotene supplementation and cancer risk: A systematic review and meta-analysis of randomized controlled trials. *International Journal of Cancer, 127*(1), 172–184.

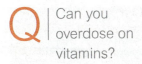

Q Can you overdose on vitamins?

Yes, you can, as more is not necessarily better. Also, short of overdosing, too high an intake of certain vitamins and minerals can harm your health—but this effect usually occurs only from taking high doses in supplement form. Because fat-soluble vitamins can be stored in the body, they pose a higher risk for overload toxicity than water-soluble vitamins do. Thus, taking megadoses of vitamins A, D, E, and K can be toxic.[22]

You can also overdose on minerals. For example, megadoses of calcium can cause digestion problems and possibly kidney damage; too much phosphorus can deplete your body's stored calcium; and overdoses of iron can be dangerous, especially in children. Excess intake of a vitamin or mineral may cause illness immediately or a create problems over time.

In part because of these risks, the Dietary Reference Intakes include a limit for certain micronutrients, called the **Tolerable Upper Intake Level (UL).** The UL is the highest level of daily intake of a nutrient that is likely to pose no risk of adverse health effects for most people (Table 8-6). The UL for vitamin A for healthy adults, for example, is 3,000 micrograms a day; for vitamin E, 1,000 milligrams a day; for calcium, 2,500 milligrams a day; and for iron, 45 milligrams a day. ULs have been set only for nutrients for which there is adequate evidence. If a vitamin or mineral does not have a UL, that doesn't mean a high intake is safe, just that an upper limit has not yet been established.

Vitamin A is a special case: High doses of vitamin A (retinol, from animal sources) can be harmful; among other concerns, high-dose retinol has been linked to birth defects in infants if consumed during pregnancy. The body can also make vitamin A from other compounds, including the carotenoids found in colorful fruits and vegetables like carrots and red peppers. These plant sources of vitamin A are not toxic in the same way as animal sources, so the UL for vitamin A applies only to retinol.

Again, it is unlikely that you could consume a toxic dose of a vitamin or mineral unless you were taking high doses in supplement form. However, it is important to note that there aren't any known benefits of consuming vitamins and minerals in amounts above recommended levels.

Tolerable Upper Intake Level (UL) One of the standards that make up the Dietary Reference Intakes; the highest level of daily intake of a nutrient that poses no risk of adverse effects in healthy people.

antioxidant A compound that protects cells from damage by free radicals by reacting with them or counteracting their effects.

Q Can I take vitamin pills instead of eating vegetables?

That's a bad idea. Although supplements can supply needed vitamins, whole foods contain hundreds of substances that may promote health and prevent disease in as-yet-unknown ways. Compounds known as **antioxidants** may protect cells from unstable molecules

TABLE 8-6 TOLERABLE UPPER INTAKE LEVEL (UL) FOR ADULTS FOR SELECTED VITAMINS AND MINERALS

	DAILY INTAKE LIMIT
CALCIUM	2,500 mg
CHLORIDE	3,600 mg
CHOLINE	3,500 mg
COPPER	10,000 µg
FLUORIDE	10 mg
FOLATE	1,000 µg*
IODINE	1,100 µg
IRON	45 mg
MAGNESIUM	350 mg*
MANGANESE	11 mg
NIACIN	35 mg*
PHOSPHORUS	4,000 mg**
SELENIUM	400 µg
SODIUM	2,300 mg***
VITAMIN A	3,000 µg****
VITAMIN B$_6$	100 mg
VITAMIN C	2,000 mg
VITAMIN D	4,000 IU
VITAMIN E	1,000 mg*
ZINC	40 mg

*From supplements or fortified foods only; there is no evidence of adverse effects of consumption from naturally occurring sources.
**Athletes and others with high energy intakes appear to be able to consume higher levels of phosphorus from food without ill effect.
***For adults with or at risk for hypertension, the UL for sodium is 1,500 mg/day.
****From preformed vitamin A (retinol) only.

Source: Food and Nutrition Board, National Academies. (2010). *Dietary Reference Intakes: UL for Vitamins and Elements* (http://fnic .nal.usda.gov/nal_display/index.php?info_center=4&tax_level=3&tax _subject=256&topic_id=1342&level3_id=5140).

known as **free radicals;** damage caused by free radicals may lead to cancer, heart attacks, and stroke. (Free radicals are produced through normal metabolism, but environmental factors such as smoking and exposure to sunlight or pollution can boost free radical production and activity.) Antioxidants such as beta-carotene, lycopene, and vitamins C and E interact with and stabilize free radicals. Antioxidants are one member of a broader class of compounds known as **phytochemicals**—chemicals found in plants that may positively affect health but have not been classified as essential nutrients.

Good sources of antioxidants and other phytochemicals include many of the nutrient-rich foods that have been mentioned throughout this chapter:[23]

- Yellow, orange, and red fruits and vegetables, including carrots, tomatoes, cantaloupe, winter squash, sweet potatoes, apricots, mangos, watermelon, papaya, pink grapefruit, raspberries, plums, and red and purple grapes
- Deep-green leafy vegetables such as spinach, collards, and chard
- Other deeply colored foods, including blueberries, blackberries, and cinnamon
- Cruciferous vegetables, including broccoli, cauliflower, cabbage, kale, bok choy, and brussels sprouts
- Members of the allium family, including onions, garlic, and leeks
- Legumes, almonds and other nuts, wheat germ; safflower, corn, and soybean oils
- Tea, red wine, and dark chocolate
- Whole grains

Current evidence supports consuming a diet high in food sources of antioxidants and other disease-protecting nutrients instead of taking antioxidant or other types of supplements. There is no evidence that multivitamin/mineral supplements prevent chronic diseases in healthy people.[24] And little is confirmed about the effects of supplements of individual nutrients—vitamins, minerals, or antioxidants. In some cases, researchers have found that high intakes from foods reduce the risk of chronic disease but intake from supplements actually increases risk. Your best bets are healthy, unprocessed foods—a variety of whole grains and colorful fruits and vegetables. And don't overdo the wine and dark chocolate. Although both contain antioxidants, you also need to consider whether the alcohol in wine and the calories in both have a place in your diet—and your life.[25]

Don't use vitamin supplements or fortified foods as an excuse to base your diet on highly processed foods. Such foods are typically devoid of vitamins and minerals, and some may even speed the loss of vitamins and minerals from your body. They also have none of the antioxidants and other phytochemicals just described. Choose nutrient-rich whole foods—processed foods should make up only a small part of your daily diet.

free radicals Unstable, highly reactive molecules created during normal metabolism and in response to environmental factors; may aid the development of cancer, cardiovascular disease, and other diseases of aging by reacting with and damaging DNA and other parts of cells.

phytochemical A naturally occurring chemical in plant-based foods that may help prevent or treat chronic disease.

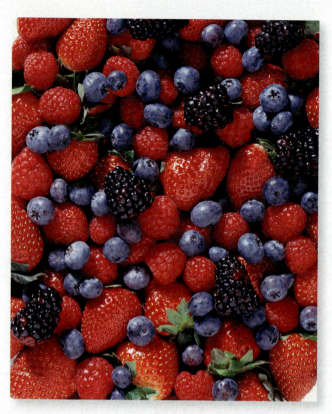

Consume foods rich in antioxidants and other phytochemicals—including whole grains and colorful fruits and vegetables—to help reduce your risk of many chronic diseases. Don't rely on supplements, which don't have all the benefits of whole foods.

Vitamins and Minerals of Special Concern

Based on recent studies, public health officials have identified one vitamin and three minerals of special concern: Americans currently consume too little calcium, vitamin D, and potassium, and too much sodium.[26]

Q | I put milk on my cereal, but that's about it for dairy. Am I short on calcium?

CALCIUM AND VITAMIN D— CRITICAL FOR STRONG BONES. You could be—the majority of Americans are short on both calcium and vitamin D. The only group whose average calcium intake meets recommended levels is males ages 19–50, and except for children and adolescent males, no group meets the recommended vitamin D intake.[27] Completing Lab Activity 8-2 will help you check your current intakes.

Calcium and vitamin D are both critical in the formation of healthy bones and teeth. Calcium is the main component of your bones, and vitamin D is necessary for your body to absorb and use calcium from your diet. Calcium deficiency

osteoporosis Loss of bone mass and density, causing bones to become fragile.

can lead to reduced bone mass and **osteoporosis,** a weakening of the bones that can cause fractures and disability later in life (see the box "Got Calcium? Tips for Reducing Your Risk for Osteoporosis"). In addition to its importance in bone health, vitamin D is also being investigated for its role in preventing a number of chronic diseases, including cardiovascular disease and certain cancers.

Everyone should pay attention to calcium and vitamin D intakes. The richest source of both is milk, which naturally contains calcium and is fortified with vitamin D. Other dairy products such as yogurt and cheese also provide calcium, but check labels to see the amount per serving. Nondairy sources of calcium include fortified soy milk and orange juice, tofu prepared with calcium sulfate, canned sardines and salmon with bones, green vegetables (broccoli, collards, spinach, and the like), almonds, edamame (green soybeans), and white beans.

Few foods naturally contain vitamin D. Oily fish such as salmon and tuna are the best sources, with smaller amounts found in liver, cheese, and egg yolks. In addition to milk, some other dairy products, breakfast cereals, and certain brands of orange juice and yogurt may also be fortified with vitamin D.

Your skin naturally produces vitamin D in response to sun (ultraviolet radiation) exposure, but many health authorities are hesitant to suggest that people spend more time in the sun due to the risk of skin cancer. Factors that reduce the skin's synthesis of vitamin D include cloud or smog cover, dark skin color, use of sunscreen, early or late time of day, winter season, and higher geographic latitudes. In the United States, there is sufficient ultraviolet radiation for year-round vitamin D production only at latitudes below a line extending between Los Angeles, California, and Columbia, South Carolina. If you live north of this line, then for at least part of the winter, the intensity of the sun's radiation is insufficient to support the synthesis of vitamin D by your skin; dietary intake is required.[28]

To reach the intake goals for both calcium and vitamin D, start by consuming more foods naturally rich in or fortified with these nutrients. If increasing your intake of food sources isn't enough, you can also consider calcium and vitamin D supplements. See pp. 297–298 for general advice and cautions on choosing supplements.

Q | I really like pretzels and other salty snacks. Is that a problem?

SODIUM AND POTASSIUM: A BETTER BALANCE FOR BETTER BLOOD PRESSURE. Salt is sodium chloride, and although sodium is an essential mineral, excess consumption is unhealthy. High intake of sodium can raise blood pressure and contribute to full-blown hypertension, an established risk factor for heart attack, stroke, and kidney disease. Blood pressure also rises with age, and more than 90 percent of U.S. adults develop high blood pressure in their lifetime—meaning that virtually everyone is at risk. Although some people are more sensitive to the effects of sodium than others, reducing sodium intake is an important goal for everyone.

Potassium intake is also key, because potassium can lower blood pressure and reduce sodium's effects on blood pressure. In fact, the widely recognized DASH diet, which is used to lower blood pressure in people with hypertension or pre-hypertension, is rich in potassium, calcium, and magnesium.

Reducing sodium intake while increasing potassium intake has been shown to reduce deaths from cardiovascular disease as well as cut medical costs. Other benefits of potassium include decreased bone loss and reduced risk of kidney stones.

Americans are currently out of balance with sodium and potassium:[29]

- *Sodium:* The suggested upper limit for sodium intake is 2,300 milligrams per day, but the average intake is nearly 3,500 milligrams per day. For much of the population—middle-aged and older adults, people with hypertension, and African Americans—an even lower intake of 1,500 milligrams per day is recommended, and many health experts recommend this lower number for everyone.
- *Potassium:* The recommended intake is 4,700 milligrams per day, but the average intake is only about 3,200 milligrams per day for men and 2,400 milligrams per day for women.

What can you do? Learn to like less salty foods! Luckily, the preference for super-salty foods is an acquired taste, and your taste buds will adjust within a few weeks or months. You can still enjoy salty foods from time to time, but make them special treats and limit your portion sizes. The vast majority of sodium in the American diet—80–85 percent—comes from salt added by food manufacturers during processing. (Naturally occurring sodium accounts for

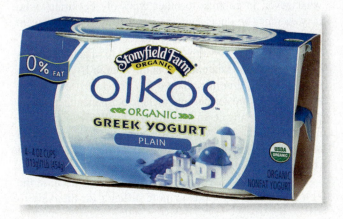

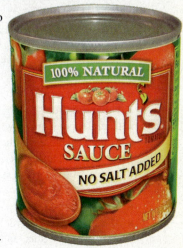

Wellness Strategies

Got Calcium? Tips for Reducing Your Risk for Osteoporosis

Q I read some things that say how bad dairy products are for you, and other things that talk about how good they are for you. How do I know what to do?

Along with other health benefits, calcium, which dairy products richly provide, is critical in the development of optimal bone density and the prevention of osteoporosis. *Osteoporosis* by definition means "porous bone" and is a sign that bone has lost calcium for strength and matrix for support. Consequently, the bone becomes fragile and can easily fracture, especially from a fall but in severe cases even after something as simple as a sneeze. Among seniors, fractures are a major cause of disability and often lead to the loss of the ability to live independently. About 25 percent of hip-fracture patients over age 50 die in the year following their fracture.

Bone loss accelerates during aging, especially in postmenopausal women. Because women start out with less bone mass than men and then lose it more rapidly, women are more likely than men to develop osteoporosis. However, the condition occurs in both sexes, and about 20 percent of the 10 million Americans with osteoporosis are men.

To reduce your risk of developing osteoporosis, build maximum bone mass in your young adult years and then work to maintain it with these strategies:

- Get your recommended intakes of calcium and vitamin D.
- Eat sufficient fruits and vegetables.
- Consume adequate amounts of protein.
- Engage in regular weight-bearing exercise, activities in which you are supporting your own weight, like walking, jogging, dancing, and resistance training.
- Avoid smoking and excessive alcohol intake.

Sources: National Institute of Arthritis and Musculoskeletal and Skin Diseases. (2009). *Osteoporosis overview* (http://www.niams.nih.gov/Health_Info/Bone/Osteoporosis/default.asp). National Osteoporosis Foundation. (2010). (http://www.nof.org).

---

about 10 percent, and salt added at the table or during cooking accounts for the remaining 5–10 percent.) So, be sure to check food labels for sodium content and make choices accordingly. Reducing the sodium in the American diet to recommended levels will likely also require a broad public health effort—perhaps with mandatory reductions in the sodium content of certain types of foods.

Increasing your potassium intake, however, is more straightforward—there are many rich food sources. Americans are low in potassium because they don't eat enough fruits and vegetables. Try some of the following good sources of potassium:

- White and sweet potatoes
- Legumes
- Tomatoes, tomato sauce, and tomato juice
- Bananas
- Oranges and orange juice
- Papaya, apricots, and peaches
- Cantaloupe, honeydew, and watermelon
- Many vegetables, including beet greens, spinach, brussels sprouts, artichokes, broccoli, collards, cucumber, celery, kale, snap beans, turnip greens, carrots, corn, red peppers
- Yogurt
- Many types of fish, including halibut, rockfish, haddock, salmon, tuna, and cod

Special Recommendations for Specific Groups

Q My girlfriend is a vegetarian. Does she need supplements?

Is she a vegan? If not, it is unlikely she will experience any real vitamin deficiencies. The popularity of vegetarian diets has risen in recent years, along with an interest in avoiding meat and meat products for environmental, philosophical, or health reasons. However, there has not been a parallel increase in vitamin deficiencies.

Vegans are vegetarians who eat no animal products whatsoever, in contrast to other types of vegetarians who may eat dairy products, eggs, and/or fish and just avoid meat and poultry (see Chapter 9 for more on vegetarian diets). Vitamin B_{12} is a concern with respect to vegans, because only animal foods naturally contain vitamin B_{12}. Although it takes a long time for vitamin B_{12} deficiency to develop, the symptoms are serious and include permanent neurological damage. Many cereals are fortified with vitamin B_{12}, so many vegetarians get their intake that way. Vegans who do not consume any foods fortified with vitamin B_{12} should consider taking a dietary supplement.

Iron can also be a concern for vegetarians, because the iron found in plant foods is more difficult for the body to

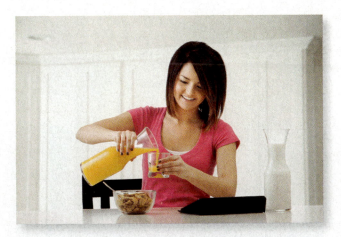

Plant sources of iron are more difficult for the body to absorb, and strict vegetarians need to consume about twice as much iron as people with nonvegetarian diets. Eating vitamin C–rich foods along with iron-rich foods is a wise practice because vitamin C helps the body absorb iron.

absorb than the iron found in meat and poultry. Vegetarians need to consume extra iron to make up for the lower absorption. Vitamin C helps the body absorb iron, so consuming vitamin C–rich foods along with iron-rich foods is beneficial. Problems with low iron are seen mostly in women of reproductive age, especially women with a heavy menstrual flow. Iron deficiency can lead to **anemia,** or low levels of hemoglobin, the component of blood that transports oxygen. This is particularly problematic during pregnancy, when the blood needs to deliver oxygen to the fetus as well as the mother. Iron deficiency may also hinder athletic performance in endurance events, which require oxygen delivery over a sustained period.

Also, regardless of her dietary choice, your girlfriend should be consuming adequate folic acid to minimize her risk of delivering a baby with serious birth defects, even if she is not planning to get pregnant soon. See Table 8-7 for more information about this and other recommendations for specific groups or circumstances.

Choosing and Using Supplements

Q How do I know which supplements to take and where to buy them?

The best approach is to obtain your essential nutrients from food rather than relying on supplements. Whole foods have the benefits of antioxidants and other phytochemicals as well as dietary fiber. Most people can achieve recommended intakes of all micronutrients by consuming nutrient-rich foods.

There is no evidence that supplements prevent chronic diseases in the general, healthy population. For some special population groups, particular supplements may be beneficial, but in

anemia Below-normal number of red blood cells or lack of sufficient hemoglobin, resulting in reduced oxygen-carrying capacity of the blood; most often caused by insufficient iron, which is needed to produce hemoglobin.

TABLE 8-7 DIETARY REFERENCE INTAKE ADJUSTMENTS FOR SPECIAL CIRCUMSTANCES

GROUP	RECOMMENDATION
WOMEN OF CHILDBEARING AGE	**Folic acid:** All women capable of becoming pregnant should consume 400 μg of folic acid from fortified foods or supplements in addition to naturally occurring food folate from a varied diet. Folate reduces the risk of neural tube defects, including spina bifida, in a developing fetus. Because the neural tube develops very early in pregnancy, before a woman may know she is pregnant, the recommendation applies to all women of reproductive age.
SMOKERS	**Vitamin C:** People who smoke should consume an additional 35 mg/day of vitamin C over that needed by nonsmokers.
PEOPLE OVER AGE 50	**Vitamin B$_{12}$:** Many older adults cannot absorb vitamin B$_{12}$ from foods, so people over 50 should meet their recommended intake by consuming fortified foods or supplements.
VEGETARIANS	**Iron, zinc, and vitamin B$_{12}$:** If plant foods are the only source of iron and zinc, then the iron and zinc requirements are approximately twice those of nonvegetarians. Vegans also need to consume vitamin B$_{12}$ (found naturally only in animal foods) from fortified foods or supplements.
ATHLETES ENGAGING IN REGULAR INTENSE EXERCISE	**Iron:** Average iron requirements are 30%–70% higher for athletes than for people engaging in typical levels of physical activity.

Source: Adapted from Food and Nutrition Board, National Academies. (2006). *DRI: Dietary Reference Intakes: The essential guide to nutrient requirements.* Washington, DC: National Academies Press.

other cases, nutrient supplements can be harmful (recall the box "Beta-Carotene and Smokers" on p. 292).

Review the results of the dietary assessment you complete in Lab Activity 8-2. If you are short on any nutrients according to the Dietary Reference Intakes (DRIs) recommendations for you, make changes in your diet first and then reassess your status before going ahead with a supplement.

If you cannot obtain enough of a particular nutrient through dietary sources, or if medical tests indicate a problem such as iron-deficiency anemia, then a supplement of a particular nutrient may be appropriate for you. But take care: Some supplements can interact with drugs or other supplements. For example, calcium reduces the effectiveness of certain antibiotics and medications used to treat seizure disorders. Follow the directions for use carefully, and check with your health care provider if you are taking any prescription or over-the-counter drugs.

Avoid high-dose supplements unless prescribed by your physician to treat a specific deficiency. There is no need to exceed the DRI, and high-dose supplements may be ineffective or even harmful. For example, your body absorbs calcium best in doses of 500 milligrams or less, so higher-dose supplements can be a waste of money. Also be sure to consider your combined intake from all supplements plus fortified foods; if you don't pay attention, you might consume a particular nutrient above the Tolerable Upper Intake Level (UL) set by the Dietary Reference Intakes (see Table 8-6).

Supplements are not intended to diagnose, treat, or prevent disease, so manufacturers cannot claim they are effective for any of those functions. Don't take vitamins because you think they can do things like increase muscle mass, keep you awake when you're sleepy, reduce stress, or prevent the common cold. Such effects have not been proven.

With respect to the quality of supplements, that is complicated to determine because supplements are not regulated by the Food and Drug Administration (FDA) the way drugs are. Therefore, knowing the best place to purchase supplements is difficult. Unlike over-the-counter and prescription drugs, supplements do not have to be proven to be safe or effective before they can be sold. If a supplement is found to be unsafe, then the FDA can remove it from the market.

The FDA doesn't analyze the content of supplements. However, it does set manufacturing standards designed to ensure that supplements contain

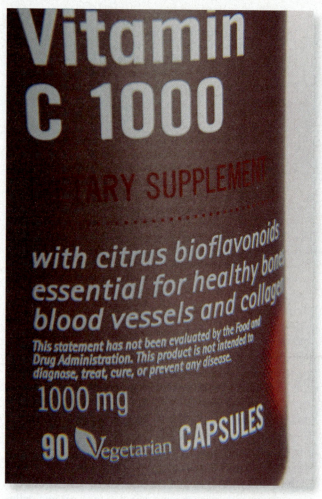

Dietary supplements are not regulated in the same ways as drugs and foods. Although they may carry claims about the product's effects on health, they must also print a warning that these claims have not been evaluated by the FDA.

the ingredients listed on the label, are not contaminated, and are appropriately packaged and labeled. If you take vitamin supplements, buy them from well-known companies, which usually have the highest quality control. You can also look for "seals of approval" from independent organizations that test supplements for proper manufacturing and accurate labeling. These seals do not guarantee that a supplement is safe or effective, but they do offer some assurance that they contain what is listed on the label. Organizations that offer product certifications include ConsumerLab.com (http://www.consumerlab.com/seal.asp), U.S. Pharmacopeia (http://www.usp.org/USPVerified/dietarySupplements), and NSF (http://www.nsf.org/business/dietary_supplements).

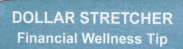

DOLLAR STRETCHER
Financial Wellness Tip

Don't buy unnecessary supplements, especially those in expensive specialty beverages, bars, and powders. Use only supplements you truly need, and start by checking cereal boxes. Many fortified ready-to-eat cereals offer high nutrient density and value.[30]

Food Labels: An Important Tool for Consumers

Q What do the percentages on food labels mean?

The percentages refer to **Daily Values (DVs),** a set of standards used on food labels to help you place the food in the context of your overall daily diet. The Daily Values are based on a diet of 2,000 calories per day, and although you may need more or less, the DV is a good benchmark. For some nutrients, including fiber, calcium, and iron, the DV is a goal. For others, including sodium and saturated fat, the DV is a limit, and the less you eat of these substances, the better.

Only certain nutrients are required to be listed on food labels—those that are considered most important for consumers when they evaluate foods. See Figure 8-7 for tips to help you use food labels to make healthier choices.

Q Are the listings on food labels actually facts? How accurate are they?

Food labels should be accurate. Manufacturers are responsible for ensuring the accuracy of food labels on their products, but the FDA

Daily Values (DVs)
Nutrient-intake standards used on food labels that quantify the nutrients as percentages in a 2,000-calorie-per-day diet.

Nutrition Facts

Serving Size 1/2 package (285g)
Servings per Container 2

Amount per Serving

Calories 300   Calories from Fat 60

	% Daily Value*
Total Fat 6g	9%
Saturated Fat 2.5g	13%
Trans Fat 0g	
Cholesterol 30mg	10%
Sodium 600mg	25%
Potassium 420mg	12%
Total Carbohydrate 45g	15%
Dietary Fiber 5g	20%
Sugars 12g	
Protein 15g	

Vitamin A 40%	•	Vitamin C 15%	
Calcium 10%	•	Iron 8%	

*Percent Daily Values are based on a 2,000 calorie diet. Your daily values may be higher or lower depending on your calorie needs.

		Calories	2,000	2,500
Total Fat	Less than		65g	80
Sat Fat	Less than		20g	25g
Cholesterol	Less than		300mg	300mg
Sodium	Less than		2,400mg	2,400mg
Total Carbohydrate			300g	375g
Dietary Fiber			25g	30g

Calories per gram:
Fat 9 • Carbohydrate 4 • Protein 4

Check serving size, number of servings, and calories
- The label information is based on ONE serving, but many packages contain more. Look at the serving size and how many servings you are actually consuming. If you consume double the serving size, then you must double everything listed on the label, including calories.
- Fat-free doesn't mean calorie-free. Lower-fat items may have as many calories as full-fat versions.

Limit saturated fat, trans fat, cholesterol, sodium, and added sugars
- For heart health, limit unhealthy fats and sodium. Check ingredient list for hydrogenated fats, which are the source of artificial trans fats.
- Limit foods with added sugars, which add calories but not other nutrients.

Look for foods rich in potassium, dietary fiber, vitamins A and C, calcium, and iron
- Get the most nutrients for your calories. Look for foods that are high in healthy nutrients and low in calories, unhealthy fats, and sodium.
- Potassium isn't required to be listed on all food labels, but it should appear on foods that have significant amounts. Look for it.
- A food that has 20% or more of the Daily Value is high in a nutrient.

Choose lean protein sources
- When evaluating a food for its protein content, make choices that are lean, low-fat, or fat-free. Compare how much protein a serving of the food provides with the total fat and calories. Get the most protein for your calories and fat.

Remember the Daily Values
- The % DV is a general guide to help you link nutrients in a serving of food to their contributions to your total daily diet. Foods may be high (20% DV or more) or low (5% DV or less) in particular nutrients.
- The % DV is based on a 2,000-calorie diet; you may need more or less.

Don't forget to check the ingredients list
- For whole-grain foods, a whole grain should appear first on the list.
- To limit added sugars, make sure that sugars are not among the first few items in the list.
- If hydrogenated fats appear on the list, the food contains at least some trans fats.

Figure 8-7 Nutrition Facts label. The information on food labels can help you make healthier choices. Use labels to evaluate individual foods and to compare different brands or types of similar foods.

Source: Adapted from U.S. Department of Agriculture. (2006). *Nutrition facts label* (http://www.fda.gov/Food/ResourcesForYou/Consumers/NFLPM/ucm274593.htm).

conducts random tests and can take action if a company is in violation of the regulations.

Consumers should keep three points in mind about food labels. First, numbers can be rounded off on food labels. A product that contains fewer than 5 calories per serving can be called "calorie-free," and perhaps most importantly, a product that has less than 0.5 milligrams of trans fat per serving can be said to contain zero trans fat. If you consume a lot of these products with small amounts of trans fat, your total intake can add up. To be sure that a product really has no trans fat, check the ingredient list for hydrogenated fats; if you see them on the list, the product contains some trans fats.

Second, use caution when reading the claims and other information on the front of food packages. Some aspects of packaging and some types of claims are more closely regulated than others. For example, a food package can have a picture of fruit on the front but not actually contain fruit. The label "low fat" is regulated and specifically means 3 grams of fat or less per typical serving, whereas the labels "low carb" and "low glycemic index" are not regulated and don't have consistent meanings. For more on the complex world of food-label regulations, visit the FDA Web site (http://www.fda.gov/Food/LabelingNutrition/LabelClaims).

Finally, consider the full profile of a food. A breakfast cereal that prominently labels itself as low in fat and sodium isn't necessarily a healthy choice if it includes a huge amount of added sugar. Potato chips that have no trans fat are still high in overall fat, salt, and calories. Fat-free isn't calorie-free, and fat-free also doesn't guarantee anything about nutrient density. Your best bet is to limit your consumption of highly processed foods and eat more fruits, vegetables, and whole grains.

Assessing Your Diet for Energy and Nutrient Intakes

Q | How do I know if I'm eating the right amounts of the right things? Is my diet good, bad, or OK?

There are different ways to assess your diet. The lab activities for this chapter will help you estimate how many calories you need to maintain your weight, as well as how your current diet stacks up against the nutrient recommendations. In Chapter 9, you'll learn more about different eating plans—another way to look at your diet. As you complete the tracking needed to assess your diet, take time to be accurate in your listing of what you eat and how much. Recall that many people underestimate their portion sizes and energy intakes, and such mistakes can affect nutrient analysis. A few days of careful data collection will give you a realistic picture of your typical diet. Then you can determine if you need to make changes to bring your diet in line with the recommendations for lifelong health and wellness.

Summary

A healthy diet will help you feel good, maintain a healthy body weight, and minimize your risk for many chronic diseases. A healthy diet also allows you to be physically active and reach all of your fitness goals. Make good choices, enjoy your food, and live well.

Choose a healthy balance of protein, carbohydrate, and fat to meet your daily energy needs. Favor nutrient-rich foods, and avoid energy-dense foods that provide little besides calories. Give special priority to foods rich in nutrients for which you fall short of recommended intakes. For many Americans, these nutrients include dietary fiber, vitamin D, calcium, and potassium.

To meet your nutrient needs within appropriate energy intakes, focus on the advice from the *Dietary Guidelines for Americans, 2010:* Balance your calories, choose nutrient-rich foods, and reduce your intake of sodium, saturated and trans fats, cholesterol, added sugars, and refined grains.

Assess your diet periodically to help yourself stay on track. Eat well and be well!

More to Explore

Dietary Guidelines for Americans, 2010
   http://health.gov/dietaryguidelines/
Interactive Dietary Reference Intakes
   http://fnic.nal.usda.gov/interactiveDRI
National Institutes of Health, Office of Dietary Supplements
   http://ods.od.nih.gov
Nutrient-Rich Foods Coalition
   http://www.nutrientrichfoods.org
Nutrition.gov
   http://www.nutrition.gov
U.S. Department of Agriculture
   http://www.choosemyplate.gov/
U.S. Food and Drug Administration: Food Labeling
   http://www.fda.gov/Food/LabelingNutrition/ConsumerInformation
U.S. Food and Drug Administration: National Nutrient Database
   http://www.nal.usda.gov/fnic/foodcomp/search

LAB ACTIVITY 8-1 Determining Energy and Macronutrient Intake Goals

COMPLETE IN connect

NAME	DATE	SECTION

This lab includes instructions for making several calculations:

- Daily calorie requirement
- Daily protein requirement
- Estimated target macronutrient intake (percentages and grams)

You can use the information from this lab to help you set important nutrition goals.

Daily Calorie Requirement

If your weight is stable, your current daily energy intake is the number of calories you need to maintain your weight at your current activity level. However, people often underestimate the size of their food portions, and so energy goals based on estimates of current calorie intake from food records can be inaccurate. You can also estimate your daily energy needs using formulas developed as part of the Dietary Reference Intakes.

Equipment

- Weight scale
- Tape measure or other means of measuring height
- Calculator (optional)

Preparation: None

Instructions

Measure your height (in inches) and weight (in pounds), and then identify the appropriate physical activity coefficient (PA) from the table below. Plug these values, along with your age, into the appropriate formula for your sex.

Height: [_____] in.   Weight: [_____] lb

PHYSICAL ACTIVITY COEFFICIENTS FOR ENERGY NEEDS CALCULATION

		PHYSICAL ACTIVITY COEFFICIENT (PA)	
PHYSICAL ACTIVITY LEVEL	DESCRIPTION*	MEN	WOMEN
Sedentary	Activities of daily living	1.00	1.00
Low active	Activities of daily living plus the equivalent of about 30 min/day of moderate activity	1.12	1.14
Active	Activities of daily living plus the equivalent of about 60–90 min/day of moderate activity	1.27	1.27
Very active	Activities of daily living plus the equivalent of about 150–240 min/day of moderate activity	1.54	1.45

* 30 min of vigorous activity is equivalent to about 60 min of moderate activity.

Formula for Men

[864 − (9.72 × age)] + {PA × [(6.44 × weight) + (12.78 × height)]}

Step 1. 9.72 × age [   ] years = [   ]

Step 2. 864 − result from step 1 [   ] = [   ] *(Result may be a negative number.)*

Step 3. 6.44 × weight [   ] lb = [   ]

Step 4. 12.78 × height [   ] in. = [   ]

Step 5. Result from step 3 [   ] + result from step 4 [   ] = [   ]

Step 6. PA (from table) [   ] × result from step 5 [   ] = [   ]

Step 7. Result from step 2 [   ] + result from step 6 [   ] = [   ] **cal/day**

Formula for Women

[387 − (7.31 × age)] + {PA × [(4.94 × weight) + (16.78 × height)]}

Step 1. 7.31 × age [   ] years = [   ]

Step 2. 387 − result from step 1 [   ] = [   ] *(Result may be a negative number.)*

Step 3. 4.94 × weight [   ] lb = [   ]

Step 4. 16.78 × height [   ] in. = [   ]

Step 5. Result from step 3 [   ] + result from step 4 [   ] = [   ]

Step 6. PA (from table) [   ] × result from step 5 [   ] = [   ]

Step 7. Result from step 2 [   ] + result from step 6 [   ] = [   ] **cal/day**

Results

Daily calorie requirement for weight maintenance: [   ] **cal/day**

Daily Protein Requirement

The Dietary Reference Intakes also provide a formula you can use to calculate the amount of protein you should average daily to meet your body's needs.

Equipment

- Weight scale
- Calculator (optional)

Preparation: None

Instructions

Measure your weight (in pounds) and plug in the appropriate value from the table below.

Weight: [   ] lb

DIETARY PROTEIN REQUIREMENTS BY AGE AND LIFE STAGE AGE/LIFE STAGE

AGE/LIFE STAGE	GRAMS OF PROTEIN PER POUND OF BODY WEIGHT
Ages 14–18	0.39 g/lb
Ages 19 and older	0.36 g/lb
Pregnant	0.50 g/lb
Breastfeeding	0.59 g/lb

For athletes engaged in heavy training: The Dietary Reference Intakes state that athletes need no additional protein, but the American College of Sports Medicine recommends a somewhat higher protein intake for both endurance athletes (0.54−0.64 g/lb) and resistance athletes (0.54−0.77 g/lb). Use a value in one of these ranges if you feel it is appropriate for you.

Protein requirement = weight: ⬚ lb × value from table ⬚ g/lb = ⬚ g

Results

Daily protein requirement: ⬚ **g/day**

Estimated Target Macronutrient Intakes

After calculating your daily calorie and protein requirements, your next step is to set intake goals for all three classes of macronutrients—protein, fat, and carbohydrate.

Equipment: Calculator (optional)

Preparation: None

Instructions

You can allocate your total daily calories among the three classes of macronutrients to suit your preferences. Just make sure that your values fall within the Acceptable Macronutrient Distribution Ranges (AMDRs) set by the Food and Nutrition Board of the National Academies, that the three percentages you select total 100%, and that the percentage you set for protein is sufficient to meet the protein need you calculated in the previous section of the lab.

NUTRIENT	AMDR (% OF TOTAL DAILY CALORIES)	YOUR GOALS (% OF TOTAL DAILY CALORIES)
Protein	10%–35%	⬚ %
Fat	20%–35%	⬚ %
Carbohydrate	45%–65%	⬚ %
TOTAL		100%

To translate your percentage goals into daily intake goals expressed in calories and grams, multiply the percentages you've chosen by your total calorie intake and then divide the result by the corresponding calories per gram. Use the total daily calorie goal you calculated in the first part of this lab activity and the percentage goals you set in the chart above.

Nutrient	Total calories per day	×	Macronutrient percentage goal (EXPRESSED AS A DECIMAL)	=	Calories per day of macronutrient	÷	Calories per gram of macronutrient	=	Grams per day of macronutrient
Protein*		×	0.	=	cal/day	÷	4 cal/g	=	g/day
Fat		×	0.	=	cal/day	÷	9 cal/g	=	g/day
Carbohydrate		×	0.	=	cal/day	÷	4 cal/g	=	g/day
Sample for carbohydrate	2,000	×	0.50	=	1,000 cal/day	÷	4 cal/g	=	250 g/day

* Check the value calculated for protein to ensure it is at or above the protein requirement you calculated in the previous section of the lab. If it is below that number, adjust your target macronutrient percentages (raise protein, lower fat or carbohydrate or both) until your protein consumption meets the DRI.

Summary of Results

Total Daily Energy Intake: [ ] cal/day

MACRONUTRIENT	PERCENT OF TOTAL DAILY CALORIES	GRAMS PER DAY
Protein	%	g/day
Fat	%	g/day
Carbohydrate	%	g/day

Reflecting on Your Results

Are you surprised with your results? Was the value calculated for your total daily calorie requirement what you expected? If not, is it higher or lower? Do your results match what you thought about your energy intake and nutrient requirements?

Planning Your Next Steps

To determine how close you are to meeting your personal intake goals, keep a running tally over the course of the day. For packaged foods, food labels list the calories and the number of grams of fat, protein, and carbohydrate. Nutrition information is also available in many quick-service restaurants, in grocery stores, in nutrition analysis software, and online. By checking these resources, you can track your total intake of calories, fat, protein, and carbohydrate and assess your current diet. (Lab Activity 8-2 will take you through a detailed analysis of your diet, including energy, macronutrients, and key vitamins and minerals.) As a first step here, describe the strategies you'll use to track your current diet to determine how it compares to the goals and requirements you calculated in this lab activity.

Source: Formulas, calorie, and protein requirements, and AMDRs from Food and Nutrition Board, Institute of Medicine, National Academies. (2002). *Dietary Reference Intakes: Energy, carbohydrate, fiber, fat, fatty acids, cholesterol, protein, and amino acids.* Washington, DC: National Academy Press.

COMPLETE IN connect

NAME	DATE	SECTION

In this lab you'll analyze one day's diet. For a more complete and accurate assessment of your diet, average and then analyze the results from several different days, including a weekday and a weekend day.

Equipment

Access to the energy and nutrient content of your foods and beverages. Information is available from food labels, restaurant nutrition guides, and the free online USDA food composition database (http://www.nal.usda.gov/fnic/foodcomp/search).

Preparation: None

Instructions

Record the foods you consume over the course of the day; be as accurate as possible in determining your portion sizes for the "Amount" column. Use the chart printed here, a nutrition analysis software program, or the free online nutrition analysis at ChooseMyPlate.gov, which is part of the *Dietary Guidlines for Americans, 2010.* If you are performing the analysis by hand using the chart in this lab, do the best you can to include complete information on everything you eat.

DAY OF THE WEEK (CIRCLE): M T W TH F SA SU

Food	Amount	Calories	Protein (g)	Carbohydrate (g)	Fiber (g)	Added sugars (g)*	Fat (g)	Saturated fat (g)	Cholesterol (mg)	Sodium (mg)	Potassium (mg)**	RAE	Vitamin C (mg)	Calcium (mg)	Iron (mg)
Sample: Wheat bread	1 slice	70	4	12	2	2	1	0.2	0	135	70	0	0	30	1

* Added sugars: Don't include naturally occurring sugars from fruit and milk in this column. Sugar content information for a food usually doesn't distinguish between naturally occurring sugars and added sugars. However, if a food doesn't include any fruit or milk products, then the sugar in the product likely all comes from added sugars. Track the major sources of added sugars in your diet.

** Potassium: Not listed on every food label, but potassium content is given if the food contains a significant amount.

Results

Calculate your totals: Complete the following chart by totaling the values in each column. (If you used MyPlate Tracker or another digital tool, copy your day's totals into the chart.) In addition, calculate the percentage of total daily calories for protein, carbohydrate, fat, and saturated fat using the following formula:

$$\frac{(\text{number of grams of energy source}) \times (\text{number of calories per gram of energy source})}{\text{total daily calories}}$$

Note: Fat and saturated fat provide 9 cal/g; protein and carbohydrate provide 4 cal/g. For example, if you consume 60 total g of fat and 2,000 cal, the percentage of total calories from fat is:

$$\frac{(60 \text{ g of fat}) \times (9 \text{ cal/g of fat})}{2,000 \text{ cal}} = 27\% \text{ total daily calories as fat}$$

Fill in the recommended totals or limits: Use the calorie and macronutrient values from Lab Activity 8-1 or choose values from Table 8-2 and the boxes "Recommendations for Macronutrients" and "Tips for Meeting Dietary Fat and Cholesterol Recommendations" on pp. 275 and 286. For vitamins and minerals, select the appropriate recommendations from Tables 8-4 and 8-5. The "reference recommendations" in the chart are basic DRI and AMDR guidelines for young adults; your individual recommendations may differ. For personalized recommendations, you can also visit the Interactive DRI website (http://fnic.nal.usda.gov/interactiveDRI).

	Calories	Protein (g)	Protein (% of total calories)	Carbohydrate (g)	Carbohydrate (% of total calories)	Fiber (g)	Added sugars (g)	Fat (g)	Fat (% of total calories)	Sat. fat (g)	Saturated fat (% of total calories)	Cholesterol (mg)	Sodium (mg)	Potassium (mg)	Vitamin A (μg RAE)	Vitamin C (mg)	Calcium (mg)	Iron (mg)
Your totals																		
Recommended totals or limits																		
Reference recommendations			10–35%		45%–65%	14 g/1,000 cal			20%–35%		<10%	<300 mg	<2,300 mg	4,700 mg	900 or 700 mg	90 or 75 mg	1,000 mg	8 or 18 mg

Reflecting on Your Results

How did your diet stack up against the recommendations? Were there any areas of concern—nutrients for which you consumed more or less than the recommended amounts? The recommendations are averages, so you don't have to meet every guideline every day, but your analysis does provide a benchmark. Were you at all surprised by the results?

Planning Your Next Steps

Choose one nutrient for which you could improve your intake—either increase or decrease—in order to bring it in line with the guidelines. Develop at least three strategies for improving your intake of that nutrient. Looking at the daily food record you used for your analysis, what foods might you add, subtract, or substitute?

If your typical daily diet meets all the recommendations, congratulations—and keep it up!

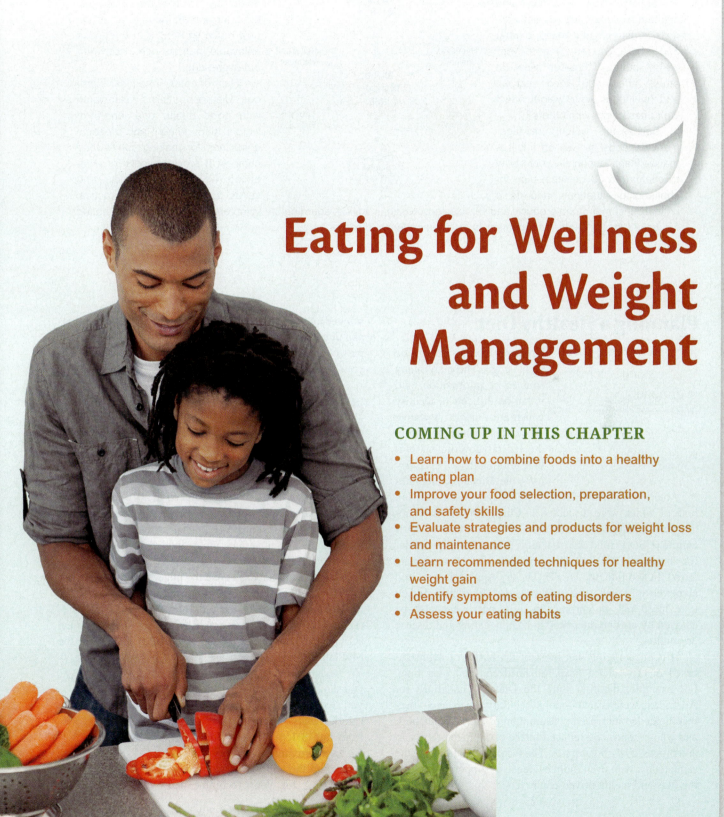

9

Eating for Wellness and Weight Management

How do eating and weight management relate to wellness? A healthy body weight is important for physical wellness, including optimal physical function and a reduced risk for chronic diseases. Body weight and eating behavior affect self-esteem, self-efficacy, and emotional and spiritual wellness, too. Social wellness is also closely linked to what and where you eat and to your weight status. Consider: How do others affect your food choices, and how does your weight affect your interactions with others?

Successful weight management depends as well on intellectual wellness, especially your ability to evaluate food choices, plan for challenging situations, and be a critical consumer of the products and services advertised for weight loss. Weight management is also dependent

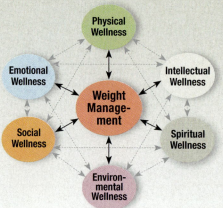

on the environment, as we live in a culture that regularly challenges even the most disciplined eaters.

Individually, it's important to take charge of your own food choices and to keep in mind that a diet isn't temporary; it's a lifestyle. Two key goals are to become a mindful eater, paying attention to what and how much you eat, and to choose enjoyable, nutrient-rich foods without overeating.[1]

This chapter introduces various dietary patterns associated with good health and long-term weight management and presents guidelines for making sound food choices. It provides tools for evaluating weight-loss products and services. It closes with practical advice regarding the symptoms and treatments of eating disorders.

Planning a Healthy Diet

 With all the contradictory information out there, how can I know what to eat and what to avoid?

Knowing what to eat can be a challenge. There are many sources of information, and it can be difficult to identify which are reliable. A couple of well-researched tools from the federal government provide information for everyday use—the Dietary Guidelines for Americans and the Dietary Reference Intakes (DRIs), both of which were discussed in Chapter 8. In this chapter, we'll examine MyPlate, the U.S. Department of Agriculture (USDA) food plan that aims to be a simple reminder for healthy eating (USDA, http://www.choosemyplate.gov/). In addition, the DASH (Dietary Approaches to Stop Hypertension) diet is a well-regarded food plan linked to reduced risk of chronic diseases, but it can also be enjoyed by anyone interested in healthy eating and disease prevention.

It is encouraging that most of the basics of evidence-based dietary advice have remained constant over time. For example, the first time the Dietary Guidelines for Americans were issued—more than thirty years ago—they recommended increased consumption of fruits, vegetables, and whole grains and reduced intake of saturated fats, salt, and processed carbohydrates. The recommendations are the same today, with even more evidence to support them. It is the fads and media-driven controversies that obscure good

science and conscientious healthy eating recommendations and that make for mass confusion. Stick to the basic principles of eating moderate portions of nutrient-rich foods and your wellness will prosper.

USDA's MyPlate

 Is there still such a thing as food groups?

Yes, dietary recommendations are still based on food groups. The USDA's **MyPlate** food guide, introduced in 2010, includes six basic food groups—grains, vegetables, fruits, protein, dairy, and oil (Figure 9-1). The primary graphic for MyPlate depicts a dinner plate divided across 4 groups (fruits, vegetables, grains, and protein), with dairy products indicated in a glass above the plate. Oils are discussed in as much detail as the other food groups but not depicted in the graphic. Unlike the old food "pyramid" that preceded MyPlate, the plate graphic does not show physical activity, but that is one of the key tabs at the top of the MyPlate home page.

To determine the amount of food you should consume from each group, you first need to calculate your daily calorie needs. Refer to your results from Lab 8-1 (or look at Table 8-2) for an approximation of those needs. Next, find the appropriate column in Figure 9-2 for your recommended

MyPlate The USDA-recommended eating plan based on six food groups—grains, vegetables, fruits, protein, dairy, and oil; designed to ensure a balanced intake of essential nutrients within energy intake limits.

Behavior-Change Challenge

Junking Junk Food

Your meals have taken a serious turn for the worse since you got a new roommate with a passion for pizza and pop. With these temptations surrounding you, you've put on 10 pounds, and your jeans are nipping at your waistline. Looking ahead to a spring break getaway, you want to end the madness and get back to eating healthy foods—and being fit and trim.

Meet Edgar

Edgar is a college student who wants to improve his diet by eating less junk and fast food and by choosing smaller portions. He'd like to change because he plans to do personal training and wants to be in better shape than his prospective clients; he's also thinking about how he'll look at the beach during the sum-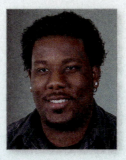mer. Edgar's challenges include his motivation level and the fact that he loves the convenience of fast food and dislikes most vegetables. View the video to learn more about Edgar and his plan. As you watch, consider:

- What strategies and techniques would you suggest to help Edgar overcome the challenges and roadblocks he faces? Think about the stages of change and techniques described in Chapter 2.
- How can you apply these or other approaches to your own goal to lose those 10 pounds and get back in shape?
- What can you learn from Edgar's experience that will help you in your own behavior-change efforts?

VIDEO CASE STUDY   WATCH THIS VIDEO IN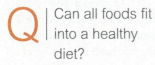

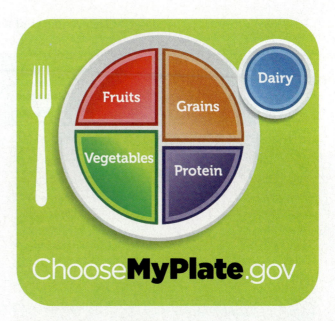

Figure 9-1 USDA's MyPlate. MyPlate includes six main food groups—grains, vegetables, fruits, protein, dairy, and oil. Its key messages are:
- Make half your grains whole.
- Vary your veggies.
- Focus on fruits.
- Know your fats.
- Get your calcium-rich foods.
- Go lean with protein.

Source: U.S. Department of Agriculture. (2012). *MyPlate* (http://www.choosemyplate.gov).

food intake pattern. You can also visit ChooseMyPlate.gov and use the electronic diet (and physical activity tracking) system, which is free and allows you to personalize your eating and activity plan. After you enter your profile, you will receive a recommended daily amount for each of the food groups, with specific details including food suggestions and amounts.

Q | Can all foods fit into a healthy diet?

All foods can fit into a diet, but naturally some foods are healthier than others. At the same time, totally eliminating any particular food, regardless of nutrient content, may be difficult to tolerate

and may undermine an otherwise healthy diet. There are also issues related to portion size and frequency, especially for sweets and treats. The rule is, not too much and not too often.

Ultimately, it's the overall quality of your diet that matters, and a good dietary plan is one that is sustainable and enjoyable and provides a variety of healthy foods. The majority of your diet should be healthy, nutrient-rich foods—but there's room for fun foods as well. Thinking that you will never again eat a favorite food makes eating a chore and sets you up for failure. Chocolate chip cookies, Grandma's apple pie, and chips and salsa can have a place in a healthy diet, even if a small and limited place. Even *Sesame Street*'s Cookie Monster knows that "a cookie is a sometime food."

Q | How much should I be eating, and from which food groups?

How much you should eat largely depends on your current body weight, your desire to change or maintain your weight, and your level of physical activity. In step with your personal goals, MyPlate and USDA strongly recommend that you base your daily diet on these simple

Daily Amounts of Food from Each Group

Food Group	Allowance on 2,000 calories/day, appropriate for a female age 19–30 years	Allowance on 2,400 calories/day, appropriate for a male age 19–30 years
Grains	6 oz/day	9 oz/day
Whole grains	≥3 oz/day	≥4½ oz/day
Vegetables	2½ cups/day	3½ cups/day
Dark green	1½ cups/week	2½ cups/week
Red/orange	5½ cups/week	7 cups/week
Beans and peas	1½ cups/week	2½ cups/week
Starchy	5 cups/week	7 cups/week
Other	4 cups/week	5½ cups/week
Fruits	2 cups/day	2 cups/day
Dairy	3 cups/day	3 cups/day
Protein foods	5½ oz/day	6½ oz/day
Seafood	8 oz/week	10 oz/week
Oils	6 tsp/day	8 tsp/day

Food group amounts are shown in cup or ounce equivalents (oz eq). Oils are shown in grams (g) and approximate teaspoons (tsp). Vegetable subgroup amounts are per week. Quantity equivalents for each food are:

- Grains, 1 ounce equivalent: ½ cup cooked rice, pasta, or cooked cereal; 1 ounce dry pasta or rice; 1 slice bread; 1 small muffin (1 oz); 1 ounce ready-to-eat cereal.
- Fruits and vegetables, 1 cup equivalent: 1 cup raw or cooked fruit or vegetable, 1 cup fruit or vegetable juice, 2 cups leafy salad greens. Legumes can count toward the daily meat and beans total *or* as vegetables.
- Protein foods, 1 ounce equivalent: 1 ounce lean meat, poultry, fish; 1 egg; ¼ cup cooked dry beans; 1 Tbsp peanut butter; ½ ounce nuts/seeds.
- Milk, 1 cup equivalent: 1 cup milk or yogurt, 1½ ounces natural cheese, or 2 ounces of processed cheese.

Figure 9-2 MyPlate food intake patterns based on daily calorie intake.

Source: Adapted from Dietary Guidelines Advisory Committee. (2010). *Report of the Dietary Guidelines Advisory Committee on the dietary guidelines for Americans, 2010* (http://www.cnpp.usda.gov/DGAs2010-DGACReport.htm; p. B2–20).

principles, which promote healthy eating and good weight management:

- Choose nutrient-rich foods from each group.
- Stay within the limit for empty calories.
- Watch your portion sizes.

Most of the recommended food choices found on MyPlate center on nutrient-rich foods, with a preference for low-fat or nonfat foods and for no added sugars. This is where many Americans get into trouble, however, as there is a tendency to consume too many calories as solid fats, added sugars, and even alcohol—and thereby to exceed a healthy calorie intake and squeeze out the essentials (Table 9-1). If you fall into this trap, you'll gain weight and be short on nutrients.

As you consider your food choices, don't focus just on what you need to limit—that can make you feel deprived.

Instead, think about all the great-tasting foods you can enjoy every day.

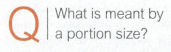 **What is meant by a portion size?** If you are like many people, you may significantly underestimate the amount of food you eat. Do you put a teaspoon of margarine or butter on your baked potato or more like ¼ cup? Is your serving of pasta ½ cup or 2 cups? And just how big was that bagel? To retrain your eye to be more accurate at estimating portion sizes, take time to check food labels, measure foods with a measuring cup or spoon, and pay attention what you have in your hand or on your plate (Figure 9-3). Practice monitoring your portions for a few days or a week, and you'll get much more accurate. Using visual cues can help you eat less, especially when you are faced with large portions.

Fast Facts

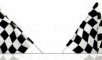

The Expanding American Food Supply

In the past 40 years, the amount of food available to Americans has increased substantially. More food is produced than people should consume. The increase has occurred primarily in foods that should be limited for wellness and weight management.

	Approximate per capita daily calories	
	1970	**2010**
Food supply (total)	3,200	3,900
Food supply (adjusted total)*	2,175	2,700
Added fats and oils and dairy fats	400	650
Flour and cereal products	425	625
Caloric sweeteners	400	450
Everything else (meat, eggs, nuts, dairy, fruits, vegetables)	925	950

*Adjusted for spoilage and waste

- What are some calories you can eliminate without making your diet unpleasant?
- What type of food most makes you overeat?

Source: USDA Economic Research Service. (2010). *Food availability (per capita) data system* (http://www.ers.usda.gov/Data/FoodConsumption).

1 cup cereal, fruit, vegetables, or cooked rice or pasta

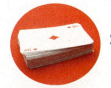

3 ounces meat, fish, or poultry

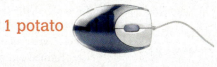

2 tablespoons peanut butter

1 potato

1½ ounces natural cheese

1 teaspoon oil or fat

Figure 9-3 Visual guide to portion sizes. Train your eye to estimate portion sizes accurately by comparing them to everyday objects such as a baseball, a golf ball, a deck of cards, a computer mouse, and dice.

TABLE 9-1 TYPICAL AMERICAN DIET VERSUS MYPLATE, ADJUSTED TO A 2,000-CALORIE/DAY DIET FOR COMPARISON

	MYPLATE RECOMMENDATION	TYPICAL DIET
GRAINS	6.0 cups	6.4 cups
WHOLE GRAINS	3.0 cups	0.6 cup
VEGETABLES	2.5 cups	1.6 cups
FRUIT	2.0 cups	1.0 cups
DAIRY	3.0 cups	1.5 cups
PROTEIN	5.5 oz eq	5.1 oz eq
OILS	27 g (6 tsp)	18 g (4 tsp)
SOLID FATS	16 g (~1 Tbsp)	43 g (~3 Tbsp)
ADDED SUGARS	32 g (~2½ Tbsp)	79 g (~6 Tbsp)
ALCOHOL	—	10 g (~¾ of a beer or glass of wine)

Source: Dietary Guidelines Advisory Committee. (2010). *Report of the Dietary Guidelines Advisory Committee on the dietary guidelines for Americans, 2010* (http://www.cnpp.usda.gov/DGAs2010-DGACReport.htm) and (https//www.choosemyplate.gov/SuperTracker).

It's not just estimating the portion sizes for home-cooked food that is difficult. It's also a challenge to figure out product and serving sizes in stores and restaurants. What passed for one portion 20 years ago could be two or three times that today. In fact, today's bagels are at least 350 calories (with nothing on them) compared to only about 150 calories 20 years ago. Similarly, a restaurant portion of spaghetti with meatballs used to be about 500 calories yet now regularly comes in at more than 1,000 calories.

Let's take a look at each of the food groups in MyPlate and identify good choices and appropriate portion sizes.

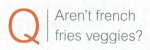 What's the big deal about whole grains? Are they really better for me?

GRAINS: MAKE HALF YOUR GRAINS WHOLE. Whole grains are recommended over refined grains because they have more fiber, vitamins, minerals, and phytochemicals, or, simply put, because they are nutrient rich. The alternative to whole grains is refined grains, which provide calories and little else. Whole-wheat bread or pasta, whole-grain cereal, brown rice, and so on are great choices for ensuring that at least half your daily grain intake comes from whole, nutrient-rich sources.

MyPlate eating patterns give recommendations for grain intake in terms of ounce equivalents. In the standard 2,000-calorie diet, six 1-ounce equivalents of grains are recommended, with at least three of those coming from whole grains (although making more than half of your grains whole is even better). Each of the following represents a 1-ounce equivalent, some whole and some refined:

- 1 slice of bread or half an English muffin
- 1 small muffin, roll, or biscuit (2- to 2½-inch diameter)
- 1 cup cereal flakes
- 1/2 cup cooked pasta, rice, or cereal
- 1 small tortilla (6-inch diameter)

As with most foods, you need to check ingredient lists to know what you are getting, especially when trying to determine whether a grain product is "whole." If it is, a whole grain will be the first ingredient on the list; otherwise it is not a whole-grain product but just sounds like one.

Breakfast is the meal when most people get lots of whole grains (and fiber), especially when eaten at home and consisting of foods like cereal (hot or cold), whole-grain toast, and juice or fruit. Healthy home-prepared breakfasts are in stark contrast to the jumbo cinnamon roll picked up on the way to work or school that, while it looks so good, is packed with up to 800 calories, 30 grams of fat, and about 50 grams of added sugars; with lots of calories and nothing else, that is one energy-dense food. A cinnamon roll can be

an occasional "fun food," but if you stick to the at-home breakfast most days of the week, your wellness and your wallet will both benefit.

Aren't french fries veggies? **VEGETABLES: VARY YOUR VEGGIES.** Technically speaking, french fries *are* vegetables—in fact, they're one of the most consumed vegetables in the United States.[2] But consider that although french fries are potatoes, and potatoes are vegetables, most of the calories in fries come from added fats. French fries are not a nutrient-rich choice from the vegetables group, and a single serving of fast-food fries will likely use up your day's discretionary calorie budget (and a good deal of the day's sodium limit). French fries should be a once-in-a-while food choice.

If you're like most Americans, you need to eat more vegetables and choose ones with little added fat. For a 2,000-calorie diet, MyPlate recommends a total of 2½ cups of vegetables per day. The following count as 1 cup of vegetables:

- 1 cup of raw or cooked vegetables—sliced, chopped, or mashed
- 2 cups raw leafy greens
- 1 large ear of corn (8–9 inches)
- 1 medium sweet or white potato (2½- to 3-inch diameter)

MyPlate also includes specific recommendations for variety to ensure that you get all the vitamins, minerals, fiber, protein, and phytochemicals that the vegetable food group has to offer:

- Dark-green vegetables: Broccoli, spinach, collards, mustard greens, turnip greens, kale, raw leafy greens that are dark in color (romaine, escarole, watercress)
- Orange and red vegetables: Carrots, pumpkin, sweet potato, winter squash, tomatoes

Mind Stretcher
Critical Thinking Exercise

We all overeat occasionally, but have you ever thought about what situations are most likely to make you overeat? If not, next time you overeat, take note of whom you are with, where you are, what foods are available, how hungry you were in advance, and what time of day the overeating occurred. Also, were you feeling particularly happy, sad, or mad when you last overate? How can you use this information to reduce instances of overeating in the future?

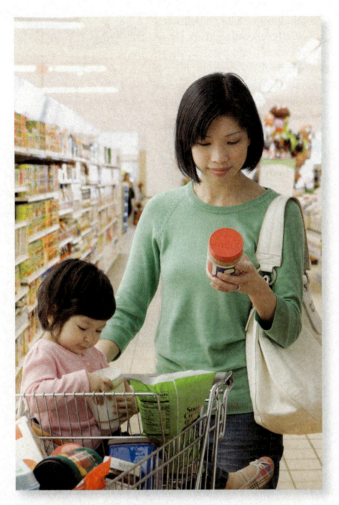

To get all your nutrients within your calorie budget, choose nutrient-rich foods from every food group.

is that they have a much longer shelf life. When you use regular canned vegetables, remember to drain and rinse the veggies to reduce the sodium content.

 Is a fruit "drink" the same thing as juice?

FRUITS: FOCUS ON FRUIT. Probably not. Only beverages that are 100-percent fruit juice can be labeled *juice* without some type of qualifier. So beverages called *fruit juice drink, fruit punch, fruit cocktail,* or *fruit-ade* have something in them besides fruit juice—typically, added sugars. Any beverage that contains juice should be labeled with the percentage: for example, "50-percent juice."

- Legumes (dry beans and peas): Black-eyed and split peas, chickpeas; black, kidney, pinto, and white beans, as well as soybeans (for MyPlate, a serving of legumes can be counted either as a vegetable or as a meat alternative)
- Starchy vegetables: White potatoes, green peas, yellow or white corn
- Other vegetables: Cabbage, cauliflower, celery, cucumbers, green beans, head lettuce, mushrooms, onions, summer squash

You don't have to include each subgroup every day, but choose vegetables from several of them daily and you'll meet the weekly recommendations. Americans currently consume a fair amount of starchy vegetables, iceberg lettuce, and tomatoes, so adding more legumes and dark-green and orange vegetables would be beneficial. To find other creative ways to add color to your vegetable choices, visit the *Fruits and Veggies Matter* Web site (http://www.fruitsandveggiesmatter.gov) for ideas and recipes.

Many people don't realize that most canned and frozen vegetables are as good a choice as fresh vegetables, especially if little or no salt or fat has been added; an advantage

Fast Facts

Quick Tips for Avoiding Weight Gain in College

One strategy for avoiding putting on the pounds is to *eat breakfast.* About 300–500 calories of nutrient-rich food consumed within an hour of waking will keep you from feeling starved later in the day and from bingeing on less healthy foods. You will also feel more attentive in class.

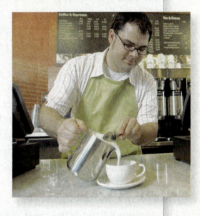

Another tip is to *avoid the barista.* Many coffee drinks are notoriously high in calories, to say nothing of cost. Beyond coffee drinks, also limit sports and energy drinks, full-calorie sodas, excessive alcohol, and juice-flavored drinks, which also carry lots of calories and usually no nutrients. Be cautious with 100-percent fruit drinks, too, as these pack significant calories. Drink water freely, milk regularly, and low-calorie flavored drinks occasionally.

Another tactic for keeping weight gain at bay is to *lose the pizza delivery number.* Pizza, a fourth meal, and almost anything else eaten late at night tend to be energy-dense, nutrient-sparse food choices. Eat well throughout the day to avoid late-night hunger, and plan ahead for situations when others might tempt you late at night.

- Do you incorporate nutrient-rich foods into your breakfast? If not, what easy changes can you make to improve your intake of these important foods?
- What simple, healthy, nutrient-rich foods can substitute for nutrient-sparse last-night snacks?

You can count juice toward your daily MyPlate fruit servings if it is 100-percent juice; such juices are nutritionally similar to whole fruits.[3] However, it's best to consume whole fruits, too, because they have fiber and are often lower in calories than juice. For example, a medium orange is the caloric equivalent of 4 ounces (1/2 cup of juice)—and most people typically drink larger servings of juice. Over time, those extra calories from juice can add up, so it is wise to choose whole fruits for a good portion of your fruit intake. Limit fruit drinks and punches with their large amounts of added sugars.

For a 2,000-calorie diet, MyPlate recommends a total of 2 cups of fruit per day, using any combination of the following examples:

- 1 cup of fresh, canned (in juice or water), or frozen fruit
- 1 cup of 100-percent fruit juice
- ½ cup dried fruit
- ½ grapefruit; 1 small apple; 1 medium pear; 1 large peach, banana, or orange

Fresh fruit can be expensive, as well as inconvenient to store and eat—two potential barriers for college students trying to eat well. In addition, the short shelf life of fresh fruit makes it difficult to get enough fruits every day. Strategies for increasing fruit intake include:

- Purchase prepackaged bags of fresh fruits with a long shelf life, such as apples and oranges.
- Freeze fresh fruit that you can't eat before it's too ripe, or buy fruit frozen; fruit lasts a long time in the freezer and is a delicious addition to cereal, yogurt, and smoothies and also great eaten alone as snacks.
- Buy canned fruit on sale, choosing fruit packed in juice or water rather than syrup.
- Watch for sales and check around your campus or community for the most inexpensive places to buy fruits and vegetables, including farmer's markets.
- Pool your fruit buying and eating with several students or neighbors to save time and money.

Q | How can hamburger and pinto beans count as the same thing?

PROTEIN FOODS: GO LEAN WITH PROTEIN. Both hamburger and pinto beans provide protein, so they do belong in the protein foods group of MyPlate. Also in this group are poultry, fish, pork, eggs, tofu, nuts, and seeds. Pinto beans and other legumes can count either toward your daily vegetable intake or toward your intake from the

protein group. Plant proteins are especially encouraged as long as you don't add fats, as they are particularly high in fiber and various other nutrients. Animal sources of protein tend to provide a more complete protein source but sometimes carry lots of saturated fat. Choose meats that are low in saturated fat, such as very lean ground beef, which is a wiser choice than, say, high-fat sausage.

Because so many types of foods are included in the protein group, MyPlate provides recommendations in terms of ounce equivalents. For a 2,000-calorie diet, 5½ ounce equivalents are recommended from the group. Each of the following counts as a 1 ounce equivalent:

- 1 ounce cooked lean meat, poultry, or fish
- 1 egg
- 1 tablespoon peanut or almond butter
- 2 tablespoons hummus
- ¼ cup legumes or tofu
- ½ ounce (1 tablespoon) nuts or seeds

Q | I don't like milk. Do I have to drink it?

DAIRY: GET YOUR CALCIUM-RICH FOODS. MyPlate recommends 3 cups of milk or the equivalent per day. Other calcium-rich foods that contribute to the dairy group include:

- 1 cup of milk or yogurt
- 1½ ounces of natural cheese (cheddar, Swiss, Parmesan)
- ⅓ cup shredded cheese
- 2 ounces of processed cheese (American)
- ½ cup ricotta cheese

Cottage cheese also counts as a calcium-rich food, but it is lower in calcium and therefore requires a larger portion size (2 cups) to equal 1 cup of milk. Ice cream, too, is a dairy product, but its fat and added sugars count toward your discretionary calorie total, thereby making ice cream less than ideal as your primary dairy source. Instead, use it as an occasional fun food. The same goes for certain other dairy foods; flavored milk and

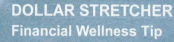

DOLLAR STRETCHER
Financial Wellness Tip

When food shopping, compare the unit cost and not just the price of the package (for example, 4 pounds for $8 is better than 2 pounds for $5). In addition, look at the top and bottom shelves and the ends of aisles for the best values. The most expensive items are usually at or just below eye level midway down the aisle. Make sure you are getting the best value for your grocery money.

yogurt, for example, tend to have added sugar, and high-fat cheese, milk, and yogurt are obviously high in fats.

Lactose-free products are also available, as are enzyme preparations that make milk and dairy products more digestible (see Chapter 8). If you avoid all dairy products, other foods—including calcium-fortified beverages like orange juice and soy milk—can provide enough calcium, although you may miss out on some of the other nutrients in dairy products.

Q | Is it a good idea to eliminate oil since it's pure fat?

OILS: RECOGNIZE AND CHOOSE HEALTHY FATS. No, absolutely not. As described in Chapter 8, fats are necessary for life. The oils recommended in MyPlate are considered good fats—those that provide the essential fats for your diet without a lot of the unhealthy saturated and trans fats that cause health problems. You need at least the equivalent of a few teaspoons of liquid oils each day to meet your need for fats in the diet. These can come from vegetable oils used in cooking, from salad dressings or mayonnaise, or from the oils in foods like fish, nuts, and avocados. Monounsaturated and polyunsaturated fats have a place in your daily diet; for a 2,000-calorie diet, 27 grams or about 6 teaspoons of oils per day are recommended. Table 9-2 provides a guide to the amount of oils in some common foods. Check food labels to identify the types and amounts of fats in processed foods.

The daily requirement for oils is easy to meet but also easy to exceed, especially with unhealthy fats. As a reminder, the unhealthy fats are those that remain solid at room temperature, like butter and shortening and the fats in animal products such as beef, chicken, and pork. All these solid fats count toward your discretionary calorie total. Unhealthy trans fats are from hydrogenated vegetable oils; try to avoid all non-natural sources of trans fats in your diet.

Q | What's the easiest way to know if I'm eating well?

MAKING MYPLATE WORK FOR YOU. The best way to assess your eating pattern is to do an analysis. Although tracking your food intake might not sound like much fun, eating well is important. You might even end up enjoying the tracking, especially as you meet your dietary goals. MyPlate is designed to help you meet all nutrition goals—appropriate energy and nutrient intakes and chronic disease prevention—so assessing your diet against the food-intake pattern for your calorie level is a good place to start.

You can use the tracking form in Lab Activity 9-1 or an online tool such as the free one at ChooseMyPlate.gov. MyPlate asks for specific food items and amounts but has an extensive database to make your calculations simple and quick. The more days you track, the more accurate the dietary information. Try to include at least one weekday

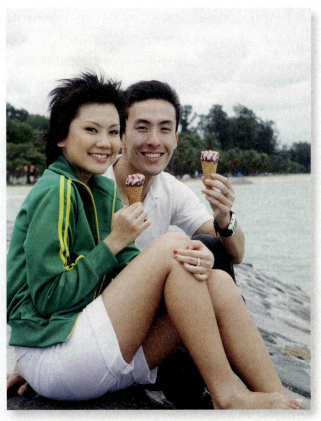

All foods can fit in a healthy diet, even sweet treats—for the latter, just not too many and not too often. Make a healthy overall dietary pattern a priority, and commit to being a mindful eater.

and one weekend day, because eating patterns often differ. It's also important to put in *everything* you eat and drink, not just the items you think will make your diet look good.

With some practice, you won't have to worry about tracking your diet, as you'll know which foods are nutrient rich and how much is reasonable to eat. See the box "Making Nutrient-Rich Food Choices" on p. 317 for guidance. The MyPlate Web site also includes sample menus and recipes to help get you started.

Q | Why is skipping breakfast so bad?

We've all heard that breakfast is the most important meal. There is some truth to that, but realistically, all meals are important. Breakfast presents its own challenges, if for no other reason than many people can't seem to find the time to have breakfast, or at least not a reasonably healthy breakfast. Skipping breakfast, however, is a sure-fire way to be really hungry and to have trouble concentrating later in the morning. Research has shown that skipping breakfast makes you much

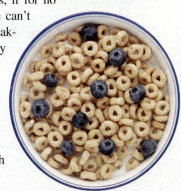

TABLE 9-2 OIL CONTENT OF COMMON FOODS

FOOD	AMOUNT OF FOOD	AMOUNT OF OIL
VEGETABLE OIL	1 Tbsp	1 Tbsp (14 g)
SOFT (TRANS-FAT-FREE) MARGARINE	1 Tbsp	2½ tsp (11 g)
MAYONNAISE	1 Tbsp	2½ tsp (11 g)
MAYONNAISE-TYPE SALAD DRESSING	1 Tbsp	1 tsp (4 g)
ITALIAN DRESSING	2 Tbsp	2 tsp (8 g)
THOUSAND ISLAND DRESSING	2 Tbsp	2½ tsp (11 g)
OLIVES, RIPE, CANNED	8 large	1 tsp (4 g)
AVOCADO	½ medium	3 tsp (15 g)
PEANUT BUTTER	2 Tbsp	4 tsp (16 g)
PEANUTS, DRY ROASTED	1 oz	3 tsp (14 g)
ALMONDS, DRY ROASTED	1 oz	3 tsp (15 g)
SUNFLOWER SEEDS	1 oz	3 tsp (14 g)
SALMON STEAK	3 oz	2 tsp (8 g)
TUNA, CANNED IN OIL	3 oz	1 tsp (5 g)

Source: ChooseMyPlate.gov. (2010). How much is my allowance for oils? (http://www.choosemyplate.gov/food-groups/oils-allowance.html#).

more likely to gain weight and more likely to make poor nutritional choices when you do get around to eating (see the box "Moderate, Regular Eating and Reduced Obesity" on p. 318).[4] Vending machines and convenience stores become the default breakfast choice but usually provide energy-rich, nutrient-poor choices—not a good use of your money.

Bacon, sausage, pancakes, waffles, sugary cereals, and other foods with a lot of fat or sugar should be saved for special occasions—and then consumed only in modest portions. And don't overdo the caffeinated coffee and tea—too much caffeine can leave you jittery and unable to focus—and the typical add-ons of cream and sugar.

At the table or on the road, eat 300–500 calories of healthy foods within about 2 hours of waking; otherwise, you'll be dragging through those early classes and ravenously hungry by midday. Good foods to pack are whole-grain bagels or bread with peanut butter, whole fruit, nonfat yogurt, and dry packaged whole-grain cereals. Most residence dining halls will pack a meal for you if you have a meal plan, so you can just stop by on your way to class and pick up your morning meal. If you live off campus, plan ahead and pack your own breakfast.

Q What are some easy snacks that are also healthy?

In the preceding answer there are suggestions for breakfast snacks to have "on the road." At-home healthy snacks can also be a positive part of your eating plan—just take care not to stock your refrigerator and cupboards with energy-dense, nutrient-poor packaged baked goods, chips, sweetened beverages, and candy. Good snack options include moderate portions of the following foods:

- Whole-grain crackers—plain or with peanut butter, salsa, or hummus or another bean dip
- Low-fat microwave popcorn
- Fruit (fresh, canned, or dried)
- Carrot and celery sticks, bell pepper strips, broccoli florets
- Nonfat yogurt with fruit (if you have a blender, make a smoothie from nonfat yogurt and frozen fruit chunks)

Wellness Strategies

Making Nutrient-Rich Food Choices

Q What are superfoods? What foods are a MUST? You know . . . nutritionally rich, full of fiber, things like that. How do I incorporate them into my diet?

Superfoods are foods packed with disease-busting and wellness-promoting nutrients. Superpower your diet with superfoods from the main food categories.

Grains

- Choose whole grains at least half the time. Look for whole-grain cereals, bread, and pasta.
- Watch your portion sizes. Commercially prepared baked goods such as muffins and bagels are often supersize, to your detriment.
- Limit sweetened carbohydrates. Try unsweetened varieties of breakfast cereals and reduced-fat granola topped with cut-up fruit. Also restrict consumption of grain-based products high in fat and sugar, such as pastries and croissants.
- For pasta sauces, think red, not white. Use red sauce (marinara) on your pasta instead of cheese or white sauce (Alfredo). Add veggies for extra goodness.

Vegetables

- Paint a rainbow. Choose a colorful variety of vegetables and load up your plate.
- Boost your veggies. Add extra vegetables to omelets, sandwiches, soups, salads, and pizzas.
- Ditch the fryer. Try steamed, roasted, or oven-baked vegetables.

- Top it off. Instead of cheese or white-sauce toppings for potatoes, broccoli, and other vegetables, try herbs, lemon juice, or salsa.

Fruits

- Skin is in. Nearly all fruits are nutrient-rich choices. Choose fresh fruit and 100-percent fruit juice most of the time. Even the skin is loaded with nutrients.
- Not so sweet. Instead of sweetened applesauce and canned fruit packed in syrup, try unsweetened apple-sauce and canned fruit packed in juice.
- Keep it fresh. Limit the number and portion size of fruit desserts like pies and pastries. Choose whole fruits most of the time.

Meat and Beans

- Grow your protein. Legumes and other plant protein sources are nutrient-rich choices.
- Meat is neat. Nutrient-rich animal proteins include beef (loin, round) with the fat trimmed off, chicken without skin, fish, low-fat lunch meats, and Canadian bacon.

Dairy

- Be a plain Jane. Instead of sweetened fruit yogurt, try plain fat-free yogurt with fresh or frozen fruit.
- Skim it. Instead of whole milk and full-fat cheeses, try low-fat or fat-free types.

Source: Adapted from USDA. (2011). 10 tips nutrition education series. ChooseMyPlate.gov. (http://www.choosemyplate.gov/healthy-eating-tips/ten-tips.html). Last accessed January 2012.

- Single-serving containers of unsweetened applesauce or fruit juice—or pack your own in reusable containers for a less expensive option that also helps reduce trash
- Nuts and seeds
- Cereals, especially whole-grain varieties with little or no added sugar
- Homemade trail mix, made from cereal, nuts, seeds, and dried fruit
- Hard-cooked egg
- 100-percent fruit juice
- Cup of vegetable soup

Energy, protein, and granola bars are also easy to carry, but read the labels carefully before you buy them because some are very high in calories, saturated fat, and added sugars.

Many companies now make snacks in 100-calorie bags, and these might be a good way to practice portion control. But don't choose a snack just based on the number of calories; make sure it also is nutrient rich.

Vegetarian Diets

Q I'm a vegetarian. Can I still use MyPlate?

Yes. MyPlate has information for all types of eaters, including vegetarians, children, pregnant women, and lactating mothers. There are vegetarian options in each food group, depending on what type of vegetarian diet you follow. **Vegans** eat only plant foods and avoid all animal products. Other vegetarians avoid flesh foods but include dairy *(lacto)* or egg *(ovo)* products or both. Thus, **lacto-vegetarians** eat plant foods and dairy products, and **lacto-ovo-vegetarians** eat plant foods, dairy products, and eggs.

About 5 million Americans consistently follow a vegetarian diet, and many more consume vegetarian meals

vegan A dietary pattern composed exclusively of plant foods, with no animal products.

lacto-vegetarian A dietary pattern composed of plant foods and dairy products.

lacto-ovo-vegetarian A dietary pattern composed of plant foods, eggs, and dairy products.

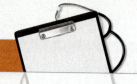

Research Brief

Moderate, Regular Eating and Reduced Obesity

If you think you can lose weight by skipping meals, think again. A recent study showed that people who eat more frequently during the day have almost half the incidence of obesity than people who eat less often. About 500 people were asked to report their diets five times over 1 year. Those who ate four or more times a day (generally three meals and a snack) were *45 percent less likely to be obese* than those who ate three or fewer meals daily.

People who regularly skipped breakfast were *450 percent more likely to be obese* compared to regular breakfast eaters. There was no indication that eating at night contributed to greater weight, after taking into account total calories. Eating breakfast or dinner away

from home, however, was associated with higher weight, potentially due to larger portions and more fat in restaurant food.

Analyze and Apply

- What does this study tell you about the benefits of the frequency of eating? How could someone on a weight-loss program apply this information?
- Why do you think skipping breakfast is related to an increased likelihood of obesity?

Source: Ma, Y., Bertone, E. R., Stanek III, E. J., Reed, G. W., Hebert, J. R., Cohen, N. L., Merriam, P. A., & Ockene, I. S. (2003). Association between eating patterns and obesity in a free-living U.S. adult population. *American Journal of Epidemiology, 158*(1), 85–92.

---

at least some of the time; this latter group is sometimes referred to as *partial vegetarians*.[5] Common reasons for choosing a vegetarian diet include health concerns, economic and ethical considerations, religious beliefs, and concern for the environment and animal welfare. Vegetarian diets tend to be lower in saturated fat and cholesterol and higher in fiber, potassium, folate, and other micronutrients and phytochemicals; these differences may help explain lower rates of heart disease, hypertension, and type 2 diabetes among vegetarians.

Healthy vegetarian protein sources include eggs (for ovo-vegetarians), legumes, nuts and nut butters, and various soy products, including tofu, tempeh, and veggie burgers. By selecting a variety of plant proteins over the course of the day, vegetarians can obtain all the essential amino acids (see Chapter 8).

Lacto- and lacto-ovo-vegetarians can follow the general guidelines for selecting foods from the milk group—choosing low-fat and nonfat options most of the time. Vegans

can choose non-dairy sources of calcium. As described in Chapter 8, vegetarians need to take special care to consume adequate amounts of iron, zinc, and vitamin B_{12}. Recall that consuming vitamin C–rich foods along with iron-rich foods can help the body absorb iron. Vitamin B_{12} is found only in animal foods and so must be obtained from fortified foods or supplements.

Other helpful websites for vegetarians include Medline Plus's Vegetarian Diet (http://www.nlm.nih.gov/medlineplus/vegetariandiet.html) and the Vegetarian Resource Group (http://www.vrg.org).

DASH and Other Dietary Plans

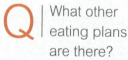 **Q** What other eating plans are there?

Many eating plans are available—in books, online, from weight-loss programs—and some are better options than others. Two eating patterns that the *2010 Dietary Guidelines for Americans* links to reduced risk of chronic disease are the DASH (Dietary Approaches to Stop Hypertension) diet and some Mediterranean-style diets.[6]

The **DASH diet,** as its full name indicates, was originally developed to help people reduce blood pressure by emphasizing whole grains, vegetables, fruits, and low-fat dairy products. DASH also includes poultry, seafood, and nuts and limits red meat, sweets, sodium, and sugar-containing beverages. The DASH diet can be customized for those at risk for high blood pressure.

Research has found that the DASH diet, especially its low-sodium version, significantly reduces blood pressure and improves heart function. Blood pressure goes down within just a few

DASH diet Dietary Approaches to Stop Hypertension, a dietary pattern designed to reduce blood pressure. Emphasizes potassium-rich vegetables and fruits and low-fat dairy products; includes whole grains, poultry, fish, and nuts; limits sodium, red meat, and added sugars.

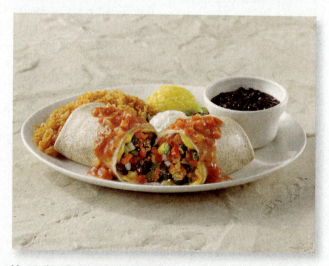

Vegetarian diets can meet all nutrient needs. But just as for a non-vegetarian diet, nutrient-rich choices from each food group are key.

weeks of starting on the DASH plan. When combined with exercise and weight loss, the DASH diet has even more benefits, including greater reductions in blood pressure, improved cognition, reduced insulin sensitivity, and improved cholesterol levels.[7] Like MyPlate, the DASH diet can be a healthy weight-reducing diet and is a good choice for everyone (http://www.nhlbi.nih.gov/health/public/heart/hbp/dash/dash_brief.htm).

Q | What's the Mediterranean diet? It sounds exotic.

The **Mediterranean diet** is not so much a diet plan but a pattern of eating associated with the traditional cuisine of the cultures bordering the Mediterranean Sea. Although diets vary among and within these countries, they have some common features, which are referred to as the Mediterranean diet (Figure 9-4):

- Staples include unrefined grains, vegetables, legumes, fruits, nuts, and seeds, with high overall fiber intake.
- Fish and (in non-Islamic countries) wine are often served at meals.
- Olive oil is the primary source of added fats.
- Consumption of saturated fat, meat, and full-fat dairy products is limited.

Many aspects of this dietary pattern are consistent with the recommendations in MyPlate and DASH. The Mediterranean diet has a total fat consumption near or over the limit suggested by the Dietary Reference Intakes, but most of that fat is from healthy, unsaturated oils. It is primarily a plant-based diet and is linked to lower rates of several chronic diseases—another healthy choice for you.

Mediterranean diet A dietary pattern associated with cultures bordering the Mediterranean Sea; the pattern emphasizes whole grains, fruits, vegetables, legumes, nuts, seeds, fish, and olive oil and limits meat, saturated fat, and full-fat dairy products.

Developing Practical Food Skills

Now that you know the basics of the eating patterns associated with good health, it's time to put that knowledge to work in everyday life. To do that, you need to develop skills at planning meals, shopping, cooking, and selecting foods when eating out. You also need the basics on food safety so that you can prepare meals and eat leftovers without worrying about foodborne illness, toxins, or allergens.

Meal Planning and Preparation

Q | What am I supposed to do if I don't know how to cook? Help!

Not having any cooking experience can be a roadblock. Most everyone can put together simple breakfasts and meals—cereal with fruit, basic sandwiches—that don't require much, if any, cooking. But for more complex meals, you may feel stuck. If you don't have access to a campus dining hall or a friendly roommate who cooks, you may have to rely more on prepared foods while you learn some cooking basics.

In terms of planning meals, think about your goals according to MyPlate. Most Americans don't eat enough whole grains, low-fat dairy, fruits, and vegetables. Here are quick tips for easy meal prep:

- For breakfast have whole-grain cereal or toast, fruit, and milk or yogurt.
- Have at least two servings of vegetables at lunch and dinner. They can be canned, frozen, or raw and fresh. Rinse any canned vegetables you use; otherwise these take no real prep skills. Recipes can be found on most veggie cans if you want to explore different options and try out some new cooking skills.
- Snack on fruit. No cooking skills are involved, and you can add fruit to many different items, so let your imagination run wild.

Meats and sweets
Less often

Wine
In moderation

Poultry, eggs, cheese and yogurt
Moderate portions daily to weekly

Fish and seafood
Often, at least two times per week

Drink water

Fruits, vegetables, grains (mostly whole), olive oil, beans, nuts, legumes, seeds, herbs and spices
Base every meal on these foods

Illustration by George Middleton   © 2009 Oldways Preservation and Exchange Trust   www.oldwayspt.org

Be physically active; enjoy meals with others

Figure 9-4 Mediterranean Diet Pyramid. The Mediterranean diet is based on minimally processed foods from plant sources, with olive oil as the principal type of fat. For more information on the Mediterranean diet and tips for incorporating it into your daily diet, visit the Oldways Web site (http://www.oldwayspt.org).
Source: © 2010 Oldways Preservation and Exchange Trust. *Mediterranean Diet Pyramid* (http://www.oldwayspt.org/mediterranean-diet-pyramid).

■ Choose lean protein sources, such as sliced turkey in a sandwich or legumes in your salad. You don't have to get fancy—just put a few things on whole-wheat bread or toss some lettuce, veggies, and low-fat cheese into a bowl.

See the box "Resources for Meal Planning and Cooking" for more ideas on easy and healthy meal preparation.

Most grocery stores now carry a vast line of breakfasts, lunches, and dinners that just need to be heated. Of course, many of these foods have a lot more sodium and fat than home-cooked versions—and they are more expensive—but they can be helpful in a pinch, especially if you buy them on sale. Read the nutrition labels and comparison-shop in terms of both price and nutrition, keeping in mind that even options that call themselves healthy may not be. You can also enrich any pre-made meal with additional vegetables, whole grains, or low-fat cheese to enhance the taste and the nutrition. To reduce the high levels of sodium in rice mixes, frozen stir-fry meals, and similar foods, use only half the seasoning packet and add your own spices to boost the flavor with less sodium. For convenience foods that call for the addition of butter or margarine, use only half the amount to reduce fats.

In the meantime, purchase a few basic pots, pans, and utensils, maybe at a yard sale, and start collecting interesting recipes. Maybe your campus offers a cooking class—a worthwhile investment of time for learning an important life skill. Visit any number of Web sites or YouTube videos to find recipes and learn the art of cooking. Don't let the fear of cooking keep you from eating well; food is too fun to avoid.

Eating Away from Home

Q | I live on campus. What kind of food should I eat in the dining hall?

The same as you would eat anywhere else: nutrient-rich foods in moderate portions with an occasional treat. Your dining hall likely offers plenty of these healthy choices but also many less nutritious "treats," so choose wisely. For example, it's up to you to opt for whole-grain cereals or egg-white omelets instead of chocolate-chip waffles, bacon, or Danish.

If you don't know which dining-hall choices are healthy, just ask, as that information is readily available. Many campuses now post nutritional information for each meal, making it even easier to choose good options.

Healthy dining-hall options include the following:

■ Whole-grain cereals, breads, and pasta; beware, though, that just because a bread looks brown doesn't mean it's a whole-grain bread

■ Oatmeal (without a lot of added sweeteners) and egg-white omelets for hot breakfasts

■ Fresh fruit—always a wise choice

■ Salads topped with fresh vegetables, legumes, and seeds; limit high-fat toppings like croutons and cheese, and select a low-fat or oil-based salad dressing served on the side

■ Vegetable or broth-based soups; having a cup of soup or a glass of water before you eat can help fill you up and keep you from overeating

■ Sandwiches and wraps containing some combination of lean meat, low-fat cheese, and lots of veggies; use salsa, vinegar, or mustard for flavor

■ Lean chicken and beef dishes; grilled, broiled, or baked fish

■ Vegetarian pasta and bean dishes with tomato-based sauces and little added fat

■ Just about any vegetable fixed without added fat—load up your plate

■ Nonfat yogurt

Q | What are the best fast-food choices? What about other types of restaurants?

Fast-food restaurants are tempting because they are efficient, relatively inexpensive, and consistent—you always know exactly what you'll get. However, many classic fast-food choices are high in calories, total and saturated fat, and sodium, as well

Fast Facts

Dorm Food: 22,000 Calories and Counting

A recent study inventoried food and beverages in the dorm rooms of college students. The researchers found an average of about 50 food items per room, representing more than 22,000 calories. The most common items were salty snacks, cereal or granola bars, main dishes, desserts or candy, and sugar-sweetened beverages. Few students had low-calorie beverages, 100-percent fruit or vegetable juices, dairy products, fruits, or vegetables. Items purchased by parents were higher in calories and fat than items purchased by students.

■ What foods do you like to keep handy in your dorm room or apartment?

■ Who purchases the majority of foods in your room or apartment? How does that influence what foods are around?

Source: Nelson, M. C., & Story, M. (2009). Food environments in university dorms: 20,000 calories per dorm room and counting. *American Journal of Preventive Medicine, 36*(6), 523–526.

Wellness Strategies

Resources for Meal Planning and Cooking

Q | What's the easiest way to avoid fast foods and instead find easy and practical recipes?

The Web sites listed here are a good place to look for ideas. Not every recipe at every site is a healthy choice, but you can use your knowledge of nutrition to make wise choices.

MyPlate Menu Planner: Helps you plan menus for a day or a week using the MyPlate recommendations for you or your family.

www.choosemyplate.gov/healthy-eating-tips/sample-menus-recipes.html

National Heart, Lung, and Blood Institute's Deliciously Healthy Eating Recipes: Includes recipes as well as an illustrated food-preparation glossary.

http://hp2010.nhlbihin.net/healthyeating

National Heart, Lung, and Blood Institute's recipe booklets: Includes heart-healthy recipes, the DASH eating plan, and Latino and African American dishes.

www.nhlbi.nih.gov/health/public/heart/obesity/lose_wt/recipes.htm

University of New Hampshire Health Services: *Good Eats: Quick & Easy Food for Busy College Students:* Includes recipes like "Breakfast Bulgur While You Shower," "Five-Minute Quesadillas," and "Starving Student's Simple Supper."

www.unh.edu/health-services/good_eats

Iowa State University Extension: Spend Smart, Eat Smart: Provides suggestions for saving money on food purchases.

www.extension.iastate.edu/foodsavings/

Centers for Disease Control and Prevention: Fruits and Veggies Matter: Go to the recipes section to find ways to use just about any fruit or vegetable.

www.fruitsandveggiesmatter.gov

Nutrient Rich Foods Coalition Recipes: A database of recipes that meet the Coalition's criteria for nutrient richness; you can search the database by ingredient, meal, total time, or difficulty level.

www.nutrientrichfoods.org/recipes

USDA Recipe Finder: A database of recipes organized not only by ingredient, meal, and cost but also by specific nutrition goals (e.g., less saturated fat) and preparation time.

http://recipefinder.nal.usda.gov

Eat Better America: This commercial site recommends specific brands in some recipes, but you can use whatever brands you find locally; the recipes follow recognized dietary guidelines and include nutritional information.

www.eatbetteramerica.com

YumYum Student Recipes: Not every recipe on this site is a healthy choice, but the site also includes student-oriented tips and how-to information.

www.yumyum.com/student

---

as low in fiber and many micronutrients. In other words, these foods are typically nutrient poor and calorie dense. Although many fast-food restaurant chains are experimenting with healthier options, it's best to approach fast food with caution and to consume it as infrequently as possible.

Among the better choices available at most chain fast-food restaurants are salads, grilled chicken, and fresh fruit. Buyer beware, however: At one popular fast-food chain, a Caesar salad with grilled chicken has only 190 total calories and 5 grams of saturated fat, whereas the "premium" salad with fried chicken (often described as "crispy") contains 490 calories and 21 grams of saturated fat. Prepackaged salad dressing can add up to 190 calories and 3.5 grams of saturated fat to the total, so don't be led to believe that a salad is by definition a healthy choice.

A regular fast-food hamburger typically has 250 calories and 3.5 grams of saturated fat; a cheeseburger, 300 calories and 6.0 grams of fat. However, adding a medium order of french fries (380 calories and 2.5 grams of saturated fat) and a medium regular soda (210 calories) suddenly makes this an almost 850-calorie, and quite unhealthy, meal. The most offending fast-food sandwiches can exceed a whopping 1,000 calories. Choosing one of these along with supersize fries and a drink can easily push the meal close to 2,000 calories, with extremely high levels of saturated fat and sodium and little in the way of nutrients.

Also crisscrossing the United States are many "fast-casual" food chains catering to a variety of ethnic tastes, among them Mexican, Chinese, Japanese, and Italian. These chains, like the basic fast-food eateries, offer menu items of varying nutritional value. Almost all fast-food and fast-casual restaurants have nutritional information available for their customers in the store and online. When convenient, it is best to check the menu online in advance for healthy options; that way, you might avoid falling into the trap of arriving at the restaurant and allowing the smells and visual cues to tempt you into making a nutrient-poor selection. Some fast-food chains post the calorie values right on the overhead menu so that you know what you are getting when you are choosing. Others print the nutrition information on the tray liner, where you can see it only after you have ordered. Lots of good that does for your diet!

For additional guidance on eating at fast-food and traditional sit-down restaurants, see the box "Tips for Eating Out." Many of the strategies suggested for dining-hall eating also apply to restaurants.

Food Safety and Technology

Food safety is often in the news. We hear frequently about recalls of contaminated foods and outbreaks of **foodborne illness,** sickness caused by contaminated foods or beverages. Food safety is a concern for both large-scale commercial food producers and people cooking at home. Technological developments affect our food supply as well, and consumers must make decisions about whether to purchase particular types of foods, including those certified organic. Food allergies are also an important issue for some people.

Q | Is food safety a worry at home?

FOODBORNE ILLNESS. Food safety is for everyone. Although many people worry about pesticides and other chemicals in their food, the biggest threats come from **pathogens**—viruses, bacteria, and other disease-causing microorganisms—that can contaminate food and cause foodborne illness. Each year, foodborne illness affects more than 75 million Americans, causing 325,000 hospitalizations and about 5,200 deaths.[8] Most cases of foodborne illness, also called food poisoning or stomach flu, last only a few days and are characterized by nausea, vomiting, diarrhea, and fever. For otherwise healthy people, these symptoms are unpleasant but not serious. Higher-risk populations (older adults, pregnant women, infants and children, and people with compromised immune

foodborne illness An illness caused by consuming foods or beverages contaminated with disease-causing organisms.

pathogen A microorganism that causes disease, such as a virus or bacterium.

DOLLAR STRETCHER
Financial Wellness Tip

These good-eating ideas are also time- and money-savers.
- Take advantage of sales, use coupons, and buy non-perishables in bulk.
- Share shopping and cooking responsibilities with roommates and friends; start a dinner club to share costs.
- Cook a big batch of a dish that freezes well—for example, a soup, stew, or pasta; save the leftovers to reheat later in the week.
- Cook from scratch to reduce your reliance on expensive convenience foods and to gain control over fat, salt, and sugar.
- Join Groupon or another local saving site for meals out or for regular groceries.

---

function), however, can suffer much more serious outcomes. If you become ill with symptoms of foodborne illness, drink plenty of fluids and wash your hands frequently to avoid spreading the infection; consult a health care provider if you have a high fever or your symptoms are very severe and don't improve within three days.

The most common causes of foodborne illness are the bacteria *Salmonella*, *Campylobacter*, and *E. coli* O157:H7 and the group of viruses called *norovirus*. These pathogens are present on many foods when you purchase them, especially animal products and fresh produce. However, cross-contamination can taint most any other food; your hands, cutting boards, kitchen counters, knives, and refrigerator shelves are all places where a pathogen can travel from one food to another. You cannot see or smell these pathogens on food.

There is no way to ensure that all the food coming into your home is free of pathogens, so you need to practice safe food handling and storage to prevent illness, just as commercial food facilities are required to do. Figure 9-5 summarizes the basic four steps for food safety: clean, separate, cook, and chill. Here are some additional tips:

- Wash fruits and vegetables under running water just before eating, cutting, or cooking. Wash them even if you plan to peel them. Scrub firm produce, such as melons and cucumbers, with a clean produce brush.
- Remove and discard the outermost leaves of a head of cabbage or lettuce.
- Keep foods at a safe temperature until served. Cold foods should be held at 40°F or below. Hot foods should be kept at 140°F or above.
- Don't eat unsafe foods, including unpasteurized milk or juice, cookie dough containing raw eggs, or raw or undercooked eggs, fish, oysters, hamburgers, and other meats.
- Clean your refrigerator regularly.

Researchers who have studied college students' food-handling practices have found that the majority don't follow the recommendations.[9] To reduce the risk of foodborne illness for yourself and the people around you, take a few extra minutes to carry out the basic steps for food safety.

Q | What about leftovers—can I still eat the pizza from Friday night?

Assuming that the pizza has been refrigerated and it isn't yet Tuesday, you're probably OK, because leftover pizza can safely last for 3 or 4 days. Refrigeration is key for leftovers, because pathogens can multiply

Wellness Strategies

Tips for Eating Out

Q What are some healthy choices available at fast-food and other restaurants?

- For sandwiches, choose whole-grain bread, rolls, or pita with lean meats and lots of vegetables; pickles, onions, hot peppers, lettuce, tomatoes, mustard, and fat-free dressings add flavor without fat.
- Skip the chips in favor of fruit (if available), or have pretzels instead.
- Skip the fries, order the kid's portion, or share them with a friend.
- For pizza, get the thin crust and ask for half the amount of cheese and twice the vegetables instead of meat toppings.
- Order salads with lots of vegetable toppings and a low-fat dressing on the side; avoid or limit creamy full-fat dressings, full-fat cheese toppings, and croutons.
- Drink water, 100-percent juice (small size), unsweetened tea, or low-fat milk instead of a milk shake or regular soda.
- Have frozen yogurt or a fruit salad for dessert rather than pie, cookies, or a milk shake.

Sit-Down Restaurants

- If you know where you're going, look for the menu online and plan what you'll order.
- Don't skip lunch if you're going out to dinner, because you'll be more likely to make poor dinner choices if you're super hungry; have a small lunch or snack.
- Always ask about how foods are prepared if you are unsure. Good wait staff will be happy to tell you.

Fast-Food Restaurants

- Order small burgers or grilled chicken sandwiches without cheese, mayonnaise, or "special" sauces.

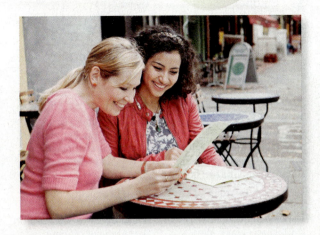

- Avoid buffets, as they are a trap for overeating.
- Skip appetizers unless you want to order one instead of an entrée or unless you at least share your entrée with others.
- If portions are large, share with a friend or take half home; ask for the to-go box when you order and place half the food in it as soon as you're served.
- Ask for salad dressing, gravy, and sauces to be served on the side.
- Choose grilled, broiled, roasted, baked, flame-cooked, or steamed dishes instead of foods that are fried, stuffed, or covered with cheese (for example, au gratin, scalloped) or a cream sauce (for example, Alfredo, hollandaise); the latter are high in calories and unhealthy fats.
- Have a water-based soup or a tall glass of water at the start of your meal as a strategy to avoid overeating—or enjoy an apple on your way to dinner.
- Try fresh fruit or sherbet for dessert.

---

rapidly at temperatures between 40°F and 140°F. Foods should be eaten within 2 hours of being taken out of the refrigerator. Table 9-3 on p. 325 provides guidelines for how long it's safe to store food in the refrigerator and freezer. These guidelines assume that your refrigerator is cold enough. Researchers studying food safety practices among college students found that the average refrigerator was above the maximum recommended temperature of 40°F, increasing the risk for foodborne illness.[10]

Have you checked your refrigerator's temperature? Use an inexpensive appliance thermometer to ensure that the refrigerator is kept at an appropriate temperature. It's also a handy tool after a power outage to determine whether the food in the fridge is still safe to eat.

Q My mom checks a roast with a meat thermometer, but I don't have one. Is it really necessary?

The best way to determine if meat is cooked to a safe temperature is to use a meat thermometer to measure its internal temperature. "Done" according to color or time in the oven isn't necessarily the same thing as "safe." Research has shown that neither color nor time adequately indicates that meat is completely cooked. The color of roast or ground beef, for example, is no longer considered a safe indicator. Similarly, for whole poultry, checking whether the juices from the bird are clear, the meat is no longer pink, or the legs easily pull away from the

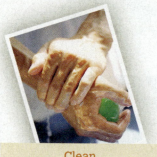

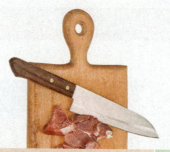

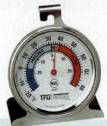

Clean	Separate	Cook	Chill
• Wash hands with soap and warm water for 20 seconds before and after handling food. If soap isn't available, use an alcohol-based gel. • Run cutting boards and utensils through the dishwasher or wash them in hot soapy water after each use. • Keep countertops clean by washing with hot soapy water after preparing food.	• Use one cutting board for raw meat, poultry, and seafood and another for salads and ready-to-eat food. • Keep raw meat, poultry, and seafood and their juices apart from other food items in your grocery cart. • Store raw meat, poultry, and seafood in a container or on a plate so juices can't drip on other foods.	• Use a food thermometer; you can't tell food is cooked safely by how it looks. • Stir, rotate the dish, and cover food when microwaving to prevent cold spots where bacteria can survive. • Bring sauces, soups, and gravies to a rolling boil when reheating.	• Cool the fridge to 40°F or below, and use an appliance thermometer to check the temperature. • Chill leftovers and takeout foods within 2 hours, and divide food into shallow containers for rapid cooling. • Thaw meat, poultry, and seafood in the fridge, not on the counter; don't over-stuff the fridge.

USDA Recommended Safe Minimum Internal Temperatures

Beef, veal, lamb, steaks, and roast	Fish	Pork	Beef, veal, lamb, ground	Egg dishes	Turkey, chicken, and duck, whole, pieces, and ground
145°F	**145°F**	**160°F**	**160°F**	**160°F**	**165°F**

Figure 9-5 Four basic steps for food safety. For additional information, visit http://www.foodsafety.gov and http://BeFoodSafe.gov

Sources: Adapted from U.S. Department of Agriculture. (2007, September). *Four easy lessons in safe food handling* (http://www.fsis.usda.gov/be_foodsafe/BFS_Brochure_Text/index.asp). U.S. Department of Agriculture. (2011, June). *"Is it done yet?"* (http://www.fsis.usda.gov/is_it_done_yet).

body are common but inaccurate techniques. The *only* safe way is to use a meat thermometer. Reusable thermometers cost a few dollars, and checking the temperature takes only 10–30 seconds. See Figure 9-5 for recommended safe internal temperatures.

Q So, is everyone allergic to peanuts these days?

FOOD ALLERGIES. Maybe not everyone, but peanuts are one of the most common food **allergens**—substances that are capable of producing an allergic reaction in the body's immune system—and cause severe reactions in some people. About 6–8 percent of children under age 4 and 3–4 percent of adults have some form of food allergy, and exposure to the allergen can have serious consequences. Food allergies are different from food intolerances such as lactose intolerance (see Chapter 8). In a food *allergy,* the body's immune system mistakenly identifies the food as a harmful substance and releases histamine and other chemicals into the

allergen A substance that is capable of producing an allergic reaction in the body's immune system; most food allergens are proteins.

bloodstream. A food *intolerance* has a different underlying cause—such as the absence of an enzyme needed to digest a food fully (as in lactose intolerance) or a sensitivity to a substance (such as MSG)—and is usually less severe than an allergy.

Symptoms of food allergies include coughing or wheezing, flushed skin, rash or hives, tingling or itchy sensations in the mouth, swelling of the lips or tongue, nausea, abdominal cramps, and diarrhea. In some cases, a severe reaction known as *anaphylaxis* occurs, characterized by constriction of the airways in the lungs, swelling of the throat causing suffocation, and severe lowering of blood pressure and shock. Anaphylaxis is a medical emergency. Prompt treatment with the hormone epinephrine during the early stages of anaphylaxis can slow and reduce the severity of the allergic reaction. People with severe allergies may carry an auto-injector with epinephrine (for example, an EpiPen) for this purpose.

To help reduce accidental exposure to allergens, people with food allergies typically read food labels carefully and ask questions before eating food from a restaurant or a dining hall. By law, any food that may contain one or more of eight major food allergens—milk, eggs, fish, shellfish, tree

TABLE 9-3 SAFE REFRIGERATOR AND FREEZER STORAGE FOR FOODS

CATEGORY	FOOD	REFRIGERATOR (≤40°F)	FREEZER (≤0°F)
LEFTOVERS	Cooked meat or poultry	3–4 days	2–6 months
	Chicken nuggets or patties	3–4 days	1–3 months
	Pizza	3–4 days	1–2 months
	Quiche with filling	3–4 days	1–2 months
SALADS	Egg, chicken, ham, tuna, macaroni salads	3–5 days	Don't freeze
HOT DOGS	Opened package	1 week	1–2 months
	Unopened package	2 weeks	1–2 months
	Opened package or deli sliced	3–5 days	1–2 months
LUNCHEON MEAT	Opened package or deli sliced	3–5 days	1–2 months
	Unopened package	2 weeks	1–2 months
BACON, SAUSAGE MEAT	Bacon	7 days	1 month
	Sausage, raw (chicken, turkey, pork, beef)	1–2 days	1–2 months
HAMBURGER, OTHER GROUND MEATS	Hamburger, ground beef, turkey, veal, pork, lamb, mixtures	1–2 days	3–4 months
FRESH BEEF, VEAL, LAMB, PORK	Steaks	3–5 days	6–12 months
	Chops	3–5 days	4–6 months
	Roasts	3–5 days	4–12 months
FRESH POULTRY	Chicken or turkey, whole	1–2 days	1 year
	Chicken or turkey, pieces	1–2 days	9 months
FISH	Lean fish	1–2 days	6 months
	Fatty fish	1–2 days	2–3 months
	Cooked fish	3–4 days	4–6 months
SOUPS, STEWS	Vegetable or meat added	3–4 days	2–3 months
EGGS	Raw in shell	3–5 weeks	Don't freeze
	Hard-cooked	1 week	Don't freeze
MAYONNAISE	Opened jar	2 months	Don't freeze
DAIRY	Milk	1 week	3 months
	Yogurt	1–2 weeks	1–2 months
	Cheese, hard, opened	3–4 weeks	6 months

Source: Adapted from FoodSafety.gov. (2010). Storage times for the refrigerator and freezer. *Keep Food Safe* (http://www.foodsafety.gov/keep/charts/storage times.html). Last accessed January 2012.

nuts (such as walnuts and almonds), peanuts, wheat, and soybeans—must list the allergens on the label. If you have a reaction to a food and are unsure whether it's due to intolerance, allergy, or foodborne illness, talk with your physician.

Q Fish is supposed to be healthy, but doesn't it contain mercury?

FISH AND MERCURY. Some fish does contain mercury, a metallic element that is a concern for human health. Mercury gets into the water from human activities (the burning of gas and other fossil fuels) and from natural sources such as volcanic eruptions. It is picked up by microorganisms that are then eaten by larger and larger organisms in a process known as *bioaccumulation.* Large predatory fish such as sharks and swordfish contain the highest levels of mercury.

In terms of your health, you have to balance the risks from mercury in fish with the benefits of consuming fish. On the plus side, fish and shellfish contain high-quality protein; they are low in saturated fat; and many types contain heart-healthy omega-3 fatty acids (see Chapter 8). Nearly all fish and shellfish contain traces of mercury, which for most people poses little health risk because the body can eliminate it. On the minus side, some varieties contain higher levels of mercury, which can be harmful to an unborn baby or a young child's developing nervous system. Because of this threat to human health, the Food and Drug Administration (FDA) and the Environmental Protection Agency (EPA) make these recommendations for women who are or may become pregnant, for nursing mothers, and for young children:[11]

- Do not consume shark, swordfish, king mackerel, or tilefish; these fish contain the highest levels of mercury.
- Limit consumption of albacore ("white") tuna to no more than 6 ounces per week; it has more mercury than canned light tuna.
- Do eat up to 12 ounces per week of a variety of fish and shellfish that are lower in mercury, including salmon, pollock, catfish, canned light tuna, and shrimp.
- For local, recreationally caught fish, pay attention to fish-consumption advisories issued by federal, state, and local governments (http://www.epa.gov/mercury/advisories.htm).

Q Are organic foods better than regular foods?

ORGANIC FOODS. This question has been and will be debated for a long time—and the answer may depend on your definition of *better.* Organic farming began in the late 1940s and has recently become quite popular. After every outbreak of foodborne illness, there tends to be a spike in interest in organic food. But is organic safer or more nutritious?

Organic refers to how the food is produced—without use of genetic engineering, ionizing radiation, chemical fertilizers, hormones, pesticides, and sewage sludge, and only by using tillage and cultivation practices such as crop rotation, cover crops, and fertilization with properly treated crop and animal wastes.[12] Advantages of organic compared to typical commercial farming include conservation of water and soil resources, recycling of animal waste, release of fewer chemicals, improved soil fertility, promotion of crop diversity, and protection of farm workers, livestock, and wildlife from potentially harmful pesticides. However, organic foods can be contaminated by pesticides from nearby conventional farms and by viruses and bacteria, especially if farms do not follow USDA rules about use of animal manures.[13]

Other differences between organic and conventional foods include:[14]

- *Nutrition:* Research results have been mixed, with some studies finding higher levels of nutrients in organic foods and others uncovering no differences between organic and conventional crops. Weather, soil, and growing conditions also affect the nutritional content of foods. However, it appears that organic foods are at least as nutritious as non-organic foods.
- *Chemical residues:* Organic foods contain fewer pesticide residues in terms of both the number and the overall amount of chemicals. However, both organic and nonorganic foods must not exceed government-set safety thresholds for pesticide residues, so both organic and nonorganic are deemed safe. In general, domestically grown fruits and vegetables have lower chemical residues than imported crops.

Fast Facts

Food Allergies

- Children with food allergies: 6–8 percent
  - The most common food allergens among children: eggs, cow's milk, peanuts, tree nuts
    - Adults with food allergies: 3–4 percent
    - The most common food allergens among adults: shellfish, peanuts, tree nuts, fish, eggs
  - Annual episodes of food-induced anaphylaxis: 30,000
- Annual deaths from food-induced anaphylaxis: 100–200
- Leading causes of fatal and near-fatal food-allergic reactions: peanuts and tree nuts
- Percentage of people with food allergies experiencing an unintended exposure during a 2-year period: 50 percent

Source: National Institute of Allergy and Infectious Diseases. (2010). Quick facts. *Food Allergy* (http://wwww.niaid.nih.gov/topics/foodallergy/understanding/pages/quickfacts.aspx).

- *Foodborne illness:* Research findings have been inconclusive. On the one hand, opting for organic meat products reduces the risk of exposure to certain chemical residues and prion diseases (*prions* are pathogenic agents able to affect cellular proteins found most abundantly in the brain; when altered, they become fatal, often quickly). On the other hand, some organic production requirements may inherently increase the risk of certain types of bacterial or fungal contamination.

- *Cost:* Organic foods usually cost more—sometimes slightly more, sometimes substantially more—due to increased production costs and in some cases lower crop yields. In addition, because they have no preservatives, organic foods may have a shorter shelf life.

- *Taste:* Again, research findings have been mixed, with some people stating they can tell the difference and prefer the taste of organic foods and other people noticing no taste differences.

It's up to you to weigh the pros and cons of organic foods and decide what's right for you. *Consumer Reports* and the Organic Center (http://www.organic-center.org) make specific recommendations about the foods with the highest pesticide residues based on government test data. If you want to purchase organic foods, note that they are labeled in three different categories:

- *100% Organic:* Foods contain all organic ingredients.
- *Organic:* Foods must contain at least 95 percent organic ingredients.
- *Made with Organic:* Foods must contain at least 70 percent organic ingredients.

Foods in the first two categories can display the USDA Organic seal.

Q | Do irradiated foods give off radiation?

FOOD IRRADIATION. No. *Food irradiation* is the process of exposing food to ionizing radiation in order to kill bacteria, viruses, and other disease-causing and spoilage-causing organisms. The food does not become radioactive, and although there may be small chemical changes, the nutritional value of the food is essentially unchanged and the shelf life may actually increase.[15] In fact, medical devices are frequently sterilized with similar technology to eliminate infection risk. Even NASA uses irradiation to help prevent astronauts from getting foodborne illness in space—which would be really unpleasant! The effects of irradiation on food and on animals and people eating irradiated food have been studied extensively, with many benefits and few if any risks identified.

The Centers for Disease Control and Prevention (CDC) states that food irradiation is a safe and effective means of preventing many serious foodborne diseases that are transmitted through meat, poultry, fresh produce, and other foods. Traditionally, U.S. consumers have responded negatively to the idea of food irradiation, but attitudes may be changing as foodborne illness becomes a greater concern.

Foods treated with irradiation can be identified by the radura symbol. One caution: The fact that a food has been irradiated doesn't mean that you can relax your home food-safety measures. If a food is exposed to pathogens, it can still become contaminated, irradiated or not.

Making Changes for the Better

Q | What are the best ways to break bad eating habits?

Applying basic techniques of behavior change along with sound nutrition principles is the best way to change for the better. Start by assessing your diet and your commitment to change. Is improving your diet a real priority? It needs to be if you want to make lasting changes in your eating habits. Do you already have a good idea what eating patterns you'd like to change, and are these changes realistic? Have you recently tracked what you eat and considered what else is going on that might influence what and how much you are eating—where you generally are, whom you are with, what time of day you eat, and how you feel?

Assess your dietary pattern against MyPlate (see Lab Activity 9-1), and then set an appropriate SMART goal. For example, if your analysis shows that your fruit intake is very low, you might tackle that first. Turn your general goal—"eat more fruit"—into a specific one: "In the next 2 weeks, I will purchase at least 3 servings of fruit each time I go to the grocery store". There is no point in making a goal to eat more fruit if you don't first make a goal to purchase it.

Next, start on the path to change with strategies and interim goals such as these:

- Make a list of the fruits you like that are available at the local market, campus cafeteria, or snack truck, along with their prices. Then develop a plan specifying fruits to buy or select at the start of your program.
- Set specific behavioral goals—for example, "I will eat fruit with my breakfast on at least 3 days during each of the next 3 weeks" or "I will carry an apple or an orange for an afternoon snack each day this week." or "Instead of a regular soft drink, I will have water or diet soda during my afternoon work break today."
- Change your environment to make success more likely. For example, you may need not only to buy fruit but also to put it in the front of the refrigerator or on the counter to remind yourself of the change you're trying to make. If you usually buy a sweetened drink from a particular vending machine or mini-market, don't go near those places for a little while to help avoid the temptation. And if snacks, especially unhealthy ones, are within arm's length during most of your day, move them to a less convenient spot, because that strategy alone is likely to reduce the temptation.

Small measurable changes are quite achievable. Once you get started with a sound plan, you are more likely to experience early successes that will encourage you to keep moving forward. After a while, your new, healthier, eating will become a habit that you don't have to think much about.

Healthy Weight Loss and Maintenance

If you're like most Americans, maintaining a healthy weight will be a challenge at some point in your life. Although the basics of weight change are simple—calories in versus calories out—the complex factors affecting your eating and exercise patterns are much more difficult. For successful weight management, you need strong commitment, clear goals, and as many strategies and supports as you can make use of. And you need to stick with it. A diet for weight management isn't a temporary thing—it's a lifelong eating pattern.

Focus on Energy Balance

Think back to the energy balance concept introduced in Chapter 7, with its "energy in" and "energy out" sides. This energy balance has neutral, positive, and negative dimensions, as follows:

- *Neutral energy balance* means that you're taking in the same number of calories that you're using and your weight will remain stable.
- *Positive energy balance* means that you're consuming more calories than your body is using and you will gain weight.
- *Negative energy balance* means that you're consuming fewer calories than your body is using and you will lose weight.

Fundamentally, changes in weight result from changes on one or both sides of the energy balance equation. Today there are many incentives for increased calorie intake, among them supersize items, special restaurant "deals," and buffets. There are also plenty of reasons for decreased calorie output: Think about the labor-saving devices and conveniences that surround you. These environmental and social factors conspire to make it difficult for many individuals to effect lasting changes in their diet and activity level.

Q My weight's fine right now, so why should I worry?

It's great if your current weight is healthy and stable—and you should strive to maintain it since it's much easier to prevent weight gain than to lose weight after you've gained it. However, if you are like most American adults,

you will put weight on over time, normally about 1–2 pounds each year starting in your early twenties. So, if you don't want to arrive at your 20th high school reunion 40 pounds overweight, you'll need to take steps now to keep your weight in check. The Dietary Reference Intakes (DRI) recommend a decrease of 7–10 calories per day for each year starting around the mid twenties. This deficit may not sound like much, but it can add up over time.

Your level of physical activity is another key dimension to be aware of, as it can heavily influence your calorie output. It's often hard to fit in exercise once you're out of college and into an 8-to-5 job, but without finding the time, your body weight is likely to creep up. Make the effort now—you'll reap the rewards not only today but long into the future.

Q How many calories does it take to lose weight?

Weight gain results from a positive energy balance, and weight loss comes from a negative energy balance. It sounds simple, and in theory it is. But to lose weight, you must overcome powerful internal and external forces that shape your eating and activity habits (see the box "Is Whom We Eat with Just as Important as What We Eat?" for more information).

A pound of body weight is equivalent to 3,500 calories, so to lose a pound, you need to create a negative energy balance of 3,500 calories. Experts recommend weight loss at a pace of 1–2 pounds per week, which for most people can be accomplished with a daily negative energy balance of 500–1,000 calories achieved through a combination of taking in fewer calories and doing more exercise. Concretely put, replacing 300 calories worth of chips with 100 calories or so from an apple or a banana, along with modestly increasing your physical activity, goes a long way toward getting your scale pointed downward.

Usually, creating a negative energy balance is relatively easy at first and becomes more difficult as time goes on. Therefore, it's best to make the calorie deficit small and reasonable so that it can be sustained until your weight-loss goals are met.

Fast Facts

Is the "Freshman 15" for Real?

Do many (or most) students truly gain 15 pounds during their first year in college, as popular thinking would have us believe? Studies have indeed consistently found weight gain among freshmen—but the average gain is only 2–5 pounds. However, if the trend of putting on weight continues beyond the freshman year, it could turn into a problem. So, while you're studying and negotiating all the challenges that come with college, don't forget to choose nutrient-rich foods in moderate portions—and to get regular exercise.

- Have you and/or any friends gained weight since starting college? What has been the main cause?
  - What concrete steps would help you shed those extra pounds?

Source: Vella-Zarb, R. A., & Elgar, F. J. (2009). The "freshman 5": A meta-analysis of weight gain in the freshman year of college. *Journal of American College Health, 58*(2), 161–166.

Q | Can I use MyPlate as a weight-loss plan?

REDUCING ENERGY IN. Yes, MyPlate can help you create an eating pattern that reduces calorie intake and yet ensures that you still get all your essential nutrients. Once you know your target energy intake, you can select many different plans. For example, if you currently consume 2,400 calories and want to cut that by 400 calories per day, follow the 2,000-calorie-per-day plan. Consume the recommended amount of food from each food group *and* keep your discretionary calories below the limit. You can also use MyPlate to track your daily physical activity, with extra credit given for moderate or vigorous exercise.

Q | Which causes more weight loss—cutting carbs or cutting fat?

In general, cutting *calories* is what causes weight loss, and being more active is what helps sustain the weight loss. Research investigating whether cutting some specific combination of fat, protein, and carbohydrate is best for weight loss is inconclusive and to date indicates that no one food regimen is best.[16]

Too drastic a cut in calories is not recommended either. Experts advise cutting just a few hundred calories a day to ensure that the new diet can be maintained over time.[17]

The bottom line is that if the new eating plan is so different or difficult that it can't be maintained, then no matter what the claims or success of others, it is not likely to work. For example, if you really enjoy carbohydrate-rich foods, it might be difficult to adopt a low-carb diet. Instead, approach a new diet with moderation in mind. Cutting back a few hundred calories a day shouldn't be too hard. In fact, most people don't even notice taking in 100–300 fewer calories in any given day—and if they can sustain that calorie reduction, their weight-loss efforts will be successful regardless of whether they are cutting carbs, protein, fat, or some combination.

Q | Is there such a thing as cutting calories too much?

Significantly cutting back on your calories may make intuitive sense for weight loss, and it may work—but if it does, it will be effective for only a short time. Extreme calorie cutting also comes with extreme hunger, which usually causes a dieter to gain all the weight back. The reason is that extreme calorie restriction is almost always followed by calorie overcompensation, which is directly followed by putting back all the weight lost—and possibly more. This is just one of the many reasons to use moderation in your calorie-cutting plan. The lowest daily calorie intake recommended is 1,200 calories for women and 1,500 calories for men.

Some popular diets recommend an occasional fast, but this approach has its own worrisome drawbacks. Fasting leads to dehydration, lethargy, difficulty concentrating, sleeplessness, irritability, and more—none of which help you succeed in the classroom, on the job, or anywhere else for that matter. Fasting produces weight loss mostly from losing water, which the body quickly restores. Also, coming off a fast may stimulate an eating binge.

To develop a good sense of how many calories you are eating or cutting, seek out calorie-count information. Campus dining halls post nutritional information, including calorie counts, and fast-food chains include it on site in their restaurants for all to see (or you can look online in advance). Most quick-serve sit-down restaurants also post calories on site and online. Unfortunately, locally owned sit-down restaurants rarely offer nutritional information.[18]

When reading labels, pay attention to serving sizes (see the box "How Food Cues and Portion Size Impact Eating"

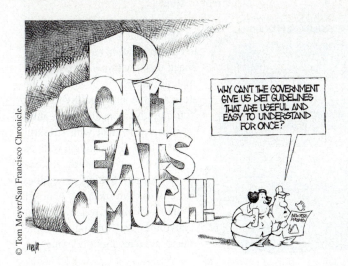

WHY CAN'T THE GOVERNMENT GIVE US DIET GUIDELINES THAT ARE USEFUL AND EASY TO UNDERSTAND FOR ONCE?

DON'T EAT SO MUCH!

© Tom Meyer/San Francisco Chronicle.

Research Brief

Is Whom We Eat with Just as Important as What We Eat?

Researchers recently set out to learn which external influence has the greatest effect on eating behavior: the behavior of others, taste, or hunger. In two studies by the same group of researchers, about 200 participants were tested for specific factors in eating, such as the presence of other people and the behavior of those individuals. These variables were manipulated in order to influence the amount of food that individuals consumed. The participants were asked afterward if it was the behavior of others, the food itself (taste), or their own hunger that drove their eating behavior. Across the two studies, researchers found that the amount of food participants ate

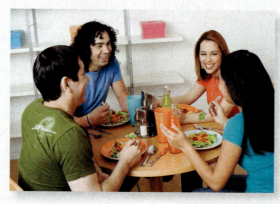

was influenced by being part of a group and also by observing their dining partners engage in certain behaviors. Interestingly, the participants' *subjective* ratings in both studies indicated that taste and hunger were the only driving factors to influence their eating.

Analyze and Apply

- What specific factors influence your eating?
- Who are the people you normally eat with, and how might they influence what and how much you eat?

Source: Vartanian, L. R., Herman, C. P., & Wansink, B. (2008). Are we aware of the external factors that influence our food intake? *Health Psychology, 27*(5), 533–538.

for an intriguing study). The label on the microwave popcorn box might say 180 calories per serving but also state that there are three servings per bag; if you eat the entire bag, that's 540 calories. Calorie content information is also available at ChooseMyPlate.gov.

Checking the calorie content of food—and keeping track of it—is a great weight-management strategy.[19] Studies of people who've lost weight and successfully kept it off show that self-monitoring works: One recent study found that those who tracked what they ate lost twice as much weight as those who did not; the record-keeping was most effective when done frequently, in detail, and close to meal and snack times.[20]

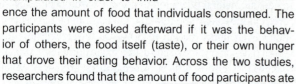

Q How can I not eat junk when I'm stressed out?

This question raises an important issue for weight management—the fact that we often eat for reasons other than hunger. These include stress, boredom, fatigue, and the desire or pressure to socialize. How can you avoid eating the wrong foods— and eating for the wrong reasons? Tracking your food habits and your motivations for eating can help.

This practice will make you more mindful—more aware of how your thoughts, emotions, and surroundings affect your eating habits. The goals are to develop food-free strategies to deal with stress and to opt for healthier snacks for times when you are feeling added pressure.

A sound strategy is to stock your room or kitchen with healthy snacks and place them in front of all the other foods. In fact, it's a good idea to avoid having less healthy snacks around at all; instead, make it so that if you really want them, you have to go to the store to get them. That way, you are forced to choose between having a healthy snack that's within your reach and making the effort to head to the store for the less healthy choice. You can also consider non-eating alternatives to deal with stressful times, including taking a walk as soon as you get home, instead of eating; texting or calling a friend to distract yourself and to make it tougher to eat anything; and turning on some music and dancing or relaxing.

DOLLAR STRETCHER
Financial Wellness Tip

Make your own snack packs—you'll save money, juice up your nutrient intake, and reduce your hunger. Package small servings of fruit, raw vegetables, yogurt, whole-grain crackers, and low-fat granola in little portable packs. Just make sure to keep them to a reasonable calorie count, 150 or less.

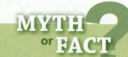

MYTH or FACT?

As a general rule, avoid eating after 9 p.m., because those calories are usually stored as body fat.

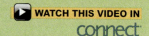

WATCH THIS VIDEO IN connect

See page 477 to find out.

Research Brief

How Food Cues and Portion Size Impact Eating

Researchers have tried to determine whether food portion size would have an explicit effect on both absolute amounts eaten and perceived amounts eaten. Fifty-four participants were invited in groups of four to eat soup, with two of the four bowls in each group designed to refill automatically and slowly so that they were never empty. Participants were randomly assigned to eat from either a self-refilling soup bowl or a regular soup bowl that emptied naturally as the individual ate. The final results also took into account the participants' body mass index (BMI).

The results showed that individuals eating from the self-refilling bowls consumed 73 percent more soup than those eating from regular bowls yet perceived themselves to have eaten the same amount as people eating from regular bowls. In addition to believing that they had consumed the same amount as those eating from regular bowls, the participants who ate from self-refilling bowls did not report feeling any fuller compared to those who ate from regular bowls, even after eating quite a bit more soup.

The researchers concluded that the visual cue of food—in this case, a bowl that was never empty—prompted individuals to keep eating because it altered their perception of expectation. In essence, we expect that as we eat, our bowl or plate should become emptier, and if it does not, we keep eating until it does. Therefore, a second conclusion was that the portion size also influenced the participants' ability to self-monitor their intake, including their perception of food consumed and their feelings of fullness.

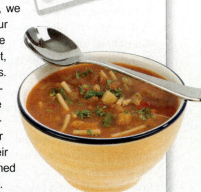

Analyze and Apply

- What do the results of this study suggest about the size of the dishes one uses for meals?
- How might you modify the dishes you use as a strategy to eat less food or more food?

Source: Wansink, B., Painter, J. E., & North, J. (2005) Bottomless bowls: Why visual cues of portion size may influence intake. *Obesity Research, 13*(1), 93–100.

A related challenge is dealing with the overabundance and easy availability of less healthy food. Such food is available almost everywhere. Vending machine treats, fast food, buffet meals, meeting snacks, holiday goodies—the list goes on and on. Even many campus dining halls offer buffet-style all-you-can-eat meals, including unlimited desserts.

The abundance and variety of food surrounding us are reason to establish good control over our food environment. Whenever possible, choose nutrient-rich over calorie-rich foods; avoid settings where you are likely to overeat; and focus on what you are eating—and how much. Keep healthier choices in plain view and easy to grab. And be aware of other influences on your eating habits—from television ads to the arrangement of foods in the grocery store and dining hall—to lessen their impact on you.

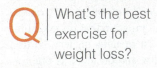

Q Why does weight loss seem to plateau?

It's not uncommon for the rate of weight loss to slow down over time. At the start of a weight-loss program, you may quickly lose some fluid weight, after which you will shed weight more slowly. Weight lost after the first few weeks is likely to be body fat—so although the losses may be smaller, they're the type of losses you want. Also, calorie intake can slowly creep up over time, thereby offsetting the negative energy balance. Try monitoring your food intake closely to see what's going on.

Consider, though, that a plateau can be OK, especially when it indicates that you have reached a comfortable weight. It is unrealistic to think that once you start losing weight, you can or should go on forever. It is important to keep in mind both safe weight minimums and the benefits of taking a reasonable, healthy approach to food and weight management. It is all too easy to become obsessed with weight loss and to slip into patterns of disordered eating, excessive exercise, or both.

The goal should be to achieve a balanced state of weight management, which requires a lifelong commitment. Ultimately, if you monitor your food intake and get enough exercise, the weight will take care of itself.

Another reason for weight loss to plateau is the drop in the body's metabolic rate, which is about 8 calories per pound lost per day. This translates into about 80 fewer calories burned by the body per day if you've already lost 10 pounds.[21] Therefore, the more you lose, the harder it becomes to lose more. This reality is yet another good reason to prevent weight gain in the first place.

Q What's the best exercise for weight loss?

INCREASING ENERGY OUT. The best exercise program for weight loss is the one you'll keep doing. Preferably it will include both aerobic exercise and strength training. Exercise uses energy ("energy out") and should be an important part of your

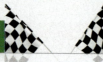

Fast Facts

Mindless Eating

Americans can be mindless eaters. Consider these facts. Research shows that movie-goers will happily eat stale popcorn as long as they are distracted by the movie—and the bigger the bucket, the more they eat. We eat half of a month's worth of bulk snack foods in the first 7 days after purchase; the rest tends to get thrown out. Short, wide drinking glasses make us pour more of a beverage than do tall, skinny glasses; most of us focus on the height of the beverage as their guide.

People tend to overeat more at a deli than in a fast-food restaurant. Fast food doesn't pretend to be anything it isn't, but some deli foods can give the impression of being healthy. At the deli counter, most individuals underestimate their calories by almost half. And when food comes in a great deal of variety (think candy), people are visually attracted to it and therefore eat much more.

- What are some unusual American eating habits you are aware of?
- What are some times you eat without being aware of what or how much you are consuming?

Source: Wansink, B. Mindless Eating. Bantam. NY, NY. 2006.

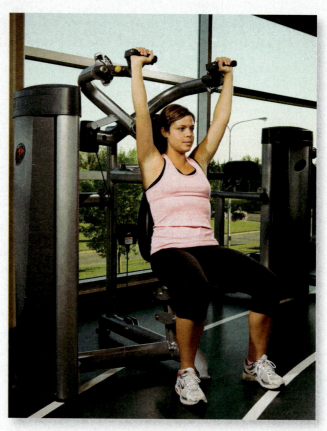

Exercise is a vital part of a healthy lifestyle for weight management. Endurance activities burn calories, and strength training maintains muscle mass and helps reduce the drop in metabolic rate that comes with weight loss.

negative energy balance equation along with reasonable dietary portion control. See the box "Tips and Techniques for Successful Weight Management."

The amount of exercise needed to lose weight and maintain weight loss varies from person to person, but many people need more than 300 minutes per week of moderate-intensity aerobic exercise (or 150 minutes of vigorous exercise) in order to maintain weight loss. Participants in the National Weight Control Registry—an ongoing study of people who have lost a substantial amount of weight and kept it off—engage in an average of 1 hour of exercise per day, which amounts to about 2,600 calories (energy) used per week through moderate-intensity exercise.[22] The 2008 physical activity guidelines suggest at least 150 minutes per week of moderate exercise but also clearly state that this is not likely to produce any significant weight loss. Greater exercise durations and/or greater intensities are needed for weight loss and weight-loss maintenance. You can try different amounts and intensities of exercise to determine what works best for you. Any amount of exercise is better than none, so develop a program that fits your life.

What type of exercise is best remains unclear, so find one or more activities you enjoy and do them as often as you can. Walking is popular, but there is no reason why you can't do or try any number of activities. And don't forget strength training to maintain your muscle mass, which

will otherwise decrease as you begin to lose weight. There really isn't a magic exercise, just consistency. You might find good motivation in the ChooseMyPlate.gov page for calories burned by different exercises.

In addition to helping with weight loss, exercise has many other direct health and wellness benefits. A program that combines a reduction in calories with an increase in exercise will yield the best results for your overall health.[23]

Lab Activity 9-2 will help you develop your weight-management program. Once you've got your plan in place, you're ready to get started!

Weight-Loss Plans, Products, and Procedures

Stores are full of plans and products promising easy weight loss. But just because a diet book has been advertised or a supplement has made it to store shelves doesn't mean it's safe and effective for weight loss.

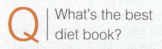

Q | What's the best diet book?   There are many, but keep in mind that any diet that sounds too good to be true probably is. Evaluate all diet plans critically. Avoid those that promise rapid, easy weight loss or say that there's no

Wellness Strategies

Tips and Techniques for Successful Weight Management

Q | What are some realistic, practical techniques for weight loss?

Create Realistic Goals and Plans

- Set a realistic SMART goal, such as preventing or stopping weight gain or achieving a small, maintainable weight loss.
- Break your long-term goal into small steps.
- Create an eating plan that won't leave you terribly hungry; allow at least 1,200 calories per day for women or 1,500 calories per day for men.

Monitor Your Behavior and Progress

- Track your food intake and physical activity.
- Weigh yourself regularly, as doing so is associated with better outcomes. (Some may need to skip this practice if it is too stressful.)

Manage Portion Sizes and Hunger

- Check food labels for the calories per serving and the total number of servings in the package.
- Measure and weigh your food portions using a measuring cup and spoon and a food scale until your "eye" is accurate.
- Serve food on small plates and in small bowls to make small servings seem more generous.
- When you eat at home, don't keep the serving dishes on the table.
- Start meals with a glass of water, a cup of vegetable soup, or a high-fiber food to help fill you up.
- Eat slowly to give the hunger center of your brain the 15–20 minutes it needs to catch up with what you've eaten. (Take small bites, chew your food, and pay attention to the flavors.)
- When you finish, clear the table and put the leftovers away; don't linger and pick at the food.
- Don't eat chips, crackers, and cookies out of the bag or box. Take a moderate portion and serve it in a dish.
- Eat four or five regular snacks and meals daily, including breakfast, spreading your food intake across the day. Eat small snacks between meals to avoid getting overly hungry.

Make Healthy Dietary and Activity Changes

- Choose foods that are nutrient rich, not calorie dense.
- Cut back on added sugars, solid fats, alcohol, and some refined grains. Maintain or increase your intake of fruits, vegetables, whole grains, and lean protein and dairy foods.
- Eat at home when you can. Prepare healthy, flavorful foods you enjoy.
- Exercise regularly. Even small increases in physical activity help.

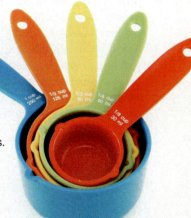

Change Your Environment

- Remove energy-dense foods from your residence; stock up on healthy foods and snacks.
- Place nutrient-rich choices in front of less healthy options.
- Keep food away from the TV and computer; having it in easy reach leads to mindless overeating.
- Avoid settings where you typically overeat. Identify cues for overeating, such as the break room at your job, and change or avoid them.

Take Care of Yourself

- Get adequate sleep.
- Manage your stress through exercise, relaxation techniques, and/or talking with friends.
- Develop strategies for dealing with other emotional triggers for eating, including anger and boredom.
- Maintain a positive body image; see Chapter 7 for tips.
- Engage in positive self-talk about your weight-management efforts; enjoy your food and imagine the beneficial effects of healthy food choices on wellness.
- Get support from friends and family.

---

need to cut calories or to exercise. Also steer clear of diets that involve extreme or gimmicky eating patterns, such as special food combinations, very rigid or complex eating rules or menus, or very limited food selections. Any healthy dietary approach should advocate variety and moderation. Visit the Academy of Nutrition and Dietetics Web site for consumers (http://www.eatright.org/public) and look for the section on "Diet Reviews" to read reviews of over 100 diet books. If you need help in developing a

personalized weight-loss plan, talk with your physician or a registered dietitian.

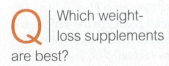

Q | Which weight-loss supplements are best?

The truth is that none of the countless weight-loss supplements that are available have been proven safe and effective for weight loss. A recent study of a variety of weight-loss supplements found

Many new weight-loss apps are available for smartphones and tablet computers such as the iPad. If you're thinking about trying a weight-loss app, here are some things to consider. Are you willing to pay for an app (some pretty good ones cost less than $5.00)? Are you interested in an app that allows you to interact with others who are trying to lose weight? What drawbacks and benefits might there be in using a weight-loss app as opposed to a more traditional weight-loss program? Will you actually use the app—and use it faithfully? A weight-loss app can provide many of the benefits seen in commercial weight-loss programs at a fraction of the cost, but it all comes down to your being willing to use it.

that none appeared to work any better than a placebo for weight loss.[24]

Most advertised weight-loss supplements contain products, natural or synthetic, that attempt to increase your metabolism or suppress your appetite. Although on the surface this approach may seem logical, it is not. In fact, inundating your body with unregulated chemicals is potentially harmful. Marketers, however, like to note that these products are "natural," implying that they must be good for you. The truth is that natural isn't always good, that some supplements are contaminated with other compounds, and that in certain cases and combinations, supplements can be dangerous or even fatal. In 2004, for example, the FDA banned the sale of dietary supplements containing ephedra, stating that the products carried unacceptable health risks, including high blood pressure, insomnia, irregular heart rate, heart attack, stroke, and death. While on the market, products containing ephedra—a "natural" substance derived from a plant—made up less than 1 percent of all dietary supplement sales but accounted for 64 percent of adverse events associated with supplements.[25]

As described in Chapter 8, supplements are not regulated the same way as prescription or over-the-counter drugs are, and they do not have to be proven safe or effective before being sold. Some supplements are believed to carry risks, and the long-term effects of many are unknown.[26] Although ingredients are listed on the label, there is no guarantee that the supplement contains those ingredients in those proportions. In addition, there have been high-profile cases of supplement contamination. The FDA has found that supplements promoted for weight loss, bodybuilding, and sexual enhancement make claims that have no scientific evidence to support them and should be used with extreme caution.[27]

Q | Can I take a pill, eat whatever I want, and still lose weight?

No. A number of prescription drugs have come and gone from the retail market intended for weight loss, however, none allow for unlimited eating. Prescription drugs are usually recommended only for individuals with a BMI over 30, although they may be appropriate for those with lower BMIs if they have significant obesity-related health problems.[28]

As of mid-2012, there are only two prescription drugs used to treat obesity, including phentermine, which suppresses appetite, and orlistat (brand name Xenical), which keeps some dietary fat from being absorbed by the intestine. Orlistat is also sold in a lower dose over-the-counter version as Alli.

In July 2012, the FDA granted approval of a third weight-loss drug, lorcaserin (brand name Belviq), which is the first to work on brain chemistry to initiate feelings of fullness. Unlike orlistat, which inhibits the absorption of up to 30 percent of the fat you consume, meaning that those calories aren't absorbed, lorcaserin makes you feel full sooner, thereby causing you to eat less. Studies have found modest weight loss among orlistat users—after 12 months, about 6 pounds on average for those taking the drug[29], and preliminary trials of lorcaserin show similar weight loss.

One other similarity between these two drugs is the stated need to eat wisely and exercise regularly, as no one drug can be expected to "do it all." Having a healthy lifestyle, with or without pharmaceutical help, is the key to long-term wellness.

In 2010, the FDA warned users of orlistat and Alli of a rare but serious side effect—liver failure—in a small number of people using the drugs.[30] At the same time, lorcaserin has shown an increased risk in heart valve failure[31], but the FDA deems that risk inferior to the potential benefits of lost

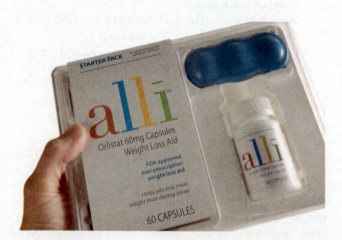

In order to be successful, all medical treatments for obesity—prescription and over-the-counter drugs and surgery—also require lifestyle changes, including a reduced-calorie diet and exercise.

weight. For anyone considering use of a weight-loss medication, the health risks from the drug must be balanced against the risks from overweight or obesity. For some people, use of prescription medications can help jump-start their weight-loss efforts and reduce the health risks associated with obesity. But as with any other weight-loss method, the key is to stick with the lifestyle changes—reduced-calorie diet, increased physical activity—over the long term.

Q What are gastric bypass and liposuction? Which is a better choice for losing a lot of weight?

Gastric bypass is a surgical procedure for the morbidly obese. It is recommended only when other approaches to weight loss have failed, and performed after a thorough medical and psychological evaluation. Gastric bypass is typically restricted for those with a BMI of at least 35 or 40 and experiencing serious health problems such as diabetes, hypertension, and heart disease. Gastric bypass involves creating a small pouch by stapling or removing portions of the stomach to reduce the amount of food that can be eaten. The surgery also bypasses part of the small intestine, thereby preventing the absorption of some calories and nutrients. (A related procedure involves placing an adjustable band around the top of the stomach to allow only a small amount of food to enter.) *Liposuction* is quite different: It's an elective cosmetic procedure that is not intended to produce any significant weight loss but instead to "reshape" certain areas of the body by removing primarily subcutaneous fat.

Neither of these surgeries is something you should consider just to lose weight. Both entail risks, including complications such as bleeding, infection, and blood clots. Although gastric bypass makes the stomach smaller, it's still possible for those who have undergone the surgery to regain a considerable amount of weight if they do not maintain dietary changes. Liposuction has no significant weight-loss benefits, and the aesthetic gains will quickly disappear if there isn't a change toward healthier eating and increased physical activity.

For more on surgery and other approaches to weight loss, visit the Web site of the Weight-control Information Network (http://win.niddk.nih.gov).

Healthy Weight Gain

Q I need to gain some weight but I don't want flab. Do I just eat more?

You do need to eat more, but you must be careful about the foods you choose—and you need to exercise. Although many Americans are concerned with being overweight, some people are underweight. Being underweight can result from an eating disorder or a chronic disease, but it can also be a concern for athletes and naturally thin people who wish to be bigger, stronger, and more muscular. In addition, elderly people may become underweight due to a gradual loss of taste and smell or the inability to prepare healthy meals.

Although being underweight isn't usually thought of as a health risk, people who are significantly underweight (BMI under 18.5) have much higher rates of premature death. Older people who are underweight are at higher risk for falls and broken bones, often the result of osteoporosis. Also, at any age, men who are chronically underweight are at greater risk for erectile dysfunction.

Even though you need to increase your calorie intake to gain weight, those calories should come from healthy, nutrient-rich foods. Eating more empty calories (energy-dense foods) will cause you to gain weight but also increase your risk for a number of chronic diseases. You need to eat 3,500 extra calories to gain a pound, so be sure to aim for healthy choices. There is no need for expensive supplements.

Here are some weight-gain strategies:

- Eat five or six times a day—regular meals and snacks. Don't drink a big glass of water or other beverage right before or while you're eating; leave room in your stomach for more healthy food.
- Add concentrated sources of calories, such as nuts, nut butters, and nonfat milk powder, to some of your typical foods.
- For breakfast, have an extra slice of whole-grain toast or a whole-grain muffin topped with peanut butter. Make hot cereals with milk instead of water, and add dried fruits and nuts.
- Top salads with legumes, sunflower seeds, avocados, and dressings made with unsaturated vegetable oils.
- For dinner, try larger portions of baked chicken or fish and whole-grain pasta or rice.
- Opt for healthy snack choices such as whole-grain crackers with peanut butter, nuts and seeds, dried fruit, yogurt, and low-fat granola.

One other important note: Be realistic about your goal. Body size and muscularity are partly determined by your genes. If everyone in your family has a thin body type, you will be limited as to how much muscle you can add.

Q What kind of workout should I do to gain weight? Avoid cardio?

Not exactly. Exercise is critical for healthy weight gain—and you want to gain weight in the form of increased muscle size and not increased fat stores. Although you shouldn't completely avoid endurance exercise, resistance training is more important, to increase muscle size. Keep doing cardio training, but put more emphasis on strength training because burning too many calories through aerobic exercise can slow down weight gain.

To increase muscle size, regularly apply the overload principle. That means working hard each time you work out. Chapter 5 has more specific details on strength training, with recommendations from the American College of Sports Medicine.[32] Be patient—adding muscle and gaining weight takes time to do right. And recall that men have a greater capacity for hypertrophy than women.

Eating Disorders

This chapter has emphasized choosing a moderate, nutrient-rich diet for wellness and weight management. Although you need to be concerned about your body composition and weight in terms of your health, your weight-management goals need to be realistic and must take into account your genes, lifestyle, and personal circumstances. For someone who is overweight, even a small amount of weight loss has significant health benefits. It's important to focus on good health—and not to be overly concerned with body weight and shape.

The truth is that many body sizes and shapes are associated with good health, and a positive body image is also important for wellness. The reality, however, is that our cultural ideals for body type and weight have been moving away from the size and shape of the average American for decades; and the media's emphasis on unattainable body types can hurt body image. A negative body image detracts from emotional wellness and can contribute to the development of an **eating disorder,** a severe disturbance in eating behavior involving insufficient or excessive food intake.

The challenge is to avoid comparing yourself to perceived cultural and media ideals. Instead, set body-weight goals according to what is healthy and realistic for you. See the suggestions in Chapter 7 for maintaining a positive body image.

Q | My roommate hardly ever wants to have dinner with us and never goes out to eat with us. Should I be worried?

Eating disorders are pretty common during college, particularly in females. Although your roommate's behavior is suspicious, it may be unrelated to disordered eating.

There are three primary types of eating disorders:

- **Anorexia nervosa,** characterized by extreme thinness and intense fear of gaining weight
- **Bulimia nervosa,** characterized by frequent bouts of binge eating following by purging or excessive exercise to compensate for the extra calories consumed
- **Binge-eating disorder,** characterized by binge eating without compensatory purging

Each type of eating disorder is distinguished by specific behaviors and risks (Table 9-4). All are dangerous, especially anorexia, which has one of the highest death rates of any psychological disorder.[33]

According to the National Institute of Mental Health, women and girls are most likely to develop eating disorders, but about 5–15 percent of people with anorexia or bulimia and 35 percent of those with binge-eating disorder are male.[34] Many individuals with eating disorders have other psychological problems, including depression, anxiety, or substance abuse. Eating disorders most often develop during adolescence or young adulthood, but they can also arise in childhood or later in adulthood.

For some people, eating disorders develop after a period of dieting, but the underlying causes are complex. Individuals with low self-esteem, feelings of inadequacy or lack of control, and extremely negative body image may be more likely than others to develop an eating disorder. People with bulimia are often impulsive, whereas those with anorexia tend to be controlling or perfectionist. Additional risk factors for eating disorders include a history of being teased about body shape or weight, a history of physical or sexual abuse, past failed attempts at dieting, relationship problems, and involvement in a sport or an activity (such as dance or modeling) that emphasizes thinness. Cultural ideals and social influences on eating patterns can also play a role. For a person with an eating disorder, behaviors such as extreme dieting, bingeing, and purging may provide a sense of control or a way to deal with stress and other painful emotions.

Q | How can I tell if a friend has an eating disorder?

Someone with anorexia will be extremely thin or rapidly losing weight. Other behaviors associated with anorexia include repeatedly weighing oneself, skipping meals or avoiding eating in front of others, taking tiny portions, and eating in a ritualistic way such as counting out food items or bites. People with anorexia may also shop and cook for friends but not eat themselves. And individuals with anorexia may be unaware they have an eating disorder and may vehemently deny that they are too thin.

People with binge-eating disorder or bulimia are usually of normal weight or overweight, so they are more difficult to identify. Binge eaters are usually aware and ashamed of their behavior and try to hide it, concealing food and eating in secret. In the case of bulimics, others may notice large stashes of food that seem to disappear

eating disorder A severe disturbance in eating patterns and behavior involving insufficient or excessive food intake.

anorexia nervosa An eating disorder characterized by extreme thinness, intense fear of gaining weight, distorted body image, and disturbed eating behaviors.

bulimia nervosa An eating disorder characterized by frequent binge-purge cycles, or rapid consumption of an unusually large amount of food followed by compensatory purging through vomiting, fasting, excessive exercise, or use of laxatives or diuretics.

binge-eating disorder An eating disorder characterized by binge eating, in which an individual rapidly consumes an unusually large amount of food; binges are not followed by purges, and most people with the disorder are overweight.

TABLE 9-4 EATING DISORDERS: CHARACTERISTICS AND RISKS

	CHARACTERISTICS	SYMPTOMS AND RISKS
ANOREXIA NERVOSA	■ Emaciation, relentless pursuit of thinness, and unwillingness to maintain a normal, healthy weight ■ Distorted body image (seeing oneself as overweight even when dangerously thin) ■ Intense fear of gaining weight ■ Extremely disturbed eating behavior ■ Weight loss through excessive diet and exercise, use of self-induced vomiting, or misuse of laxatives, diuretics, or enemas ■ Lack of menstruation	■ Thinning of bones ■ Brittle hair and nails ■ Dry and yellowish skin, growth of fine hair over body ■ Anemia, muscle weakness and loss ■ Severe constipation ■ Low blood pressure, slowed breathing and pulse, lethargy ■ Drop in internal body temperature ■ Depression, anxiety, obsessive behavior ■ Death from complications (cardiac arrest, electrolyte and fluid imbalances, suicide)
BULIMIA NERVOSA	■ Recurrent, frequent binge-purge cycles: eating an unusually large amount of food followed by compensatory purging (vomiting or use of laxatives or diuretics), fasting, or excessive exercise ■ Feeling a lack of control over eating ■ Fear of gaining weight ■ Unhappiness with body size and shape ■ Disgust or shame about eating behavior ■ Normal weight or slightly underweight	■ Electrolyte imbalance ■ Gastrointestinal problems (reflux disorder, irritation from laxative abuse) ■ Worn tooth enamel and decaying teeth from exposure to stomach acids ■ Chronically inflamed and sore throat ■ Kidney problems from diuretic abuse ■ Dehydration from purging fluids ■ Depression, social withdrawal ■ Death from complications (cardiac arrest from irregular heartbeat)
BINGE-EATING DISORDER	■ Recurrent, frequent episodes of binge eating; no compensatory purging ■ Feeling a lack of control over eating ■ Disgust or shame about eating behavior ■ Overweight or obesity	■ Risks from excess body weight, including high blood pressure and type 2 diabetes ■ Depression

Source: Adapted from National Institute of Mental Health. (2009). *Eating disorders* (http://www.nimh.nih.gov/health/publications/eating-disorders/complete-index.shtml).

quickly, frequent trips to the bathroom after meals, excessive and rigid exercise regimens, discolored teeth (from vomiting), and withdrawal from usual activities and friends.

Eating disorders are serious, sometimes life-threatening conditions that require medical and psychiatric treatment. If you suspect someone has an eating disorder, talk to her or him. Communicate your concerns in a caring way, and offer specific examples of your friend's eating or exercise behaviors that you've noticed and that you're worried about. Express your support and offer to help find a counselor, nutritionist, or other health care professional.

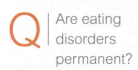

Q | Are eating disorders permanent?

No, but this doesn't mean they are easy to treat. The first step in treating an eating disorder is acknowledging its presence, which can be difficult, especially for someone with anorexia.

A troubling recent development has been the spread of pro-eating-disorder Web sites that describe, endorse, and support anorexia and bulimia. These sites provide tips for behaviors like purging and hiding rapid weight loss from others. By providing advice and support, these sites may normalize what are actually extreme and dangerous behaviors, making them appear safe and also making it more difficult for individuals to confront the severity of their condition.[35]

Once a problem is recognized, the person needs to seek help from a health care professional with training and experience in treating eating disorders. Referrals are available from the National Eating Disorders Association (800-931-2237; http://www.nationaleatingdisorders.org). The treatment plan depends on the nature of the symptoms and any physical problems. For example, someone with anorexia who is extremely thin and experiencing an irregular heart rhythm will likely need to be treated in the hospital, at least to start. In other cases, outpatient therapy can be appropriate. Treatment may involve medication, psychotherapy, and nutritional counseling.

If you suspect someone has an eating disorder, including yourself, it's best to address the issue, not avoid it. Eating disorders can be life threatening, but when they are acknowledged, they can be successfully treated. No one has to struggle with an eating disorder—help is available.

Summary

A healthy diet is one that allows you to meet your nutrient needs, enjoy your food, and maintain a healthy body weight. Several dietary patterns can meet the goals of a healthy diet, including the USDA's ChooseMyPlate, the DASH diet, the Mediterranean diet, and a variety of vegetarian eating patterns. For most Americans, bringing their current diet in line with a healthy dietary pattern requires eating more fruits, vegetables, whole grains, lean meats, fish, and low-fat dairy while limiting intake and portion sizes of foods and beverages high in calories from solid fats, added sugars, and alcohol.

Strategies that can help you maintain a healthy eating pattern include preparing foods at home, making wise choices when eating out, and using sound food-safety practices. Successful weight loss and maintenance require permanent changes to eating and exercise habits.

Most weight-loss products do not promote safe and effective long-term results. Prescription drugs or surgery should be considered only when other weight-control measures have been unsuccessful and body weight is causing significant health problems. Like severe obesity, eating disorders are serious medical conditions that require treatment.

Put weight management in the proper perspective—it is important but it should not be all that you think about. Eating should be a pleasurable activity. Be adventurous and try different foods; just make sure to do everything in moderation, including regular exercise. Enjoy your food, eat well, and be happy.

More to Explore

American Dietetic Association
 http://www.eatright.org/Public

DASH Eating Plan
 http://www.nhlbi.nih.gov/hbp/prevent/h_eating/h_eating.htm

FoodSafety.gov
 http://www.foodsafety.gov

Health Canada: Food and Nutrition
 http://www.hc-sc.gc.ca/fn-an/index-eng.php

MedlinePlus: Weight Control
 http://www.nlm.nih.gov/medlineplus/weightcontrol.html

MyPlate
 http://www.choosemyplate.gov

National Eating Disorders Association
 http://www.NationalEatingDisorders.org

Nutrition.gov
 http://www.nutrition.gov

Weight-control Information Network
 http://win.niddk.nih.gov

NAME	DATE	SECTION

This lab asks you to compare your diet to the pattern recommended by MyPlate. You can complete the analysis for 1 day, but for a more complete and accurate assessment of your diet, average and then analyze the results from 3 days, including a weekday and a weekend day.

Equipment: None

Preparation: None

Instructions

Fill in the target total intake goals for each food group for your energy level from Figure 9-2. Make as many copies of the log as you need, depending on the number of days you're assessing. Track the amount of foods from each food group you consume over the course of the day in terms of ounce equivalent, cups, and so on. Complete the analysis using the following log or the free online nutrition analysis available at MyPlate Tracker (http://www.myplate tracker.gov). If you complete the analysis online, you can repeat it periodically to see how your diet changes.

Day of the week (circle): M T W Th F Sa Su

☐ = 1 cup or ounce equivalent ▷ = ½ cup or ounce equivalent

GROUP / AMOUNTS		CHECK NUMBER CONSUMED	MY TOTAL	TARGET TOTAL*
Grains (1 oz eq = 1 slice bread, 1 cup dry cereal, ½ cup cooked rice or pasta)	Whole-grain	☐ ☐ ☐ ☐ ☐ ☐ ☐ ▷	oz eq	oz eq
	Other	☐ ☐ ☐ ☐ ☐ ☐ ☐ ▷	oz eq	oz eq
Vegetables (1 cup raw or cooked vegetables, 2 cups leafy greens)		☐ ☐ ☐ ☐ ☐ ☐ ☐ ▷	cups	cups
Fruits (1 cup fruit or juice, ½ cup dried fruit)		☐ ☐ ☐ ☐ ☐ ▷	cups	cups
Dairy (1 cup milk/yogurt, 1½ oz natural cheese, 2 oz processed cheese)		☐ ☐ ☐ ☐ ☐ ▷	cups	cups
Protein (1 oz eq = 1 oz meat, 1 egg, ¼ cup legumes, 1 Tbsp peanut butter, ½ oz nuts/seeds)	Low-sat-fat	☐ ☐ ☐ ☐ ☐ ☐ ☐ ▷	oz eq	oz eq
	High-sat-fat	☐ ☐ ☐ ☐ ☐ ☐ ☐ ▷	oz eq	oz eq
Oils (tsp)		☐ ☐ ☐ ☐ ☐ ☐ ☐ ▷ ☐ ☐ ☐ ☐ ☐ ☐ ☐	tsp	tsp

*Target total from Figure 9-2 or http://www.choosemyplate.gov.

Additional information

Number of vegetable subgroups consumed (dark green, orange/red, starchy, legume, other): ☐
Other foods eaten that don't fit into the groups:

Comments (including environmental cues—locations, people, day/times—that triggered overeating or poor choices):

___

Results

Complete the following chart by averaging your totals for the number of days you tracked and then comparing them to the recommended MyPlate totals for each group. (If you used SuperTracker or another digital software tool, copy your results into the chart.)

GROUP / AMOUNTS		MY AVERAGE TOTAL	TARGET TOTAL*
Grains	Whole-grain	oz eq	oz eq
	Other	oz eq	oz eq
Vegetables		cups	cups
Fruits		cups	cups
Dairy		cups	cups
Protein	Low-sat-fat	oz eq	oz eq
	High-sat-fat	oz eq	oz eq
Oils		tsp	tsp

Average number of vegetable subgroups consumed (dark green, orange/red, starchy, legume, other): ___

Other foods eaten that don't fit into the groups:

___

Reflecting on Your Results

How did your diet stack up against the recommendations? Were there any areas of concern—food groups for which you consumed more or less than the amounts recommended for you? The recommendations are averages, so you don't have to meet every guideline, every day, but your analysis does provide a benchmark. Were you at all surprised by the results?

___

Planning Your Next Steps

Choose one food group for which you could improve your intake—either increase or decrease your overall intake or improve the quality of your choices—in order to bring it in line with the guidelines. Develop at least three strategies for improving your intake from that food group. Consider the foods you ate during your analysis: Where could you make changes? What foods might you add, subtract, or substitute?

___

If your typical daily diet follows the MyPlate pattern, congratulations—and keep it up!

COMPLETE IN connect

NAME	DATE	SECTION

Equipment: None

Preparation: None

Instructions

Identify the Pros and Cons of Weight Loss for You

PROS	CONS

Set a SMART Goal

If you set a body-weight goal in Lab Activity 7-2 based on body-composition assessment, you can use that as your long-term goal. You can also set a lifestyle or behavior goal. Make sure your goal meets all the SMART criteria.

Calculate a Negative Calorie Balance

If you've set a body-weight goal, you will need to maintain a negative calorie balance for a period of time. Use the formulas below to determine your daily negative-calorie-balance goal and the number of weeks you will need to meet this goal.

1. Current weight ☐ lb − target weight (from Lab 7-2) ☐ lb = total weight to lose ☐ lb

2. Total weight to lose ☐ lb ÷ weekly weight loss* ☐ lb = time to achieve target ☐ weeks

3. Weekly weight loss target ☐ lb × 3,500 cal/lb = weekly negative calorie balance ☐ cal/week

4. Weekly negative calorie balance ☐ cal/week ÷ 7 days/week = daily negative calorie balance

    ☐ cal/day

*A loss of no more than 1–2 lb/week is recommended for most people.

You can achieve a daily negative calorie balance by taking in fewer calories (eating less) or expending more energy (being more active), or both. Most people find that pursuing both strategies at the same time is most effective.

Strategies for Reducing Energy In

Identify at least three strategies for reducing calorie intake. You might eliminate certain items from your typical daily diet (sweetened beverages, high-calorie snacks) or substitute lower-calorie choices (low-fat milk instead of whole milk). You can identify exactly how many empty calories a food contains using the MyPlate Super-Tracker Food-A-Pedia (https://www.choosemyplate.gov/SuperTracker/foodapedia.aspx). Be realistic. Calculate the total calories saved by your strategies.

1.	
2.	
3.	
Others:	Total calories cut: _____

Strategies for Increasing Energy Out

Identify at least three realistic strategies for increasing calorie expenditure, and calculate the total extra calories burned by your strategies. Use the activity calorie costs in Table 7-4.

1.	
2.	
3.	
Others:	Total calories expended: _____

Strategy Check

Add up your calories cut and calories expended [   ]

Have you met your negative calorie balance goal? If not, go back and make additional adjustments.

Changes to Habits or Environment

Develop strategies to help make your targeted change; look for ideas in the Wellness Strategies boxes throughout the chapter. For example, if reducing portion sizes is part of your plan, you might measure your portions for a week or use a smaller plate. Identify at least three strategies to make changes to your habits or environment to support your behavior-change efforts.

1.
2.
3.
Others:

Monitoring

Tracking some part of your effort—what you're eating and/or your physical activity—boosts your changes of success. Develop a plan for self-monitoring and briefly describe what you'll do.

Confidence Check

Your plan is in place, and you're ready to start. How confident do you feel that you can engage in the strategies you've selected and stay on track? Rate your confidence level from 1 (least confident) to 10 (most confident). If your confidence is shaky, why is that? Identify a key roadblock or possible derailment, and identify a way to address it. Review the behavior-change techniques in Chapter 2 if needed.

Confidence level (1–10): _____
Key challenge and method for addressing it:

Results, Reflection, and Planning for the Future

Follow your plan for a week, and see how it goes; then review your progress. Did you meet your goals? Did you try all the strategies you planned? Which ones, if any, did you skip? Why? After you review your progress, identify at least one change to your plan that will help you be more successful going forward.

Progress to date:
Change to plan to boost success:

Keep trying and stick with it. Your efforts over the long term are what matters.

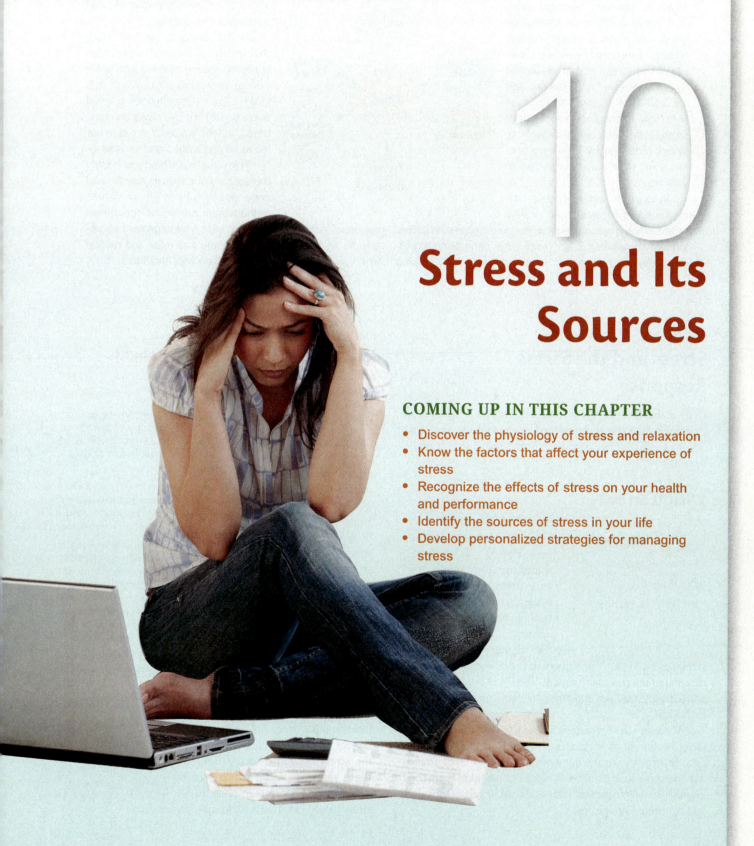

10

Stress and Its Sources

COMING UP IN THIS CHAPTER

- Discover the physiology of stress and relaxation
- Know the factors that affect your experience of stress
- Recognize the effects of stress on your health and performance
- Identify the sources of stress in your life
- Develop personalized strategies for managing stress

How does stress relate to overall wellness? Your physical status can be a cause of stress if you are ill, fatigued, or unfit. Taking action to improve your physical wellness—through exercise, healthy eating, and adequate sleep—significantly lessens stress effects. Emotional wellness both influences stress and is influenced by it. Optimism, enthusiasm, and the ability to express feelings all help you manage stress. Positive spiritual wellness can also facilitate stress reduction by helping you to focus on what's truly important in your life.

In terms of social wellness, having supportive others is healthy, whereas being around negative people increases life stress. Intellectual wellness is also involved in decreasing stress, especially as it relates to managing your time, making wise financial decisions, and addressing life's challenges. And don't forget environmental wellness: Are your typical environments loud, demanding, and stressful, or are they comforting and pleasing to the senses?

In this chapter, you will learn that stress can be positive (as in the cases of getting married and graduating) or negative (as when one loses a job or experiences a loved one's death) but can never be eliminated. In fact, we *need* stress in our life to be challenged and to grow.

This chapter will help you identify the sources of stress in your life and cope positively with stress. Stress management is essential for optimal wellness. You'll learn effective stress-management strategies as well as techniques to help you relax and recoup when you feel the world's weight on your shoulders.

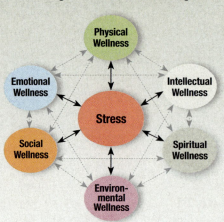

Stress and the Stress Response

One of the first steps for successful stress management is recognizing the physical and emotional changes that occur when you are stressed. Sometimes, they can be dramatic.

What Is Stress?

Q | I don't get it. Everyone else is stressed out about finals, but I feel fine. Is stress overrated?

Stress affects nearly everyone, and while your friends are stressed about finals, something else might trigger stress for you—say, money, work, family, friends, relationships, or time management. Specific events that trigger stress are called **stressors**—physical or emotional demands from your external or internal environment. The list of potential stressors is nearly endless, and stressors vary from individual to individual.

We know stress when we have it. By definition, **stress** is the collection of physical and emotional changes we experience in response to the demands of stressors. Your friends may perceive final exams as a source of potential harm (bad grades), so they experience stress and all its related physical and emotional symptoms.

The Stress Response: Fight or Flight

Q | When I'm feeling especially stressed, my cheeks get hot and my palms sweat. Is this normal?

Almost any response to stress can be considered normal, and hot cheeks and sweaty palms are quite typical. Under normal circumstances, your body is in a fairly relaxed and stable state of functioning, called **homeostasis.** Your breathing and heart rates are relatively low and steady, and other body processes function at a "normal" level—maintaining body temperature, digesting food, producing energy, and so on.

Everything changes when you are exposed to a stressor that you perceive as a threat—a state of **acute stress.** Through a series of rapid physiologic reactions that occur outside conscious control, collective changes known as the **stress response** or the **fight-or-flight response** occur, which prepare the body for a physical response to the stress (see Figure 10-1). Many systems

stressor A specific physical or psychological event, condition, or demand that triggers stress.

stress The collective physical and emotional changes experienced in response to a stressor.

homeostasis A stable state of physiological functioning (metabolic equilibrium) actively maintained by complex biological mechanisms that operate via the autonomic nervous system.

acute stress A state of stress experienced in response to an immediate perceived threat, real or imagined.

stress (fight-or-flight) response Physiological changes in reaction to a stressor that prepare an individual for a physical response (to fight or to flee).

Behavior-Change Challenge
De-Stress with Success

You work full time and are taking night courses toward your business degree. Your wife works at home, where she also cares for your twin toddlers. As if your life isn't pressurized enough, your roof is leaking and needs repair. Your anxiety about your professional, academic, and home responsibilities is sky-high. You begin to wonder: Is there anything I can do to relieve my stress?

Meet Peter

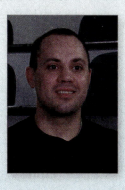

Peter is a full-time corrections officer. Along with his wife, he also attends school. Peter recognizes that he is stressed about his job and his many commitments, and he wants to deal more effectively with stress. View the video to learn more about Peter, his behavior-change goals and strategies, and his achievements over the course of his program. As you watch, consider:

- What are Peter's chief sources of motivation and support, and what are his specific behavior-change strategies? Are these sufficient for his program to be successful? Explain.
- Where will you find motivation and support for your desired behavior change?
- What can you learn from Peter's experience that will help you in your own behavior-change efforts? What strategies that he adopted will work for you?

VIDEO CASE STUDY **WATCH THIS VIDEO IN**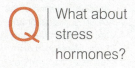

increase their functioning, while some nonessential systems slow or stop, to conserve or redirect critical resources.

The stress response prepares the body for a physical reaction to a threat regardless of whether a physical reaction is required or whether the perceived threat is real or imagined. However, if you're only imagining something stressful or if the stressor doesn't require a physical response—an upcoming exam or a specific social situation, for example—then the fight-or-flight response isn't appropriate. Moreover, chronic exposure to the stress response can harm your health.

Q | What about stress hormones?

The stress response involves many body systems, and several hormones play key roles. When the brain senses a stressor, it activates the **autonomic nervous system (ANS),** which provides unconscious controls of critical internal body processes, such as heart and breathing rates and digestion. The two branches of the ANS play different roles in the body's response to stress: The **sympathetic nervous system** generates the fight-or-flight response, and the **parasympathetic nervous system** helps return the body to homeostasis once the threat has passed.

When a stressor activates the sympathetic nervous system, it releases the hormones **adrenaline** (epinephrine) and **cortisol,** two chemical messengers that bind to cells and trigger the fight-or-flight response. Although beneficial for that brief period of need, sustained high levels of these hormones can have negative health effects, including a dampening of the immune system.[1]

Another stress hormone is **oxytocin,** which acts as a neurotransmitter in the brain. (A *neurotransmitter* carries information from one nerve cell to another.) Women release oxytocin during labor to assist in cervical dilation and also during breastfeeding to "let down" their milk.[2] However, oxytocin also suppresses the stress response.

autonomic nervous system (ANS) Branch of the nervous system that provides unconscious control of basic body processes; consists of two divisions, sympathetic and parasympathetic.

sympathetic nervous system A division of the autonomic nervous system that quickly generates the fight-or-flight response in reaction to a perceived threat; it accelerates key body processes to prepare the body for physical action.

parasympathetic nervous system A division of the autonomic nervous system that balances the actions of the sympathetic nervous system by slowing body processes, returning the body to homeostasis once a stressor has passed.

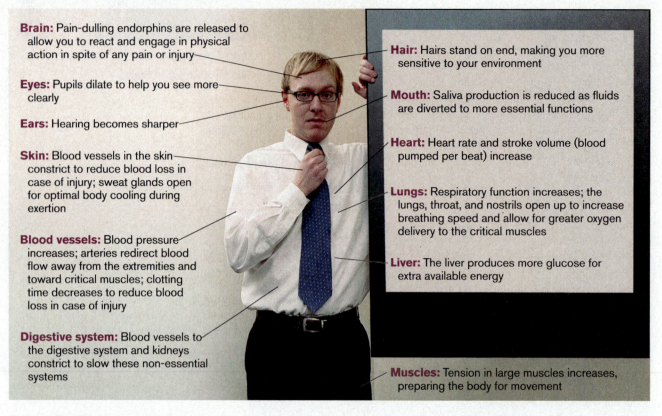

Brain: Pain-dulling endorphins are released to allow you to react and engage in physical action in spite of any pain or injury

Eyes: Pupils dilate to help you see more clearly

Ears: Hearing becomes sharper

Skin: Blood vessels in the skin constrict to reduce blood loss in case of injury; sweat glands open for optimal body cooling during exertion

Blood vessels: Blood pressure increases; arteries redirect blood flow away from the extremities and toward critical muscles; clotting time decreases to reduce blood loss in case of injury

Digestive system: Blood vessels to the digestive system and kidneys constrict to slow these non-essential systems

Hair: Hairs stand on end, making you more sensitive to your environment

Mouth: Saliva production is reduced as fluids are diverted to more essential functions

Heart: Heart rate and stroke volume (blood pumped per beat) increase

Lungs: Respiratory function increases; the lungs, throat, and nostrils open up to increase breathing speed and allow for greater oxygen delivery to the critical muscles

Liver: The liver produces more glucose for extra available energy

Muscles: Tension in large muscles increases, preparing the body for movement

Figure 10-1 **The fight-or-flight response.** The stress response prepares the body for a physical response to a stressor.

Counterbalancing Fight or Flight: A Return to Homeostasis

Once the stress crisis passes, the body usually returns to a relatively unstressed state, or homeostasis.

Q How do I know when I'm finally relaxed again?

From a physiological perspective, your body will experience a decrease in metabolism, heart rate, and blood pressure; as well, your muscles will relax and your breathing will slow, all moving back to what is normal for you. It doesn't take much, however, for the fight-or-flight response to kick in again. If your body doesn't return to homeostasis on its own, you can use relaxation techniques to elicit the *relaxation response*; see pp. 370–372.

The Stress Emotions: Anger and Fear

Anger and fear are the primary emotions associated with stress. When the stress response kicks in, you may feel yourself becoming angry (the urge to "fight") or fearful (the urge to run, or "flight").

Q What's wrong with getting angry? Everybody does it.

ANGER. Anger may be a helpful response in some situations, but in others, it can be inappropriate or even harmful. Anger is a natural response to a perceived threat, whether real or imagined. Types of threats that produce anger include betrayal, injustice, and jealousy. Anger can be caused by an external event, such as a traffic jam, or an internal event, such as a personal financial problem.

Anger, as a primitive survival emotion, produces both emotional and physiological changes. Anger can be useful in certain situations. For example, in the face of imminent danger, it can provide the courage to defend yourself or a loved one. But anger can also be problematic, especially if your emotions rage out of control and lead to physical harm to you or others. Harmful manifestations of anger include the following:

- Shouting at people or using violent words
- Being unable to deal with difficult situations without anger
- Using or being tempted to use aggression or violence
- Using anger to make you feel better

adrenaline A hormone secreted by the adrenal glands, which sit on top of the kidneys; it binds to body cells and helps trigger the immediate changes of the fight-or-flight response, including increases in heart rate, blood pressure, and energy supplies.

cortisol A hormone secreted by the adrenal glands, which sit on top of the kidneys; it is secreted in response to stress and helps trigger the changes of the fight-or-flight response, including increased blood glucose, altered immune function, and reduction in nonessential body functions.

oxytocin A hormone that acts as a neurotransmitter in the brain; in women, it facilitates dilation of the cervix during labor and the letdown reflex during breast-feeding; it also facilitates trust, empathy, and social bonding.

Wellness Strategies

Dealing with Anger

Q | Sometimes I get pretty angry. What can I do?

If you feel yourself becoming angry in a situation in which expressing your feelings is inappropriate or unhelpful, then you need to find a positive way to deal with your anger. Try the following strategies:

- Reason with yourself: Engage in self-talk to calm yourself.
- Convert anger into a more constructive behavior. If getting angry isn't going to improve the situation, what will? If the problem can't be solved, what else could you do right now that would be useful?
- Step back or remove yourself from the situation; take a time-out.
- Use deep breathing or another relaxation technique to diffuse your anger.

If you find yourself regularly needing to manage your anger, you may want to keep a journal of the circumstances that produce it. It won't be long before you begin to recognize certain patterns, and this awareness in turn can help you better manage your anger.

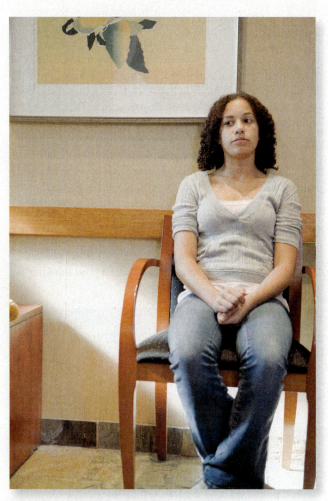

The fight-or-flight reaction prepares the body for a physical response to a stressor, whether such a response is needed or not. Physical and emotional changes occur until the crisis or challenge is over, and then the body returns to homeostasis.

- Being recognized as an angry person and feared or avoided by others
- Avoiding situations because you fear your own temper

People who are frequently and inappropriately angry are also at increased risk for anger-linked health problems, including hypertension, heart disease, and a decrease in immune functioning.[3]

Q | Should I just vent when I'm feeling angry?

Common wisdom tells us to blow off steam, or vent, when we're angry, but this is rarely a good approach. Releasing anger in an uncontrolled way reinforces and escalates the feeling rather than addressing the situation or helping to restore emotional composure.

What about suppressing anger? That can also have a negative impact if anger remains uncontrolled. People who hold in their angry feelings may develop a hostile, cynical attitude and try to get back at others indirectly—this is known as *passive-aggressive behavior*. These patterns of thinking and behavior can damage health and relationships.

Because anger is a normal emotion, it's important to learn to manage it in positive ways (see the box "Dealing with Anger"). If you feel your anger building, ask yourself these three questions:[4]

1. Is this situation important enough to get angry about?
2. Am I justified in getting angry?
3. Will expressing my anger make a positive difference?

If the answer to all three questions is yes, then a calm expression of your anger may be appropriate. This means stating your feelings or needs in an assertive but not aggressive or demanding manner. Assertive communication involves respecting the feelings and views of everyone—leading to a

Mind Stretcher
Critical Thinking Exercise

Think about the last time you got terribly angry. Who was the target of your anger? What specific situation caused the anger? Who else was around at the time? What were you doing just before you became so angry? Were you especially hungry or tired? Make a list of all the different aspects of the anger event. What triggers do you recognize? How can you avoid or minimize them in the future?

calming of tempers rather than an escalation of anger. If you answer no to any of the three questions, then you need to find a way to calm yourself.

Q What's the difference between fear and anxiety? Can anxiety be useful?

FEAR AND ANXIETY. The word *fear* is often used interchangeably with the word **anxiety,** which refers to a persistent state of worry, unease, and nervousness not directed at any particular threat. Fear or anxiety may be categorized as rational (useful) or irrational (useless). Rational fear or anxiety is a reaction to real events that are life threatening and require a response to avoid or survive the danger. For example, being trapped inside a burning building elicits fear that is rational and useful because it will help you try to get out quickly. This fear will usually disappear when the stressor is eliminated.

Irrational (useless) fear or anxiety is unreasonable or excessive. An irrational fear can take the form of a **phobia,** which is a persistent, unreasonable, intense fear of a specific object, activity, or situation. Irrational fear can be so powerful that it interferes with daily functioning and causes a variety of mental, emotional, and physical problems. *Social phobia*—the fear of embarrassment or humiliation in social situations—may lead to avoidance of all social interaction, creating social isolation.

The fear reaction is also altered in people who have *post-traumatic stress disorder (PTSD).* Anyone can develop PTSD after a frightening event, but it is most common among veterans of war and survivors of abuse, disasters, and other crises. People with PTSD feel fearful or stressed even when there is no danger; they may be constantly on edge and experience nightmares and flashbacks of the trauma. PTSD is usually treated with psychotherapy or medication or both.

The difference between normal and disordered fear or anxiety is how frequently it occurs and whether it disrupts everyday functioning. For example, after hearing about a shooting at a university on the other side of the

anxiety A persistent state of worry, unease, and nervousness not directed at any particular threat; can be a normal reaction to stress or, if excessive, may indicate a psychological disorder.

phobia A persistent, intense, irrational fear of a specific object, activity, or situation; a form of anxiety disorder.

country, the average person might feel temporary unease and worry. A person with disordered anxiety or fear, however, might be unable to sleep for days, worrying about a worst-case scenario in which his or her university is attacked—and maybe even taking excessive preventive measures.

If your fear or anxiety is so constant that it interferes with your ability to function and relax, you may have what is known as *generalized anxiety disorder.* Maybe you worry excessively about things that are unlikely to happen or you feel tense and anxious all day long for no real reason. Maybe you worry about the same things that other people do—money, relationships, family problems, difficulties at work or school—but you take these worries to a higher level: "The economy is in the tank; I'm sure I will get fired" or "She hasn't handed our tests back yet; I must have done terribly." A constant, excessively high level of anxiety can cause physical problems, such as body aches, insomnia, and exhaustion. It also can lead to difficulty in maintaining a normal lifestyle and can make relaxation almost impossible.

Q What should I do to stop worrying so much?

"If you can solve your problem, then what is the need of worrying?" asked an eighth-century Buddhist scholar named Shantideva. "If you cannot solve it," he continued, "then what is the use of worrying?" The easy answer in both cases is that there is no need to worry. But it can be hard to stop worrying. Different strategies are appropriate for different people. For some, substituting planning and problem solving for worrying can help; for others, a relaxation technique is most beneficial. Self-help doesn't work for everyone, but here are some relatively effective psychosocial techniques any worrier can try:

- *Self-monitoring* involves noticing when you start to feel anxious and recording when and where the feelings began, their intensity, and the symptoms. Become familiar with your patterns of worry to better prepare for worrisome situations and to adjust your thinking.

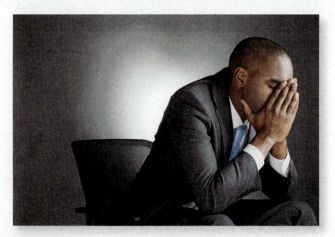

Worry—about grades, money, relationships—is perfectly normal. But if anxiety is so severe or constant that it disrupts your daily functioning and prevents you from ever relaxing, you may have an anxiety disorder.

- *Cognitive therapy* attempts to make thought patterns more positive—to reappraise worry. Creating more positive and realistic thoughts ("I can help the situation get better") reduces worrisome thoughts.
- *Worry exposure* may be the most challenging technique. It involves being presented with situations and ideas that create worry in order to become used to the worry and to see that worry and anxiety do not cause negative events—or help things get better.

If your worries are interfering with your daily life, talk to a counselor or another health professional. See the box "Smartphone Stressing You?" for additional insight on stressors.

Factors Affecting the Experience of Stress

Q Why do we all respond so differently to stress?

Personality, life experience, social setting, typical patterns of thinking, and even biological sex all have an effect on how each of us responds to life's ups and downs. Stress is an individualized experience. Don't feel bad—or make someone else feel bad—if you aren't stressed out by the same things as your friends or family members.

Personality

Q Personality-wise, who are the most stressed people?

It's not entirely clear, but some researchers have looked at collections of characteristics, called *personality types,* and others have studied particular *traits,* such as those you might use to describe a friend or family member (for example, honest, intelligent, shy, assertive, hard-working, low-key) to see who is most stressed. **Personality** is a collection of qualities or traits that characterize an individual, including emotional, intellectual, and social factors. Personality may be expressed in patterns of thinking, feeling, and

personality The collection of emotional, intellectual, and social qualities or traits that characterize an individual.

Research Brief

Smartphone Stressing You?

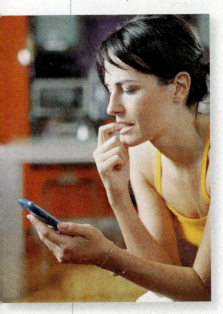

Compulsively checking your smartphone may not actually be that smart and in fact may be part of a pattern indicating increased personal stress. Recent research suggests that those of us who relentlessly check our phones for e-mails, tweets, and texts may be experiencing stress at dramatically higher levels than those who do not. The research seems to show that this pattern is not necessarily a problem for professionals checking their work phones but instead for the personal users who feel that they have to keep tabs on everything—constantly.

Researchers in England wanted to explore how the use of iPhones, Androids, Blackberries, and other similar hand-held devices may elevate stress. They conducted various types of stress tests among more than 100 participants, including university students, retail workers, and public-sector employees, with all of them completing a smartphone-use survey. One of the big findings was that most people do in fact purchase smartphones for work-related reasons. It is only after using them for a while that certain people begin to favor the device for its ability to maintain control over all aspects of their communication and relationships, particularly the personal ones. This development in turn creates a dependency on the phone to stay in touch or to remain in control, which leads to higher levels of stress from the constant bombardment of information and the need to control it.

Ultimately, the more a person checks his or her phone, for any reason, the more the individual's stress rises. The researchers even documented cases where smartphone users perceived incoming alerts (rings, vibrations, and so on) when in fact there were none. The researchers described these as extreme cases of highly stressed smartphone users.

Analyze and Apply
- How often do you check your smartphone?
- In what ways, if any, does using your phone cause you to feel stress?
- What strategies can you use to reduce your dependency on your phone?

Source: Balding, R. (2012). Presented at the British Psychological Society meeting, Chester, U.K. (http://www.healthfinder.gov/news/newsstory.aspx?Docid=660651&source=govdelivery) Last accessed January 2012.

behavior; in approaches to different situations; and in interactions with others.

Researchers in the 1950s developed a model of personality based on two patterns of behavior:

- **Type A personality:** Being rushed, ambitious, impatient, time conscious, goal driven, competitive, aggressive, and quick to anger; having difficulty relaxing
- **Type B personality:** Being patient, easygoing, and adaptable to changing circumstances

Although widely used in the popular media, the type A/type B model of personality has been criticized as an oversimplification. Of more recent vintage, and similarly controversial, are the concepts of type C and type D personalities. *Type C* individuals tend to be introverted, respectful, eager to please, and compliant; disease-related outcomes have not yet been substantiated in this population. *Type D* individuals experience increased levels of anxiety, irritation, and depressed mood, along with elevated cortisol, and evidence from close studies shows that Type D's can have a threefold increased risk for future cardiovascular problems.[5]

While you cannot change your personality, you can change patterns of thinking and behavior that might be causing problems for you. Your personality is the result of heredity as well as social, psychological, and behavioral factors. The prenatal environment may also play a role in the development of personality and responses to stress: If a mother has a high level of cortisol during pregnancy, the fetus has a similarly high level.[6] This exposure to excess cortisol in the womb can affect the receptors for stress-related substances in the brain, thereby making the baby more susceptible to stressors later in life (see the box "The Negative Consequences of Prenatal Stress").

type A personality
A personality type characterized by traits of urgency, impatience, hostility, excessive competitiveness, and drive for success.

type B personality
A personality type characterized by traits of relaxation, patience, and adaptability.

Research Brief

The Negative Consequences of Prenatal Stress

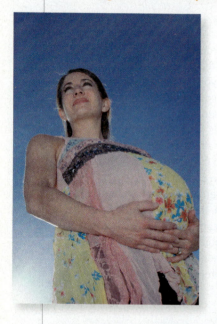

Behavioral and biological researchers have long recognized that women who experience stress during pregnancy tend to have offspring with slower physical development, difficulties in learning and attention, and symptoms of anxiety and depression. These kinds of outcomes attributed to prenatal stress have been difficult to measure objectively. Most of the past evidence was based on women's ability to recall stressful events that had occurred during their pregnancy, and these recollections were likely biased by the reality of having a child with developmental or emotional delays. Issues encountered prenatally that the women may not have thought stressful at the time became magnified in light of their belief that their prenatal stress may have somehow caused the delays and symptoms observed in their children.

Interestingly, recent, well-controlled laboratory research in rats has demonstrated a strong relationship between prenatal stress and developmental and/or emotional delays. Specifically, this research showed that when pregnant female rats were subjected to stressful situations, their offspring were later shown to have impaired learning and memory abilities, less capacity to cope with stressful situations (such as food deprivation), and symptoms of anxiety and depressive behavior as compared to rats in control groups that had been born to unstressed mothers. All of these outcomes are similar to those noted in children born to stressed human mothers. The rat research also points to the hormone cortisol as the underlying problem, because its presence is necessary during acute stress yet detrimental if chronically present, as it was in the rats and is believed to be in humans. In fact, in pregnant women, above-normal cortisol levels can also stimulate the release of a particular hormone from the placenta that will cause premature birth, which is another factor that can affect normal development.

Analyze and Apply

- Prior to the rat research, why was it difficult for researchers to measure the developmental outcomes that were suspected to be linked to prenatal stress?
- What strategies can a woman use to minimize chronic stress during pregnancy?

Source: Weinstock-Rosin, M. (2008). The long-term consequences of prenatal stress. *Neuroscience and Biobehavioral Reviews, 32*, 1073–1083.

Experience also plays a significant role in individual personality development. Every situation you are exposed to from birth on helps to form your personality, and how you respond to different events provides you with experience in handling stressful situations. Think about the personality traits of your parents and siblings and the ways they react to stress. Not everyone in a family has a similar personality or deals with stressors in the same manner. But by observing others and being aware of your own thoughts and behaviors, you can learn about why you react the way you do. With strategies such as self-talk and relaxation techniques, you can reshape problematic responses to stressors even if you can't change your basic personality traits.

Gender and Biological Sex

Do men and women handle stress differently? Consider the following example:

Together, Jaymes and Maisha have been trying to start a custom furniture business while still in school. Jaymes has worked with furniture his whole life, and Maisha is majoring in business, so this seems like a logical extension for them and a plan for their future. Their days are long and pressured, and both feel the constant strain of balancing school, work, and their 18-month-old daughter, Bailey. Yet despite equally tension-filled lives, Maisha and Jaymes handle the stress in totally different ways. "When I have a bad day, I'll come home and play with Bailey, then call some friends and tell them what happened," says

Maisha. "When Jaymes has a bad day, it's so obvious, because he won't talk about anything. He internalizes everything." Maisha worries that keeping everything to himself isn't good for Jaymes.

Q | My guy friends can't deal with stress. Why do girls seem to know how to handle it?

Subtle hormonal and evolutionary differences may help explain the differences you've noticed. Researchers looking at both biological and behavioral responses to stress have found that women are more likely to deal with stress by "tending and befriending"—nurturing those around them and reaching out to others. And they've found that men are more prone to initiate a confrontation or to withdraw, similarly to what happens in the fight-or-flight response.[7]

Women and men's differing responses may be due to cultural differences in what is considered gender-appropriate behavior, but there is also a biological component. In the initial response to stress, men and women release the same stress hormones, cortisol and adrenaline. Women, however, also secrete oxytocin, which mitigates the production of cortisol and adrenaline. Men also produce oxytocin during stressful times, but its effects are diminished by testosterone, which men produce in significantly greater quantities than women. Therefore, oxytocin may enhance relaxation in women and provide some protection from the damaging effects of stress hormones.

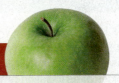

Wellness Strategies

You Are What You Think

Q | How can a person think more positively when feeling totally stressed?

People who think that they won't succeed are usually right. In contrast, those who are confident that they can succeed, within reason, usually do. The latter attitude is often referred to as positive thinking. *Positive thinking* is a combination of things, including believing in yourself, surrounding yourself with supportive people, and focusing on the good that can come from a situation.

How do thought patterns affect stress? Consider that if you choose to think that things will always work out for the worst or that nobody likes you, even when the evidence says otherwise, you are likely to feel much more stress than others. In addition, as a negative thinker, you may not be the kind of person with whom others like to spend a lot

of time. Instead, channel your thinking to create a positive outlook. Successful people almost always think positively but also realistically, and they spend very little time worrying about things they can't control or feeling stressed by disapproval and rejection.

Analyze and Apply

Here are some typical negative thoughts that college students experience. How can you turn them into positive statements?

1. I can't ever make the Dean's list.
2. I'll never get an A in this class.
3. I'm switching majors because this one is too hard.
4. That teacher hates me—that's why I'm failing.
5. I know I'll never find a job.
6. My friends think this is a terrible major for me.

Gender and sex differences in response to stress may have a profound effect on wellness and may be one of the reasons why women typically enjoy a longer life expectancy than men. Higher levels of oxytocin facilitate social interaction and feelings of attachment.[2] The increased oxytocin level and associated "tend-and-befriend" behavior pattern increase relaxation and reduce hostility, thereby decreasing the health risks from anger. They also help women build and maintain strong social networks, another factor linked to improved health and greater life expectancy. Although women are three times more likely to suffer from depression related to stress, they seem to have stronger coping mechanisms for stress than do men.

These gender and biological differences may have their roots in evolution. Females traditionally tended to their offspring in the face of danger rather than fighting, which was left to the males. Additionally, socializing might have been a protective measure, because the bigger the social circle, the greater the protection from physical harm. These differences are still seen today. Reports show that on days women report high stress at work, their children report that their mothers are especially loving and nurturing; men, however, tend to withdraw from their family on high-stress days. Further, on the days men face particularly stressful days at work, they also report having more stress at home.[8]

With respect to stress, men might be well advised to act more like women. To seek social support—to tend and befriend—is health protective.

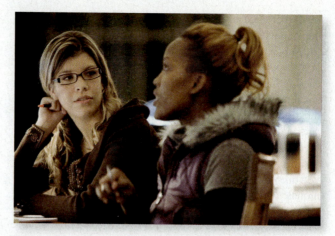

Women are more likely than men to respond to stressors with a tend-and-befriend pattern of behavior, which reduces anxiety, increases feelings of attachment, and helps women build and maintain social support networks.

Ways of Thinking: Cognitive Patterns

Cognitive factors play an important role in determining your responses to a stressor and the ways you cope with it.

Q | Why does it seem my friends handle stress so differently than I do?

THEORIES ABOUT STRESS RESPONSES. On the surface, it can seem that everyone handles stress differently. However, when you look closely, you'll notice that people often follow the same series of steps when they are confronted with a stressor. This cognitive process, known as the **transactional model of stress,**[9] outlines how we all assess and approach a stressful situation:

Step 1: *Primary appraisal* is the initial reaction to a stressor, when you determine whether the stressor presents harm ("am I OK, or am I in trouble?"). If you think you're OK, then you are likely to move on. If you think you're in trouble, then you intuitively go to the next step.

Step 2: *Secondary appraisal* allows you to determine how much control you feel you have over the threat ("what can I do now?"). If you feel lots of control, then you will have minimal stress. Perceiving that you have no control means lots of stress and going to step 3.

Step 3: *Coping* is deciding what to do about the threat. You base this decision on the situation and everything around you—people, material resources, thoughts, emotions, cost versus benefit of different actions, and so on.

Step 4: *Reappraisal* occurs after you have addressed the stressor. At this point, you decide whether the threat still exists. If so, you begin the appraisal process again; if not, you move on.

transactional model of stress A four-step framework for evaluating a person's ability to cope with a stressor before deciding how to respond and then assessing whether the response was successful.

Fast Facts

Society Under Stress

Feeling stressed out? If so, you have a lot of company, as these results from surveys by the American Psychological Association reveal:

- 30 percent of Americans feel that stress affects their ability to get things done at least once a week.
- 47 percent of Americans say that they have lain awake at night due to stress.
- 52 percent of Americans are concerned about the level of stress in their life.
- 64 percent of young adults indicate that their relationships are a significant source of stress.
- 69 percent of Americans say that work has a significant impact on stress levels.
- 71 percent of Americans name money as the number-one factor that affects their stress level.

Sources: American Psychological Association. (2009). *Stress in America 2009* (http://www.apa.org/news/press/releases/2009/11/stress.aspx). American Psychological Association. (2008). *Stress in America 2008* (http://www.apa.org/news/press/releases/2008/10/stress-women.aspx).

attribution theory A theory of about how an individual explains success or failure after a stressful event—whether the outcome is due to external or internal factors.

According to transactional theory, we all follow a similar pattern of thinking when we deal with stress, even if it doesn't seem so from the outside.

Attribution theory provides another window into our responses to stress; it focuses on how we assess our success or failure after a stressful event.[10] This theory asserts that the more successful we are in coping with stress, the more likely we are to take full responsibility for our actions ("I aced the test because I worked hard at it"). Conversely, if we can't effectively deal with a stressor, we attribute it to some external force ("I failed the test because I have a terrible teacher"). Interestingly, when we fail at something, we are likely to attribute our failure to an external force. However, when rivals fail, we typically attribute their failure to a cause within them.

Q | Why do I get so down on myself when I'm stressed?

COPING WITH STRESS. Certain thought patterns and ways of thinking—including ideas, beliefs, expectations, and perceptions—can contribute to your stress level and have a negative impact on your health (in other words, you are what you think). However, there are two types of coping strategies for dealing with negative self-talk and stressors: problem-focused coping and emotion-focused coping.[11]

Problem-focused coping involves attempting to do something practical and constructive about the stressor—for example, finding a tutor to help prepare for a math test; participating in mock job interviews at the career center. *Emotion-focused coping* entails attempting to regulate emotions elicited by a stressful event—to feel less anxious and upset about the stressful circumstance. However, this should not be confused with attempting to deal with emotions through avoidance or denial, which does nothing to deal with the impact of a stressor. More effective emotion-focused coping techniques involve positive self-talk, talking with others, and journaling. These approaches should be used cautiously, however, because it can have negative health effects for people who tend to dwell on negative thought patterns and emotions.

We all have a tendency to choose coping methods that are familiar, regardless of their effectiveness. The reason is that change is uncomfortable, so we stick with what we know, even if it isn't good for us. The best advice is to recognize your stress and to try different coping strategies, giving each a chance to work. In doing so, keep in mind that it may take time to build your problem-solving skills or to obtain the benefits from emotional-approach coping.

Stress and Wellness

Stress comes in all shapes and sizes. If they are not effectively addressed, so do the associated problems. Stress affects your physical and mental performance, your risk for cardiovascular and other chronic diseases, and the functioning of your immune system.

Stress and Performance

The link between stress and performance is often highlighted during sporting events, especially big competitions like the Super Bowl, Wimbledon, and the Olympics. Some athletes do well under this pressure; think of quarterback Tom Brady, tennis great Serena Williams, and Olympic sprinter Usain Bolt. Others don't perform as expected. Stress affects performance at all levels of sport—college, high school, and even peewee. Why some athletes rise to the occasion while others never seem quite "on" on the big day is often related to how they handle stress. They are all physically well conditioned, but as coaches are fond of saying, "Winning is 10 percent physical and 90 percent mental."

Performance isn't just about sports. Your ability to "perform" under stress is also about taking tests, speaking in public, job interviews, dating, and much more.

Q | I'd rather drop a class than give a presentation in it. Why does stress make public speaking so much worse for me?

As stress and anxiety increase, so do performance and efficiency, but only up to a point. The fight-or-flight response is possibly the ultimate performance enhancer—it enabled our ancestors to survive. The heightened senses, increased heart rate and blood flow, surging energy production, and other physiological changes are due to arousal. Arousal and stress, while not the same, share many traits, one being the ability to affect performance for better or worse.

Indeed, as most of us have experienced, there is a fine balance between the right amount of arousal or stress and an improved or optimal performance. Too much arousal or

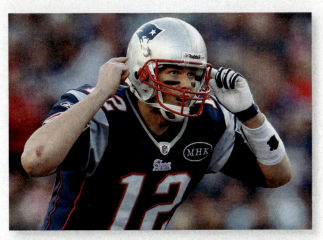

In order to succeed, Tom Brady and athletes everywhere must be able to channel their stress in ways that aid, rather than hinder, performance. Stress affects performance at all levels of sport—professional, college, high school, and even peewee.

Yerkes-Dodson law The principle that some stress (arousal) is beneficial to performance but too much is detrimental; also called the inverted U hypothesis.

or stress can cause a novice runner to start the race too fast, only to falter badly in the second half. During a speech, intense arousal or stress can impair memory, focus, and concentration so that the speaker forgets lines and can't focus on questions from the audience.

The relationship between arousal and performance, in which some is good but too much is not, is best described by the **Yerkes-Dodson law** (Figure 10-2). Also known as the inverted U hypothesis, this principle was developed in the early 1900s by psychologists Robert Yerkes and John Dodson. Note in the figure that the peak of the inverted U represents the point at which the amount of arousal (physical and mental) helps maximize performance. If there is too little or too much arousal or stress, performance is likely to suffer.

At times it may be impossible to avoid high-stress, high-importance situations in which there is a tremendous amount of arousal, such as a class speech and some types of lab-skills tests. According to the Yerkes-Dodson law, if you *overlearn* the task—that is, practice it enough so that it becomes second nature—you should be able to perform to your potential regardless of the situation.

Stress and Overall Health

Q | Can stress really make me sick?

People with unresolved chronic stress and people who handle stress poorly are at increased risk for a wide range of stress-related health problems. Conditions that can be caused or worsened by stress include cardiovascular disease, impairment of the immune system, digestive and metabolic disorders, and depression and other mental health problems.[12]

How much stress is too much? It depends on the individual and his or her coping resources. Warning signs of excess stress in each of the dimensions of wellness are listed in Figure 10-3.

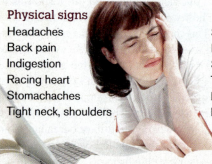

Physical signs

Headaches
Back pain
Indigestion
Racing heart
Stomachaches
Tight neck, shoulders

Sweaty palms
Restlessness
Sleep difficulties
Tiredness
Dizziness
Ringing in ears

Emotional signs

Crying
Anxiety
Anger
Overwhelming sense of nervousness
Boredom—no meaning to things

Edginess—ready to explode
Loneliness
Feeling powerless to change things
Unhappiness for no reason
Easily upset

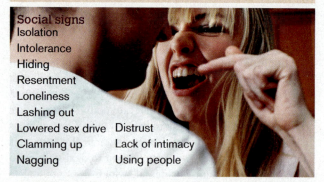

Social signs
Isolation
Intolerance
Hiding
Resentment
Loneliness
Lashing out
Lowered sex drive   Distrust
Clamming up   Lack of intimacy
Nagging   Using people

Behavioral signs

Excess smoking
Grinding teeth
Bossiness
Substance abuse

Compulsive gum chewing
Compulsive eating
Critical of others
Inability to get things done

Intellectual signs

Trouble thinking clearly
Inability to make decisions
Lack of creativity
Thoughts of running away

Memory loss
Constant worry
Forgetfulness
Loss of sense of humor

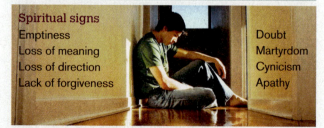

Spiritual signs
Emptiness
Loss of meaning
Loss of direction
Lack of forgiveness

Doubt
Martyrdom
Cynicism
Apathy

Figure 10-3 Stress warning signals.

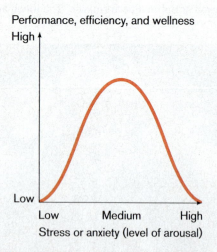

Performance, efficiency, and wellness

High

Low

Low   Medium   High

Stress or anxiety (level of arousal)

Figure 10-2 Yerkes-Dodson law: Stress and performance. Performance and efficiency are enhanced by a certain amount of stress or anxiety. A moderate amount of stress challenges people to perform at their highest level. Too little stress means too little challenge and little or no motivation or improvement. Too much stress causes both wellness and performance to decline.

Acute Versus Chronic Stress

Q | What does stress do to the body over time?

Short-term, acute stress typically results in the fight-or-flight response and its associated changes, which include a release of corticosteroids. Acute stress can have health effects—muscle tension, headache, heartburn, and so on—but these problems are usually temporary and diminish when the stress response ends and the body returns to homeostasis. In contrast, the effects of **chronic stress** can be more serious and long-lasting, particularly as corticosteroid levels remain elevated.

An early model of how chronic stress affects health is the **general adaptation syndrome (GAS),** proposed by endocrinologist Hans Selye. This model has three stages:

chronic stress Stress that lasts a long time or occurs frequently.

general adaptation syndrome (GAS) A model of the body's response to chronic stress; the three phases are alarm (fight-or-flight response), resistance, and exhaustion.

eustress A positive stressor that enhances physical or mental functioning; it is typically short term and may feel exciting or motivating.

distress A negative stressor that causes emotional pain, anxiety, or injury; it may be short or long term and cause anxiety and other unpleasant feelings.

allostatic load Cumulative physical damage of chronic exposure to the stress response, especially the effects of stress hormones.

- *Alarm reaction:* The acute reaction to a stressor (fight or flight)
- *Resistance:* The body's attempt to adapt to the demands of a persistent stressor (such as a negative work environment, chronic physical pain, an unhappy relationship)
- *Exhaustion:* The state of impaired functioning that occurs if a persistent stressor exhausts the body's resources for coping

Selye's model also distinguishes between positive and negative stress. A positive stressor, or **eustress,** enhances physical or mental functioning (for example, strength training or a challenging school project). A negative stressor, or **distress** (for example, the death of a family member or a job loss), can cause emotional pain, anxiety, or injury, especially if the stress isn't resolved effectively. Chronic exhaustion and distress are associated with increased risk for health problems, as they produce elevated corticosteroid levels that have many negative physiological consequences.

Recent research studies have focused on **allostatic load,** which is the cumulative physical damage of chronic exposure to stress hormones. A high allostatic load may result from frequent or chronic stressors, poor coping with stressors, inability to shut down the stress response, or an uneven stress response in different body systems. When people's allostatic load exceeds their ability to adapt and cope, they are at increased risk for a variety of health problems.[13]

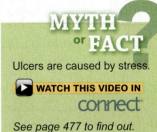

MYTH or FACT?

Ulcers are caused by stress.

▶ **WATCH THIS VIDEO IN** connect

See page 477 to find out.

Underlying Factors in Stress-Related Health Problems

Q | How does stress tear you down physically?

The links between stress and illness can be difficult to pinpoint because there is no standard measure of stress and there are significant individual differences in how people react to stressors and cope with stress. Two pathways of causality can be examined: behavioral and biological.

While under stress, people may engage in behaviors that either enhance or hurt their health. Negative health behaviors associated with stress include poor sleep, little or no physical activity, poor eating habits, smoking or drinking more, and avoiding medical care. People who are stressed and engage in unhealthy behaviors are at elevated risk for developing health problems, having worse outcomes from disease, and even experiencing higher rates of premature mortality.

As described earlier, the physiological response to a stressor involves the release of cortisol, adrenaline, and other hormones that control the fight-or-flight response. The actions of these hormones, especially cortisol, can cause problems if a person is chronically exposed. These include elevated blood pressure and cholesterol levels; hindered glucose metabolism; a suppressed immune response; and increased physiological inflammation, which is linked to many other health problems, including cardiovascular disease, allergies, and certain forms of cancer.

Mind Stretcher
Critical Thinking Exercise

What are the three most negative stressful issues that you regularly must deal with? Can you think of any stressful situations you have encountered recently that are positive? Describe the different approaches you use to deal with the positive and negative stressors. How can you apply the positive approach to help reduce the stress during negative situations?

Stress and Specific Conditions

Q | Can stress be a factor for serious physical conditions?

Stress is a risk factor for both serious chronic diseases and minor health problems. Stress can contribute to the development of cardiovascular disease; increase the risk for infections like colds; and cause headaches, skin changes, and digestive problems (Table 10-1). As described in the last section, negative health behaviors that may increase when a person is under stress—including smoking, drinking, and poor eating habits—also raise the risk for many serious health outcomes. (Unfortunately, stress can sometimes interfere with a person's attempts to improve physical health; see the box "Dieting Stress: Can It Impede Weight Loss?")

Remember, however, that some level of stress is beneficial and can even improve performance. In any case, it's impossible to avoid stress. You shouldn't fear stress or feel that any one stressful event will cause you to get sick or contract a terrible disease. In fact, the majority of people confronted with traumatic life events remain disease-free. As you'll see later in the chapter, there are many positive steps you can take to manage stress and reduce your risk of developing a stress-related health problem.

Sources of Stress

Stressors can come at you from all sides. Your friends and family, your job, your schoolwork, and even your patterns of thought and behavior can be stressors. Major

underlying causes of stress are change and fear of the unknown: "Can I handle college?" "Will I make new friends right away?" "Will I still have enough time to keep up with my job responsibilities?" When thinking about stressors, *change* is the operative word. You might think that something can't be stressful if it produces a good outcome, but that is not how stress works. Starting college is a positive occasion but quite stressful. Graduating from college is even more exciting—and can be even more stressful. It isn't necessarily the outcome that defines an event as stressful, but the type and amount of change anticipated.

Life Experiences Large and Small

Q | I understand that marriage, divorce, and losing a job are stressful, but why do little things cause so much stress?

Major life events—including marriage, a serious illness, getting or losing a job, and the death of a friend or family member—do cause stress. We all experience big life changes, most of which we can anticipate in advance. Particularly stressful, however, are big

TABLE 10-1 STRESS-RELATED HEALTH PROBLEMS

CONDITION	POTENTIAL EFFECTS OF ACUTE AND CHRONIC STRESS
CARDIOVASCULAR DISEASE	Damage to arteries from increased blood pressure, heart rate, blood-fat and glucose levels, and inflammation
INFECTIONS AND OTHER PROBLEMS RELATED TO IMMUNE FUNCTIONING	Increased risk of an acute infection or a flare-up of a chronic infection (for example, genital herpes) due to suppression and dysregulation of immunity; possible reduction in the body's ability to fight cancer due to immunity changes
BODY COMPOSITION AND FAT DISTRIBUTION	Increased body-fat storage due to the stress-related rise in glucose and insulin in the blood; weight gain and abdominal obesity resulting from long-term exposure to cortisol
DIABETES	Glucose intolerance, insulin resistance, and type 2 diabetes due to excess glucose; with acute stress, destabilization of blood glucose levels in people with diabetes
MENTAL HEALTH DISORDERS	Increased risk for development or worsening of certain psychological disorders, including depression
HEADACHES	Muscle tension in the head, neck, and shoulders linked to tension and migraine headaches
DIGESTIVE PROBLEMS	Worsening of heartburn; changes in how quickly food moves through the digestive tract, leading to diarrhea or constipation
SKIN CHANGES	Increased skin sensitivity and worsening of acne, psoriasis, and hives
SLEEP	Disruption of sleep patterns

Research Brief

Dieting Stress: Can It Impede Weight Loss?

What are the psychological and physiological effects of restricting calories or monitoring one's diet on a daily basis? Researchers at the University of California recently tried to answer this question. They asked 121 females to participate in a study to measure the effect of dietary restriction or dietary monitoring on psychological stress and blood cortisol, each of which is known to be counterproductive to weight loss.

Each woman was randomly assigned to one of four groups: (1) dietary monitoring with no calorie restriction, (2) dietary monitoring with calorie restriction, (3) no dietary monitoring with no calorie restriction, and (4) no dietary monitoring with calorie restriction. The women participated in the study for 3 weeks. Women who were assigned to monitor their diet were asked to track their calories each day. Women assigned to restrict their calories had to limit their daily intake to 1,200 calories. At the start and end of the study, each woman completed a questionnaire on her perceived stress level and also had her saliva collected for 2 consecutive days to test for cortisol.

Regardless of group assignment, women who restricted their calories showed an overall increase in the total output of cortisol. Even those who were assigned to just monitoring their daily calories reported a rise in perceived stress. The study results show that either behavior—restricting calories or counting calories—increased real (cortisol) or perceived stress levels, which can only make losing weight that much more difficult.

Analyze and Apply
- What are the implications of the study results for women who want to lose weight?
- How does it make you feel when you think about having to count or restrict calories?

Source: Tomiyama, A. J., Mann, T., Vinas D., Hunger, J. M., DeJager, J., & Taylor, S. E. (2010). Low calorie dieting increases cortisol. *Psychosomatic Medicine, 72*(4), 357–364. Doi: 10.1097/PSY.0b013e3181d9523c.

---

changes that are unexpected and that we perceive to be out of our control.

Yet even the routine aspects of our day can create stress, and so can the many unexpected, uncontrollable stressors of daily living. Homework, job deadlines, traffic jams, and bills due for payment are just some of the "little" things that we often feel are outside our control—and that cause intense stress. Over time, these day-to-day stressors add up and overwhelm our ability to cope. The busier and more successful we become, the more daily hassles we may have to face and manage.

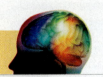

Mind Stretcher
Critical Thinking Exercise

Make a list of the daily hassles you commonly encounter, such as being awakened too early by loud neighbors, standing in a long line for lunch, and repeatedly misplacing your keys. Divide your list into two groups: avoidable and unavoidable. For each stressor that is potentially avoidable, describe a strategy for eliminating it from your life. For stressors that are unavoidable, make a list of effective coping mechanisms.

Time Pressures

Q | Time is my problem. How do I make more of it!?

Typical reasons for a time crunch include classes, work, social relationships, family, studying, sleeping, eating, parenting, and caregiving for family members. In the next section we'll explore time-management strategies that can help you get more done, minimize stress, and improve your quality of life.

Job and Financial Pressures

Q | What is rated the most stressful thing?

In typical surveys of American adults, money and work consistently top the list of stressors (Table 10-2). Chronic workplace stress has been linked to cardiovascular disease and premature mortality: Studies following thousands of workers over time found that in men, the risks for chest pain, heart attack, and death rose along with the reported incompetence of their bosses, and the risks increased the longer the study participants worked in the same stressful environment. On the positive side, the more competent the participants thought their bosses were, the lower their risk

TABLE 10-2 TOP STRESSORS REPORTED BY AMERICAN ADULTS

STRESSOR	PERCENT REPORTING STRESSOR AS SIGNIFICANT		CHANGE (2007–2011)
	2007	2011	
MONEY	73%	75%	+2%
WORK	74%	70%	−4%
THE ECONOMY	69%	67%	−2%
FAMILY RESPONSIBILITIES	60%	57%	−3%
RELATIONSHIPS	59%	58%	−1%
FAMILY HEALTH PROBLEMS	55%	53%	−2%
HOUSING COSTS	51%	49%	−2%
PERSONAL HEALTH CONCERNS	55%	53%	−2%
JOB STABILITY	42%	49%	+7%
PERSONAL SAFETY	31%	32%	+1%

Source: American Psychological Association. (2011). *Stress in America: Stress in America Press Room.* Washington, DC: APA (http://www.apa.org/news/press/releases/stress/index.aspx).

of developing heart disease.[14] Although most studies on stress, work, and disease haven't proven cause-and-effect relationships, it's reasonable to assume that dissatisfaction at work can translate into great risk for ill health or premature death. How we interact with others in the workplace is important to our health and quality of life; and because we spend so much time at work, these relationships clearly count.

Although there is no consensus about the number-one stressor for college students, concerns relating to money (such as work and loans), academics, roommates, and relationships are often near the top of the list. Job-related stressors vary: The job needs and expectations of a full-time freshman living in a residence hall differ from those of a commuting parent attending night classes part-time while holding down a full-time job. Whereas the part-time student already has an income, the new freshman may feel a desperate need to get one. However, the part-time student likely has many financial obligations, and going back to school simply adds to that burden.

Typically, students who work more than 20 hours per week have worse health profiles than those working fewer hours. Sleeping less, eating unhealthy foods, smoking and drinking more, and having a higher BMI have all been noted more frequently in students with heavy work schedules—and more students tend to work, and for more hours, as they progress through college.[15] Stress-management strategies, including time management, goal setting, and problem solving, can diminish day-to-day stressors (also see the box "Getting Through Tough Economic Times").

DOLLAR STRETCHER
Financial Wellness Tip

Creating a budget and sticking to it can greatly reduce financial stress. Start by tracking all your income and expenses for 2–4 weeks. You can use these data to help set a long-term budget. Try a free or low-cost computer program or smartphone app to track and sort expenses by category.

Q I have to work to help pay for college. What is the best job so I can still get good grades?

There is no ideal job that will pay college bills without cutting into study time, but a job related to your major area

Wellness Strategies

Getting Through Tough Economic Times

Q | How do I not let financial stress and work stress get to me?

If you are stressed out about job insecurity, job loss, or financial problems, try some of the following strategies:

- *Keep things in perspective.* Recognize the good aspects of life and retain hope for the future. Appreciate the positive things that happen every day.
- *Strengthen connections with your family and friends.* They can provide important emotional support.
- *Engage in activities* such as physical exercise, sports, and hobbies that can relieve stress and anxiety.

- *Develop new employment skills*—a practical and effective problem-focused method of coping as well as a way of directly addressing financial difficulties. Returning to school is one such strategy.
- *Volunteer in your community.* It reduces stress, gets your mind off your problems, and broadens your network.
- *Focus on making things better, not on what has gone wrong.* Don't compare your current situation with the past. If you've had a major setback, give yourself time to heal and then move on.

Source: Substance Abuse and Mental Health Services Administration. (2009). *Getting through tough economic times* (http://www.samhsa.gov/economy). Visit the Web site for additional information and advice.

of study, if available, is a good choice. Such employment can provide hands-on training, may help prepare you for classes, and can serve as a springboard to future internships and jobs. Although you will have the burden of time commitment no matter what job you choose, if it is one that helps the academic cause, you are likely to enjoy it more, plan better, and use it to be more successful. On the other hand, if you are working at a job that you dislike, or one that has terrible hours or is far from campus or home, you may be adding stressors to your already pressurized life. Some find that working on campus has the advantage of minimizing commuting time. Campus jobs may not pay as well as some off-campus jobs and may be difficult to come by (at least the really good ones), but persistence usually pays off. Also, some college faculty members have grant money available to pay students a small salary to assist with research. This can be a great way to make some money, learn more about your field, and build a relationship with your instructors.

Relationships and Families

Q | I really miss my friends from back home. How do I deal with being so homesick?

Being homesick is a common experience for most people when they leave home for the first time. But instead of homesick, the feeling might be better referred to as "friendsick" since your friends are often what you are most missing. Starting college disrupts your network of friends, with the disruption being greater the farther away from home you go—and it's a lot of work to build a new group of friends. Having a support group at the start of college helps: for example, meeting your new roommates in advance, being part of a sport or academic team, or knowing others who are headed to the same college. College and university administrators are well aware of the benefits of built-in friends, and this may be a large reason behind freshman live-in policies and residence hall learning communities. Surveys consistently show higher rates of retention for students who live on campus and get involved in learning communities[16]—not to mention the better opportunity to establish lifelong friendships. So don't get caught up worrying what your old friends are up to; instead, focus on developing new friendships at college, many of which will last forever.

Q | What about dealing with stress when you're not 19, single, and living in the dorms?

Each autumn brings newly enrolled nontraditional students (age 25 or older) to college campuses, many of whom have jobs, spouses, children, and ailing parents, to name just a few potential stressors for such individuals. In fact, women constitute a majority of both traditional (55 percent) and nontraditional (58 percent) college students and only about one-third of U.S. college students live in residence halls; but two-thirds work, and most have more than one job.[17]

Although nontraditional students are much more likely to attend college part-time, many 4-year colleges treat all students as if they were the traditional 18- to 21-year-olds, a reality that can be frustrating for older students. Two-year colleges have a much higher percentage of older and nontraditional students and also tend to provide programs and services well matched to the needs of that population.

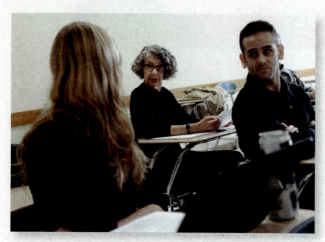

Traditional and nontraditional students may have different stressors, but both groups face challenges and changes that they must work through in order to adapt to college life and succeed in meeting their goals.

Mind Stretcher
Critical Thinking Exercise

What places always make you feel the most stressed? What is the one place you go to find the least stressful environment? List your regular environments in order from the most stressful to the least stressful, indicating one reason why you think each is stressful or not. For the stressful places, come up with at least one way to reduce the stress associated with that environment.

If you are a nontraditional student with a myriad of life responsibilities, you will need to do some creative time management and select a reasonable course load. Unlike students on the "4-year plan," you will need to focus on each course individually, making sure to make progress in small steps while keeping a sharp focus on your long-term goal. Importantly, too, you will need the support of your family and coworkers to succeed.

Social and Environmental Stressors

Your social and physical environments can also present stressors. Social stressors include interacting with new people, facing tough competition or discrimination, and using English if it isn't your first language. Stressors in the physical environments include crowded or loud residences, poor public transit, and extreme weather. Adjusting to college can be one the most difficult social and environmental challenges you will ever face. The rewards for persevering, however, are large and lifelong, as anyone who made it through will tell you.

Q I've never shared a bedroom before. How am I supposed to live with someone I've never met?

Having a roommate, a unique experience for many first-year students in 4-year colleges, may be the most stressful initial experience in college life. The situation of being thrown together with a stranger becomes even more challenging when a housing crunch forces you to have multiple roommates in a room designed for only two. Potential problems might be avoided by reaching out to your new roommates in advance, such as by visiting one another on Facebook or getting together with them during the summer before you start college.

Regardless, communication and respect are keys to living with someone new. Respecting your roommate includes common courtesy, such as not talking with others about things that happen in private space and not posting photos or unkind comments on Facebook. And as far as communication goes, start by learning about each other. What are your respective study and sleep habits (morning person or night owl)? What are your tolerances for noise and clutter? How do you want to handle visitors, shared expenses, and borrowing or using each other's clothes and food? Setting "house rules" will help things run more smoothly. Some schools even suggest roommate contracts to address misunderstandings, as minor arguments are inevitable. If concerns can't be worked out, seek out the advice of the resident assistant or advisor.

What are your top stressors? Do they include academic work or expectations; balancing work and school; a parent or child that needs special care? It's impossible to list all the stressors faced by college students, and something that was quite stressful during your first or second year may seem insignificant later on.

Managing Stress

Once you've identified your major stressors, it's time to think about coping strategies. What are you doing now to manage stress? What else could you do? In surveys, more than 90 percent of Americans report trying some form of stress-management technique (Table 10-3).

There are enough good stress-management strategies that everyone can find something helpful. What won't work is doing nothing or continuing to do what you've always done—unsuccessfully (see the box "Stress Management: What Not to Do").

Time Management

By managing your time wisely, you can minimize stress and improve your quality of life. Time-management techniques help you identify, prioritize, schedule, and

Wellness Strategies

Stress Management: What Not to Do

Q I tend to eat when I'm stressed out. Is this the wrong approach?

There are better and worse ways to manage stress. Here are some things to avoid:

Don't use tobacco, drugs, or alcohol: These substances provide temporary relief from stress, but they are highly addictive and lead to a host of health problems.

Don't binge-eat: Although eating your favorite foods may seem comforting, using food to reduce stress is bound to lead to more problems, including weight gain and possibly even eating disorders.

Don't give up emotionally: Feeling completely helpless can be both psychologically and physically damaging. Find small, practical things you can do to improve a negative situation, or try a relaxation technique.

Don't be inflexible: Holding tightly to your patterns of thinking and behavior in the face of change may be comforting, but remaining stuck in familiar but unsuccessful patterns usually creates even more stress.

Don't avoid the situation: Behavioral or cognitive avoidance will only make the situation worse the next time.

---

execute tasks, projects, and goals in a successful and satisfying way. They can help you avoid time traps, including procrastination, lack of focus, and poor multitasking. Effective time management is challenging but well worth the effort.

Q I thought computers were supposed to make me use my time better, but every time I log on, I waste tons of time! What can I do?

Going online is a journey, and one that makes many people wander off in unproductive ways. Strategies to minimize wasted computer time include setting online time limits, planning your Web destinations before logging on, and sticking to your original task (researching a term paper, for example). For social-networking sites like MySpace and Facebook, set aside a certain time each day to visit them, and don't let it compete with time designated for other work. When doing schoolwork, log out of your social sites, turn off your cell phone, and close down your e-mail. If you eliminate these temptations, you are more likely to get your work done.

Q Do I really need a planner?

Most people who effectively manage their time will tell you the secret is to have some type of planner—and to use it. Making a daily schedule is one of the most effective time-management strategies. People who use planners don't forget or miss deadlines, and they plan ahead. Some use paper-and-pencil-planners; others use a cell phone, a PDA, or a computer program.

Use your planner to prioritize. Enter your deadlines and projects, and create a to-do list to schedule and chunk your work. Divide your list into two columns or categories: Group A for the highest priority, must-do tasks, and Group B for less-important items that can wait for your attention. Break up the large projects into smaller chunks, don't wait until the last minute to get started, and make sure you know all the instructions. Review and update your list each day.

TABLE 10-3 AMERICAN ADULTS' STRESS-MANAGEMENT TECHNIQUES

TECHNIQUE	PERCENT REPORTING USE OF TECHNIQUE
Eating healthier foods	77%
Exercising more	75%
Losing weight	66%
Reducing stress	60%
Getting more sleep	58%
Reducing or eliminating alcohol	17%
Quitting smoking	13%

Source: American Psychological Association. (2011). *Stress in America: Stress in America Press Room.* Washington, DC: APA (http://www.apa.org/news/press/releases/stress/index.aspx).

Wellness Strategies

Time-Management Tips

Q How can I manage my time better?

Keep a time diary: Keep a time diary for a few weekdays and a few weekend days to see where your time goes. Use 15-minute blocks and write down everything you do. Take a close look and see where you can use your time more effectively—perhaps by reading while on the bus, electronically recording your notes, or cutting back on TV. Your time log should identify where you can save time and use time better. This clarification alone will help reduce stress and make you more productive.

Divide your time into small blocks: Use the 10-minute rule for overwhelming or difficult assignments. Work on the task for a minimum of 10 minutes, and if it is still difficult, put it down and move on. More often than not, you will find that after 10 minutes of work, the task doesn't seem so bad and the end is in sight. Regardless, breaking a task down into small blocks makes it much easier to complete.

Avoid distractions: Little distractions add up to lots of wasted time. If your apartment or dorm room has too many distractions, go to the library.

Do things right the first time: Taking the time to understand the instructions will allow you to do the job right the first time and eliminate the need to redo things. You will have more time to spend on other important tasks.

Don't try to save time by skipping healthy habits: There are some things you need to do more of, like exercise, sleep, and eat healthy foods (which usually take time to prepare).

Following a to-do list reduces stress by letting you focus on what is most important and freeing you from worrying that you should be working on something else. Your to-do list also helps you say no to distractions. While saying no is often difficult, it is a big part of managing time and reducing stress. Realize that it is better to say no and competently complete what you are working on rather than to take on too many new tasks and do them poorly, if at all. See the box "Time-Management Tips" for additional ideas.

Cognitive Strategies

Certain events may be out of your control, but regardless of the source of such potential stressors, the way you think about them ultimately determines their impact on you.

Q Does positive thinking really stop me from worrying?

ENGAGE IN REALISTIC SELF-TALK. By examining your patterns of thinking, you can better recognize self-defeating thoughts, negative statements, and irrational beliefs that undermine your mood, behavior, and health. Occasional negative self-talk ("I can't possibly get this paper done on time") is unavoidable, but once you can recognize your negative self-talk, you can begin to restructure your thoughts, making them more positive, affirming, and realistic ("It won't be easy, but I can get this paper done"). Review the discussion of self-talk in Chapter 2; also see the box "ABCDE Model for Effective Thought Remodeling" for suggestions. Many people use the ABCDE model informally, because it's a logical approach to managing stress. Try applying this model to a current stressor in your life.

Q I just can't seem to get over my bad quiz grade. What's the best way to move on?

Some of us get hung up on a bad grade, while others may be worried about paying for next semester's tuition. Moving on isn't always easy, but it's critical for reducing unhealthy stress. In addition to the ABCDE model, try focusing on the present, setting realistic goals, and developing healthy problem-solving techniques.

FOCUS ON THE PRESENT. One of the great stressors is worrying about yesterday or tomorrow and not focusing on what is happening right now. You may have done poorly on your last quiz, but where do you stand overall in the course? Have your other assignments been OK? Was it just the first quiz of the semester? Does the instructor drop students' lowest quiz score? Once you focus on where you are today, you can relax and have a more positive outlook ("She does drop the lowest quiz score, so I should be OK").

SET REALISTIC GOALS. Realistic goals are key for successful behavior change—and they are just as important for stress management. Setting too high a goal (for example, getting an A on all your assignments) is just a set-up for more stress. Instead, make your goal to get an A in the class (assuming you have a history of A-type success) rather than worrying about every assignment. Similarly, if you have never exercised before, you shouldn't plan on running a marathon this spring. Instead, attempt a local 5K. And if you've never received an A in any college course, don't shoot for straight A's this coming semester.

Wellness Strategies

ABCDE Model for Effective Thought Remodeling

Q | Are there any techniques I can use to motivate positive self-talk?

Psychologist Albert Ellis believed that people cause themselves stress and emotional pain with their belief systems. He developed the *ABCDE model,* which comprises the following steps, to help people do cognitive restructuring and engage in more positive and realistic self-talk.

A: Identify your *adversity* (for example, "I lost my part-time job").

B: Identify your instinctive *beliefs* about the adversity ("I can't pay my bills").

C: Identify the *consequences* of those beliefs ("I'll have to quit college").

D: Begin to *dispute* those beliefs ("I can certainly find another job").

E: Become *re-energized* when you successfully dispute a belief ("I can stay in school!").

Source: Ellis, A. (1985). Expanding the ABC's of rational-emotive therapy. In M. J. Mahoney & A. Freeman (Eds.), *Cognition and psychotherapy* (pp. 313–323). New York: Plenum.

Instead focus on *one class* for an A, and simply strive to do your best in all your classes.

Recognize your strengths and weaknesses and set realistic goals based on them. If writing isn't your strength, your goal could be to improve on that during the upcoming semester. If you haven't been too good at getting assignments done on time, then that could be a realistic goal. If you set small, achievable goals, you can put the pieces in place to make them happen—and thereby reduce your stress.

DEVELOP PROBLEM-SOLVING SKILLS. Problem solving is best accomplished by setting realistic goals, focusing on the present (you can't solve what has already happened), and keeping a positive outlook ("I can do this!"). Here are four basic steps in problem solving:

1. Identify the problem and describe it as accurately as you can. If it's large, break it down into manageable parts.
2. Brainstorm all possible solutions. Can you change the stressful circumstance? If not, can you change how you think about it?
3. Consider the positive and negative aspects of each potential solution, and then select the approach you think is most promising.
4. Evaluate the effectiveness of the solution you tried. If you don't think it worked, try one of your other possible solutions.

Problem-solving skills can often be developed by watching others who are successful and asking for advice. Once you know others' strategies, a little trial and error will show you which ones work best for you. See the box "Cognitive Stress-Management Techniques" for additional tips.

Healthy Relationships and Social Support

Healthy and supportive relationships have consistently been shown to reduce stress and improve overall health and well-being. However, all relationships are not equally supportive. A network of supportive friends, or even just one such friend, can be vital to well-being. See the box "How to Win Friends—and Keep Them."

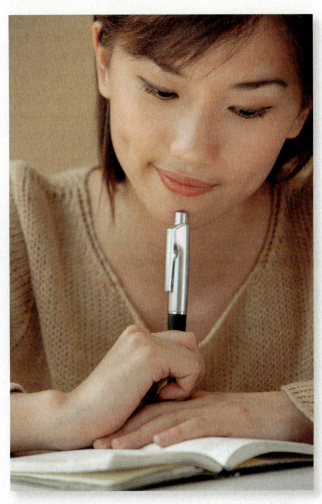

Effective problem solving involves identifying and describing a problem, coming up with and evaluating possible solutions, and then giving one a try.

Wellness Strategies

Cognitive Stress-Management Techniques

Q What are positive ways to change negative behavior and reduce my stress?

Accept things you cannot change, and find a way to work within any limitations: This is a much better approach then being forever mad about something. If math isn't your strength, don't try to tough it out. Find a math tutor (available for free on most campuses) or online help resources. Make it as pleasant an experience as possible.

Laugh a little—or a lot: Laughter makes you feel good. It may lower blood pressure, reduce stress hormones, increase muscle flexion, boost immunity, and trigger the release of the body's natural painkillers. Don't be afraid to laugh out loud, or laugh when you are alone or in a crowd. It will brighten your mood and the mood of those around you.

Slow down: Pace instead of race: Plan ahead and allow enough time to get the most important things done. College students often think they work best under deadlines. Ask any professor, however, and she will tell you that students who plan ahead and pace themselves usually do the best. Waiting until the last minute often results in many avoidable mistakes.

Let it go: The world won't end because you got a bad grade on a quiz or didn't have time to clean the kitchen. Don't beat yourself up for little things.

Q I can't seem to make any new friends. What can I do differently?

Meeting new people is the first step to making new friends. For full-time students starting college, the pool of potential friends is one of the great benefits of living in a residence hall. Getting a job, volunteering, joining an intramural club, and participating in academic group projects are all ways to meet new people. By doing the things that you find interesting, you are more likely to find people who share your interests.

The second step is to make time for your friends—don't just do things when you want to. Occasionally go out of your way for others and show them you truly care. Making time also includes showing up on time for events and remembering birthdays and special occasions. These actions go a long way toward cultivating long-lasting relationships.

Be a good listener. When under stress, your friends just want to be heard, and your listening is a meaningful gesture that creates a deep sense of personal connection. Listening is not easy for everyone, yet we can all benefit greatly from its healing power. Here are some tips for active listening:

- *Ask people about their feelings and really pay attention to what they say.* One of the easiest mistakes to make while listening is to think about what you want to say next instead of focusing on what the person is saying to you. Listen carefully and don't constantly interrupt.
- *Reflect back what you hear, so the other person knows you genuinely understand.* You might repeat key points to show that you are listening and to make sure that you have understood them correctly.

- *Focus your questions, comments, and attention on the other person.* Put your own feelings and needs aside. You want your friends to do the same for you when you are the one who needs to be listened to.

Q Some of my friends have told me I'm rude, but I don't know why they say that. How can I know?

Have you ever thought that you were saying something kind, but it turned out you offended someone? We may have good intentions with what we want to say, but it doesn't always work out that way. By taking a close look at your patterns of communication, you might find that you can make changes that will help you maintain good relationships with others.

There are three general patterns of communication:

- **Passive communication** involves failing to express feelings, thoughts, and beliefs honestly, usually in order to avoid conflict. This allows others to violate our rights, and the outcome is usually feelings of resentment and victimization.
- **Aggressive communication** involves directly standing up for personal rights and expressing thoughts, feelings, and beliefs in a way that is emotionally honest

passive communication A communication style in which the goal is to avoid confrontation; by failing to express honest feelings, beliefs, or thoughts, the individual allows his or her rights to be violated.

aggressive communication A communication style in which the individual's primary goal is to get what he or she wants, even if it requires manipulating and belittling others; needs and desires are clearly expressed but with a lack of consideration for others' feelings or welfare.

Wellness Strategies

How to Win Friends—and Keep Them

Q What's the best way to make a friend and keep a friend?

More than 75 years ago, Dale Carnegie wrote *How to Win Friends and Influence People,* one of the first self-help books. It is still in circulation today and has sold more than 15 million copies worldwide. Carnegie postulates that selling is all about making friends, and his key points include these:

- Become genuinely interested in other people.
- Smile.

- Remember that a person's name is to that person the sweetest and most important sound in any language.
- Be a good listener; encourage others to talk about themselves.
- Talk in terms of the other person's interests.
- Make the other person feel important—and do it sincerely.

Source: Carnegie, D. (1981). *How to win friends and influence people* (rev. ed.). New York, NY: Simon & Schuster. (Original work published 1936.)

---

but may make others feel humiliated, degraded, belittled, or intimidated.

- **Assertive communication** involves standing up for personal rights and expressing thoughts, ideas, feelings, needs, and beliefs in direct, honest, and appropriate ways that are sensitive to others.

Although assertive people may sometimes be seen as aggressive, there is quite a difference. Imagine a situation in which a friend is 20 minutes late. An aggressive response would be: "You're late, and you've ruined my day by making me late." An assertive response would be: "I will have to adjust my schedule now that our meeting is starting late." The difference between assertive and aggressive communication is not always so obvious. Although each lets it be known that the friend's lateness has caused a problem, the assertive expression is kinder, indicating some level of sympathy and acknowledging that everyone occasionally runs late. Assertive communication will help you maintain relationships while still expressing your thoughts and feelings. Here are some tips for communicating assertively:

- *Use confident body language:* Stand up straight, look people in the eye (but don't stare them down), and relax.
- *Use a firm and pleasant tone.*

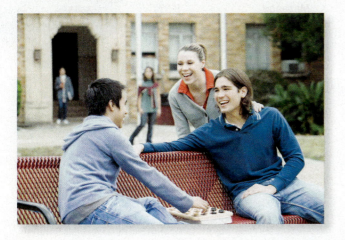

- *Don't assume that you know what other people are going to say or do:* Let them explain before you react.
- *Think win-win:* Look for a compromise or a way for everyone to get their needs met.

So, if your friends tell you that you're rude, adopt a communication style that is assertive instead of aggressive. Assertive people can go far in life for many reasons: They actively seek what they want; they consider others' feelings; and they are willing to work things out so that everyone prospers.

Q How do you tell if a friendship is worth it?

Relationships don't develop overnight, and they take conscious effort to maintain. But not everyone is meant to be friends. If you find yourself with people who make you feel bad about yourself or who are constantly negative, then they may not be the right people for you. Try to surround yourself with positive, sharing people.

High schools friends often drift apart during and after college. If a relationship fades because the people are changing, then cherish all that you had in the past and wish each other the best for the future. If a relationship is fading because one of the people is not trying, then consider the motivation behind the lack of effort before deciding to work hard to maintain it. Ask yourself these questions regarding both new and established friendships:

- Do you feel that your conversations are more forced than fluid?
- Do you feel the other person truly understands, accepts, and supports you? And do you feel that way toward that person?

assertive communication A communication style in which the primary goal is to solve a problem, finding a balance between one's own needs and the needs of others; needs and wants are clearly expressed and in a way that is respectful and sensitive to others.

- Does spending time with the other person make you feel energized—or drained?
- Do you include the other person in your life because you cherish his or her company or just to have a bigger social circle?

Listen to your feelings. Ultimately, you're the only one who knows if a relationship is worth keeping. But it's important to have a few special people you can count on in your life. Keep in mind that not everything always goes perfectly in any relationship. Feelings get hurt; people get angry at each other; and sometimes you feel pressured. These are normal occurrences, yet they should pass quickly if the relationship is healthy overall. If these difficult times happen often or don't seem to go away, it may be time to reevaluate the relationship.

Relationship violence is something that should never happen, not even one time. Violence can be physical, sexual, or psychological, but it is never OK. You should never make light of abuse or try to justify or excuse violent behavior by blaming the victim or by blaming yourself if you are the victim. Respect your friends at all times, express your feelings, and don't compromise when it comes to your own safety. If you or someone you know is in an abusive relationship, contact the Rape, Abuse, and Incest National Network (RAINN) Hotline at 1-800-656-HOPE (4673), the National Domestic Violence Hotline at 1-800-799-SAFE (7233), or your local emergency services at 911.

Healthy Lifestyle Choices: Activity, Diet, and Sleep

The more stress you feel, the more likely you are to make poor health choices. At the same time, the more poor health choices you make, the more stress you are likely to have. Break the cycle and your health will improve while your stress decreases.

Q Does working out really relieve stress?

PHYSICAL ACTIVITY. Working out is a proven stress buster. The great thing about exercise is that it doesn't take much activity to reduce your stress level. Although losing weight may take weeks or months, you can shed stress in minutes. Exercise bouts as short as 10 minutes have been shown to elevate people's moods, and the intensity doesn't need to be too high.[18] A brisk walk around the block or dancing to a song or two can often be an effective mood lifter. Further, people who exercise regularly tend to have a much milder physical stress reaction to typical stressors. See Chapters 3–5 for more on the physical and mental benefits of exercise.

Any amount of physical activity can help. If you're a regular exerciser, you should view your workouts as a means of managing stress, along with all their other health benefits. If you don't currently exercise or exercise only infrequently, try taking a brisk 10-minute walk next time you are feeling particularly stressed. Walking isn't the only exercise that can reduce stress, but it's one of the simplest, especially if you want an immediate de-stressor. If a quick walk isn't possible for you at a time of stress, try the relaxations techniques discussed later in the chapter.

Yoga and t'ai chi, along with Pilates, are all activities that can help manage stress.

- Yoga, described in Chapter 6, involves a series of physical postures and stretches emphasizing balance and breathing control.
- T'ai chi is a martial art that resembles a slow, graceful dance.
- Pilates, described in Chapter 5, includes a series of fluid movements performed in a precise manner, accompanied by specialized breathing techniques and mental concentration.

Although different in their specifics, these activities share certain characteristics: slow, purposeful movements; high levels of concentration; and focused breathing. These traits make them very effective for reducing both acute and chronic stress. However, when you use physical activity as part of a stress-management program, the type of activity is not as important as regular participation. Find an activity you like, do it often, and enjoy the benefits.

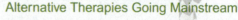

Fast Facts

Alternative Therapies Going Mainstream

Complementary and alternative therapies for stress and other health problems have become more widespread in recent years. A 2007 survey by the National Center for Health Statistics found that the following therapies are growing in popularity, with as many as one in eight American adults having practiced them.

Deep breathing	12.7%
Meditation	9.4%
Massage	8.3%
Yoga	6.1%
Imagery	2.2%
Pilates	1.4%
T'ai chi	1.0%

- Why do you think alternative therapies have become so popular?
- If you needed to de-stress, would you likely favor alternative or traditional therapies? Why?

Source: National Center for Health Statistics. (2008.) Complementary and alternative medicine use among adults and children: United States, 2007. *National Health Statistics Reports,* No. 12 (http://www.cdc.gov/nchs/products/nhsr.htm).

Q | Does what I eat affect my stress level?

EATING HABITS. The foods you eat can affect your stress level, for better or worse. A nutrient-rich diet containing a good mix of healthy fats, whole grains, lean protein sources, and fruits and vegetables keeps you healthy and can counteract the effects of stress by supporting your immune system and controlling your blood pressure.

What about foods to avoid or limit? Most people know that caffeine is a stimulant. Caffeine may help you stay awake to study, but it will make it more difficult for you to fall asleep—and sleeplessness can start a cycle of reduced sleep and increased stress. Too much caffeine can also cause jittery and anxious feelings that are similar to the stress response. Limiting caffeine intake is a wise stress-management strategy.

Fried and other fatty foods may also make falling asleep difficult, so it is best to avoid them, especially later in the evening. Sodium and sugar in the diet can also make sleep difficult or cause irritability for some people. Try keeping a journal or log that tracks your stress level, sleeping pattern, and the foods and beverages you consume. Look for a pattern linking eating habits and stress. If you reduce or eliminate the offending foods, your stress level will go down.

Q | Why do I need sleep? Does it play a role in stress management?

SLEEP. Sleep is essential for optimal wellness. Although sleep is critical to our well-being, it tends to be one of the first things neglected when we feel stressed, especially when pressured by time. Make time for sleep! You'll be healthier, and you'll function at a higher physical and mental level when you are awake (see the box "Sleep, Bad Sleep, and Really Bad Sleep").

Among adults, sleeping less than 6 or 7 hours a night leads to a host of health problems. College students often make a game of seeing how little sleep they can get, especially around exam time. Sleep deprivation, usually defined as less than about 4 or 5 hours in a 24-hour period, makes you function as if you were drunk, so why would you want to take an exam in that condition? Lack of sleep hurts your ability to concentrate and is associated with lower grades. It is also linked to increased risk of health problems, in both the short term (colds) and the long term (high blood pressure, blood glucose abnormalities, abdominal fat accumulation).[19] Furthermore, people who sleep less than 6 hours are more likely to die prematurely than those who sleep 6–8 hours a night.[20]

Periods of high stress are times when sleep is both most important and most difficult to obtain. Establishing good sleep habits early in college will serve you well during difficult times. Strive for a consistent 6–8 hours of sleep a night, depending on your needs. For tips, see the box "Getting a Better Night's Sleep."

If you regularly feel tired, you're probably not getting enough sleep. If your sleep is sufficient, you should feel rested during the day and should be able to stay focused and attentive, even in situations you might describe as boring. You should not feel fatigued or constantly irritable. You should also wake up on your own in the morning rather than being awakened from a sound sleep by your alarm. If you often doze off during the day or can't wake up without a loud alarm, you probably need more sleep. Take the Epworth Sleepiness Scale to assess your sleep status (http://www.sleepeducation.com/SleepScale.aspx).

Q | Is snoring bad for me or just annoying for other people?

Snoring is very common. It occurs when tissues in the throat relax during sleep, partially blocking the airway. As air flows past the relaxed tissues, they vibrate and produce harsh sounds. These sounds can be loud and make it difficult for others to sleep.

A more serious condition, *obstructive sleep apnea,* is linked to persistent snoring. In apnea, the throat is blocked and the person stops breathing for 10 or more seconds. Shifts in blood levels of oxygen and carbon dioxide trigger the body to wake up—the airway opens and the person takes a gasping breath. This typically happens over and over during the night, and although the person may be unaware of it, sleep is significantly disrupted. Sleep apnea can cause severe and persistent daytime sleepiness; it also increases the risk of high blood pressure and other cardiovascular problems. Anyone suspected of having sleep apnea needs to seek medical care.

For general snoring, here are some self-management measures:

- Lose weight if you are overweight.
- Sleep on your side.
- Treat any nasal congestion from a cold or allergies.
- Avoid alcohol and other sedatives, especially close to bedtime.
- Try over-the-counter nasal strips.
- Consider a dental mouthpiece that helps keep airways open during sleep.

If these strategies don't reduce snoring, get evaluated by a health care professional. You can be tested for apnea by wearing monitors at home or in a specialized sleep lab. Treatments for apnea include surgery and wearing a pressurized mask during sleep.

Q | I just can't seem to get to sleep. How can I turn my brain off?

Insomnia is a sleep disorder characterized by persistent difficulty falling asleep or staying asleep, impairing a person's ability to function normally. Many insomniacs complain that they are unable to rest their mind for more than a few minutes at a time—usually a sign that the insomnia is due to stress.

insomnia A sleep disorder characterized by persistent problems falling asleep or staying asleep.

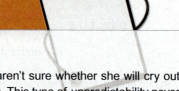

Research Brief

Sleep, Bad Sleep, and Really Bad Sleep

Many people regularly enjoy a good night's sleep, but others struggle mightily on a nightly basis. So what is a "bad" night's sleep? Physiologically, a bad night's sleep is one full of disruptions, which lead to higher levels of circulating glucocorticoids (hormones that affect metabolism). This hormonal surge fuels increased sympathetic nervous activity and decreased circulating growth hormone.

Specifically, the researchers identified a hierarchy of bad sleep. First there is continuous, uninterrupted, but insufficient sleep. This pattern, also known as *short sleep,* is common when one gets to bed late or rises early. Second is *short, fragmented sleep.* This type of sleep, though uncommon, is characterized by sleep that is interrupted on a regular basis. Third and worst is *short, unpredictably interrupted sleep.* Such a pattern can occur when people have a newborn and aren't sure whether she will cry out in 5 minutes or 5 hours. This type of unpredictability never allows for a deep healthful sleep and instead elevates glucocorticoid levels, leaving the individual feeling unrested throughout the day and at higher risk for a host of chronic diseases over time.

Analyze and Apply

- On the basis of the terms used in this study, what is your typical sleep pattern? Explain.
- If you suffer, or hypothetically were to suffer, from fragmented sleep, what could you do to improve your sleep?

Source: Sapolsky, R. (2004). *Why zebras don't get ulcers.* (3rd ed., p. 238). New York, NY: St. Martin's Griffin.

Insomnia is more than just difficulty going to sleep. It can also include difficulty returning to sleep in the middle of the night or waking too early in the morning. The pattern of insomnia often is related to the underlying cause.

Fast Facts

Hit the Hay to Raise Your GPA

Students who are early birds have GPAs a full point higher on average than night owls. Early risers may find it easier to get to class on time and to study. By going to bed earlier, they may also be less likely to drink, party, and engage in other activities that hurt academic performance. If you are a night owl, try slowly shifting your sleep schedule toward that of an early bird. Also avoid scheduling classes early in the morning if possible.

- What are some instances when insufficient sleep may have affected your grade for a course or an important exam, or your performance on some other significant occasion?

Source: Clay K., Tatum, J. I., Taylor D. J., Bramoweth, A. D., Roane, B. M., & Alloway, K. A. (2008). Morningness and eveningness relationship to college GPA. *Sleep, 31* (Abstract Suppl), A239. Research abstract presented at the annual meeting of the Associated Professional Sleep Societies.

Although psychoactive drugs, hormonal shifts, and mental disorders can all disrupt sleep, the most common causes of insomnia among college students are fear, anxiety, and overall stress.[21] In addition to stress, poor sleep habits and too much noise or light can also affect sleep, as anyone who has ever lived in a residence hall or shared an apartment with three or four roommates knows.

Because emotional stress is a primary cause of insomnia, finding effective stress reducers can help to improve sleep. Stress affects the quality and quantity of sleep, and when we sleep poorly, our stress level often rises. This cycle of poor sleep and increased stress will continue until our sleep needs are met, which often requires several nights of quality sleep. Chronic sleep deprivation cannot be made up for by just one or two good nights of sleep.[22]

Try any of the stress-management techniques suggested in this chapter to help reduce your level of stress and improve your sleep. If problems persist, keep a sleep diary of your sleeping and waking times and related information (such as caffeine intake, exercise habits, and stress level), and discuss your sleep problems with a health care professional.

Spiritual Wellness

Q | Will spirituality make me more or less stressed?

Without an awareness of personal values, we may find that our life is dictated by the demands of others—a highly stressful situation. Having a strong personal belief system makes us more resilient and therefore better able to handle stressful

Wellness Strategies

Getting a Better Night's Sleep

Q | What can I do to sleep better?

Try these strategies for ensuring that your Z's are high quality.

Maintain a regular sleep schedule: Go to bed and get up at the same time every day. Staying up later than usual and sleeping in on the weekends disrupts your regular sleep schedule. Consistency will make you feel better.

Create a sleep-friendly environment: Try to make your bedroom comfortable, quiet, cool, and dark. Soft and monotonous noise, along with room darkening, is often helpful for sleep.

Avoid caffeine, alcohol, and nicotine: Caffeine and nicotine are stimulants and may double the time it should take you to fall asleep. Alcohol induces sleepiness, but it causes poorer sleep and restlessness through the night. Also, don't eat a large or heavy meal within 2 or 3 hours of bedtime.

Establish relaxing bedtime rituals: Reading, listening to soothing music, and taking a warm bath or shower are common ways to help your mind and body associate bedtime with relaxation and peacefulness. Allow yourself time to wind down.

Exercise regularly: Any type of regular exercise helps you fall asleep and sleep better through the night. However, exercising too late in the evening may make it difficult to fall asleep.

---

situations. Spirituality, although not necessarily religiosity, helps give our life context. **Spirituality** has three general components: feeling a connectedness to ourself and to others, developing a system of personal beliefs and values,

Fast Facts

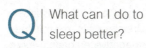

Asleep at the Wheel

More than one-third of surveyed drivers report having fallen asleep while driving on at least one occasion. Even more disturbing is that 13 percent of respondents say that they have dozed off on a monthly basis while driving, and 4 percent admit to having had an accident from sleeping at the wheel. Overall, almost two-thirds of Americans report driving while feeling drowsy at least once in the past year. Research shows that after about 20 hours without sleep, the effects on driving ability are the same as those from being legally drunk.

- If you have ever drifted into sleep or become drowsy while driving, what circumstances caused your drowsiness?
- What strategies do you use to avoid falling asleep at the wheel?

Source: National Sleep Foundation. (2010). Facts and stats. *Drowsy Driving.org* (http://drowsydriving.org/about/facts-and-stats).

and finding meaning and purpose in life. For many people, religion and religious practices such as prayer or meditation offer paths to developing spirituality. However, spirituality does not necessarily mean religion, and people can develop spirituality in other ways. Spirituality is personal and subjective; no two people have exactly the same spiritual beliefs, be they religious or not.

Self-discovery is a good way to explore your spirituality. You can begin by thinking about your relationship with yourself and then look to how you nurture relationships with people important to you. Also consider your beliefs and values—what your purpose in life is, and what you would like to accomplish. Ask yourself:

- What are the important relationships in my life?
- Where do I find comfort?
- What gives me hope? Joy?
- What do I believe will happen to me when my physical life ends, and how do I feel about it?

Spirituality has many benefits. Those who regularly engage in a spiritual practice (such as communing with nature or meditating) are better able to focus on their personal goals. By knowing what's important, you can focus less on the unimportant things, thus minimizing your stress. Spirituality also imparts a sense of connectedness and belonging and therefore helps keep you from feeling lonely. Knowing your place in the world releases you from the burden of feeling responsible for everything around you. Unburdening yourself then allows you more time to cultivate and nurture meaningful relationships and ultimately lead a healthier life, in all dimensions of wellness.

spirituality A person's system of beliefs and values, feelings of connectedness to self and others, and experience of finding meaning and purpose in life.

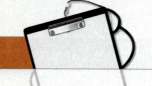

Research Brief

The Stress of Setting Life Goals

We have all been encouraged to set goals in life, but where the impetus for these goals comes from may have a big impact on our stress and happiness. Researchers followed a group of college graduates, evaluating their goals as well as factors such as self-esteem, anxiety, physical signs of stress, and overall satisfaction with life. These former students were categorized as to whether they set intrinsic or extrinsic goals. *Intrinsic goals* include having meaningful personal relationships, strong community involvement, and good physical health. *Extrinsic goals* include achieving a certain level of pay and/or a certain appearance or image (say, wealth and good looks). It turns out that intrinsic goal setters were happier,

less stressed, and more satisfied with life than extrinsic goal setters. The group with extrinsic goals, even if they achieved them, reported more negative emotions, more physical symptoms of stress and anxiety, and less life satisfaction.

Analyze and Apply

- What are some of your life goals, and where did the impetus come from?
- If your goals are extrinsic, what can you do to make them more intrinsic?

Source: Niemiec, C. P., Ryan, R. M., & Deci, E. L. (2009). The path taken: Consequences of attaining intrinsic and extrinsic aspirations in post-college life. *Journal of Research in Personality, 43*(3), 291–306.

See the box "The Stress of Setting Life Goals" for broader insight into goal setting in life.

Steps to develop spiritually include:

- *Improve your self-esteem.* Use small steps to gain confidence in what you do.
- *Engage in meaningful activities.* Express your creativity, spend time enjoying nature, or engage in a personal spiritual practice.
- *Foster relationships with the people who are important to you.*
- *Help others.* Volunteer your time or return a favor. Helping others helps you by giving you a different perspective on life and potentially boosting your motivation to achieve. Volunteering can raise your self-esteem and improve your mood.

For most people, spirituality is an ever-changing process of self-exploration. Age and life experiences will certainly make you readjust your spiritual beliefs. Ultimately, though, self-exploration will lead to greater personal fulfillment at all stages of life.

Relaxation Techniques

Relaxation techniques intended for stress reduction are popular. If practiced regularly, relaxation techniques can have lasting benefits, not only returning you to homeostasis but bringing you peace of mind and good health.

Q How does a relaxation technique actually help?

The **relaxation response** is a physiological state of deep rest that changes the physical and emotional responses to stress.[23] Just as stress causes potentially harmful physiological responses, relaxation causes potentially beneficial ones, calming the fight-or-flight response and returning the body to normal

functioning. Breathing and heart rate slow, muscles relax, and metabolism and blood pressure decrease, all producing a much healthier state of being.

BREATHING AND POSTURE. Breathing deeply relaxes muscles, quiets the mind, and gets oxygen into the blood, where it can invigorate all parts of the body, even a tired brain. However, most people use only about half of their breathing capacity at best—and less when they're under stress.

Deep, or diaphragmatic, breathing involves filling your lungs by expanding your abdomen rather than your chest. When you breathe in, the diaphragm contracts and flattens downward, creating a vacuum that draws in air. When you exhale, the diaphragm returns to its dome shape, pushing air out of the body. You can practice diaphragmatic breathing anywhere: Just rest one hand lightly on your lower abdomen so that you can feel your breath move your body. Breathe in slowly through your nose and then let go of your breath slowly through pursed lips, all while feeling your abdomen expand during inhalation and relax during exhalation. Although this breathing pattern may be unfamiliar, it is physiologically most effective. The next time you feel especially stressed, try repeating diaphragmatic breathing a few times, focusing on the movement of your abdomen. You should feel some stress relief in a matter of minutes.

Posture is also important. Good posture radiates ease and confidence and can immediately make you feel better about yourself (it can also make you look slimmer). Try improving your posture a few times during the day. You can start by standing with your back to a wall and making sure that your heels, buttocks, shoulders, and head are all touching the wall. This effort will make you stand tall. Then walk away from the wall, holding that upright posture. When you are stressed, stand or sit tall, and you should look and feel better right away.

relaxation response
A physiological state of deep rest that reverses the body's responses to stress.

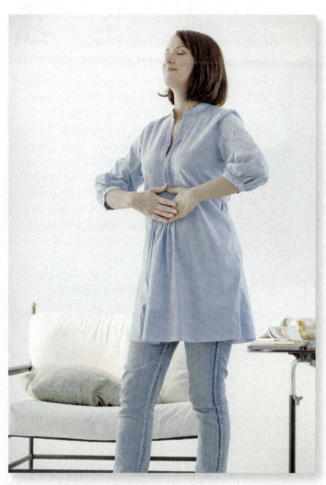

Deep breathing is a technique that can be used anywhere to induce the relaxation response. Instead of taking shallow breaths that slightly expand your chest, take deep breaths that fill your lungs and expand your abdomen.

PROGRESSIVE MUSCLE RELAXATION. A general stretching workout can help your muscles relax, but other techniques directly address muscle tension. **Progressive muscle relaxation (PMR)** involves tensing muscles and then actively reducing that tension while concentrating on your body and not your stressors. Start with a specific muscle group, say, your left calf: Inhale and gently squeeze the calf muscle until you feel some tension and hold it for 6 to 10 seconds. Squeeze gently to avoid soreness or injury. After a few seconds, release the tension and the breath to allow both physical and emotional relief. Begin each PMR session at either your head or your toes and work in the opposite direction. If time is short, focus on the large muscle groups, but be sure to perform the exercises on both sides of your body. If you have time, it is best to practice PMR daily, involving as many muscles as possible, one by one. Even with a brief PMR session, however, you should feel some immediate stress relief.

progressive muscle relaxation (PMR) A relaxation method that involves tensing and relaxing muscles in sequence.

meditation A broad group of self-directed practices that quiet and focus the mind and relax the body.

Q | What is meditation, and how does it reduce stress?

MEDITATION. Meditation, an internal state of relaxed awareness, can be a great way to ease the day's stress. You can practice meditation almost anywhere, anytime—even while commuting or going for a walk. Meditation can produce a deep state of relaxation and a tranquil mind, and this emotional calming doesn't end with the meditation session.[24] People who meditate regularly can experience long-lasting emotional and physical benefits.

There are many types of meditation, some more formal than others. Some people meditate by focusing on one object or thought, whereas others try to quiet their mind of everything. Don't be intimidated by thinking that you aren't mystical enough to meditate or don't know how. Prayer and contemplation are examples of using concentration to elicit the relaxation response. Yoga and t'ai chi include meditation in their practice, and deep breathing can also be a form of meditation.

Two general categories of meditation are exclusive meditation and inclusive meditation. To practice *exclusive meditation,* find a quiet place where you won't be interrupted for at least 10 minutes and focus on a single word or phrase while trying to eliminate all other thoughts. You can use any word or phrase that makes you comfortable. Close your eyes and breathe slowly while repeating your word or phrase. Continue for 10–20 minutes. Sounds simple, but if you are new to meditation, your thoughts will quickly wander. Once you notice that, refocus and come back to your special word or phrase. So that you can relax during meditation, set an alarm to keep your mind from worrying about the time or to wake you if you should fall asleep.

Inclusive meditation, also known as mindfulness meditation, allows your mind to wander as you observe your thoughts. The key aspect of inclusive meditation is to not judge or react emotionally to your thoughts; just observe them as an outsider might. Inclusive meditation can reduce negative-thinking patterns and help you realistically reappraise potential stressors as less threatening and challenging than they seem.

Other meditative techniques are prayer and sacred chants. Prayer is a widely practiced example of meditation and can be spoken or written. Praying can release stress because it is a recognition that help can come from many sources (a higher being, general faith, self-confidence) and that you are not on your own.

Repeating a phrase or sentence that is sacred or meaningful to you, called a *mantra,* can also be calming. Find something meaningful to you, something that calms or encourages you (such as "I am capable and strong"). You can say it to yourself quietly or out loud. Although saying it quietly may be necessary at times, it is believed that saying the mantra out loud brings the most fulfillment. Repeating your mantra while walking is a great way to reduce stress.

Take a purposeful walk and repeat your mantra, loudly if possible, focusing on the words. Time will pass as you feel your stress going away and your self-confidence increasing, and by the end of the walk, you will feel invigorated.

Q Is closing my eyes and thinking of the beach really going to help?

VISUALIZATION/MENTAL IMAGERY. Many people engage in **visualization**—a technique using all the senses to imagine a place or scene that is comfortable, soothing, and relaxing—for pleasure, without realizing they are practicing stress reduction. Have you ever imagined yourself being on a warm beach while in reality you were stuck in the middle of winter? Or have you ever thought about what it would feel like to win the lottery? Visualization temporarily removes us from reality, providing a respite from the daily grind, some mental rest and relaxation. Practicing visualization is simple. You start by finding a quiet spot and making yourself comfortable. Once you are settled, close your eyes and visualize a place you find comfortable, safe, and relaxing. Stay focused on your image. Eventually, you will feel as if you are actually there, experiencing the sights, sounds, and smells of your image. (Put the book down and try it for a few minutes. When you return, you'll feel more focused on what you're reading here.)

Visualization can also be used as a performance booster in sports and other activities. Imagine what you would like to happen—hitting a baseball, delivering a great speech, asking your boss for a raise—and use it as a form of mental rehearsal.

Q I like to listen to music when I'm upset. Does that reduce stress?

OTHER STRATEGIES FOR RELAXATION. For many people, music is a powerful mood elevator, and listening can help anyone relax. When you can, get up and dance to your music or sing out loud. It is amazing how quickly your stress level will drop. Other things to try:

- *Keep a journal:* Journaling allows you to explore your thoughts and emotions, work through your worries, and revisit the good things in your life. It can increase your awareness of your

visualization For stress management, a technique using all the senses to imagine a place or scene that is comfortable, soothing, and relaxing.

Fast Facts

Music Soothes the Savage . . . Student?

Researchers have found that listening to music that is soothing or that people select for themselves can often reduce anxiety, improve mood, and quiet the physical stress response. These positive changes have been seen among patients in hospital waiting rooms and in students who have just taken a challenging exam. In addition, listening to loud music with a fast tempo increases blood pressure and heart and breathing rates. Pick music to match your mood, level of energy, and level of stress.

- Under what stressful circumstances have you listened to music to reduce stress? Did it work?

typical patterns of thinking in response to stressors and serve as a good problem-solving tool.

- *Read:* Reading a book or some poems, especially when it is by choice and for pleasure, allows you to clear your mind for 30 minutes or so and come back to your routine tasks more invigorated.
- *Get a massage:* Massage can reduce physical discomfort and mental stress.
- *Spend time with a pet:* Pets provide relief from stress and loneliness and their own particular type of social support. Walking and playing with a dog are also opportunities for physical activity.
- *Take a humor break:* Laughter improves both emotional and physical wellness. Find ways to make yourself and those around you laugh more frequently—read or watch cartoons; post funny pictures around your residence or as your computer screensaver; play a silly game.

When Stress Becomes Too Much: Getting Help

Q My stress is killing me. Should I see someone?

We all experience stress, but for some of us, it may seem truly overwhelming. Constant or excessive stress can lead to increased anxiety, panic attacks, depression, and, in worst-case scenarios, even suicide. Because it can be hard to know when your stress has reached a point that you can no longer deal with it alone, it is better to take action too soon rather than too late.

Stress becomes dangerous when it interferes with your ability to live normally. If you feel out of control or don't know what to do, then your stress is becoming a danger to you and you should seek help. Unfortunately, many students don't know where to turn, are ashamed of their feelings, or don't think anyone can help them.

Virtually all colleges and universities provide free counseling—a valuable yet underutilized service. Seeking assistance from the counseling center or calling a stress hotline can help. Even talking with a close friend or family member can help bring you back to a place of greater stability. For many people who are feeling too stressed, talking to someone about their worries can help tremendously. Talking can put worries into perspective, identifying which are controllable and can be addressed and which cannot be controlled and need to be let go of. Your friends and family may be able to help you with stress, but if you are experiencing anxiety attacks, feel depressed, or have considered suicide, seek professional help immediately.

Q When are sad feelings just being "down in the dumps," and when are they serious depression?

Everybody experiences times of feeling sad, blue, or down in the dumps. Ups and downs are normal. Maybe you didn't turn in a paper on time or didn't get the work shift you wanted. Maybe you found out that your car needs a lot of repair work. Such situations can make anyone feel down. Typically, though, these feelings pass in a few hours or days, and we move on. However, when the depressed mood continues for many days or weeks, and especially if it interferes with daily activities and responsibilities (socializing, parenting, job, school), you might be suffering from **depression** (Figure 10-4).

Unfortunately, many people, especially men, never seek treatment for these symptoms. Maybe they rationalize that their feelings are only temporary ("I'll feel better tomorrow") or justified ("Everyone feels down when they do badly on an exam"). Maybe they're ashamed ("People in my family don't get depressed"). But depression is a serious illness with serious consequences, which can include suicide. Male or female, it's important to be honest with yourself if you recognize symptoms of depression in yourself. Don't think these feelings will just go away; they probably won't. Seeking help is the best thing you can do for yourself and those around you.

If you're depressed, it is also important to realize that feelings of exhaustion and helplessness are part of the illness rather than an accurate reflection of your circumstances. These negative feelings will fade with treatment. See the box "Living Well with . . . Depression" for more information.

depression A psychological disorder characterized by feelings of sadness and hopelessness, loss of interest in activities that were once enjoyable, poor concentration, and physical symptoms such as fatigue, sleeping problems, and poor appetite.

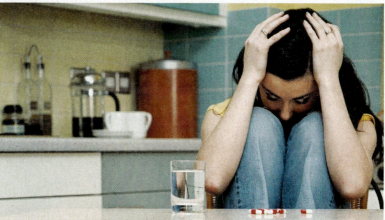

Symptoms of depression

Ongoing sad, anxious, or empty feelings

Feelings of hopelessness

Feelings of guilt, worthlessness, or helplessness

Feeling irritable or restless

Loss of interest in activities or hobbies that were once enjoyable

Feeling tired all the time

Difficulty concentrating, remembering details, or difficulty making decisions

Sleep disturbances: insomnia, waking in the middle of the night, or sleeping all the time

Overeating or loss of appetite

Thoughts of suicide or suicide attempts

Ongoing aches and pains, headaches, cramps, or digestive problems that do not go away

Risk factors for suicide

Previous suicide attempts

History of depression or other mental illness

Alcohol or drug abuse

Family history of suicide or violence

Physical illness

Impulsive or aggressive tendencies

Feeling isolated, cut off from other people

Unwillingness to seek help

Figure 10-4 **Symptoms of depression and risk factors for suicide.** Not everyone suffering from depression will have all these symptoms. Visit the site for the American Association of Suicidology (http://www.suicidology.org) for more on recognizing and responding to suicide warning signs.
Sources: National Institute of Mental Health. (2012). *Depression* (http://www.nimh.nih.gov/health/topics/depression). Centers for Disease Control and Prevention. (2012). Suicide prevention. *Violence Prevention* (http://www.cdc.gov/violenceprevention/suicide).

Living *Well* with . . .

Depression

Depression is a common and potentially serious illness that can interfere with a person's daily life and relationships. Some people experience bouts of severe symptoms (*major depression*), and others experience long-term but less severe symptoms (*dysthymic disorder*). Depression can run in families, and symptoms usually start between ages 15 and 30. Depression is more common in women than in men, but men have higher rates of suicide.

Overall, about one in twenty Americans report current symptoms of depression, although only about 30 percent of those affected have sought treatment. This is unfortunate, because even in severe cases, depression is highly treatable. The first step for a person experiencing symptoms (see Figure 10-4) is to visit a health care professional for an evaluation.

Once diagnosed, depression is typically treated with medication, psychotherapy, or both. Antidepressant medications affect levels of neurotransmitters such as serotonin and norepinephrine. Medications affect different people in different ways, so almost everyone needs to try more than one before finding the most effective choice. Psychotherapy can help people change negative patterns of thinking and behaving that contribute to their depression; it can also help them work through problems in personal relationships. Depression symptoms may last or recur, so long-term management of the condition is often needed.

Self-help measures can accompany professional treatment. The National Institute of Mental Health recommends the following:

- Engage in mild physical activity or exercise.
- Go to a movie or sporting event, or engage in another activity that you once enjoyed.
- Participate in religious, social, and other activities.
- Set realistic goals for yourself.
- Break up large tasks into small ones, set priorities, and do only as much as you can.
- Don't isolate yourself; spend time with people and confide in a trusted friend or relative.
- Expect your mood to improve gradually, not immediately; do not expect to suddenly "snap out of it." During treatment, sleep and appetite may begin to improve before mood.
- Postpone important decisions, such as changing jobs, until you feel better; discuss decisions with others whom know you well and who have a more objective view of your situation.
- Remember that positive thinking will replace negative thoughts as your depression responds to treatment.

Source: National Institute of Mental Health. (2012). *Depression* (http://www.nimh.nih.gov/health/topics/depression). Last accessed January 2012.

Q | What should I do about a friend who seems depressed or suicidal?

It is very serious when someone appears to be suicidal, and you should not take it lightly. If the threat seems imminent, call 911. If you aren't sure, call, or encourage your friend to call, the National Suicide Prevention Lifeline (1-800-273-TALK). Don't try to talk your friend out of it unless you are a trained counselor. If you called 911, do your best to keep your friend calm until help arrives. Follow these guidelines: Listen; let your friend express his or her feelings, and don't make any judgments.

If the threat is not imminent, talk to your friend using the same approach:

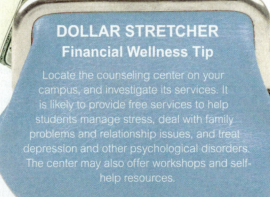

DOLLAR STRETCHER
Financial Wellness Tip

Locate the counseling center on your campus, and investigate its services. It is likely to provide free services to help students manage stress, deal with family problems and relationship issues, and treat depression and other psychological disorders. The center may also offer workshops and self-help resources.

listening, showing empathy, and not judging. It's OK to ask your friend to talk about his or her suicidal thoughts, plans, and timeline. Strongly recommend that your friend seek professional help. Check back with him or her frequently: Did she follow up with a counselor? Is she still harboring suicidal thoughts? Is he taking prescribed medications? Has his mood improved?

Addressing potentially suicidal thoughts in a friend or loved one is difficult, but it must be done. If you misinterpreted your friend's intentions, you risk upsetting him or her with your suspicions. However, the risk of doing nothing is much greater. Don't hesitate to act if you suspect suicidal thoughts.

Summary

Stressors are all around you, so you need to know how to manage stress—your physical and emotional reactions to those stressors. Although your body automatically prepares you for a physical response to stress, most stressors do not require such a reaction. If the stress response occurs too often or for extended periods, it can take a serious physical and emotional toll. Factors that affect your response to stressors include personality traits, gender, biological sex, and typical thinking patterns. Although the top sources of stress vary from person to person, common stressors include major life changes; minor daily hassles; relationships; environmental factors; and time, job, and school pressures.

Many techniques can help you manage stress. Some (time management, problem solving) allow you to change the stressful circumstances. Others (relationships, exercise, sleep, healthy diet, spiritual practices) help maintain your resilience against the effects of stress. Still others (meditation, deep breathing, progressive muscle relaxation, visualization) directly induce the relaxation response. If stress becomes severe or signs of depression occur, seek professional help.

More to Explore

American Psychological Association Help Center
http://www.apa.org/helpcenter/

Benson-Henry Institute for Mind Body Medicine
http://www.massgeneral.org/bhi

Go Ask Alice! Emotional Health
http://www.goaskalice.columbia.edu/Cat4.html

National Institute of Mental Health: Health Topics
http://www.nimh.nih.gov/health/index.shtml

National Sleep Foundation
http://www.sleepfoundation.org

Student Counseling Virtual Pamphlet Collection
http://www.dr-bob.org/vpc

LAB ACTIVITY 10-1 What's Stressing You?

COMPLETE IN connect

NAME	DATE	SECTION

This lab includes a checklist of common stressors encountered by many college students. Identifying your stressors is the first step in successful stress management.

Equipment: None

Preparation: None

Instructions

Check each event or situation that you have experienced in the past 12 months.

___ Death of close family member

___ Death of close friend

___ Divorce

___ Marital separation

___ Marriage

___ Pregnancy

___ Miscarriage

___ Birth of a child

___ Parents divorce or remarry

___ Starting or ending an intimate relationship

___ Sexual difficulties

___ Dating problems

___ Change in health of close family member

___ Spouse changing careers or going back to school

___ Major incident with the law

___ Jail term

___ Personal injury or illness

___ Chronic car trouble

___ Holidays or vacation

___ Major dental work

___ Major change in eating habits

___ Major change in sleeping habits

___ Major change in physical activity habits

___ Change in social activities

___ Change in religious activities

___ Change in recreation

___ Change in financial state

___ Change in jobs

___ Change in work hours or responsibilities

___ Trouble with boss at work

___ Trouble getting along with coworkers, classmates, or teammates

___ Change in residence

___ Starting, transferring, or dropping out of college

___ Changing academic majors

___ Dropping a course

___ Failing a course

___ Attempting to get a job or internship

___ Significant personal achievement

Results

Count up the total number of events checked and look for patterns and trends. Are most of your stressors things you have some control over and therefore can change (for example, not getting enough sleep, failing a course, changing eating habits)? Or are your stressors major life events that lie out of your control (such as divorce of parents or a death in the family) and require you to find some effective techniques for coping and relaxation? This lab focuses on the first group, but you should take all your stressors seriously and take steps now to make things better. See Lab Activity 10-2 for more on handling high levels of stress.

Total number of checked events

☐

Number of events that can be eliminated, changed, or improved

Number of events that are out of your control

The more events you check, the more likely you are dealing with unusual amounts of stress. Also, people often don't realize all the stress accumulating in their lives. Although major stressors are easy to recognize (such as divorce and death), the little stressors can add up and have just as damaging an effect on our overall wellness. This list helps you keep track of all your stressors, just as keeping a diary helps you see patterns in your daily life.

Reflecting on Your Results

Are you surprised by the total number of stressful events in your life? Did your responses to this quiz match your impression of how much stress you are dealing with?

Planning Your Next Steps

Everyone has stressors they can eliminate or improve through changes in behavior or thinking patterns. Look at the stressors on the list above that you identified as events or situations that you have some control over. Then consult the chapter for tips and techniques on how you might eliminate one or more of those stressors or reduce their impact on you. Consider time management, social support, realistic goal setting and self-talk, and problem solving. Choose a technique you find interesting and appealing, and try it out for a week. Report on your experiences.

Stress-management technique. Describe specifically what you plan on doing during the week to eliminate or improve a stressor:

Results of trying technique. What effect, if any, did the technique you tried have on your stress level? Do you think it changed how you felt or how you acted regarding the stressors you focused on?

LAB ACTIVITY 10-2

NAME	DATE	SECTION

Do you handle stress well, or do you fly off the handle? How we deal with stress goes a long way toward determining our stress-related health outcomes. Handle it well (use appropriate responses, have good levels of social support, regular sleep and exercise, eat well, and so on), and you are likely to minimize your risk of negative health outcomes. Handle your stress poorly (get angry, hold a grudge, resent others, don't get enough sleep or exercise, overeat, and so on), and you are at greater risk for negative health outcomes. This quiz will help you determine how well you are handling the stress in your life.

Equipment: None

Preparation: None

Instructions

Answer the following questions yes or no.

Yes/No

_____ **1.** Do other people frequently irritate you?

_____ **2.** Are you easily irritated when you can't complete a task?

_____ **3.** Do you notice yourself worrying a lot, especially about things you can't influence?

_____ **4.** Do you normally use alcohol, tobacco, or drugs to relax, especially after a hard day?

_____ **5.** Do you often have trouble falling asleep or sleeping through the night?

_____ **6.** Do you frequently experience an upset stomach, which then keeps you from enjoying your food?

_____ **7.** Are you worried about how others judge you?

_____ **8.** Are you always concerned about passing your classes?

_____ **9.** Do you think you will never graduate, or never get a job if you do graduate?

_____ **10.** Do you struggle with letting others contribute to group projects, instead wishing you could do it all yourself?

Results

Although there is no "right" number of yes or no answers, you should take a careful look at your responses and note any patterns.

_____ TOTAL NUMBER OF YES ANSWERS

If you answered yes to a majority of these questions, then you probably struggle to manage your stress, and others might even see you as someone not so pleasant to be around.

Reflecting on Your Results

Were you surprised by the number of yes answers? Did your responses to this quiz match your impression of how well you handle stress in your life?

Planning Your Next Steps

If you need to work on how you handle stress, look back through this chapter for techniques and tips on managing stress, especially the ones that use physical relaxation. Choose one you find interesting and appealing, and try it out for a week. Report on your experiences.

Stress-management technique. Describe specifically what you did during the week:

Results of trying technique. What effect, if any, did the technique you tried have on your stress level? Do you think it changed how you felt or how you acted?

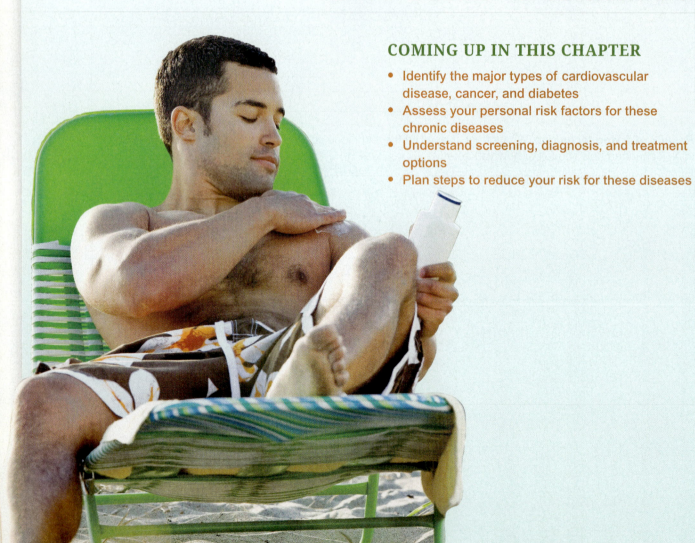

11

Chronic Diseases

COMING UP IN THIS CHAPTER

- Identify the major types of cardiovascular disease, cancer, and diabetes
- Assess your personal risk factors for these chronic diseases
- Understand screening, diagnosis, and treatment options
- Plan steps to reduce your risk for these diseases

How do chronic diseases relate to overall wellness? The physical wellness component is straightforward: Chronic diseases have physical signs and symptoms and affect physical functioning. In terms of emotional wellness, the diagnosis of a chronic disease can be devastating, just as test results showing no disease can be a tremendous relief. Even if a chronic disease is in an early stage, the stress of medications, treatments, and lifestyle changes can be overwhelming. It is therefore crucial to seek support from family and friends or other sources.

When faced with a chronic disease, it is also important to make intellectually sound decisions based on second opinions and information from reliable sources. Friends and family can help you evaluate your options. Your spiritual wellness is also a consideration—your values and beliefs may contribute to your treatment options and decisions, as well as provide comfort and direction.

Environmental factors may play a part as well. Did your environment contribute to your problem? Can the environment be a part of your solution? Perhaps exploring the beautiful outdoors will help you cope with chronic disease and improve your overall wellness.

A diagnosis of cardiovascular disease, diabetes, or cancer can be very frightening because these chronic diseases sometimes mean death or at least very difficult times. More than 100 million Americans are living with cardiovascular disease, cancer, or diabetes, and each year these diseases kill about 1.5 million people, accounting for nearly 70 percent of all U.S. deaths (Table 11-1). Yet it is vital to keep in mind that many other people do not die—at least not right away. Many forms of cardiovascular disease, diabetes, and cancer are treatable and manageable. Further, these chronic diseases in many instances are preventable.

This chapter introduces the different types of cardiovascular disease, cancer, and diabetes and their major risk factors. You'll have opportunities to assess your own disease risk and learn about common treatment options and prevention measures.

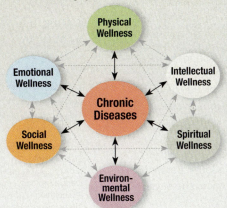

Cardiovascular Disease

Q What is cardiovascular disease? How many people die from it?

Cardiovascular disease (CVD) is not a single disease but rather a broad collection of many diseases that affect the heart (*cardio*) or blood vessels (*vascular*) or both. According to the American Heart Association, approximately 80 million Americans have some form of cardiovascular disease (see Table 11-1). And although deaths due to cardiovascular disease have declined in the last 20 years, CVD is still responsible for one in every three deaths in the United States. By 2030, over 40 percent of the U.S. population is projected to have some form of CVD.[1]

When working as it should, the heart pumps blood throughout the body, delivering oxygen and nutrients and removing carbon dioxide and cellular waste products via a network of strong and elastic blood vessels. Any problem with the heart or blood vessels decreases the quality of life and increases the risk of death. Chapter 4 described the functioning of a healthy cardiovascular system.

cardiovascular disease (CVD) Any disease that affects the heart (*cardio*) or blood vessels (*vascular*) or both.

Types of Cardiovascular Disease

Q Heart attacks and strokes affect different parts of the body, so why are they always lumped together?

Heart attacks and strokes are both forms of cardiovascular disease (CVD). As previously mentioned, CVD is a group of diseases that affect the heart or blood vessels or both. Although a stroke isn't directly related to the heart, it stems from vascular problems, so it is classified as a form of cardiovascular disease.

Mind Stretcher
Critical Thinking Exercise

Have you ever thought about your personal risk for cardiovascular disease, cancer, and diabetes? What risk factors do you have? Have you taken steps to lower your risk for any of these chronic diseases? Why or why not? Are any of your daily health habits influenced by the goal of reducing your future risk of chronic diseases?

Behavior-Change Challenge
Stopping Diabetes in Its Tracks

Imagine that you've been experiencing unusual thirst and fatigue and having occasional blurred vision. You reason that you are simply eating too many salty snacks (gaining several pounds along the way), not working out (though your workouts always made you feel better), and studying too many hours. But when the symptoms do not let up during spring break, you check with your doctor. You discover that you have prediabetes—higher-than-normal blood glucose levels that can develop into full-blown type 2 diabetes. You're sick with worry. Fortunately, your doctor tells you about certain lifestyle changes that might spare you from advancing to type 2 diabetes. Eating healthier foods, exercising regularly, and losing about 7 percent of your body weight can make a difference, she says.

Meet Josh

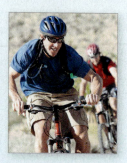

You resolve to take action while knowing that change will be hard. You join a support group led by a wellness coach, Josh, who has overcome his own prediabetes. How? For starters, by replacing the junk food in his diet with healthy meals, Josh lost the extra 10 pounds he'd carried around. Now Josh has begun bicycling regularly again, with the goal of participating on a local team for the Tour de Cure cycling events that will raise funds for the American Diabetes Association.

In thinking about your behavior-change goals, consider:

- How might you specifically apply Josh's experience to modify your diet?
- What is significant about Josh's return to cycling? What are some ways you can motivate yourself to get back into an exercise routine?

In fact, stroke is one of the most common types of CVD, responsible for over 100,000 deaths in the United States each year. Other common types of CVD are coronary artery disease, hypertension, heart failure, and peripheral artery disease (Figure 11-1). As you read about the various types of CVD in this section, note how they relate to one another. The different types of CVD do not occur in isolation, and unfortunately having one type of CVD sometimes leads to the development of other types.

TABLE 11-1 ESTIMATED PREVALENCE AND ANNUAL MORTALITY FROM CARDIOVASCULAR DISEASE, CANCER, AND DIABETES

	PREVALENCE	MORTALITY
CARDIO-VASCULAR DISEASE	82,600,000	811,940
CANCER	11,958,000	577,190
DIABETES	25,800,000	71,382

Sources: American Cancer Society. (2012). *Cancer facts & figures 2012.* Atlanta, GA: American Cancer Society. American Cancer Society. (2011). Cancer prevalence: What is cancer prevalence? (http://www.cancer.org/cancer/cancerbasics/cancer-prevalence). American Diabetes Association (2011). Diabetes basics: Diabetes statistics (http://www.diabetes.org/diabetes-basics/diabetes-statistics/). Roger, V. L., and others. (2012). Heart disease and stroke statistics 2012 update: A report from the American Heart Association. *Circulation, 125,* e2–e220.

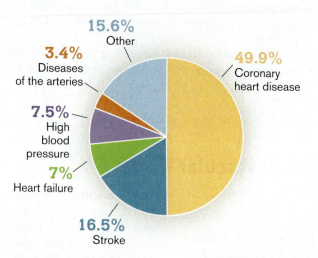

15.6% Other
3.4% Diseases of the arteries
7.5% High blood pressure
7% Heart failure
16.5% Stroke
49.9% Coronary heart disease

Figure 11-1 Percentage breakdown of U.S. deaths from cardiovascular disease.
Source: American Heart Association. (2012). Heart disease and stroke statistics 2012 update: A report from the American Heart Association. *Circulation, 125e.*

Q What type of cardiovascular disease kills the most people?

CORONARY ARTERY DISEASE. Coronary artery disease (CAD), also sometimes referred to as coronary heart disease (CHD), is the single leading cause of death in the United States. CAD occurs when blood flow in the arteries that feed the heart is inhibited. The most common cause of CAD is **atherosclerosis,** the buildup of fats, cholesterol, and other cellular waste

coronary artery disease (CAD) Disease of the arteries of the heart characterized by the buildup of fats and other substances and reduction of blood flow.

products on the lining of the arteries (Figure 11-2). Known as *plaque,* this buildup narrows the arteries, reducing blood flow. If the plaque becomes large or it ruptures and creates a clot, the artery may be completely blocked. A partial or full blockage is known as an *occlusion.* Atherosclerosis typically begins in childhood and can worsen with age. It can lead to **arteriosclerosis**—a general hardening, or loss of elasticity, in the arteries.

When atherosclerosis occurs in the *coronary arteries*—the arteries that supply blood to the heart—the result is coronary artery disease. Atherosclerosis can also affect arteries in other parts of the body. If an artery leading to the brain is affected, the result is a stroke; if an artery in a limb is affected, the condition is called peripheral artery disease. Both of these forms of CVD are described below.

Coronary artery disease often has no symptoms as it develops. When the condition reveals itself, it may be in one of the following ways:

- **Angina pectoris** is chest pain that typically results from reduced blood supply to the heart. The pain often occurs with exercise or stress because the heart isn't receiving enough blood for the demands of increased exertion; the pain quickly subsides with rest. Angina may feel like pressure or a squeezing chest pain that may also radiate to the shoulders, arms, neck, jaw, or back.

- **Heart attack,** also called a **myocardial infarction (MI),** occurs when the blood supply in one of the coronary arteries is blocked, thus depriving a part of the heart of needed oxygen (see Figure 11-2). Unlike angina, the pain associated with a heart attack may occur without exertion, and it doesn't resolve with rest; the pain is also usually more severe than that of angina. Immediate medical attention can help limit the damage to the heart muscle.

- **Arrhythmia** is a change in the normal pattern of the heartbeat. The rhythm may become irregular or too slow or fast. Although some types of arrhythmias are harmless, others prevent the heart from pumping blood effectively and can cause sudden cardiac death. Sudden cardiac death, or **cardiac arrest,** is characterized by a sudden loss of responsiveness, pulse, and blood pressure. It is different from a heart attack, in which the heart usually keeps beating. Cardiac arrest is usually fatal unless treated immediately with CPR or an electrical shock to the heart. Coronary artery disease is a common underlying cause of dangerous arrhythmias.

atherosclerosis Buildup of plaque in the inner lining of arteries, leading to narrowing, reduction of blood flow, and possible blockage.

arteriosclerosis A chronic disease characterized by abnormal thickening and hardening of the arteries, resulting in loss of elasticity.

angina pectoris Chest pain caused by a reduced blood supply to the heart.

heart attack (myocardial infarction) Damage or death of heart muscle due to insufficient blood supply, usually caused by a blockage in a coronary artery that deprives part of the heart of oxygen.

arrhythmia Abnormal heart rhythm.

cardiac arrest Sudden temporary or permanent cessation of heartbeat.

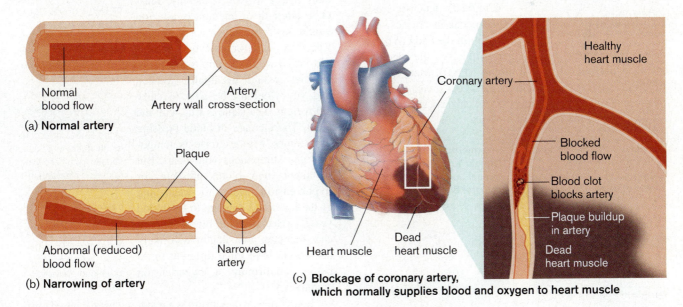

(a) **Normal artery**
Normal blood flow
Artery wall Artery cross-section

(b) **Narrowing of artery**
Plaque
Abnormal (reduced) blood flow
Narrowed artery

(c) **Blockage of coronary artery, which normally supplies blood and oxygen to heart muscle**
Coronary artery
Heart muscle
Dead heart muscle
Healthy heart muscle
Blocked blood flow
Blood clot blocks artery
Plaque buildup in artery
Dead heart muscle

Figure 11-2 Atherosclerosis and heart attack. Plaque deposits can accumulate and narrow the interior space of an artery, reducing blood flow. If a clot forms and blocks a coronary artery, the results are a heart attack and heart muscle damage.

Sources: Adapted from National Heart, Lung, and Blood Institute. (2011). What is atherosclerosis? *Diseases and conditions index* (http://www.nhlbi.nih.gov/health/dci/Diseases/Atherosclerosis/Atherosclerosis_WhatIs.html). NHLBI. (2011). What is a heart attack? *Diseases and conditions index* (http://www.nhlbi.nih.gov/health/dci/Diseases/HeartAttack/HeartAttack_WhatIs.html).

Risk factors and strategies for preventing coronary artery disease are described later in the chapter.

Q | Is stroke caused by a blocked artery or a burst artery?

STROKE. Either one. Strokes are the number-three cause of death in America and are a leading cause of serious disability. A **stroke,** or "brain attack," occurs when the blood (and oxygen) supply to a part of the brain is suddenly interrupted. If blood flow stops for more than a few seconds, brain cells can die, causing permanent damage (Figure 11-3). There are two major categories of stroke:

- *Ischemic stroke,* in which an artery supplying blood to the brain is blocked by a blood clot. Atherosclerosis is the most common cause of ischemic stroke.
- *Hemorrhagic stroke,* in which a blood vessel bursts, causing blood to leak into the brain. Some people are born with or develop defects in blood vessels that make a hemorrhage more likely to occur.

Sometimes people have **transient ischemic attacks (TIAs),** or "mini-strokes," which are caused by a temporary blockage and typically do not cause lasting damage. However, a TIA is a warning sign for a more serious stroke. Strategies for recognizing symptoms of TIAs and strokes are presented later in the chapter.

Q | Can I really get CVD in my arms and legs?

PERIPHERAL ARTERY DISEASE. Yes. As previously described, atherosclerosis can occur in arteries anywhere in the body. When it occurs in the limbs, most commonly the legs, the condition is called **peripheral artery disease (PAD).** Many people have mild or no symptoms from PAD, but it can cause leg pain when walking, leg numbness or weakness, and coldness

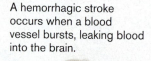

An ischemic stroke occurs when a blood vessel supplying the brain becomes blocked, as by a clot.

A hemorrhagic stroke occurs when a blood vessel bursts, leaking blood into the brain.

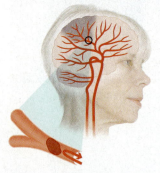
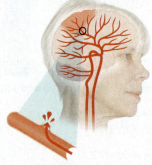

Figure 11-3 Stroke.
Source: National Institute of Neurological Disorders and Strokes. (2009). *Stroke: Challenges, progress, and promise.* NIH Publication No. 09-6451.

or paleness of the limb. Untreated, PAD can lead to severe infections, causing tissue death and sometimes requiring amputation of the affected limb. Because atherosclerosis in the limbs is typically associated with plaque buildup in other parts of the body, people with PAD are also at increased risk for heart attack and stroke.

Q | If my blood pressure goes up naturally when I exercise, why is high blood pressure so bad?

HIGH BLOOD PRESSURE. Temporary increases in blood pressure are usually fine; consistently high blood pressure is not. *Blood pressure* refers to the force of blood pushing against the walls of your blood vessels. It is typically reported using two numbers, such as 110/70 mm Hg, with *mm Hg* standing for "millimeters of mercury," the unit used to measure blood pressure. The first, or top, number is the **systolic blood pressure,** which is the force produced when the heart contracts. The second, or bottom, number is the **diastolic blood pressure,** which is the force between beats, when the heart is at rest.

Your heart plays a huge role in controlling your blood pressure, and the heart, like any other muscle, typically gets stronger when it is exercised. Consider a comparison to weight lifting. You lift a moderately heavy weight to increase muscular strength or endurance, but you would never consider carrying that weight around for extended periods of time. It would be impossible. Your muscles would eventually weaken and you wouldn't be able to carry the weight. The same is true with the heart. The increase in blood pressure that comes with exercise is temporary and strengthens your heart. But sustained high blood pressure, or **hypertension,** leads to weakening of the heart and damage to the blood vessels. (Because your blood pressure can fluctuate, your doctor will likely test you at least three different times before confirming a hypertension diagnosis.)

Sometimes hypertension is a result of other conditions, such as kidney or adrenal gland problems. In these cases, addressing the underlying cause often eliminates the related hypertension. However, in the majority of cases (90–95 percent), the direct cause of hypertension is unknown.

stroke Interruption of the blood and oxygen supply to part of the brain; caused by a blocked artery (ischemic stroke) or a ruptured blood vessel (hemorrhagic stroke).

transient ischemic attack (TIA) Temporary blockage of one or more arteries in the brain; doesn't typically cause lasting damage but is a warning sign for a full-blown stroke.

peripheral artery disease (PAD) Damage or dysfunction of arteries in the limbs, most commonly in the legs; usually caused by atherosclerosis and resulting in reduced blood flow.

systolic blood pressure Force of blood on the vessel walls during the contraction of the heart; the top number in a blood pressure reading.

diastolic blood pressure Force of blood on the vessel walls when the heart is at rest (between contractions); the bottom number in a blood pressure reading.

hypertension Sustained high blood pressure.

There is strong correlation with atherosclerosis and other vascular conditions: As blood vessels affected by atherosclerosis become less elastic, they are less able to expand and thus resist the flow of blood the heart is pumping. Blood pressure increases, straining both the heart and the blood vessels.

Hypertension is a common form of cardiovascular disease. It is also one of the forms of CVD that can lead to other diseases, including heart attack, stroke, and heart failure.

Q | For blood pressure, how high is too high?

For adults, recommended systolic pressure is less than 120 and diastolic pressure less than 80 (Table 11-2). If your systolic or diastolic blood pressure number is too high, your blood pressure is classified according to that number. It's important for young adults to achieve healthy blood pressure levels because blood pressure tends to rise with age. Luckily, there are many strategies you can adopt to help keep your blood pressure in the healthy range throughout your life.

Although less common, some people have low blood pressure (hypotension), which is classified as a systolic pressure below 90 or diastolic pressure below 60, or both. Consistently low blood pressure can be normal for some and is usually considered a problem only if it causes a symptom such as dizziness or fainting or if it's due to an underlying medical condition. Consistently low blood pressure is different from a sudden drop in blood pressure due to something like bleeding or an allergic reaction; such a drop would be considered dangerous.

Q | Is heart failure the same as a heart attack?

HEART FAILURE. No, but a heart attack can lead to **heart failure,** which basically means that your heart isn't doing its job adequately. It's still pumping, but it isn't able to get enough blood to the body's organs and tissues. This lack of blood supply often leads to shortness of breath, fatigue, and fluid buildup. The fluid buildup can cause swelling in the ankles or other parts of the body. It can also affect the ability of the kidneys to eliminate fluid, leading to additional swelling as well as fluid buildup in the lungs, which impedes breathing. Heart failure complicated by fluid buildup is referred to as *congestive heart failure.*

Heart failure can develop suddenly or over time. It often results from complications of other forms of cardiovascular disease.

heart failure A condition in which the heart is unable to pump blood at a sufficient rate or volume, resulting in insufficient blood flow to the organs and tissues and, in some cases, fluid buildup.

OTHER FORMS OF CARDIOVASCULAR DISEASE. A number of other conditions can also affect cardiovascular health. Some people are born with defects in their heart or major blood vessels; such problems may be repaired with surgery during infancy or may not be discovered until many years later. In other cases, problems may develop as result of infection or underlying atherosclerosis.

Q | What can be done to eliminate a heart murmur?

In most cases, a so-called heart murmur has no ill effects, and no treatment is needed. The diagnosis of "heart murmur" refers to a variety of conditions involving the valves in the heart. Normally, heart valves work in a coordinated fashion—they open to let blood flow in or out of the heart and then close to stop blood from flowing backward. If a valve doesn't open all the way, blood flow is blocked or reduced. If a valve doesn't close all the way or tightly enough, blood can leak back through the valve in the wrong direction.

Valve problems can result from inherited defects, infections, or heart disease. The most common problem, affecting about 2 percent of adults, is with the *mitral valve,* located between the left atrium and left ventricle. If the valve is floppy or bulges (prolapses) slightly, a physician listening to the heart may hear a murmur. In most people, *mitral valve prolapse (MVP)* is harmless and requires no treatment or lifestyle changes. People with severe MVP or

TABLE 11-2 BLOOD PRESSURE CLASSIFICATION FOR ADULTS AGE 18 AND OLDER

CATEGORY	SYSTOLIC (TOP NUMBER)		DIASTOLIC (BOTTOM NUMBER)
NORMAL	LESS THAN 120	AND	LESS THAN 80
PRE-HYPERTENSION	120–139	OR	80–89
HYPERTENSION, STAGE 1	140–159	OR	90–99
HYPERTENSION, STAGE 2	160+	OR	100+

Source: National Institutes of Health, National Heart Lung and Blood Institute. (2011). *What is high blood pressure?* (http://www.nhlbi.nih.gov/health/health-topics/topics/hbp/).

other more serious valve problems may be treated with medication or surgery. Antibiotics used to be recommended before certain dental and medical procedures for all people with MVP to prevent infection of the heart valve; however, antibiotics are currently recommended for only a small proportion of people with MVP. If you have any questions about your own situation, check with your physician.

Q | What causes varicose veins, and how can I avoid them?

Varicose veins are the product of improper valve function leading to blood accumulation and the twisting and enlargement of affected veins. The resulting decreased oxygen supply causes the veins to appear blue. This condition typically occurs on the inside of the legs from the groin to the ankle or on the back of the calves down to the feet. Many of the causes of varicose veins, such as aging, heredity, and hormone changes, are not controllable. The best prevention measures are exercise (movement) and avoidance of excess weight.

Assessing Your Risk for Cardiovascular Disease: Factors You Cannot Control

Because one in three Americans dies from cardiovascular disease, everyone is at risk in some way and to some degree. However, some people are at much higher risk than others. As a rule, people with a family history of cardiovascular disease (CVD) are more at risk that those without, men are more at risk than women, African Americans are at greater risk than Caucasians, and people over 65 are more at risk than those who are younger. These are not the only factors contributing to CVD risk, and it's extremely important to evaluate which of your risk factors you can change (modify or alter) and which you cannot. This section describes factors over which you have little control,

including heredity, age, sex, and ethnicity. The next section describes factors that you can change, such as diet, smoking, alcohol consumption, and stress.

Q | Is there any way you can reverse genetically predisposed heart problems?

HEREDITY/GENETICS. You can't reverse your familial predisposition to heart disease, and some risks factors are not modifiable at all. Yet there are still many things you can do. It has been long known that people with a family history of cardiovascular disease are more likely than others to develop CVD themselves. That's one of the reasons it's important to know your family health history. In recent years, specific genes have been identified that are responsible for some inherited cardiovascular disorders.[2] Types of CVD that may be caused by inherited traits include certain forms of *cardiomyopathy* (enlarged and weakened heart muscle), arrhythmia, and aneurysm, as well as *Marfan's syndrome,* a connective tissue disorder that may affect the heart.

Treatment for inherited forms of CVD is the same as for other forms. The advantages to knowing if you have a genetic predisposition for CVD are that you can seek early treatment and prevention of additional forms of CVD and that your family members can be tested for potential CVD problems. Consult these resources for information on collecting and organizing your family health history: https://familyhistory.hhs.gov/fhh-web/home.action and http://www.geneticalliance.org/fhh. For various reasons, though, not everyone has access to a family history. A common reason for missing information is adoption. If you or someone you know is adopted, use these resources for ideas on researching family health history: http://www.genetichealth.com/resources_adoptees_and_genetic_information.shtml and http://www.talkhealthhistory.org/family/faq_13.shtml.

Q | Why does getting older make a person more likely to have CVD?

AGE. According to the American Heart Association, the prevalence of CVD rises with age, from less than 15 percent among those under age 40 to over 70 percent among those over age 60.[3] This increased prevalence is primarily due to wear and tear on the heart and blood vessels. Over time, there are changes in the structure and functioning of the heart and in the ability of blood vessels to relax and contract.[4] These changes contribute to all forms of cardiovascular disease; for example, Figure 11-4 shows the increasing prevalence of high blood pressure with age.

The association between aging and CVD doesn't mean that it is inevitable or that older people can't have a healthy heart and live active, productive lives. It just means that there is no denying that time and use take a toll.

Fast Facts

Circulatory Highways

The adult body contains billions of arteries, veins, and capillaries. If all the blood vessels were laid end to end, they would extend about 100,000 miles—enough to encircle the earth four times.

- Given the large number of human blood vessels, what is the significance of a partial or full blockage?
- Why are some blockages worse than others?

Source: Franklin Institute. (n.d.). Blood vessels. *The human heart* (http://www.fi.edu/learn/heart/vessels/vessels.html).

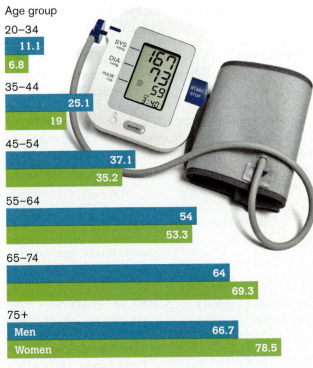

Age group

Age group		
20–34	Men 11.1	Women 6.8
35–44	Men 25.1	Women 19
45–54	Men 37.1	Women 35.2
55–64	Men 54	Women 53.3
65–74	Men 64	Women 69.3
75+	Men 66.7	Women 78.5

Percent of population

Figure 11-4 **Prevalence of high blood pressure among adults age 20 and over, by age and sex.** The risk of hypertension rises steadily with age. Hypertension is defined as having systolic blood pressure of 140 or over, having diastolic blood pressure of 90 or over, taking antihypertensive medication, or being diagnosed with hypertension twice by a medical professional.
Source: American Heart Association. (2012). Heart disease and stroke statistics 2012 update: A report from the American Heart Association. *Circulation, 125e.*

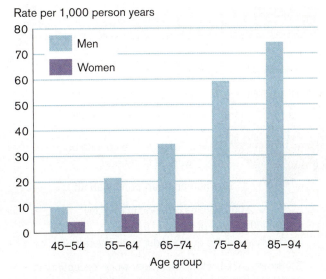

Rate per 1,000 person years

Figure 11-5 **Incidence of cardiovascular disease among adults age 20 and over, by age and sex.** The rates here include coronary artery disease, stroke, heart failure, and intermittent claudication (leg pain during walking or other exercise, due to insufficient blood flow to muscles).
Source: American Heart Association. (2012). Heart disease and stroke statistics 2012 update: A report from the American Heart Association. *Circulation, 125e.*

Q | Why do more men have heart attacks than women?

BIOLOGICAL SEX. More men develop and die from cardiovascular disease than women—and they do so at younger ages (Figure 11-5). There isn't a single clear reason for this discrepancy. Researchers attribute the differences to a number of factors, including higher rates of smoking, excess alcohol consumption, and other negative lifestyle choices among men. There may be biological causes as well. Premenopausal women tend to have better cholesterol profiles than men, and although the cause for this tendency is still being studied, increased estrogen levels and other hormonal differences are thought to play a key role.[5] Long before signs of CVD appear, these hormonal differences affect the cardiovascular system. (See p. 390 for more on cholesterol.)

Notably, although more men than women have heart attacks, women are more likely to die from them.[6] Because women typically have heart attacks later in life, they tend to be sicker and to have more risk factors and other diseases, and these factors can complicate diagnosis and treatment. Certain medications also appear to work better for men than women.

Additional research is under way to determine other possible reasons for the difference in CVD prevalence and mortality among men and women. Studies examining the differences in heart physiology and rhythms and hormone fluctuations, as well as research focusing on differences in diagnosis and treatment mechanisms, are on the horizon.

Q | How does ethnicity affect cardiovascular disease? What group or groups are most at risk?

ETHNICITY. Studies have found different rates of CVD and associated risk factors among different ethnic groups. African Americans have a higher prevalence of CVD overall and of high blood pressure and strokes in particular; in fact, African American adults have the highest rate of hypertension in the world.[7] Asian Americans and Latinos have a lower prevalence of heart disease than other groups, and Asian Americans have a significantly lower prevalence of stroke. As a group, American Indians and Alaska Natives have the highest prevalence of stroke.

The reasons for the differences among ethnic groups are complex, but socioeconomic factors, as well as significant differences in modifiable CVD risk factors, may play a role. For example, Latinos have a significantly lower rate of smoking than African Americans or Caucasians, but American Indians and Alaska Natives have a higher rate of smoking than other groups. Latinos, African Americans, and American Indians and Alaska Natives have higher rates of diabetes. Rates of leisure-time physical activity are low among all groups but particularly low among Latinas.[8]

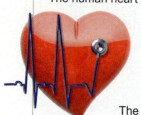

Fast Facts

Heart at Work

The human heart beats about . . .

- 70 times per minute
- 100,000 times in one day
- 35 million times in a year
- 2.5 billion times during an average lifetime

The human heart pumps about . . .

- 2,000 gallons of blood in one day
- 700,000 gallons of blood in a year
- 50 million gallons of blood during an average lifetime

Consider: What other muscles work exceptionally hard? How do you think the effort of these muscles compares to that of the heart?

Source: NOVA Online. *Cut to the heart: Amazing heart facts* (http://www.pbs.org/wgbh/nova/heart/heartfacts.html).

(These and other modifiable risk factors are discussed in more detail in the prevention section of the chapter.)

There may also be biological differences among the groups. For example, researchers have found higher levels of salt sensitivity among African Americans, meaning that their blood pressure goes up in response to salt consumption.[9] These findings have led to a lower recommended sodium intake target for African Americans; see Chapter 8 for more information.

Cardiovascular Disease Prevention

Unlike the unchangeable factors of heredity, sex, age, and ethnicity, you can modify factors related to your lifestyle in order to reduce your risk of CVD and high blood pressure. For example, you can eliminate use of tobacco, alcohol, and drugs and manage your stress. And you can get your blood pressure and cholesterol levels checked regularly. The lifestyle factors discussed in this section, because they can be changed or modified, are both risk factors and prevention strategies. As is the case with other areas of your health, when it comes to preventing CVD, your lifestyle choices have the greatest impact.

Q Are people who can eat all they want and not gain weight still at risk for cardiovascular disease?

CHOOSE A HEALTHY DIET AND ACTIVITY LEVEL AND CONTROL YOUR WEIGHT. Yes, because body weight and food choices are only part of what affects the risk for cardiovascular disease. Beyond the factors of genes, age, biological sex, and ethnicity, physical activity also counts. Even for someone who doesn't seem to gain weight, weight maintenance isn't possible unless energy intake is balanced with energy output.

In addition, being physically active directly reduces one's risk for CVD. Regular moderate exercise increases cardiovascular capacity by strengthening the heart and improving the elasticity of the arteries. Regular exercise also helps control cholesterol, high blood pressure, diabetes, and body weight, thus providing a combination of benefits for reducing CVD risk. See Chapter 4 for more on setting up a program for developing cardiorespiratory fitness.

Q If you have excellent cardiovascular fitness but CVD runs in your family, do you have a greater risk than someone with no family history of CVD?

This is a tough question to answer because to consider only fitness and genetics ignores other important factors that affect risk: How old are the two people? What sex? Do they smoke? How much do they drink? What foods do they consume? These factors, along with a number of others, will give a more complete picture of risk. Although an increased level of fitness certainly helps to prevent CVD, it may or may not balance out the other factors.

You are a sum of all of your risk factors—those that can be modified and those that can't—so examining only part of the equation can't give an accurate answer. It's like trying to see the full picture when you've only matched the first couple of pieces in the puzzle.

To assess your overall risk for cardiovascular disease, complete Lab Activity 11-1.

Q What types of foods should I avoid and eat to help prevent cardiovascular disease?

Salt can affect cardiovascular disease by raising blood pressure in salt-sensitive people. The effect of salt on blood pressure is one of the reasons the Dietary Reference Intakes set a limit for sodium (see Chapter 8). CVD risk can also be affected by fat intake; for heart health, it's recommended that you choose unsaturated fats and limit your intake of saturated and trans fats.

The best food plan for CVD prevention is balanced and moderate. Eat more fiber-rich whole grains, fruits, vegetables, legumes, fat-free and low-fat dairy products, and seafood. Limit excess calorie intake from added sugars, unhealthy fats, cholesterol, and highly processed foods. If you drink alcohol, keep your intake moderate. See Chapters 8 and 9 for more on limiting salt intake and putting together a healthy dietary plan. The DASH diet is especially recommended for people who are salt sensitive or have high blood pressure.

Q | If I'm overweight, is my risk a lot higher?

Yes. Added weight places added stress on the heart. The degree of extra stress depends on how overweight you are—the greater the weight, the greater the stress on the heart. If you're just a few pounds overweight, the stress is not as extreme. However, you would still decrease your risk if you lost the extra weight. If you're severely overweight, your risk is considerably higher. The risk for cardiovascular disease increases by about 37 percent in people who are moderately overweight. Among people who are obese, CVD risk goes up 81 percent.[10] See Table 7.2 for more about what qualifies as overweight.

People with excessive body fat are more likely to develop cardiovascular diseases even if they have no other risk factors. Unfortunately, other risk factors often accompany overweight or obesity. Excess body fat is linked to increased cholesterol and blood pressure levels and elevated risk for type 2 diabetes. People with more abdominal fat (apple shape) are at greater risk than those who carry their excess fat in the hip area (pear shape).

Increased physical activity and a balanced diet are CVD-prevention strategies that have a direct effect on overweight and obesity. Remember, however, that obesity is a complex condition that may involve genetic and other factors. If you are severely overweight or obese, see your doctor before beginning additional activities or making significant changes to your diet. See Chapters 7 and 9 for more information on evaluating your body composition and setting appropriate goals.

Q | Smoking causes cancer, not cardiovascular disease—right?

AVOID TOBACCO. Wrong. Smoking not only raises cancer risk but also significantly increases risk for cardiovascular disease. Smokers have twice the risk of heart attack of nonsmokers and are more likely than nonsmokers to die suddenly from heart attacks.[11] Smoking contributes to CVD in a number of ways. Smoking affects fatty buildup in the arteries by negatively affecting good and bad cholesterol levels. Smoking also increases heart rate, contributes to arrhythmias, elevates blood pressure, reduces the oxygen level in the blood, and may trigger blood clots. Almost all cases of peripheral artery disease occur in smokers, and smokers face greater complications from the disease, including amputations, than do nonsmokers. Smoking also limits the capacity for exercise—one of the few things that might help reverse some of smoking's negative effects.

The body slowly begins to heal as soon as someone quits smoking. According to the U.S. Surgeon General, the risk of CVD falls by 50 percent after just 1 year as a nonsmoker.[12] Cardiorespiratory fitness still has to be developed through aerobic fitness, however. The length of time to restore it depends on how much and how long one smoked, as well as the frequency, intensity, and duration of physical activities.

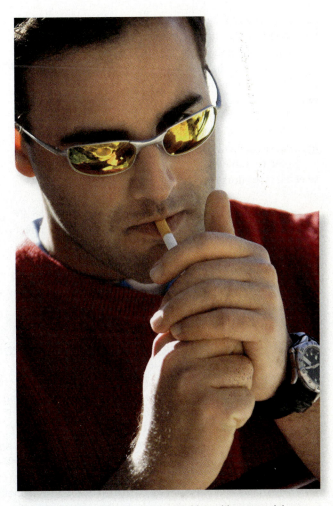

Although most people associate smoking with cancer risk, smoking is also one of the biggest contributors to cardiovascular disease. If you smoke, quit. If you've tried and failed to quit, keep trying until you succeed.

See Chapter 13 for more on the effects of smoking and strategies for quitting.

Q | Does alcohol affect cardiovascular disease? What about other drugs?

KEEP ALCOHOL USE MODERATE AND AVOID DRUGS. The effects of alcohol use can be positive or negative.[13] Research has found an association between moderate alcohol intake and reduced risk of cardiovascular disease. Moderate intake of alcohol is defined as no more than 2 drinks per day for men or 1 drink per day for women—with 1 drink being the equivalent of 12 ounces of beer, 5 ounces of wine, or 1.5 ounces of 80-proof spirits (see Chapter 13).

The underlying cause for the benefit of moderate alcohol consumption is unclear, but alcohol use is associated with a small increase in HDL (good cholesterol). Another possible effect may be reduced clot formation, which can lower the risk of heart attack and stroke. Some components in grapes and red wine, including flavonoids and resveratrol, have received special attention by researchers; these compounds act as antioxidants and may also relax the blood vessels and reduce blood pressure.[14]

On the other hand, drinking too much alcohol on a regular basis or in binge episodes has many negative cardiovascular effects. It is linked to high blood pressure, heart failure, arrhythmia, stroke, and sudden cardiac death. Excessive alcohol intake can also contribute to obesity because alcohol is relatively high in calories.

Refer to Table 11-3 for information on the effects of selected other drugs on CVD.

change heart rhythms, and over time the hormones associated with uncontrolled stress may alter glucose and blood-fat levels. However, the strongest link between stress and health may be in how we choose to manage stress—especially if we do so in a negative way. See the box "Don't Worry, Be Happy." Without good coping skills or appropriate stress-management techniques, people may choose negative outlets for stress such as overeating and increasing tobacco or alcohol use. These actions, in turn, have a direct negative impact on cardiovascular health. See Chapter 10 for healthy ways to manage your stress.

Q | Is stress a major factor in cardiovascular disease?

MANAGE YOUR STRESS IN HEALTHY WAYS. The direct cause-and-effect relationship between stress and cardiovascular disease is still being studied, but there are a number of likely connections. The acute stress response can raise blood pressure and

Q | How often do I have to get my blood pressure and cholesterol checked?

HAVE REGULAR SCREENINGS. Regular screenings are very important, but blood pressure and cholesterol aren't the only things you should have checked. You should also have regular screenings for triglycerides and diabetes.

TABLE 11-3 DRUGS AND RELATED CARDIOVASCULAR DISEASE COMPLICATIONS

ANABOLIC STEROIDS (NONMEDICAL USE)	Abuse can lower HDL and raise LDL; increase the risk of atherosclerosis, hypertension, stroke, and heart attack; and may also cause blood clots and enlargement of the ventricles of the heart.
CAFFEINE	Probably safe in moderate amounts, according to the American Heart Association. Research studies on the links between caffeine and CVD have yielded conflicting results.
COCAINE	Use can lead to overstimulation of the heart, resulting in increased risk for heart attack, stroke, high blood pressure, heart failure, blood clots, enlargement of the heart, and infections of the heart lining. Further complications may include aneurysm and aortic dissection (splitting of the inner wall of the aorta), both of which can be fatal.
HEROIN	Injection use can cause permanent damage to veins. Users are also more susceptible to blood vessel blockages and blood clots, heart attack, stroke, and infections of the heart lining.
INHALANTS	Some types can cause rapid and irregular heart rhythms, leading to heart failure; other types reduce the oxygen-carrying capacity of the blood and harm the heart muscle.
MARIJUANA	Use increases heart rate and blood pressure and reduces the oxygen-carrying capability of the blood, which can strain the cardiorespiratory system. Some research suggests that heart attack risk is four times greater within 1 hour of smoking. Marijuana smoke contains some of the same harmful chemicals as cigarette smoke, and research points to a possible increased risk for heart attack and stroke among heavy users and older users.
METHAMPHETAMINE	Use increases heart rate and blood pressure and can lead to atherosclerosis, heart attack, stroke, or heart failure.

Sources: Adapted from American Heart Association. (2012). *Cocaine, marijuana, and other drugs and heart disease* (http://www.heart.org/HEARTORG/Conditions/Cocaine-Marijuana-and-Other-Drugs_UCM_428537_Article.jsp). American Heart Association. (2012). *Caffeine and heart disease* (http://www.heart.org/HEARTORG/GettingHealthy/NutritionCenter/Caffeine_UCM_305888_Article.jsp). Baggish, A. L., & others. (2010) Long term anabolic-androgenic steroid use is associated with left ventricular dysfunction. *Circulation: Heart Failure, 3*(4), 472–476. Cleveland Clinic. (2008). *Heroin: Abuse and addiction* (http://my.clevelandclinic.org/disorders/heroin_addiction/hic_heroin_abuse_and_addiction.aspx). National Institute on Drug Abuse. (2010). *Research report series inhalant abuse* (https://www.drugabuse.gov/sites/default/files/rrinhalants.pdf). National Institute on Drug Abuse. (2010). *Research report series marijuana use* (https://www.drugabuse.gov/sites/default/files/rrmarijuana.pdf). Richards, J. R., and others. (2011). *Methamphetamine toxicity.* Medscape Reference (http://emedicine.medscape.com/article/820918-overview).

Research Brief

Don't Worry, Be Happy

Researchers have looked at psychological and social influences on cardiovascular disease risk. In one recent large-scale study, adults were followed for 10 years and assessed for symptoms of depression, hostility, and anxiety as well as for the expression of positive emotions—happiness, enthusiasm, joy, and contentment. The researchers found that the happiest people had a lower risk of angina and heart attacks compared to those who were moderately happy and, especially, those who were unhappy, anxious, and depressed. In a separate study, researchers noted an association between negative emotions and heart disease in healthy individuals as well as in the risk of mortality among individuals with established heart disease. Furthermore, positive emotions were protective for both groups. Uniquely, this study adjusted for other risk factors in the study participants.

How do positive emotions reduce CVD? Researchers speculate that the happier, more satisfied people may handle stress better, sleep better, and practice more heart-healthy lifestyle behaviors. All these differences can contribute to better heart health.

Analyze and Apply

- What do the studies described in this Research Brief suggest about the importance of positive emotions?
- What do you do now to try to be happy? What else could you do?

Sources: Davidson, K. W., and others. (2010). Don't worry, be happy: Positive affect and reduced 10-year incident coronary heart disease: The Canadian Nova Scotia Health Survey. *European Heart Journal, 31*(9), 1065–1070. Pedersen, S. S., and others. (2011). Heart and mind: Are we closer to disentangling the relationship between emotions and poor prognosis in heart disease? *European Heart Journal 32*(19), 2341–2343.

Regular, however, doesn't mean the same frequency for each of these factors.

- *Blood pressure:* Unless your doctor advises otherwise, the American College of Physicians recommends that blood pressure be measured in adults every 1–2 years. Your doctor may recommend a different frequency based on your results.
- *Cholesterol and triglycerides:* For adults over 20, cholesterol should be checked every 5 years unless your doctor advises more frequent screening due to high levels or other risk factors.
- *Diabetes:* Screening is recommended for all adults age 45 and older and for younger people who have risk factors, including overweight.

You can use the results of your screening tests to take appropriate action, if needed, to reduce your risk for CVD.

Q | What can I do to lower my blood pressure?

REDUCE ELEVATED BLOOD PRESSURE. There are many steps you can take to lower your blood pressure if it is high (see the blood pressure classifications in Table 11-2). It's important to address blood pressure even if it's only slightly elevated, in the pre-hypertension range. Young adults with pre-hypertension are more likely to develop atherosclerosis over time than those with healthy blood pressure.[15]

You'll notice that blood pressure has come up many times in this chapter—it keeps reappearing because it is so important. First, hypertension is a type of cardiovascular disease. Second, it is a risk factor for other types of CVD. And third, addressing hypertension is a prevention strategy because keeping your blood pressure in check can help prevent CVD and complications from many conditions.

Other prevention strategies described in this section can have a positive effect on blood pressure. Eating a balanced, low-sodium diet, engaging in regular physical activity, maintaining a healthy weight, limiting alcohol consumption, and avoiding smoking can all help reduce your risk for hypertension. If you can't maintain healthy blood pressure with lifestyle measures, many types of medications are available.

Q | How does the fat in the foods I eat affect my cholesterol levels?

MAINTAIN HEALTHY CHOLESTEROL AND TRIGLYCERIDE LEVELS. Cholesterol and triglycerides are found both in foods and in your blood, but the connections between the foods

DOLLAR STRETCHER
Financial Wellness Tip

If you don't have a regular source of medical care, take advantage of free blood pressure screening. Many campuses and community health departments offer no-cost blood pressure checks, as well as free glucose tests and other screenings. Check with your campus health center. Free screening is also available at many supermarkets and pharmacies.

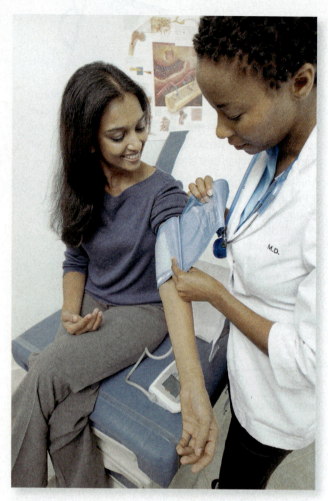

High blood pressure often has no symptoms, but even slightly elevated blood pressure harms the cardiovascular system. It is important to get blood pressure checked regularly and to take steps to reduce it if it is elevated.

you eat and the fats (*lipids*) in your blood are complex. **Cholesterol** is a waxy substance that occurs naturally in all cells of the body. It is produced by the liver and obtained in the diet; it is carried by the blood and is used to maintain cell walls and to produce certain hormones. Although it's a needed substance, excess cholesterol can build up on artery walls and increase your risk for cardiovascular disease.

To understand how cholesterol affects your risk for CVD, recall the types of cholesterol that were introduced in Chapter 8:

- **Low-density lipoprotein (LDL)** is known as bad cholesterol because it tends to deposit cholesterol on artery walls, thus limiting blood flow and increasing the risk for CVD.
- **High-density lipoprotein (HDL)** is known as good cholesterol because it carries excess cholesterol back to the liver so that the body can eliminate it.

The goal is a low level of LDL and a high level of HDL. **Triglycerides** are another common fat that is found in both foods and the body; high blood levels of triglycerides are also linked to increased CVD risk.

To assess a person's risk for CVD, blood-fat screening is recommended every 5 years for adults. The screening is a blood test done after 9–12 hours of fasting. The results typically include values for total cholesterol, HDL, LDL, and triglycerides (Table 11-4). Based on the results, your physician may recommend specific lifestyle strategies.

Elevated LDL levels may be caused by genetic factors that affect the liver's production of cholesterol, or they may stem from excessive intake of dietary cholesterol or, especially, saturated and trans fats. (Eating saturated and trans fats encourages the body to produce more total cholesterol and LDL; trans fats also decrease HDL.)

Triglyceride levels tend to increase with age, but high levels can occur in people of any age. Risk factors for high triglyceride levels include overweight, inactivity, cigarette smoking, excessive alcohol use, and diets very high in carbohydrate. A high level of triglycerides, like elevated cholesterol, appears to facilitate the development of atherosclerosis.

To improve cholesterol and triglyceride levels, experts recommend the following lifestyle measures:

- Choose unsaturated fats over saturated and trans fats.
- Eat fish, especially oily fish, two or more times per week (see Chapter 8 for more on the omega-3 fatty acids in fish).
- Consume the recommended amounts of dietary fiber while keeping intake of refined carbohydrates and added sugars low.
- Avoid excess alcohol consumption.
- Maintain a healthy weight.
- Be physically active.
- Avoid tobacco.

Because elevated cholesterol levels are sometimes genetic, prevention strategies may have a limited effect for some people. But "limited effect" does not mean "no effect," and these strategies are vital for overall good health.

Young adults may not be likely to have a heart attack within the next few years, but that doesn't mean they can ignore their cholesterol and triglyceride levels. Those with unhealthy blood lipid levels are much more likely to have buildup in their arteries when they reach middle age than their age peers without abnormal levels.[16] Don't wait to adopt healthy eating and exercise habits—what you do in your younger years matters.

cholesterol A fat, waxy substance produced by the liver and consumed from animal products; excess cholesterol in the bloodstream can be deposited on artery walls.

low-density lipoprotein (LDL) A type of lipoprotein that circulates in the blood and deposits cholesterol on artery walls, increasing the risk of cardiovascular disease; also known as bad cholesterol.

high-density lipoprotein (HDL) A type of lipoprotein that circulates in the blood and carries excess cholesterol back to the liver for elimination from the body; also known as good cholesterol.

triglycerides The most common form of fat in foods and in the body; high blood levels of triglycerides increase risk for CVD.

TABLE 11-4 CHOLESTEROL AND TRIGLYCERIDE CLASSIFICATION

	RISK CATEGORY
TOTAL CHOLESTEROL LEVEL	
LESS THAN 200 MG/DL	Desirable
200–239 MG/DL	Borderline high
240 MG/DL AND ABOVE	High blood cholesterol
LDL CHOLESTEROL LEVEL	
LESS THAN 100 MG/DL	Optimal
100–129 MG/DL	Near or above optimal
130–159 MG/DL	Borderline high
160–189 MG/DL	High
190 MG/DL AND ABOVE	Very high
HDL CHOLESTEROL LEVEL	
LESS THAN 40 MG/DL (MEN) OR 50 MG/DL (WOMEN)	A major risk factor for heart disease
60 MG/DL AND ABOVE	Considered protective against heart disease
TRIGLYCERIDE LEVEL	
LESS THAN 150 MG/DL	Normal
150–199 MG/DL	Borderline high
200–499 MG/DL	High
500 MG/DL AND ABOVE	Very high

Note: These values apply to healthy adults. For people with heart disease or diabetes, the targets for LDL cholesterol and triglycerides may be lower.

Source: American Heart Association. (2011). *What your cholesterol numbers mean* (http://www.heart.org/HEARTORG/Conditions/What-Your-CholestrolLevels-Mean_UCM_305562_Article.jsp).

Mind Stretcher
Critical Thinking Exercise

Have you had the recommended screening tests for CVD, cancer, and diabetes? Why or why not? If not, what could you do to make them a priority and obtain them at recommended intervals?

Q Why does diabetes affect the heart?

CONTROL DIABETES. People with diabetes are two to four times more likely to develop cardiovascular disease than nondiabetics, and at least 65 percent of people with diabetes die from some form of heart disease or stroke.[17] Over time, elevated blood glucose levels associated with diabetes damage nerves and blood vessels and contribute to atherosclerosis. Diabetes is often accompanied by other CVD risk factors, including hypertension, high lipid levels, and increased weight. Elevated blood glucose levels can harm the cardiovascular system even if they aren't high enough for a diagnosis of full-blown diabetes. High blood glucose levels are one of the five traits that define **metabolic syndrome,** a cluster of medical conditions that puts people at risk for both heart disease and type 2 diabetes. A person who has at least three of the five traits listed in Table 11-5 is classified as having metabolic syndrome.

Following the CVD prevention strategies described earlier will help to reduce your risk for diabetes and metabolic syndrome. Diabetes will be discussed in more detail later in the chapter.

Symptoms, Diagnosis, and Treatment of Cardiovascular Disease

Q Would I know if I had CVD?

Maybe, but maybe not. Some forms of cardiovascular disease have no visible symptoms. Even if there are observable symptoms, you may still need testing to determine whether you have CVD.

Q Does cardiovascular disease hurt? Would it affect my everyday activities?

SYMPTOMS. It depends. Different types of cardiovascular disease have different symptoms. Some are painful and some are not. For example, hypertension typically doesn't have any

metabolic syndrome
A group of risk factors linked to overweight and obesity that increase the chance of heart disease, diabetes, and stroke: large waistline, low HDL, and elevated triglycerides, fasting blood sugar, and blood pressure.

TABLE 11-5 METABOLIC SYNDROME*

TRAITS/MEDICAL CONDITIONS	DEFINITION
LARGE WAIST CIRCUMFERENCE	■ 40 inches (102 cm) or more in men ■ 35 inches (88 cm) or more in women
ELEVATED LEVELS OF TRIGLYCERIDES	■ 150 mg/dl or higher
LOW LEVELS OF HDL (GOOD) CHOLESTEROL	■ Below 40 mg/dl in men ■ Below 50 mg/dl in women
ELEVATED BLOOD PRESSURE LEVELS	■ 130 mm Hg or higher for systolic blood pressure **or** ■ 85 mm Hg or higher for diastolic blood pressure
ELEVATED FASTING BLOOD GLUCOSE LEVELS	■ 100 mg/dl or higher

*Metabolic syndrome is defined as having three or more of the traits/conditions listed.

Source: Pub Med Health. (2011). *Metabolic syndrome* (http://www.ncbi.nlm.nih.gov/pubmedhealth/PMH0004546/).

TABLE 11-6 WARNING SIGNS OF HEART ATTACK AND STROKE

HEART ATTACK WARNING SIGNS	STROKE WARNING SIGNS
■ **Chest discomfort:** Most heart attacks involve discomfort in the center of the chest that lasts for more than a few minutes, or goes away and comes back. The discomfort can feel like uncomfortable pressure, squeezing, fullness, or pain. ■ **Discomfort in other areas of the upper body:** Can include pain or discomfort in one or both arms, the back, neck, jaw, or stomach. ■ **Shortness of breath:** Often comes along with chest discomfort, but it also can occur before chest discomfort. ■ **Other symptoms:** Breaking out in a cold sweat, nausea or light-headedness.	■ **Sudden numbness** or weakness of face, arm, or leg, especially on one side of the body. ■ **Sudden confusion,** trouble speaking or understanding. ■ **Sudden trouble seeing** in one or both eyes. ■ **Sudden trouble walking,** dizziness, loss of balance or coordination. ■ **Sudden severe headache** with no known cause.
For more information about detecting and responding to a heart attack, go to http://www.heart.org/idc/groups/heart-public/@wcm/@hcm/documents/downloadable/ucm_304575.pdf.	For a quick way to remember stroke warning signs and to find more information, go to http://www.stroke.org/site/PageServer?pagename=symp.

Source: American Heart Association. (n.d.). *Heart attack, stroke, and cardiac arrest warning signs* (http://www.heart.org/HEARTORG/General/Heart-Attack-Stroke-and-Cardiac-Arrest-Signs_UCM_303977_SubHomePage.jsp).

noticeable symptoms, but heart attacks and strokes can be very painful. Other types of CVD, such as heart failure, have longer-lasting complications that may or may not be painful. Shortness of breath or swelling of the legs and ankles, for example, may make day-to-day activities difficult or even painful. Signs of CVD include chest pain, fatigue, shortness of breath, leg pain, *palpitations* (the sensation of irregular or forceful heartbeat), and light-headedness and fainting.

Q | How can you tell if a person is having a heart attack or a stroke?

Each has clear warning signs that you can learn to recognize—and it's important to react appropriately if you do spot any symptoms. Call 911 or the appropriate emergency number if you detect any of the signs listed in Table 11-6. Prompt treatment can increase the chance of survival and limit the damage caused by the heart attack or stroke. Women may be less likely to believe or recognize they're having a heart attack and more likely to delay treatment. As it is for men, the most common heart attack symptom for women is chest pain or discomfort. But women are somewhat more likely than men to experience other symptoms, including shortness of breath, nausea, and back or jaw pain.

Q | When are you supposed to use CPR?

Cardiopulmonary resuscitation, or CPR, is a form of artificial blood circulation and respiration. Basic CPR consists of chest compressions alternated with rescue breathing (mouth-to-mouth respiration) at a ratio of 30 compressions to two breaths. Compression-only CPR, with chest compressions delivered at the rate of 100 per minute without any rescue breaths, has been found to be an equally effective technique and is now also endorsed by the American Heart Association.[18]

CPR is used for victims of cardiac arrest, which occurs when the heart suddenly stops beating or beats so irregularly that oxygenated blood isn't pumped to the brain and the rest of the body. Victims typically become suddenly unresponsive and may also stop breathing. If these signs are present, call 911 and then begin CPR right away.

CPR doesn't usually restart the heart, but it can temporarily maintain circulation, providing the opportunity for a successful resuscitation while limiting damage to the brain and heart from lack of blood flow. Resuscitation usually requires advanced care with *defibrillation,* a procedure in which an electronic device administers an electrical shock to the heart. Some locations now have automated external defibrillators (AEDs) designed for use by laypeople. AEDs are relatively simple to use; they automatically detect arrhythmias and deliver a shock that may correct the heart rhythm.

AEDs can be used in conjunction with CPR, and training for both is available. Most classes can be taken in a single day. Contact a local health care provider, the American Red Cross, or American Heart Association to find a class near you. CPR and use of AEDs are easy skills to learn and could mean the difference between life and death for someone you love.

For more information about performing CPR and using an AED, go to http://www.mayoclinic.com/health/first-aid-cpr/FA00061 or http://www.mayoclinic.com/health/automated-external-defibrillators/HB00053.

DIAGNOSIS. CVD may be diagnosed before you have symptoms, and you can take early steps to control it. Everyone should get recommended screening tests, including those for blood pressure and cholesterol, as well as regular health checkups.

There are many diagnostic tests to recognize and assess problems with the heart and blood vessels. Your physician may conduct multiple tests to rule out other possible causes for your symptoms as well as to confirm a CVD diagnosis. Table 11-7 describes some of the relevant tests.

Q | What kinds of medicine and help are available?

TREATMENT. A diagnosis of cardiovascular disease can be scary, but many successful forms of treatment are available. Lifestyle changes are always the first line of defense and can be used to both prevent and treat CVD. A variety of medications are available to help when lifestyle changes fall short; the type of medication depends on the type of CVD. Commonly used drugs include those that lower blood pressure or cholesterol, prevent clots from forming, increase the pumping strength of the heart, and relax blood vessels.

Unfortunately, lifestyle changes and medications aren't always successful at controlling CVD. In some cases, surgery or other procedures may be needed. *Coronary angioplasty* is a procedure in which a catheter is inserted into blocked coronary arteries. When the blockages are reached, a small balloon is used to push through the blockage. Often a *stent,* a small wire tube, is inserted to assist in keeping the artery open. If coronary artery blockages are too severe, *coronary bypass surgery* may be needed. During bypass surgery, a blood vessel taken from elsewhere in the body is grafted to the heart, producing a bypass, or detour, around the blocked artery to create a new route for blood flow. Blockage of several arteries may require multiple bypasses.

A *pacemaker* is an electrical device that regulates heartbeat. The advanced models now available can increase heart rate in response to activity, as well as detect and regulate irregular heart rhythms. The device is typically implanted in the upper chest near the collarbone, using local anesthesia. In most instances, the procedure is considered minor surgery, and patients go home within a day.

If a heart valve malfunction is too severe to treat with medication, open heart surgery may be necessary for *heart valve repair* or *replacement.* Repairing the valve or valves is the preferred choice, but repair is not always possible. Replacement valves may be tissue valves (human or animal) or mechanical valves made from plastic or metal.

When the heart can no longer perform its job of getting oxygenated blood to the body's tissues and there is risk for death, a heart transplant may be the option. A *heart transplant* involves replacing the diseased heart with a healthy heart from a human donor. A heart transplant is now considered a relatively simple operation. According to the U.S. Department of Health and Human Services Organ Procurement and Transplantation Network, more than 2,000 Americans per year receive a new heart (http://optn.transplant.hrsa.gov/latestData/rptData.asp).

TABLE 11-7 TESTS FOR DIAGNOSING AND MONITORING CARDIOVASCULAR DISEASE

ELECTROCARDIOGRAM (ECG OR EKG)	Electrodes are placed on the skin to detect the heart's electrical signals, which are recorded; the test can show problems with heart rate or rhythm and detect underlying damage to the heart.
EXERCISE STRESS TEST	An electrocardiogram is performed while the person is exercising on a treadmill or stationary bike; the test monitors the response to exercise and detects problems with the cardiovascular system during physical effort.
CORONARY ANGIOGRAPHY	A catheter is threaded though an artery, typically in the leg, and dye is injected into the arteries of the heart; special X-rays are then used to identify blockages. A similar procedure can be done to visualize the brain's blood vessels.
BLOOD TESTS	In addition to checking cholesterol and glucose levels, blood samples can be analyzed for enzymes and proteins in the blood that indicate heart-muscle damage.
CHEST X-RAY	Ionizing radiation creates pictures of the heart, lungs, and blood vessels that can be used to determine the size and shape of the heart as well as to detect fluid buildup or damage.
ECHOCARDIOGRAM	A small device called a *transducer* transmits ultrasound waves into the chest, which are converted into computerized images of the heart; the test can show the heart's size, structure, and motion, as well as blood volume and speed and direction of blood flow.
NUCLEAR SCAN; POSITRON EMISSION TOMOGRAPHIC (PET) SCAN	In both tests, small amounts of radioactive tracer materials are injected into the bloodstream; special imaging equipment monitors blood flow to the heart, as well as the heart's efficiency in pumping blood, and checks for heart-muscle damage.
COMPUTED TOMOGRAPHY (CT) SCAN	A special X-ray machine takes cross-sectional images that are used to create three-dimensional models of organs. Scans can be used to detect problems in blood vessels in both the heart and the brain.
MAGNETIC RESONANCE IMAGING (MRI)	A special scanner uses radio waves, magnets, and a computer to create images of organs and tissues; MRIs can evaluate the condition of the heart and blood vessels and detect the presence and size of aneurysms and malformed blood vessels that are potential causes of hemorrhagic stroke.
ELECTROENCEPHALOGRAM (EEG)	Electrodes are placed on the scalp, and the electrical activity of the brain is monitored for any indications of problems.

Q How likely is it that someone will survive and recover from CVD? Is there a cure for it?

Because one in three Americans dies from some type of cardiovascular disease, it's hard to talk in terms of a cure. However, most people who die from CVD are older. Some younger people do develop and die from CVD, but it's much less common. It's important to realize that many forms of CVD are treatable. Many people not only survive but live long and productive lives when they appropriately manage their CVD.

Cancer

Cancer is common and potentially deadly. In their lifetimes, about one in two men and one in three women will develop some form of cancer. Luckily, there are many

Fast Facts

Chronic Disease by the Numbers

The average lifetime probability of developing a chronic disease is fairly high. But remember—these are averages. Your risk could be much higher or lower depending on your personal risk factors, including your lifestyle choices.

Cancer
Men: 1 in 2
Women: 1 in 3

Diabetes
Men: 1 in 3
Women: 2 in 5 (Hispanic women: 1 in 2)

Cardiovascular disease
Men: 2 in 3
Women: 1 in 2

- What family members or friends of yours have one of these chronic diseases?
- What lifestyle changes have they made to reduce their risk of future complications?

Sources: American Cancer Society. (2012). *Cancer facts & figures 2012.* Atlanta, GA: American Cancer Society. Roger, V. L., and others. (2012). *Heart disease and stroke statistics 2012: A report from the American Heart Association. Circulation, 125,* 2e–220e. Centers for Disease Control and Prevention. (2011). *CDC statements on diabetes issues lifetime risk for diabetes mellitus in the United States* (http://www.cdc.gov/diabetes/news/docs/lifetime.htm).

things you can do to reduce your risk of developing cancer, and many forms of cancer are very treatable, especially when discovered in the early stages.

Q What is cancer? What is the difference between malignant and benign tumors?

Like cardiovascular disease, **cancer** is not one disease but rather a broad category of disease, all varieties of which are characterized by uncontrolled growth of cells. Typically cells grow and divide in a controlled and orderly fashion, and rates of new cell growth and old cell death are balanced. If a damaging mutation occurs in a cell, under normal circumstances, the cell will either undergo repair or self-destruct.

If something affects this cycle, abnormal cells may grow and reproduce in an uncontrolled manner (Figure 11-6). Mutated cells often divide more quickly than surrounding tissues and may "clump" into masses known as **tumors.** It usually takes many mutations before a cell becomes cancerous and begins to divide uncontrollably.

Most tumors are **benign,** or noncancerous. Benign tumors do not invade other tissues and are typically not harmful unless they interfere with bodily functions. For example, uterine fibroids, which are benign tumors, are relatively common in women of childbearing age. They can vary from the size of a seed to the size of a grapefruit or larger, but they typically don't interfere with day-to-day function. However, benign brain tumors put pressure on sensitive areas of the brain and cause serious symptoms, so they typically are removed.

Malignant tumors are known as cancer. Not only can these tumors invade nearby healthy cells and organs, they can also **metastasize,** or spread, to other parts of the body through the

cancer A group of diseases characterized by uncontrolled growth and spread of abnormal cells.

tumor Mass of cells with no physiological function that arises from uncontrolled cellular growth; may be benign or malignant.

benign Noncancerous.

malignant Cancerous.

metastasize To spread from the original site to other parts of the body.

Normal cell division and growth control

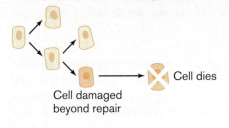

Cell damaged beyond repair → Cell dies

Cancer cell division and loss of growth control

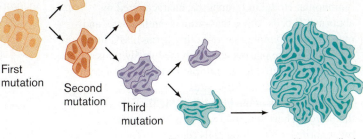

First mutation → Second mutation → Third mutation → Fourth or later mutation → Uncontrolled growth

Figure 11-6 Normal cell division versus cancer cell division. Normal cells divide in a controlled fashion and will self-destruct if they are damaged beyond repair. Cancer usually involves multiple mutations, after which cancer cells will grow and divide uncontrollably.

Source: Adapted from National Cancer Institute. (2009). *Understanding cancer series: What is cancer* (http://www.cancer.gov/cancertopics/understandingcancer/cancer/allpages).

blood and lymphatic systems. Tumors that have metastasized are known as *secondary tumors,* and the original, or first, tumor is considered the *primary tumor.*

Some benign tumors undergo changes and become malignant. For example, benign tumors in the colon are known as *polyps,* and they can be easily removed with minor surgery. However, if left in place, polyps can become malignant over time, and colon cancer can invade surrounding tissues and organs and then spread to other parts of the body.

Q | How many Americans have cancer?

The American Cancer Society estimates that nearly 12 million Americans with a history of cancer are alive today. This figure includes both people who are currently undergoing treatment and those who are now considered cancer-free.[19] About 1.6 million new cancer cases are diagnosed each year, and cancer claims more than 570,000 lives per year, or more than 1,500 a day. Though still large, the number of new cases of cancer occurring each year has begun to decline slightly.

Types of Cancer

Scientists estimate there are hundreds of types of cancer. Cancers are classified according to the body location where they originate and by the kind of tissue or fluid from which they develop. Though some cancers are mixed types, most fall into one of the following general groupings:[20]

- *Carcinoma* arises in skin or in tissues that line or cover internal organs, glands, or other body structures such as breasts, lungs, bladder, and skin; it accounts for 80–90 percent of all cancer cases.
- *Sarcoma* arises from connective or supportive tissues such as bone, cartilage, fat, muscle, blood vessels, and tendons; sarcoma is less common than carcinoma but often much more dangerous.
- *Lymphoma and myeloma* originate in the cells of the immune system. There are two major types of lymphoma: Hodgkin lymphoma, characterized by abnormal B cells (those that produce antibodies), and non-Hodgkin lymphomas (all other forms). Myeloma originates in the plasma cells of bone marrow; it is commonly referred to as multiple myeloma because it typically occurs at multiple sites.
- *Leukemia* occurs in the blood-forming tissues of the body such as bone marrow. It is characterized by abnormal white blood cells (needed to fight infection), red blood cells (needed to carry oxygen), and platelets (needed to minimize excessive bruising and bleeding) rather than the solid tumors of most other cancers.
- *Central nervous system cancers* begin in the tissues of the brain or spinal cord.

Q | What is the most common type of cancer? Which type is most severe?

The most frequently diagnosed cancers in the United States are two types of skin cancer—*basal cell carcinoma* and *squamous cell carcinoma*—for which 2 million people are treated each year. Because most cases of these cancers are noninvasive and highly curable, they are not included in cancer registries and statistics.

In terms of cancers that are potentially invasive, lung cancer is the leading cause of cancer deaths in both men and women, accounting for about 30 percent of all such deaths (Table 11-8). With regard to incidence, men develop more lung and prostate cancers than any other cancers, and women experience more lung and breast cancers.

Overall cancer deaths in the United States have decreased slightly in recent years. But some cancers, such as lung, liver, and pancreatic cancers, still have poor survival rates because they are typically diagnosed at an advanced stage. Table 11-8 shows the 5-year survival rates for common cancers.

Assessing Your Risk for Cancer

Q | What are my chances of getting cancer?

Anyone can get cancer. There's no way to tell for sure who will develop cancer or when it might happen, but some general patterns of risks are associated with cancer. Overall cancer risks can be viewed in two ways. *Lifetime risk* is the probability of developing or dying from cancer in your lifetime, and *relative risk* refers to the extent of the relationship between a risk factor and a specific kind of cancer. For example, women in the United States have a one-in-three lifetime risk of developing cancer.[21] A woman who smokes has a relative risk of lung cancer of 12, meaning that she is twelve times more likely to develop lung cancer than a nonsmoker. Specific risk factors, some of which are controllable and some of which are not, are described in the next sections.

Q | If someone in my family has cancer, am I likely to get it too?

HEREDITY/GENETICS. Because cancer is uncontrolled cell growth, and cell growth is controlled by genes, all cancers involve some type of genetic mutation (damage). These mutations can take many forms, so diseases as different as leukemia and lung cancer are both considered cancers.

Most genetic mutations are random, occurring as a result of a genetic mistake when a cell divides or in response to environmental factors such as sunlight, chemicals, and tobacco. Only about 5–10 percent of all cancers are linked

TABLE 11-8 MOST FREQUENTLY DIAGNOSED CANCERS IN THE UNITED STATES, 2012 ESTIMATES

SITE OR TYPE	ESTIMATED NEW CASES	ESTIMATED DEATHS	5-YEAR SURVIVAL RATE, ALL STAGES
LUNG AND BRONCHUS	226,160	160,340	16%
PROSTATE	241,740	28,170	99%
BREAST, FEMALE*	226,870	39,920	89%
COLON AND RECTUM	143,460	51,690	64%
BLADDER	73,510	14,880	78%
MELANOMA	76,250	9,180	91%
NON-HODGKIN LYMPHOMA	70,130	20,130	67%
KIDNEY	64,770	13,570	70%
THYROID	56,460	1,780	97%
UTERINE CERVIX	12,170	4,220	69%
UTERINE CORPUS (ENDOMETRIUM)	47,130	8,010	82%
PANCREAS	43,920	37,390	6%
LEUKEMIA (ALL TYPES)	47,150	23,540	67%
ORAL CAVITY AND PHARYNX	40,250	7,850	61%
LIVER	28,720	20,550	14%
OVARY	21,880	13,850	46%

*Male breast cancer is rare, accounting for about 1% of all breast cancers; risk factors include increased estrogen levels, radiation exposure, heavy drinking, and a family history of breast cancer.

Source: American Cancer Society. (2012). *Cancer facts & figures 2012*. Atlanta, GA: American Cancer Society.

to inherited genetic mutations—those that an individual is born with. As a rule, hereditary cancers tend to occur at an earlier age than those due to other causes.

In evaluating your own risk, consider how many family members have had a particular type of cancer and whether any were diagnosed at a young age. Let your health care provider know about any family history of cancer. Depending on your circumstances, earlier or more frequent screenings for particular cancers may be recommended. For some forms of cancer, specific genetic tests are available; see the box "The Ups and Downs of Genetic Testing: Things to Know" for more information.

Q Is cancer common in young adults? What types of cancer should I worry about now, when I'm 20?

AGE. The likelihood of being diagnosed with cancer rises with one's age. Although cancer can occur at any age, 77 percent of all cancers are diagnosed in people age 55 or older.[22] Over time, genetic mutations from internal and environmental factors can build up. Increased exposure along with the body's decreasing ability to repair damaged cells makes us more susceptible to cancer as we age. It's important

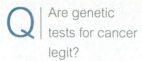

Wellness Strategies

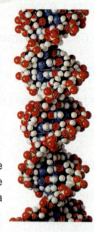

The Ups and Downs of Genetic Testing: Things to Know

Q Are genetic tests for cancer legit?

Genetic testing is available for some types of cancer, including cancers of the breast, colon, ovary, thyroid, kidney, and prostate. This screening has both limitations and benefits.

Limitations of Testing

- An accurate gene test will indicate if a certain mutation is present. However, having the mutation does not guarantee that cancer will develop—and people without the mutation can still get cancer.
- Current tests look only for the most common mutations; other cancer-causing mutations are not detected. And most cancer cases are not due to inherited mutations.
- Determining that one is at a higher risk for disease can cause psychological stress, affect child-bearing decisions, and influence family communication.
- State-of-the-art diagnostics and therapies to keep up with the identification of mutant genes are seriously lacking, according to the National Cancer Institute.

Benefits of Testing

- A negative result can provide tremendous relief and eliminate the need for additional frequent and expensive testing.

- A positive result can lead people to take prudent risk-management strategies, including lifestyle changes, more frequent testing, and other measures prescribed by their physician.
- Testing is becoming more accurate, and more mutations are being identified.

Genetic testing is also available to screen for genes that increase the risk of CVD and diabetes, as well as a number of other diseases and disorders. Tests have been developed for more than 2,000 diseases, but researchers have identified only a small portion of the genetic mechanisms of most diseases. Importantly, use caution when evaluating information about genetic tests, especially those that are marketed directly to the public. To learn more about genetic testing, visit the website of the National Human Genome Research Institute at http://www.genome.gov/19516567.

Sources: Centers for Disease Control and Prevention. (2011). *Public health genomics—genomic testing* (http://www.cdc.gov/genomics/gtesting/). National Cancer Institute. (2006) *Understanding cancer series gene testing* (http://www.cancer.gov/cancertopics/understandingcancer/genetesting).

---

to adopt lifestyle prevention strategies early in life in order to curb susceptibility as much as possible.

Testicular cancer seems to be an exception to the tendency for cancer incidence to increase with age. Although testicular cancer is not common—about 8,500 cases and 350 deaths are reported annually in the United States—its highest rates occur in males ages 15–34. Among men in their twenties, it is the most prevalent form of cancer, followed by lymphoma. The most common cancers among women in their twenties are cancers of the thyroid, breast, cervix, and uterus and Hodgkin lymphoma. About 8 percent of cases of melanoma are diagnosed in people under age 35, so skin cancer prevention and awareness are also critical for young adults. See the box "Self-Exams for Cancer" for helpful prevention strategies.

Q Are men or women more likely to get cancer?

BIOLOGICAL SEX. An estimated half of all men and one-third of all women in the United States will develop cancer at some point in life. Data are inconclusive as to why more men than women are affected.

Many researchers attribute the differences to lifestyle factors, such as higher rates of smoking and excessive alcohol consumption, as well as to greater occupational exposure to dangerous chemicals.

Q What groups are most at risk for cancer?

ETHNICITY. According to the American Cancer Society, the highest incidence of cancer diagnoses and cancer deaths is among African Americans.[23] The death rate for African American females is 16 percent greater than that of white females, and for males, it is 33 percent greater. Other ethnicities have lower cancer rates overall but higher rates of specific cancers, including those of the cervix, uterus, liver, and stomach. Asian American and Pacific Islander men have the highest rate of liver cancer (twice that of African Americans), and Latinas have the highest rate of cervical cancer.

These disparities can be attributed to a number of factors. Low income is associated with limited access to health care and insurance. Cultural dietary practices and preferences for early marriage and childbirth affect cancer risk. Genetic

Wellness Strategies

Self-Exams for Cancer

Q What self-exams for cancer should I do, and how often?

Several self-exams can help spot different kinds of cancer, including those that sometimes strike younger people:

- *Testicular self-exam* can be performed monthly to check for lumps that could indicate early cancer. WebMD Testicular Self-Exam (http://www.emedicine health.com/testicular_self-exam/article_em.htm).
- *Breast self-exam* has both benefits and limitations, and the American Cancer Society recommends it as a nonmandatory option for checking for changes in the breasts. If performed, it should be done carefully and correctly.

WebMD Breast Self-Exam (http://women.webmd.com/breast-self-examination).
- *Skin self-exam* can be performed check for problems; a record such as a body mole map can help determine if changes occur over time.
American Academy of Dermatology: How to Examine Your Skin (http://www.aad.org/skin-conditions/skin-cancer-detection/about-skin-self-exams).

Check out available apps for self-exam tracking and monitoring systems. In all cases, if you notice anything unusual during a self-exam, have your health care provider evaluate it.

---

carcinogen A substance or agent that causes cancer.

factors may also play a role in the more aggressive forms of breast cancer in African American women and the elevated risk of prostate cancer among African American men. For more on cancer disparities, visit the Web sites for the American Cancer Society (http://www.cancer.org) and the National Cancer Institute (http://www.cancer.gov).

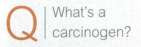

Q What's a carcinogen?

EXPOSURE TO CANCER-CAUSING AGENTS. A **carcinogen** is any substance that causes cancer. Carcinogens include solvents, pesticides, asbestos fibers, tobacco smoke, certain hormones and viruses, and radiation from X-rays, radon, sunlight, and tanning lamps or beds.[24] Radiation sources and risks are described in more detail below.

The news often has stories about cancer-causing pollutants in the environment. Although the risks are real, exposure to environmental chemicals isn't a major cause of cancer for most people—it's responsible for perhaps 2 percent of all cancers.[25] Lifestyle choices and other factors play a much more important role in determining cancer risk. But for people exposed to carcinogens regularly or at relatively high levels because of their jobs—chemical workers and miners, for example—carcinogenic chemicals are a significant risk factor.

Cancer Prevention

Q Is there a way to keep from getting cancer?

For most people diagnosed with cancer, the precise cause is unknown. Experts point to a combination of controllable and uncontrollable risk factors. Although you can't do anything about your family history, age, sex, or ethnicity, there are many positive steps you can take to reduce your risk. Your use of tobacco, your diet, your level of physical activity, and the other lifestyle factors discussed next can increase or reduce your risk.

Tobacco. Cigarettes contain thousands of chemicals, including more that 60 known cancer-causing agents. Smoking leads to 80 percent of lung cancer deaths, as well as most cancers of the larynx, oral cavity, pharynx, esophagus, and bladder, and it contributes to kidney, pancreatic, cervical, and stomach cancers and to cardiovascular and other diseases. Regular cigar smokers who inhale are exposed to many of the same risks as cigarette smokers. Smokeless tobacco contains 28 known cancer-causing agents and leads to increased risk of oral cancer. Second-hand smoke, also known as environmental tobacco smoke (ETS), contains more than 50 cancer-causing agents and has been linked to lung cancer, nasal sinus cancer, respiratory infections, and heart disease in exposed nonsmokers. Research findings on marijuana have been mixed, but marijuana smoke contains some of the same chemicals as tobacco smoke and has been implicated in increased risk of certain cancers.[26] For your health and wellness, avoid tobacco in all forms.

Diet, physical activity, and body weight. The American Cancer Society estimates that one-third of all cancer deaths in the United States are due to poor nutrition and physical inactivity and/or excess body weight. Obesity has been linked to breast, endometrial, colon, kidney, and esophageal cancers. Regular exercise helps control body weight; in addition, physical activity improves bowel functioning and the levels of insulin and other hormones.

Research Brief

Indoor Tanning and Melanoma

Ultraviolet rays from tanning beds and lamps are classified as a carcinogen, meaning that they cause cancer. How big is the risk? Researchers recently studied over 2,000 adults ages 25 to 59 with a history of indoor tanning. They looked at the amount of exposure—total number of tanning hours—as it related to a melanoma diagnosis. After controlling for other risk factors for skin cancer, including hair and skin color and freckling, the researchers found a significant association between indoor tanning and melanoma, as shown in the graph.

In short, indoor as well as outdoor tanning should be avoided. Indoor tanners should research sunless

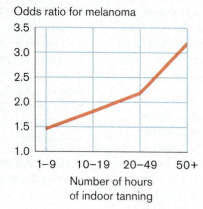

Odds ratio for melanoma

Number of hours of indoor tanning

1–9   10–19   20–49   50+

tanning options instead at http://www .webmd.com/healthy-beauty/features/ sunless-tanning.

Analyze and Apply

- What is this study's key lesson about ultraviolet radiation exposure during indoor tanning?
- Why do you think people seek out indoor tanning? What advice would you give to a close friend who has regular indoor tanning treatments?

Source: Lazovich, D., and others. (2010). Indoor tanning and risk of melanoma: A case-control study in a highly exposed population. *Cancer Epidemiology, Biomarkers & Prevention, 19*(6), 1557–1568.

Certain nutrients and foods have been linked to a lower risk of cancer. Although researchers have tried to identify specific nutrients as protective, the best evidence at present supports the consumption of a healthy overall diet. The American Cancer Society recommends a diet rich in plant-based foods, including whole grains, fruits, and vegetables. See Chapter 9 for more on planning a healthy diet.

Alcohol. More than 2 drinks per day increases the risk of cancers of the mouth, throat, esophagus, larynx, liver, and breast. For women, even just 1 alcoholic drink per day results in a very small increase in breast cancer risk. Alcohol may have direct effects on body cells, and it can also influence levels of hormones and certain nutrients. Risk increases with the amount of alcohol consumed and with tobacco use in combination with the alcohol.

Infectious agents. Infection with human papillomaviruses (HPV) is the primary cause of cervical cancer and may also be linked to other cancers. Chronic infection with hepatitis B can cause liver cancer, and *Helicobacter pylori* infection can lead to stomach cancer. Cancers from these viruses and bacteria can be prevented through vaccination, antibiotic treatment, and lifestyle choices that lower the risk of infection.

Radiation. All sources of radiation, including medical X-rays, radioactive substances, and sunlight, are potential carcinogens. Avoid unnecessary medical X-rays and imaging scans; ask how each X-ray or scan will help, and keep a record of all your X-rays to avoid duplication. Be aware that computed tomography (CT) scans use much higher radiation doses than standard X-rays, dental X-rays, and mammography. If radon (a naturally occurring radioactive gas) is a concern where you live, test your residence for

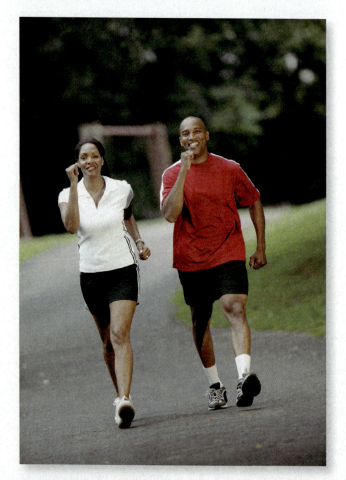

About one-third of all cancer deaths are related to physical inactivity and poor dietary choices. Regular exercise directly reduces the risk of certain cancers, including those of the breast and colon. Exercise also helps maintain healthy body weight, which further reduces cancer risk.

radon and take appropriate steps if levels are high. For more on radon, visit the Web site for the Environmental Protection Agency (http://www.epa.gov/radon).

Sunlight, tanning lamps and booths. Ultraviolet (UV) rays from any source—sunlight, sun lamps, or tanning booths—cause early aging of the skin and skin damage that can lead to melanoma, the most dangerous form of skin cancer. Getting a "base tan" isn't healthy and doesn't protect your skin from sun damage—a tan *is* damage. Use sunscreen when you're outdoors, and don't use tanning lamps or booths (see the box "Indoor Tanning and Melanoma"). Although people with lighter skin tones are at higher risk for melanoma, darker skin does not eliminate risk. African Americans and Latinos have much lower rates of skin cancer than whites, but when they do develop melanoma, it is usually diagnosed at a more advanced stage and has a lower survival rate[27] (see the box "Protecting Your Skin from the Sun").

Stress. Stress activates the body's hormones, and this stimulation can cause changes in the immune system and the body's ability to protect itself against infection and diseases, including cancer. Although human studies have provided no conclusive evidence that increased stress levels lead directly to cancer, minimizing stress has other positive effects on the body, as we have seen.

Chemicals. In the United States, exposure to carcinogenic chemicals on the job is linked to many more cases of cancer than exposure to general environmental pollution. Workers exposed to asbestos, benzene, cadmium, nickel, and vinyl chloride are at increased risk for a number of cancers. Chemicals and others substances in the home—such as some cleaners, paint and solvents, motor oil, and pesticides—may also elevate risk for cancer, although to a lesser degree. Always handle and dispose of hazardous chemicals appropriately.

To identify your personal risk factors as well as strategies for prevention, complete Lab Activity 11-1.

Symptoms, Diagnosis, and Treatment of Cancer

Cancer takes many forms. Some have early warning signs and some do not. Some have screening tests and some do not. In all cases, it's better to detect cancer as early as possible. The best things you can do are to be alert for early warning signs and have preventive screenings as recommended.

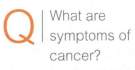 **When am I supposed to get all those cancer tests—and does everyone really need them?**

EARLY SCREENING. Early cancer screening is critical for everyone. Screening tests performed before any symptoms appear can help find cancer in its earliest and most treatable stage. Table 11-9 on p. 405 summarizes the American Cancer Society's recommendations for screening. Follow these guidelines or more specific guidelines provided by your physician based on your family history and risk factors. These tests can help detect early cancers and improve your chances of living a long and healthy life.

Q **What are symptoms of cancer?**

SIGNS AND SYMPTOMS. The initial stages of cancer often have no symptoms or very general symptoms that may indicate any number of other health issues. The acronym CAUTION can help you remember general symptoms to watch for:

- **C**hanges in bowel or bladder habits
- **A** sore that does not heal
- **U**nusual bleeding or discharge
- **T**hickening or lump in the breast or elsewhere
- **I**ndigestion or difficulty swallowing
- **O**bvious change in a wart or mole
- **N**agging cough or hoarseness

Also remember to check your skin for the ABCDEs of melanoma; see Figure 11-7 on p. 406. Consult your physician if you experience any of these symptoms.

Q **What tests will a doctor do to figure out if a symptom really means cancer?**

DIAGNOSIS. There is no single test to diagnose cancer. Depending on the type of cancer suspected, one or more of the following tests may be used to diagnose cancer and monitor its progress:

- *Biopsy:* Removal of a tissue sample so that the cells can be examined under a microscope for abnormalities.
- *Imaging procedures:* Use of X-rays, magnetic resonance imaging (MRI), computed tomography (CT), ultrasound, and other high-tech scans to produce visual images of abnormal masses or sites of unusual chemical activity.
- *Tumor marker and other lab tests:* Measurement of specific substances in the blood, urine, or tissues that tend to occur in high levels with certain cancers. DNA testing may also be used to look for specific genetic mutations.

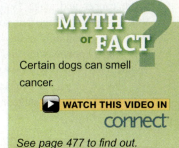

MYTH or FACT?

Certain dogs can smell cancer.

▶ **WATCH THIS VIDEO IN** connect

See page 477 to find out.

Q **What does it mean when they say someone has stage IV cancer?**

When someone is diagnosed with cancer, both the type of cancer and stage of development will be identified. There are a number of staging systems, but staging is typically based on factors such as the size and location of the tumor, the number

Wellness Strategies

Protecting Your Skin from the Sun

Q | How can I protect my skin from the sun?

Ultraviolet (UV) radiation can cause sunburn as well as other skin damage. Different types of UV light have different effects on the skin. *Ultraviolet B (UVB) radiation* has shorter wavelengths and affects primarily the skin's top layer, causing a sunburn you can see. *Ultraviolet A (UVA) radiation* has longer wavelengths and is more likely to infiltrate deeper into the skin and cause damage that is less immediately obvious—but over time leads to premature aging of the skin. Both UVA and UVB exposure can cause skin cancer.

The best way to avoid damage from UV radiation is to stay out of the sun, especially when the sun is most intense (between 10 a.m. and 4 p.m.). When you are out in the sun, covering up with long sleeves and a hat provides the most protection; special clothing for sun protection is also available. If your skin will be exposed to the sun, use plenty of sunscreen. Tips:

- Choose a sunscreen with an SPF (sun protection factor) of 30 or higher, which should block 97 percent of the sun's UVB rays if used correctly. SPF is a relative measure based on sun exposure; a sunscreen with an SPF of 30 should allow skin to be exposed without burning to 30 times more UVB rays than normal.

- Know your rays. As of 2012, the FDA required new testing and labeling on sun protection products. Look for a sunscreen that shields against both UVA and UVB rays—one that is labeled "broad spectrum," meaning that it has UVA protection that is equivalent to its UVB protection factor. This new labeling system also applies to sun protection cosmetics.

- Use plenty of sunscreen. The average person needs about 1 ounce to cover the body—that's one-quarter of a 4-ounce bottle.

- Apply sunscreen 30 minutes before you go outside, and reapply it at least every 2 hours.

- Use a water-resistant sunscreen if you'll be in the water or if you sweat heavily.

- Combination sunscreen and insect-repellant products are less effective, so use a higher SPF and apply it more frequently.

- Remember that UV rays are not blocked by clouds, so apply sunscreen even on cloudy or hazy days.

For more information, visit the Web sites for the Skin Cancer Foundation (http://www.skincancer.org/Sunscreen) and SkinCancerNet (http://www.skincarephysicians.com/skincancernet).

---

of lymph nodes involved, and whether the disease has metastasized (spread) to a distant location in the body. A stage of I, II, III, or IV will be designated, with stage I indicating early stage cancer and stage IV indicating an advanced cancer that has spread. Stage 0 is sometimes used to describe cancer that is found only in the layer of cells in which it began; this is also known as *in situ* (Latin for "in its place") cancer. Figure 11-8 on p. 406 shows the different stages in cancer.

The *prognosis,* or projected outcome, for survival typically decreases as the stage increases. For example, in stage I colon cancer, the tumor is small and localized, and the potential for successful treatment is high. On the other hand, in stage IV colon cancer, the malignant cells have spread to the lymph nodes and other tissues and organs, and treatment is likely to be more complicated and less successful.

Q | Once someone has cancer, what's the best way to treat it?

TREATMENT. The type and the stage of the cancer help determine the most effective treatment. The person's age, health, and lifestyle are also taken into account. Although we tend to think of cancer treatments as being used for the sole purpose of curing cancer, sometimes treatments serve to keep cancer from spreading or simply to relieve symptoms. The most common cancer treatments are chemotherapy, radiation, and surgery, and often more than one treatment type is used.

Chemotherapy is the use of drugs to kill cancer cells or to inhibit their growth. Often it is a combination of

chemotherapy Treatment involving the use of chemical agents (drugs) to kill cancer cells.

Mind Stretcher
Critical Thinking Exercise

Do you feel that you have the ability to influence your own risk of cancer? Why or why not? Has your idea about your level of control over your risk affected your health habits and your choices about screening tests?

TABLE 11-9 CANCER SCREENING GUIDELINES FOR THE EARLY DETECTION OF CANCER IN AVERAGE-RISK ASYMPTOMATIC PEOPLE

CANCER SITE	POPULATION	TEST OR PROCEDURE	FREQUENCY
BREAST	Women, age 20+	Breast self-examination (BSE)	It is acceptable for women to choose not to do BSE or to do BSE regularly (monthly) or irregularly. Beginning in their early 20s, women should be told about the benefits and limitations of breast self-examination (BSE). Whether a woman ever performs BSE, the importance of prompt reporting of any new breast symptoms to a health professional should be emphasized. Women who choose to do BSE should receive instruction and have their technique reviewed on the occasion of a periodic health examination.
		Clinical breast examination (CBE)	For women in their 20s and 30s, it is recommended that clinical breast examination (CBE) be part of a periodic health examination, preferably at least every three years. Asymptomatic women age 40 and older should continue to receive a clinical breast examination as part of a periodic health examination, preferably annually.
		Mammography	Begin annual mammography at age 40.*
CERVIX	Women, age 21+	Pap test HPV test	All women should begin cervical cancer screening at age 21. Women between the ages of 21 and 29 should have a Pap test every 3 years. They should not be tested for HPV unless it is needed after an abnormal Pap test result. Women between the ages of 30 and 65 should have both a Pap test and an HPV test every 5 years. This is the preferred approach, but it is also OK to have a Pap test alone every 3 years. Women over age 65 who have had regular screenings with normal results should not be screened for cervical cancer. Women who have been diagnosed with cervical pre-cancer should continue to be screened. Women who have had their uterus and cervix removed in a hysterectomy and have no history of cervical cancer or pre-cancer should not be screened. Women who have had the HPV vaccine should still follow the screening recommendations for their age group. Women who are at high risk for cervical cancer may need to be screened more often. Women at high risk might include those with HIV infection, organ transplant, or exposure to the drug DES. They should talk with their doctor or nurse.
COLORECTAL	Men and women, age 50+	Fecal occult blood test (FOBT) with at least 50% test sensitivity for cancer, or fecal immunochemical test (FIT) with at least 50% test sensitivity for cancer, **or**	Annual, starting at age 50. Testing at home with adherence to manufacturer's recommendation for collection techniques and number of samples is recommended. FOBT with the single stool sample collected on the clinician's a fingertip during a digital rectal examination in the health care setting is not recommended. Guaiac-based toilet bowl FOBT tests also are not recommended. In comparison with guaiac-based tests for the detection of occult blood, immunochemical tests are more patient-friendly, and are likely to be equal or better in sensitivity and specificity. There is no justification for repeating FOBT in response to an initial positive finding.
		Stool DNA test, **or**	Interval uncertain, starting at age 50
		Flexible sigmoidoscopy (FSIG), **or**	Every 5 years, starting at age 50. FSIG can be performed alone, or consideration can be given to combining FSIG performed every 5 years with a highly sensitive gFOBT or FIT performed annually.
		Double contrast barium enema (DCBE), **or**	Every 5 years, starting at age 50
		Colonoscopy	Every 10 years, starting at age 50
		CT Colonography	Every 5 years, starting at age 50
ENDOMETRIAL	Women, at menopause		At the time of menopause, women at average risk should be informed about risks and symptoms of endometrial cancer and strongly encouraged to report any unexpected bleeding or spotting to their physicians.
PROSTATE	Men, ages 50+	Digital rectal examination (DRE) and prostate-specific antigen test (PSA)	Men who have at least a 10-year life expectancy should have an opportunity to make an informed decision with their health care provider about whether to be screened for prostate cancer, after receiving information about the potential benefits, risks, and uncertainties associated with prostate cancer screening. Prostate cancer screening should not occur without an informed decision-making process.
LUNG CANCER	Men and women who meet noted criteria	Low-dose CT	Low-dose CT screening may be recommended for people who meet NLST criteria: Current or former smokers aged 55 to 74 years, a smoking history of at least 30 pack-years, no history of lung cancer. Individuals should not receive a chest X-ray for lung cancer screening. Low-dose CT screening is NOT recommended for everyone: Discuss the pros and cons with a physician. Utilize a facility that uses "best practices" for CT screening.
CANCER-RELATED CHECKUP	Men and women, age 20+		On the occasion of a periodic health examination, the cancer-related checkup should include examination for cancers of the thyroid, testicles, ovaries, lymph nodes, oral cavity, and skin, as well as health counseling about tobacco, sun exposure, diet and nutrition, risk factors, sexual practices, and environmental and occupational exposures.

*Beginning at age 40, annual clinical breast examination should be performed prior to mammography.

Sources: Adapted from American Cancer Society. (2012). *Cancer facts & figures 2012.* Atlanta, GA: American Cancer Society. American Lung Association. (2012). *Lung cancer CT screening for early detection.* Washington, DC: American Lung Association. *Screening guidelines for the prevention and early detection of cervical cancer.* Published online March 14, 2012, in *CA: A Cancer Journal for Clinicians.* First author: Debbie Saslow, PhD, American Cancer Society, Atlanta, GA.

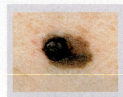

Asymmetry:
The two halves of the mole don't match

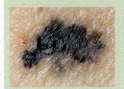

Border:
The borders are uneven and edges may be scalloped or notched

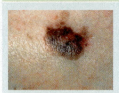

Color:
The mole has a variety of colors–different shades of brown, tan, or black or even red, blue, or another color

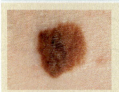

Diameter:
A size larger than a pencil eraser (¼ inch or 6 mm)

Evolving:
Changing in size, shape, color, elevation, or another trait, or any new symptom such as bleeding, itching, or crusting

Figure 11-7 ABCDEs of melanoma. Most of the spots and growths on your skin are harmless, but atypical moles can be the first sign of serious skin cancer. If any of your moles have or develop the characteristics shown here, see your physician.
Source: Skin Cancer Foundation. (2010). *Warning signs: The ABCDEs of melanoma* (http://www.skincancer.org/the-abcdes-of-melanoma.html).

drugs that may be administered intravenously, inserted into a body cavity, or taken orally in pill form. Chemotherapy is a systemic treatment because it circulates through the blood to other parts of the body in order to also reach secondary tumors. More than 50 percent of cancer patients are treated

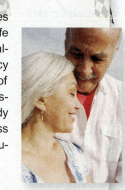
with chemotherapy. Because chemotherapy typically targets all rapidly dividing cells, including noncancerous ones, its side effects include nausea, hair loss, and anemia.

Radiation therapy, or *radiation,* is the use of high-energy rays to kill or damage cancer cells in an attempt to keep them from growing or spreading. Unlike chemotherapy, radiation is a local rather than a systemic treatment. Therapy may be administered

radiation therapy The use of high-energy rays to kill or damage cancer cells to keep them from growing or spreading; also known as radiation.

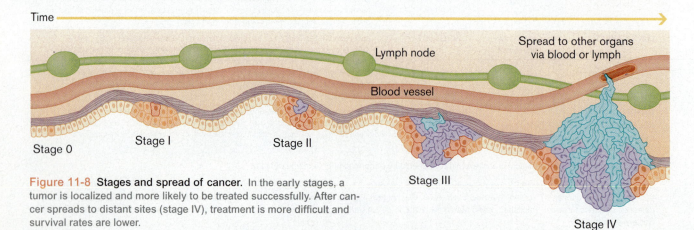

Time

Lymph node

Blood vessel

Spread to other organs via blood or lymph

Stage 0 Stage I Stage II Stage III Stage IV

Figure 11-8 Stages and spread of cancer. In the early stages, a tumor is localized and more likely to be treated successfully. After cancer spreads to distant sites (stage IV), treatment is more difficult and survival rates are lower.

externally by a machine aiming radiation directly at the tumor site or internally by implanting a small amount of radioactive material in or near the tumor. Radiation is not typically used for cancers that have spread; it may be used alone or in conjunction with chemotherapy or other types of treatment.

Surgery is also used for cancer treatment. It is the oldest form of cancer treatment and, like radiation, is a local treatment. Surgery can serve a number of purposes. It can be preventive, removing suspicious cells before they turn cancerous. It can be curative, entirely removing an early-stage cancerous growth, along with surrounding tissue. If the entire primary tumor cannot be surgically removed or if the cancer is suspected of having spread, surgery is usually combined with other treatment methods.

Diabetes

Diabetes is a serious chronic condition that affects a growing number of Americans. Overall, an estimated 25.8 million Americans, or about 8 percent of the population, have diabetes, yet more than one-quarter of them—nearly seven million people—don't know it.

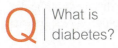 **What is diabetes?** Typically referred to simply as *diabetes*, **diabetes mellitus** is a metabolic disorder characterized by problems with the body's production or use of **insulin,** a hormone produced by the pancreas. Much of the food you eat is converted to glucose by your digestive system. Glucose is the body's main source of fuel and is transported via the bloodstream to cells throughout the body, which use it for growth and energy production. Glucose requires two things to enter a cell: *glucose transporters,* which are the doorways in cell walls that glucose can pass through, and the hormone insulin. In normal metabolism, when glucose enters the bloodstream, the pancreas responds by pumping out insulin. The insulin binds to receptors on a cell wall, signaling the glucose transporter to open and allow glucose to pass into the cell. Once most glucose is absorbed, the pancreas stops releasing insulin, and blood levels of both insulin and glucose are fairly low.

In diabetes, the pancreas does not produce enough insulin or the body's cells do not respond appropriately to the insulin that is produced. Consequently, glucose builds up in the bloodstream because it cannot be transported into cells, a condition called *high blood sugar,* or **hyperglycemia.** Eventually, blood glucose levels are so high that the excess glucose is excreted in the urine. In addition, because the cells can't obtain sufficient glucose, the body loses its main source of energy.

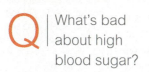 **What's bad about high blood sugar?** Prolonged hyperglycemia damages nerves, blood vessels, and other organs. Symptoms of hyperglycemia include increased thirst, frequent urination, headaches, blurred vision, weight loss, fatigue, and stomach and intestinal problems. Left untreated, hyperglycemia can lead to a life-threatening condition called *ketoacidosis,* also sometimes referred to as diabetic keto-acidosis (DKA). When elevated levels of glucose remain in the blood rather than being absorbed and utilized by the cells, the cells call on the body to release another form of fuel. The body shifts to "starvation mode" and begins to break down fats for fuel—and fats do not break down as efficiently as glucose. This "burning" of fat produces a harmful acidic by-product, *ketones,* that can build up to toxic levels in the blood. Over the long term, diabetes is associated with many serious complications, including higher rates of cardiovascular disease and lower life expectancy (Figure 11-9).

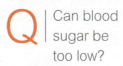 **Can blood sugar be too low?** When the amount of glucose in the blood rises, the pancreas produces more insulin in an

diabetes mellitus A disorder of carbohydrate metabolism characterized by inadequate production or use of insulin, leading to elevated blood glucose levels.

insulin A hormone produced and secreted by the pancreas that circulates in the blood and enables glucose absorption by cells.

hyperglycemia Excessively high blood glucose levels; also known as high blood sugar.

Eyes	Changes in vision; damage to the small blood vessels in the eyes; blindness
Skin	Problems ranging from rashes and blisters to bacterial and fungal infections
Mouth	Bleeding gums and frequent oral infections
Stomach	Delayed stomach emptying, leading to heartburn, nausea, and vomiting
Heart and blood vessels	Increased risk of hypertension, atherosclerosis, heart attack, stroke, and peripheral artery disease
Bladder	Urinary tract infections and bladder problems
Sexual function	Erectile dysfunction in men; problems with sexual response and vaginal lubrication in women
Kidney	Damage that, if severe, requires treatment with dialysis (artificial cleaning and filtering of the blood with a specialized machine) or kidney transplant
Lower legs and feet	Nerve and blood vessel damage leading to poor circulation, infections, and sores that don't heal; in severe cases amputation may be required, and diabetics are eight times more likely to have a lower limb amputated than those without diabetes

Figure 11-9 Possible complications of diabetes.

attempt to push the additional glucose to the cells. This increased push can leave the glucose levels in the blood low, a condition called *low blood sugar,* or **hypoglycemia.** Most cases of hypoglycemia occur in people with diabetes and are related to inaccurate use of glucose-lowering medications or irregular eating patterns. Though hypoglycemia can occasionally be caused by hormone deficiencies or other medical conditions such as cancer, it is relatively rare in healthy adults and children older than 10.

The primary danger of hypoglycemia is to the brain: Without glucose, brains cells die, potentially causing permanent brain damage or, in severe cases, death. Symptoms of hypoglycemia can include confusion, dizziness, pounding heart or racing pulse, pale skin, sweating, weakness, poor concentration, and loss of consciousness.

Q | Who is most likely to develop diabetes?

Diabetes is more common in older than younger adults—less than 1 percent of Americans under 21 years of age have diabetes. However, the number of diabetes cases continues to grow among children and teens. Additionally, an estimated 79 million American adults (age 20+) have prediabetes (more about this below).[28]

Types of Diabetes

Q | Are some kinds of diabetes more dangerous than others?

There are three primary types of diabetes: type 1, type 2, and gestational. **Type 1 diabetes** can occur at any age but appears most often in children and young adults under the age of 20. Type 1 diabetes is considered an *autoimmune disease* because it is usually caused by the body's own immune system attacking and destroying the insulin-producing cells of the pancreas. These cells, called *beta cells,* are then unable to produce insulin. Without insulin, glucose quickly builds up in the bloodstream and cells start dying from lack of an energy source. Type 1 diabetes is fatal within days or weeks if not treated.

Type 2 diabetes, which develops more slowly, is the most common type of diabetes and accounts for 90–95 percent of all diagnosed diabetes cases in the United States.[29] In

Mind Stretcher
Critical Thinking Exercise

Has anyone in your family experienced serious heart disease, cancer, or diabetes? How has it impacted their life? How has it affected your perception of your own risk and of the importance of prevention measures?

type 2 diabetes, cells don't respond properly to insulin, a condition called *insulin resistance.* When glucose enters the bloodstream, the pancreas does release insulin. However, due to problems with insulin receptors or glucose transporters, glucose is unable to enter cells. The pancreas may pump out more insulin to help overcome the resistance, and some amount of glucose is absorbed—but levels of both glucose and insulin in the blood rise. The pancreas can't produce extra insulin indefinitely, so glucose levels in the blood increase further (Figure 11-10).

When the signs of high blood glucose levels are first recognized during pregnancy, the diagnosis is **gestational diabetes.** This type of diabetes affects about 3–8 percent of pregnant women in the United States.[30] Gestational diabetes typically occurs late in pregnancy and is a result of pregnancy's many hormonal changes and the impact of those changes on insulin production and absorption. If not managed properly, gestational diabetes can cause problems for both mother and baby. Babies born to mothers with gestational diabetes may be unusually large, and their size may complicate the birth process. They may also experience chemical imbalances and respiratory problems after birth. Gestational diabetes usually disappears following the baby's birth, but women with this form of the disease are at increased risk of developing type 2 diabetes after their pregnancy.

Q | Can you have high blood sugar without having diabetes?

Before developing type 2 diabetes, people often have a condition called **prediabetes,** also known as *impaired glucose tolerance.* An estimated 54 million Americans have blood glucose levels that are higher than normal but not high enough to be classified as diabetes. People with prediabetes can suffer from many of the same complications as those with full-blown diabetes, so taking action is important if blood glucose is elevated even slightly above normal. See the section on diagnosis below for more information about glucose levels.

Assessing Your Risk for Diabetes

Q | What causes diabetes?

Different types of diabetes have different causes. Type 1 diabetes is an autoimmune condition; it is suspected that the primary triggers are genetic

hypoglycemia Abnormally low blood glucose levels; also known as low blood sugar.

type 1 diabetes Form of diabetes characterized by little or no insulin secretion; an autoimmune disease that occurs when the immune system destroys the insulin-producing cells of the pancreas.

type 2 diabetes The most common form of diabetes, characterized by impaired insulin use by the cells and, in some cases, insufficient insulin production.

gestational diabetes The form of diabetes in which high blood glucose levels occur during pregnancy.

prediabetes A condition characterized by blood glucose levels that are above normal but not yet high enough to be classified as diabetes.

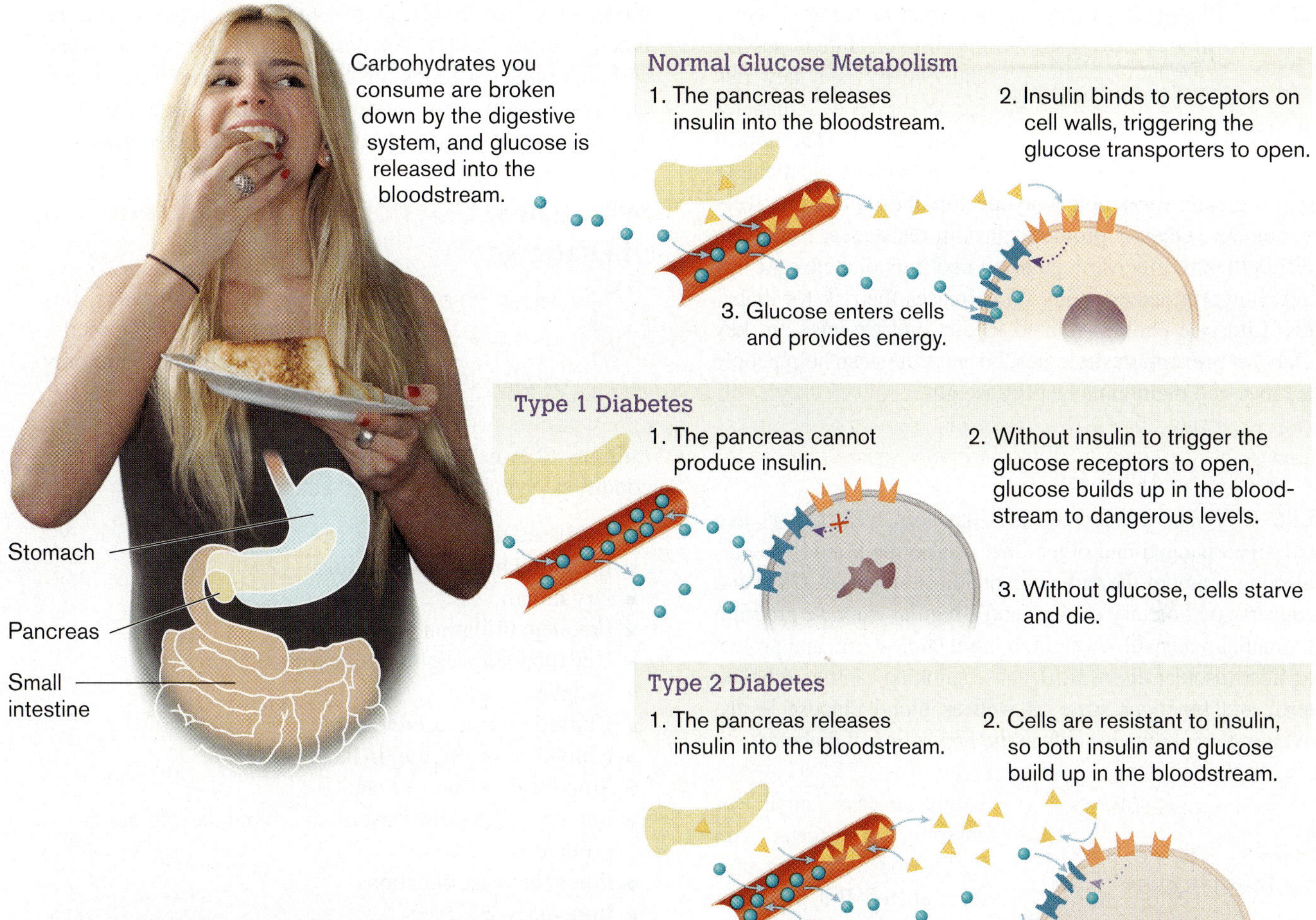

Carbohydrates you consume are broken down by the digestive system, and glucose is released into the bloodstream.

Stomach

Pancreas

Small intestine

Normal Glucose Metabolism

1. The pancreas releases insulin into the bloodstream.

2. Insulin binds to receptors on cell walls, triggering the glucose transporters to open.

3. Glucose enters cells and provides energy.

Type 1 Diabetes

1. The pancreas cannot produce insulin.

2. Without insulin to trigger the glucose receptors to open, glucose builds up in the bloodstream to dangerous levels.

3. Without glucose, cells starve and die.

Type 2 Diabetes

1. The pancreas releases insulin into the bloodstream.

2. Cells are resistant to insulin, so both insulin and glucose build up in the bloodstream.

3. Some glucose enters the cell, but the amounts are insufficient for healthy cellular function.

Figure 11-10 Normal glucose metabolism, type 1 diabetes, and type 2 diabetes. In diabetes, glucose metabolism is disrupted, and blood glucose levels increase. Cells become starved for energy and may die.

and viral, but doctors don't yet know the exact causes. This uncertainty makes pinpointing specific risk factors difficult. However, we do know that type 1 diabetes develops most often in children, occurs about equally in males and females, and is highest among non-Hispanic whites.[31]

The direct causes of type 2 diabetes are also unknown, but due the greater numbers of people with type 2 diabetes, more research has been conducted about it. Anyone can get type 2 diabetes, but according to the National Institutes of Health, those most at risk are people with one or more of the following characteristics:[32]

- Age 45 or older
- Overweight
- Not physically active
- A family history of diabetes
- High blood pressure or high cholesterol
- *Gestational diabetes*—diabetes during pregnancy—or having given birth to a baby weighing more than 9 pounds
- Blood glucose levels that are higher than normal but not high enough for diabetes

- African American, American Indian, Asian American, Pacific Islander, or Hispanic/Latino genetic heritage
- *Polycystic ovary syndrome*—a hormonal condition that leads to irregular or absent ovulation
- Dark, thick, velvety skin around the neck or in the armpits
- Blood vessel problems affecting the heart, brain, or legs

To assess your risk for diabetes, complete Lab Activity 11-1.

Q If both my dad and my grandfather have diabetes, will I get it too?

Not necessarily—although you are at higher-than-average risk for developing diabetes. A family history of diabetes, which you obviously can't change, is a risk factor for getting the disease. However, if you take a look at the other risk factors for diabetes, you'll notice most are related to lifestyle choices. Making positive choices in these areas can help you delay, and even prevent, the onset of diabetes.

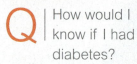

Q I keep hearing that more and more people are getting diabetes. Why is that?

As a nation, we are becoming bigger, fatter people, and obesity is a key risk factor for type 2 diabetes (Figure 11-11). The impact of overweight on diabetes risk is greater for people who develop obesity at a relatively young age. Obesity promotes insulin resistance, leading to difficulties in glucose regulation and thus diabetes. At any age, however, excess body fat increases the risk for diabetes. Lifestyle choices related to diet and exercise are key diabetes prevention strategies, because they can help people achieve and maintain a healthy weight.

Diabetes Prevention

Like CVD and cancer, diabetes has some risk factors that can't be changed and others that can be modified. Diabetes also has many of the same prevention strategies as CVD and cancer: good dietary choices and a regular exercise program to maintain a healthy weight, control cholesterol, and protect against vascular diseases. Because smoking can raise cholesterol and blood pressure as well as blood glucose levels, avoiding smoking also aids in the prevention of diabetes.

Q Does eating too much sugar cause diabetes?

Eating excess sugar, or anything in excess, can lead to obesity, a risk factor for diabetes. But the sugar itself does not directly cause diabetes. Diabetes is related to genetics and a variety of lifestyle choices.

For someone who has diabetes, a recommended dietary plan may include specific goals and limits for carbohydrate intake, because foods that contain carbohydrates raise blood glucose levels. As described in Chapter 8, some carbohydrate-rich foods are healthier choices than others. Opt for mostly whole grains and unprocessed carbohydrates; limit intake of added sugars and processed grains.

Symptoms, Diagnosis, and Treatment of Diabetes

Q How would I know if I had diabetes?

SYMPTOMS. Diabetes cannot be observed directly, and many of the symptoms of early diabetes are subtle. That helps explain why millions of Americans with diabetes are unaware of their condition. Symptoms you can watch for include:

- Increased thirst
- Increased hunger after eating
- Dry mouth
- Frequent urination
- Unexplained weight loss or weight gain
- Fatigue
- Blurred or decreased vision
- Numbness or tingling in hands or feet
- Slow-healing sores or cuts
- Itching of the skin, most often around the vaginal or groin area
- Frequent yeast infections
- Impotency
- Loss of consciousness (in rare cases)

Many of these symptoms aren't specific to diabetes, but if you experience one or more of them, you should discuss it with your health care provider.

Q Do I need to be tested for diabetes even if I don't have any symptoms?

DIAGNOSIS AND TESTING. The American Diabetes Association recommends that all adults over the age of 45 should be tested, and the tests should be repeated at least every 3 years. However, if you are at higher risk, as indicated by the risk factors above, earlier or more frequent tests may be recommended, especially if symptoms appear. Discuss any symptoms or concerns with your health care provider.

Doctors usually test for diabetes through a blood test. Three different tests are used to diagnose diabetes and prediabetes (Figure 11-12). If any of these tests indicates elevated glucose levels, a repeat test will be done for confirmation:

- *A1C test,* which provides an estimate of average blood glucose levels over the preceding 2–3 months
- *Fasting plasma glucose test (FPG),* which measures blood glucose after an 8-hour fast
- *Oral glucose tolerance test (OGTT),* which measures glucose at set intervals following ingestion of glucose-containing fluids

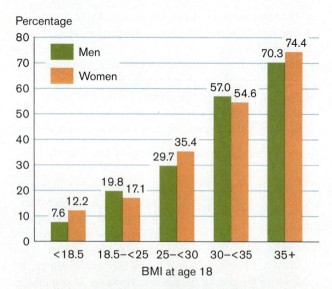

Figure 11-11 Lifetime risk of diabetes by BMI at age 18.
A person who is overweight or, especially, obese at age 18 has a very high lifetime risk for developing type 2 diabetes. Excess body fat is one of the key risk factors for diabetes.

Source: Narayan, K. M. V., and others. (2007). Effect of BMI on lifetime risk for diabetes in the U.S. *Diabetes Care, 30*(6), 1562–1566.

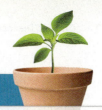

Living *Well* with . . .

Type 2 Diabetes

People with type 2 diabetes can lead long, productive lives. Managing blood sugar is the key. Here are four very important steps:

Get regular exercise: Be active at least 30 minutes on most days. Even brisk walking four or five times a week can help control blood sugar. Physical activity can also aid in reducing weight and blood pressure, improving cholesterol levels, and preventing heart and blood flow problems.

Develop regular eating habits: Treating diabetes doesn't require eliminating sugar completely from the diet. However, carbohydrates, no matter the form, have the most dramatic effect on blood sugar. For this reason, people with diabetes need to plan meals and snacks carefully. To keep blood sugar levels from fluctuating too much, they should eat something every 3 or 4 hours.

All meals and snacks should include carbohydrates but in limited amounts. A dietitian can help individuals work out an appropriate carb-counting method, but a general rule of thumb is 15–30 grams per snack and 45–75 grams per meal. Overall, meals should follow general dietary principles. The American Diabetes Association's "Create Your Plate" plan is one approach:

- Draw an imaginary line down the middle of the plate; divide one side again to make three sections.
- Fill the largest section with nonstarchy vegetables such as broccoli, carrots, tomatoes, green beans, mushrooms, peppers, cabbage, and salad greens.
- Fill one of the smaller sections with starchy foods such as whole grains, rice, pasta, cooked beans, potatoes, and corn.
- Fill the other smaller section with meat or meat substitutes such as fish, seafood, lean meats, chicken or turkey without skin, or tofu.
- Add a glass of nonfat or low-fat milk, yogurt, or a small roll, as well as a piece of fruit.

Watch the American Diabetes Association Create Your Plate video at http://www.youtube.com/watch?v=A6LZijdsGu0.

Test blood glucose: Careful blood sugar monitoring is a vital indicator of when diabetes is under control and when it isn't. A doctor or diabetes educator will provide training for using a testing device. The best times to check levels are before meals and before bed. Keeping an ongoing record of blood glucose is also important, because it will serve as a reference if unexpected symptoms should arise.

Medicate: Take any prescription medications as directed.

A local diabetes education expert and a reputable diabetes education Web site can be great resources. Seeing one's doctor regularly and always reporting changes or concerns is important. For more information, visit the Web site of the American Diabetes Association (http://www.diabetes.org) and the Centers for Disease Control and Prevention Diabetes Public Health Resource (http://www.cdc.gov/diabetes).

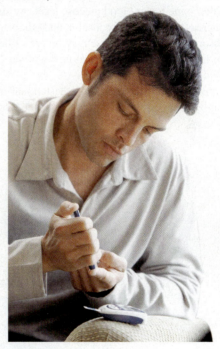

	A1C	Fasting plasma glucose (FPG)	Oral glucose tolerance test (OGTT)
Diabetes	≥6.5%	≥126 mg/dl	≥200 mg/dl
Pre-diabetes	5.7%–6.4%	100–125 mg/dl	140–199 mg/dl
Normal	<5.7%	<100 mg/dl	<140 mg/dl

Figure 11-12 Criteria for diagnosing diabetes. The numbers for the A1C test refer to the average plasma glucose concentration. The numbers for the other two tests refer to the milligrams of glucose per deciliter of blood.

Source: American Diabetes Association. (2010). Position statement: Standards of medical care in diabetes—2010. *Diabetes Care, 33*(suppl 1), S11–S61.

If you already have severe symptoms, your doctor may also order a urinalysis to help determine if you have additional complications that need to be treated. Because there is no cure for diabetes, a diagnosis can be scary. The good news is that in most instances diabetes can be successfully treated and managed.

Q I have a friend who has to give herself shots. Does everyone with diabetes have to do this?

TREATMENT. People with type 1 diabetes require daily insulin, which is usually administered by regular self-injections. Some people with this form of the disease, however, use an insulin pump, a small computerized device that injects a constant dose of insulin. The pump is typically strapped to the waist area and has a small tube with a needle that is inserted and taped to the stomach. A newer inhaled form of insulin is being studied.

Many people with type 2 diabetes can manage their condition with oral medications and lifestyle strategies such as a healthy eating plan, regular exercise, and maintenance of a healthy weight. A number of types of oral medications are available. Some lower blood glucose levels by stimulating the pancreas to release more insulin, and others improve glucose absorption by cells. These may be prescribed individually or in combination. Some people with type 2 diabetes also need to take insulin.

Most physicians prefer to manage gestational diabetes with lifestyle changes. Insulin may be needed in some cases, however.

Q What about those ads for diabetes supplies? Besides taking medication, what does someone with diabetes have to do?

For all types of diabetes, self-management is crucial. People with diabetes should work with their physicians and other health care professionals to develop an appropriate and manageable plan for diet, exercise, and medication. It is also important to learn how to self-test glucose levels accurately in order to get the optimal benefits from the diet, exercise, and medication regime—and when to test them. Another essential part of self-management is to watch for signs of diabetes complications and to report changes or concerns to the appropriate health care provider without delay. See the box "Living Well with . . . Type 2 Diabetes" for more information.

Putting It All Together for Chronic Disease Prevention

Cardiovascular disease, cancer, and diabetes are common diagnoses, but there are various strategies you can adopt to help reduce your risk. Many of these approaches are the same for all three groups of diseases. See Table 11-10, "Top Lifestyle Choices for Preventing Chronic Disease."

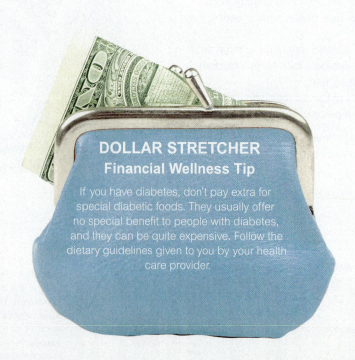

DOLLAR STRETCHER
Financial Wellness Tip

If you have diabetes, don't pay extra for special diabetic foods. They usually offer no special benefit to people with diabetes, and they can be quite expensive. Follow the dietary guidelines given to you by your health care provider.

TABLE 11-10   TOP LIFESTYLE CHOICES FOR PREVENTING CHRONIC DISEASE

	BENEFITS FOR CARDIOVASCULAR DISEASE	BENEFITS FOR CANCER	BENEFITS FOR DIABETES
1. GET REGULAR PHYSICAL ACTIVITY	■ Reduces cholesterol ■ Lowers high blood pressure ■ Decreases weight	■ Reduces incidence of and mortality from all-site cancer and some site-specific cancers	■ Helps control blood glucose, weight, and blood pressure ■ Raises "good" cholesterol and lowers "bad" cholesterol ■ Helps prevent heart and blood flow problems
2. EAT A BALANCED DIET	■ Helps lower blood pressure and cholesterol levels ■ Helps prevent obesity, diabetes, heart disease, and stroke, especially when the individual eats lots of fresh fruits and vegetables, cuts out added salt, and consumes less saturated fat and cholesterol	■ Increases intake of antioxidants and dietary fiber, especially through consumption of generous amounts of fruits and vegetables ■ Limits fat, sugar, and sodium, which are believed to be linked to some cancers	■ Prevents or delays development of type 2 diabetes in high-risk individuals by reducing fat and calorie intake and contributing to weight loss
3. DON'T SMOKE, OR STOP IF YOU DO	■ Lowers the risk of high blood pressure, heart disease, and stroke; heart attack risk decreases soon after quitting.	■ Prevents organ damage	■ Prevents increases in blood glucose, cholesterol, and blood pressure, all of which can contribute to diabetes
4. CONSUME ALCOHOL ONLY IN MODERATION	■ Can decrease risk of heart disease if consumption is limited to about 1 drink/day for women and 1–2 drink/day for men; 1 "drink" equals 1 can of beer, a glass of wine, or a shot of liquor according to the American Heart Association	■ Decreased risk of cancers of the mouth, pharynx, larynx, esophagus, liver, and breast if individuals who drink limit intake to no more than 2 drinks/day for men and 1 drink/day for women; 1 "drink" equals 12 oz of beer, 5 oz of wine, or 1.5 oz of 80-proof distilled spirits according to the American Cancer Society ■ Lowers breast cancer risk in women, especially those at high risk	■ According to still-controversial research, decreased risk of diabetes for individuals who drink a moderate amount of alcohol (about 1 drink/day for women and 1–2 drinks/day for men; 1 "drink" equals 1 can of beer, a glass of wine, or a shot of liquor). However, weigh the consequences: drinking alcohol also has negative health risks such as high blood pressure and increased weight. It is not recommended that individuals begin drinking if they do not already consume alcohol.

(continued)

TABLE 11-10 *(continued)*

	BENEFITS FOR CARDIOVASCULAR DISEASE	BENEFITS FOR CANCER	BENEFITS FOR DIABETES
5. GIVE YOUR FAMILY HEALTH HISTORY TO YOUR HEALTH CARE PROVIDER UP FRONT	■ Helps health care providers care for patients since family health history is an important part of cardiovascular disease risk assessment	■ Helps health care providers care for patients since family health history is an important part of cancer risk assessment	■ Helps health care providers care for patients since family health history is an important part of diabetes risk assessment

Sources: American Association for Cancer Research, American Cancer Society, American Heart Association, Centers for Disease Control and Prevention, National Center for Chronic Disease Prevention and Health Promotion, National Diabetes Information Clearing House, and National Institutes of Health.

Summary

Although chronic diseases are often associated with older age, everyone is susceptible. However, modifiable risk behaviors are responsible for much of the incidence of chronic disease. You can reduce your own risk by making smart choices related to tobacco use, nutrition, physical activity, and alcohol consumption. What you do as a young adult is a critical factor in whether or when you develop a chronic disease and how severe its effects will be.

Cardiovascular disease, cancer, and diabetes, though scary, are quite manageable in many cases. Understanding the nature of each disease and knowing your risk factors is crucial, as is having regular screenings. If a disease is present, early detection and appropriate treatment or management are essential. Maintaining healthy lifestyle habits, as well as a support network of friends and family, is vital to preserving or regaining your health.

More to Explore

American Cancer Society
http://www.cancer.org

American Diabetes Association
http://www.diabetes.org

American Heart Association
http://www.americanheart.org

CDC Chronic Disease Prevention and Health Promotion
http://www.cdc.gov/chronicdisease

National Cancer Institute
http://www.cancer.gov

National Heart, Lung, and Blood Institute
http://www.nhlbi.nih.gov

National Institute of Diabetes and Digestive and Kidney Diseases (NIDDK)
http://www.niddk.nih.gov

COMPLETE IN connect

NAME	DATE	SECTION

Risk factors for the major chronic diseases that affect Americans have been clearly identified. In this lab, you'll complete online risk assessments for CVD, cancer, and diabetes and then reflect on your results. Save your assessment results for future reference and to discuss with your health care provider.

Equipment

- Computer with Internet access
- Printer (optional); you can also save your assessment results to a file on your computer

Preparation: None

Instructions

Complete each of the following online risk assessments, save or print your results, and enter your information in the chart that appears in the Results section below.

- American Heart Association: My Life Check

  http://www.mylifecheck.heart.org

  In the following Results section, record your score (out of 10) and list areas where your rating for "Where You Are Now" was not excellent.

- MD Anderson Cancer Center: Cancer Risk Check

  http://www.mdanderson.org/patient-and-cancer-information/cancer-information/cancer-topics/prevention-and-screening/cancer-risk-factors/riskcheck.html

  In the following Results section, note any factors—controllable or uncontrollable—that are identified as placing you at elevated risk for cancer. The top section of the report may identify cancers for which your age or ethnicity are risk factors.

- American Diabetes Association: Diabetes Risk Test

  http://www.diabetes.org/diabetes-basics/prevention/diabetes-risk-test/

  In the Results section below, record the assessment of your current risk for diabetes. Note areas the tool identifies as risk factors that may increase your future risk of diabetes.

Results

Record key components of the results of each of your assessments. For each category of chronic disease, list at least three risk factors you have. These can be anything identified by the assessment—age, blood pressure, tobacco use, activity level, diet, and so on. For each risk factor you list, indicate whether it is modifiable.

ASSESSMENT	RISK FACTORS	MODIFIABLE?
Cardiovascular disease Overall score: [ ] / 10	1. 2. 3.	☐ yes ☐ no ☐ yes ☐ no ☐ yes ☐ no
Cancer	1. 2. 3.	☐ yes ☐ no ☐ yes ☐ no ☐ yes ☐ no

ASSESSMENT	RISK FACTORS	MODIFIABLE?
Diabetes	1.	☐ yes ☐ no
Current risk:	2.	☐ yes ☐ no
	3.	☐ yes ☐ no

Reflecting on Your Results

What commonalities do you see among your modifiable risk factors? What risk factors do you have that raise your risk for more than one chronic disease?

Are the modifiable risk factors you identified ones you were already aware of? Do the results of these assessment tests make you think more seriously about making changes? Why or why not?

Planning Your Next Steps

Choose one specific modifiable risk factor identified by the assessments you completed. Set a goal for change, and then list three strategies for achieving your goal. (If you have no modifiable risk factors, focus on strategies for addressing an uncontrollable risk factor—for example, obtaining age-appropriate screening tests.)

Give it a shot—take action today to lessen your disease risk. If one approach doesn't work, try another until you experience success. Once you've successfully changed a risk factor, try working on another. Reassess yourself periodically to see the effect your actions have on your disease risk.

Up for the challenge? Write a date for reassessment here and then record a reminder on your own calendar.

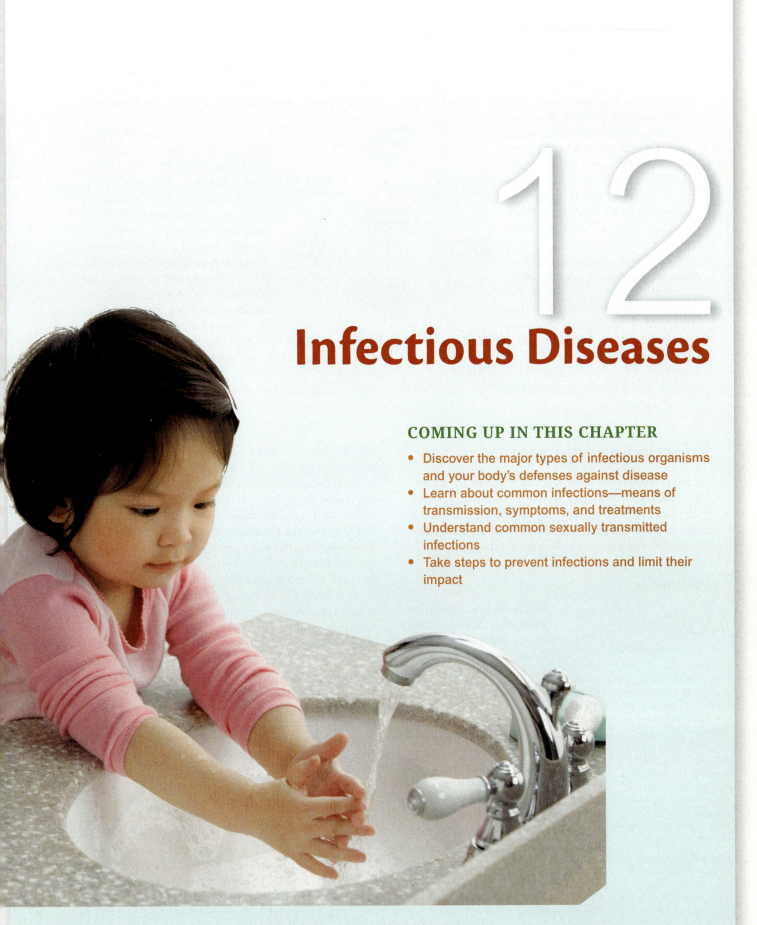

12

Infectious Diseases

COMING UP IN THIS CHAPTER

- Discover the major types of infectious organisms and your body's defenses against disease
- Learn about common infections—means of transmission, symptoms, and treatments
- Understand common sexually transmitted infections
- Take steps to prevent infections and limit their impact

How do infectious diseases relate to your overall wellness? If you're a young adult, they are a predictable cause of temporary illness and discomfort in your life. Physical wellness is diminished in the short term by even minor infections, such as head colds. However, good physical wellness and intellectually sound health choices can help protect you from infections. For example, are you applying critical thinking to try to avoid infectious diseases and to treat them safely? Do you wash your hands regularly, and are your immunizations up to date?

Emotional, social, and spiritual wellness, especially as they affect your stress levels, can make you less susceptible to infections. How are your communication and relationship skills? If you're sexually active, do you always practice safer sex?

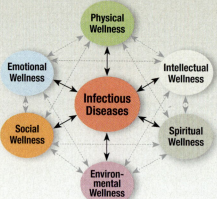

Your environment also factors into your infection risk. Water and food can spread infectious diseases, as can insects and rodents. Experiencing a natural disaster such as a flood or tornado can cause your body systems to break down, exposing you to a greater risk of infections.

As we saw in Chapter 1, infectious diseases were the number-one cause of death in the United States before 1900, and they remain a leading killer worldwide. Although U.S. death rates have dropped dramatically, infectious diseases are still a major cause of illness and lost work and school time. This chapter provides an introduction to infectious diseases, including infections that are sexually transmitted. You'll learn how to recognize and treat common diseases—and, most importantly, how to prevent them.

Infection and Immunity

An **infectious disease** is one that can be passed among people. Common infections include colds, flu, bronchitis, mononucleosis, and the many sexually transmissible infections. Some infections are easy to catch and relatively mild; others are much more serious—but often more difficult to catch.

Pathogens

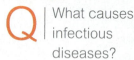

Q What causes infectious diseases?

infectious disease A disease that is transmissible from person to person through direct or indirect means; infection refers to invasion and multiplication of an organism; symptomatic disease follows if the body cannot quickly eliminate the pathogen.

pathogen A specific causative agent of infectious disease; examples include viruses, bacteria, protozoa, and fungi.

Infections are caused by **pathogens,** disease-causing agents that can be passed among people. Pathogens fall into a number of categories (Figure 12-1). Most pathogens are tiny, infection-causing viruses and bacteria often referred to as *microbes* or *microorganisms.* However, infections can also be caused by larger organisms, including lice and parasitic worms; these infections may also be referred to as *infestations.*

Many microbes live in a healthy human body and are needed to keep the body functioning normally. For example, your intestines contain types of bacteria that help digest food, destroy disease-causing microbes, and provide needed vitamins. However, even these

helpful organisms can cause illness if their numbers become unbalanced or if they gain entry into a part of the body that is normally microbe-free. For example, healthy people usually carry *Staphylococcus aureus* bacteria on their skin and in their nasal passages without suffering any illness. But *S. aureus* can cause a number of different diseases if it enters the body through a cut or sore. Similarly, antibiotics can kill friendly bacteria in the mouth, allowing fungi to grow out of control and causing a disease known as *thrush.*

It is important to distinguish between an *infection,* in which a disease-causing organism invades your body and multiplies, and a *disease,* in which you are experiencing obvious signs and symptoms. In some cases, you can have an infection without ever experiencing symptoms, as is often the case with the human papillomavirus (HPV), which we will examine later in this chapter. Your body may also be able to destroy an infectious agent before it ever causes symptoms, meaning that you had an infection but not a disease. An infectious disease with symptoms occurs when your body's defenses cannot quickly and completely fight off an invading pathogen.

Q Why are some infections more serious than others?

Many factors determine the severity of an infectious disease. For one thing, pathogens vary in their *virulence*—their innate ability to cause intense or severe symptoms. The cold viruses typically cause only mild, temporary infections affecting the upper respiratory system; but HIV (the virus that causes AIDS) and

Behavior-Change Challenge
Chilling Out with Colds and the Flu

Things are tough for you right now. You're studying every free minute for the exam that your dream job requires. You're also feeling a huge responsibility to help your lab partners meet a crucial project deadline. With your stress levels sky-high, you have come down with what feels like a terrible cold or flu. What should you do?

Meet Gabby

Gabby, who has been jug- 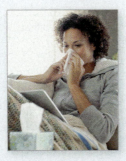 gling two jobs and many family responsibilities, arrives at work lightheaded, coughing, and sneezing. Her office colleagues urge her to go home and go to bed. Characteristically, Gabby would ignore their advice and simply redirect her nose to the grindstone while maybe planning to visit the vending machines to keep her energy up. This time, she reluctantly accepts their advice, all the while fearing a long recuperation. To her surprise, after a couple days at home, Gabby is much better. Having rested, eaten nutritiously, and drunk plenty of fluids, she resumes her daily routine with her health restored. Now Gabby sees the need to take care of herself, especially when her life pressures are mounting, so that she doesn't get sick. Consider:

- What behavior changes did Gabby make to deal with her sickness?
- When you are starting to feel sick with a cold or flu, what should you do to care for yourself?
- What have you learned from Gabby's experience?

the smallpox virus usually produce severe symptoms. For another thing, pathogens can infect different parts of the body; a bacterial infection confined to a small area of skin is likely to be less severe than an infection by the same bacterium if it gains access to the bloodstream and therefore the entire body. The amount of the pathogen you are initially exposed to can also have an impact—the less of the infectious agent in your system, the easier your body can destroy it.

Naturally, your health status is also important. The mere presence of a pathogen doesn't mean you'll become ill. Think about the times you've been around a sick person but haven't become ill yourself. Many pathogenic organisms are present on and in your body at all times, but if the agent isn't too virulent, and if your own resistance is strong, then you won't become ill. A strong immune system can fight off more infectious agents than a weak one. Some groups of people, therefore, are at relatively higher risk than others for serious effects from infections, including infants, older adults, and pregnant women. Infections that pose little risk to a healthy adult may be dangerous to individuals in these groups.

The Cycle of Infection

Q | How do you actually catch an infectious disease?

For an infectious disease to occur, a pathogen must gain entry into a host's body and start to replicate and cause symptoms. The transmission of an infection requires (1) a source of pathogens, (2) a susceptible host, and (3) a mode of transmission. Whether a person gets a disease depends on the relationship among these three factors.

- *Source of pathogens:* Infectious agents can come from another person, an animal, water, or even soil. The environment that supports a pathogen's survival and growth is called its *reservoir,* and reservoirs often contain a large community of the pathogen. For many common infectious diseases, the reservoirs are the bodies of individuals who are already infected. Many disease-causing organisms can survive only a short time once they leave their usual reservoir or host.

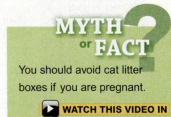

MYTH **or** FACT **?**

You should avoid cat litter boxes if you are pregnant.

▶ **WATCH THIS VIDEO IN** connect

See page 477 to find out.

- *Susceptible host:* People are more susceptible to infection if their immune system is weak or one of their natural physical defenses is compromised—such as by a cut in the skin. For example, very young children, older adults, and people with underlying health problems are all more susceptible to infections. Factors such as stress, smoking, and the use of antibiotics or other drugs affect a person's risk of infection.
- *Mode of transmission:* Understanding how pathogens are transmitted sheds light on ways to break the cycle. To cause an infection, a pathogen must exit its reservoir and then reach and enter a new host. This transmission can occur through direct and indirect contact, inhalation, and contact with a disease *vector* such as a mosquito or tick. Different pathogens have different typical modes of transmission. People can transfer pathogens from their hands, mouth, or genitals by coming into direct contact with another person—through touching, kissing, or sexual activity. Sexually transmitted infections such as chlamydia, gonorrhea, and herpes are usually transmitted through direct contact. Injection drug use can also directly transmit a pathogen into the bloodstream of a new host.

Pathogen	Effects	Diseases
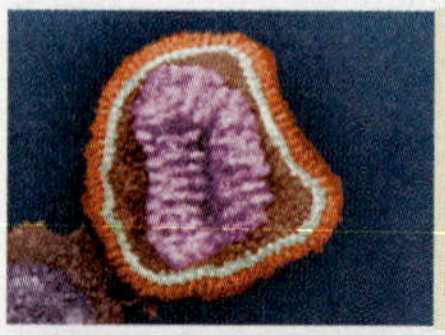 **Viruses** Tiny microbes consisting of one or more molecules of DNA or RNA surrounded by a protein coat	Viruses can enter and take over body cells, using them to rapidly produce more copies of the virus while at the same time damaging or destroying the cells.	Common cold, influenza, mononucleosis, hepatitis, cold sores, genital herpes, HIV/AIDS, genital warts, measles, mumps, rabies, polio
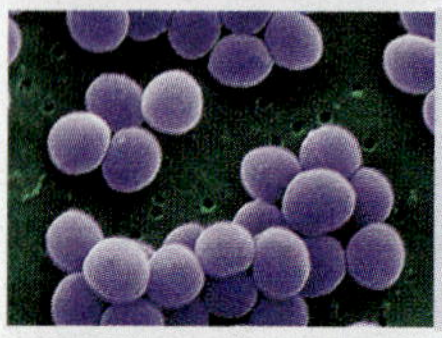 **Bacteria** Single-celled organisms that may be in the shape of rods, balls, or spirals	Bacteria may secrete toxins or enzymes that destroy cells or interfere with cell functioning.	Lyme disease, pneumonia, peptic ulcers, tuberculosis, boils, toxic shock syndrome, strep throat, meningitis, gonorrhea
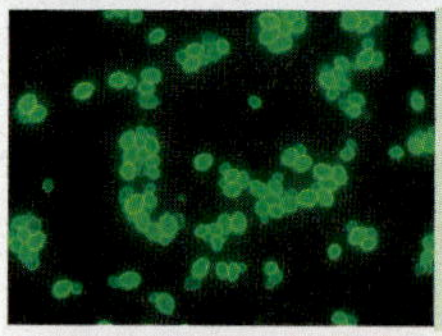 **Fungi** A primitive form of plant that may be single- or multi-celled	Fungi may release enzymes that destroy cells.	Yeast infections, thrush, athlete's foot, jock itch, certain types of pneumonia and meningitis
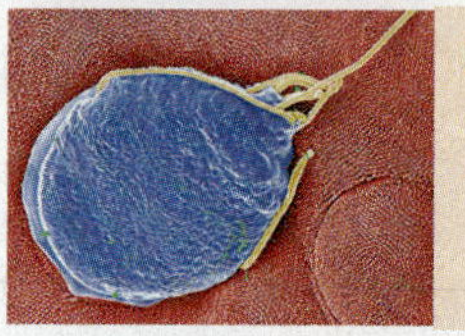 **Protozoa** Microscopic single-celled animals that can live independently of a host	In the human body, protozoa may release toxins and enzymes that destroy cells or interfere with their functioning.	Malaria, giardiasis, toxoplasmosis, African sleeping sickness
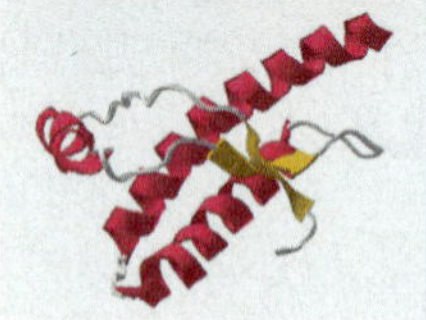 **Prions** Specific types of abnormal proteins	Prions accumulate in the central nervous system and cause degenerative diseases.	Bovine spongiform encephalopathy ("mad cow disease"), Creutzfeldt-Jakob disease
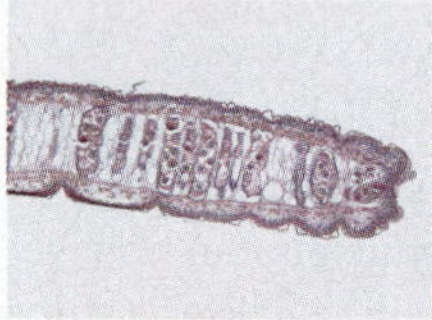 **Helminths** Parasitic worms that live in or on a host	Worms compete with body cells for nutrients and can block blood and lymph vessels or the digestive tract.	Tapeworm infection, pinworm infection, hookworm infection, swimmer's itch
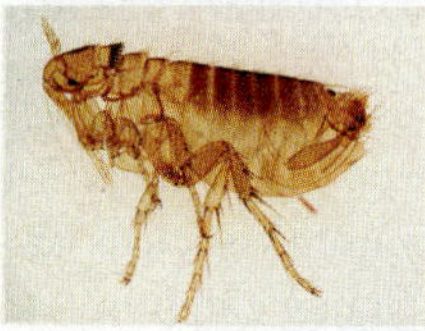 **Ectoparasites** Complex organisms that may live in or on a host's skin	Infestations may cause local irritation; in some cases, ectoparasites also transmit other types of pathogens.	Scabies; lice, tick, and flea infestations

Figure 12-1 Pathogens, effects, and associated diseases.

The viruses that cause the common cold may be transmitted directly or indirectly. If a person with a cold sneezes onto her hand and her phone, a potential new host could pick up the virus from shaking her hand or borrowing her phone—and then touching his own eyes or nose and transferring the virus.[1]

In contrast, the flu virus is most often transmitted through inhalation: A person sneezes or coughs, and the virus is sprayed into the air in tiny droplets, which other people can breathe in. These droplets can also land on surfaces in the environment. Although some pathogens die quickly after leaving their hosts, cold and flu viruses viable after many hours on surfaces such as desks and doorknobs.[2] Indirect contact can also occur when a person ingests contaminated water or food.

Finally, some pathogens are transmitted through insect or animal vectors. Malaria is an example of a vector-borne disease. A mosquito picks up the disease-causing protozoan by biting an infected person and then can pass the protozoan on to the next person it bites. Lyme disease is another example of an infection transmitted through an insect vector. The Lyme disease bacterium normally lives in mice and other small animals, but it is transferred to humans through the bite of a deer tick. Typically, the pathogens enter the

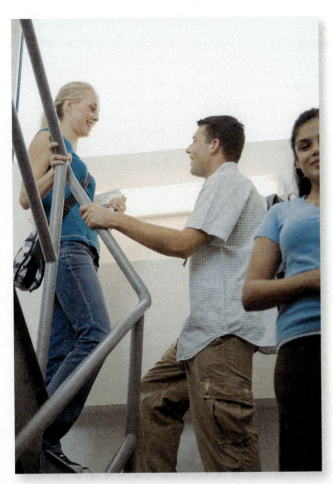

Many viruses and bacteria can be easily transmitted through direct and indirect contact. You can pick up pathogens by shaking hands or by touching shared surfaces such as doorknobs, handrails, and keyboards.

Fast Facts

Superbugs on the Loose

Many infectious diseases, including HIV-AIDS, staphylococcal infections, tuberculosis, influenza, gonorrhea, candida infection, and malaria, are increasingly difficult to treat because of the proliferation of antimicrobial-resistant organisms, or *superbugs*. Between 5 and 10 percent of all hospital patients develop an infection related to these superbugs, and about 90,000 people die each year as a result.

According to the Centers for Disease Control and Prevention, antibiotic resistance in the United States costs an estimated $20 billion a year in excess health care costs; $35 million in other societal costs; and more than 8 million additional days that people spend in the hospital. People infected with antimicrobial-resistant organisms are more likely to have longer hospital stays and usually require more complicated treatment.

- What are some reasons why hospital patients might be particular targets for superbug infections?
- What steps can you take to minimize your risk of contracting a superbug infection in the course of your daily life?

Source: National Institute of Allergy and Infectious Disease, Department of Health and Human Services (http://www.niaid.nih .gov/topics/antimicrobialResistance/Understanding/Pages/quick Facts.aspx). Last accessed January 2012.

new host through any of the body's natural openings (mouth, nose, genitals, and so on), as well as through cuts and scrapes on the surface of the skin.

The Body's Defenses

 How do I get my resistance to disease?

Although we are each born with a specific capacity to resist certain diseases, there is little consistency from one person to the next. Therefore, some people seem to never get colds or can inhale tuberculosis bacteria yet never contract the disease, while others are overly prone to colds and flus. Scientists are still trying to determine the exact causes for differences in disease resistance. Some of the resistance seems to be present from birth, yet it remains to be determined how much is inherited and how much is determined by factors such as age, illness, and nutritional status.

Our built-in defenses include the physical barrier of the skin, the body's largest organ, which most pathogens cannot penetrate unless it is damaged. Thus, you are more likely to get an infection if your skin has been scraped, cut, or burned or if passage through the skin is aided by something like an injection or a bite from a mosquito. This is also why wearing gloves when handling infectious

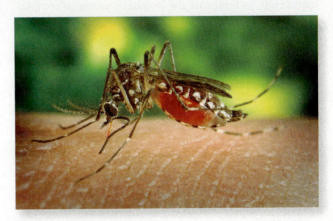

Your skin provides an effective physical barrier, but pathogens can be transmitted through cuts, scrapes, and burns, as well as injection drug use or the bites of certain animal or insect vectors. Female mosquitoes can penetrate the skin and potentially transmit infections such as malaria and West Nile virus.

agents is so important, as you may not be aware of small openings in your skin.

The mouth, nostrils, eyelids, lungs, and genitals are all lined with mucous membranes, which although delicate, provide significant protection by secreting mucus that traps pathogens. The hairs in your nose and ears also trap many pathogens. Any foreign substances that enter the lungs may be expelled through the cough reflex or by the actions of hairlike cilia in your lungs that help push particles up and out.

Just as injury to the skin increases your risk of infection, so does damage to these other physical barriers. One reason that smoking increases your risk of infection is that it destroys the cilia in the lungs. If you have a sexually transmitted infection that causes sores or blisters, you are more likely to contract another infection. For example, having genital warts or herpes infection increases your risk for contracting HIV infection.[3]

Your body also has chemical barriers, including those in the acids, proteins, and enzymes of the digestive tract, that can discourage the entry and spread of pathogens. Substances in tears can dissolve the outer coating of certain bacteria. Vaginal secretions normally produce a slightly acidic environment, which encourages the growth of some microbes and discourages the growth of others.

You can bolster your body's physical defenses through actions such as washing your hands and limiting contact with objects and surfaces used by a person who is ill.

The Immune System

Q | How do I develop my immunity?

Your **immune system** comes into play when a pathogen gets through any of the previously mentioned physical or chemical barriers. *Immunity,* the ability to resist a particular disease, derives from the overall workings of the immune system, a complex network of specialized organs, tissues, and cells that defends the body from disease-causing microbes and helps repair damaged tissue. A complete description of the immune system and the immune response is beyond the scope of this text, but here are a few key concepts to keep in mind:

- Immune cells constantly circulate through your body, ready to recognize foreign substances and take action. All cells carry protein markers on their surface; protein markers on pathogens, known as **antigens,** are recognized as being foreign and trigger the immune response.
- Some cells of the immune system respond to the damage and toxins a pathogen produces. They move to the site of the infection, "eat" the invading microbes, and destroy infected body cells. Pain and swelling at the site of an infection are often

the result of the body's battle to keep the infection from spreading.

- If an infection persists or spreads, other cells of the immune system produce large numbers of **antibodies**—specialized proteins bind to the pathogen's specific antigen and help mark it for destruction.
- The fever (elevated body temperature) that often accompanies an infection can help speed up parts of the immune response. It may also make the host a less hospitable environment for the pathogen. Fevers of 100°F or less are usually not harmful and don't need to be treated.
- For certain pathogens, once you've been exposed, the body produces specialized "memory" cells. These cells are able to recognize the antigen associated with the pathogen and respond quickly if you ever become infected with the same microbe again. In this way, you can essentially become immune to the pathogen—if you are infected, your body will quickly kill the pathogens and no disease will develop.

Although immunity occurs naturally after an infection, it can also be acquired without actually experiencing the infection, through a *vaccination* (see p. 423), which is a direct injection of antibodies. Babies can temporarily acquire immunity from their mothers through breastfeeding, because breast milk contains numerous protective maternal antibodies.[4]

One sign of an active immune system, or an *immune response,* is swollen lymph glands or lymph nodes. Your lymph glands are part of the **lymphatic system,** a collection of vessels and organs that carry out several different functions in the body. Lymph vessels pick up fluid lost from capillaries and return it to the circulatory system. The lymph vessels are similar to blood vessels, but to move fluid, they rely on compression from muscle contractions rather than the pumping action of the heart.

The lymphatic system also plays a key role in the defense against invading pathogens. The spleen, thymus, and bone marrow help produce and activate infection-fighting cells. Lymph vessels transport fluid containing foreign material and cellular debris to lymph nodes for disposal. The lymph nodes are located at intervals throughout the body; they contain many immune cells, which during an infection ingest and destroy invading pathogens.

The lymph nodes that most often become swollen are those in your neck,

immune system A complex network of organs, tissues, and cells that produce the immune response and defend the body from disease-causing agents.

antigen Protein molecules on the surface of infectious agents that the immune system recognizes as foreign, triggering the immune response.

antibody Molecule produced by the immune system that binds to a specific antigen, marking it for destruction.

lymphatic system Network of vessels and organs that returns fluid to the circulatory system; produces, activates, and transports infection-fighting cells; and plays a role in disposing of foreign material and cellular debris.

armpits, and groin. The location of a swollen gland can provide clues to the source or location of an infection. The swelling usually subsides within a few days, but it can take up to several weeks after an infection has cleared for lymph nodes to return to normal size.

The Role of Immunizations

Q | Do vaccines weaken my immune system?

Vaccines strengthen your immune system by preparing your body to fight infection; they create immunity against infections you have not previously had. Vaccines are made from killed, weakened, or incomplete pathogens and work by exposing the body to foreign antigens from the microbe, which the immune system responds to by producing antibodies. Vaccines do not cause the infectious

disease, but they do prime your body to respond to the pathogen if you are ever infected. A vaccine may also include an inactive version of a bacterial toxin so that the body can develop a defense against it as well.

However, no vaccine is completely effective, and some people have a stronger immune response to a vaccine than others do. The effects of some vaccines fade, so regular booster shots are needed to maintain immunity. The Centers for Disease Control and Prevention provides an updated list of the recommended immunizations for U.S. adults and children (http://www.cdc.gov/vaccines/recs/schedules/default.htm) that is used by most licensed physicians in the United States. See Figure 12-2 for information on recommended adult immunizations.

vaccine A preparation of weakened or killed microorganisms or inactivated toxins that is administered to stimulate immunity; it elicits an immune response that offers long-lasting protection against that particular antigen.

DOLLAR STRETCHER
Financial Wellness Tip

Wash your hands often and thoroughly to prevent illnesses that can be costly in terms of both time and money. You don't need fancy soaps, chemicals, or antibacterial formulas; plain old soap and water is just as effective. If you use liquid soap, get a refillable dispenser that squirts out just enough for a single use.

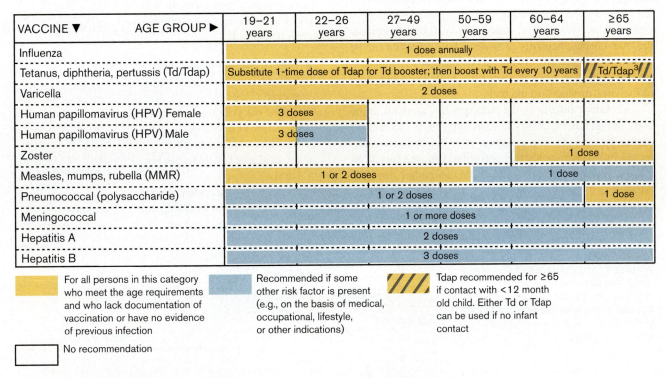

VACCINE ▼ AGE GROUP ▶	19–21 years	22–26 years	27–49 years	50–59 years	60–64 years	≥65 years
Influenza	1 dose annually					
Tetanus, diphtheria, pertussis (Td/Tdap)	Substitute 1-time dose of Tdap for Td booster; then boost with Td every 10 years					Td/Tdap[3]
Varicella	2 doses					
Human papillomavirus (HPV) Female	3 doses					
Human papillomavirus (HPV) Male	3 doses					
Zoster					1 dose	
Measles, mumps, rubella (MMR)	1 or 2 doses			1 dose		
Pneumococcal (polysaccharide)	1 or 2 doses					1 dose
Meningococcal	1 or more doses					
Hepatitis A	2 doses					
Hepatitis B	3 doses					

For all persons in this category who meet the age requirements and who lack documentation of vaccination or have no evidence of previous infection

Recommended if some other risk factor is present (e.g., on the basis of medical, occupational, lifestyle, or other indications)

Tdap recommended for ≥65 if contact with <12 month old child. Either Td or Tdap can be used if no infant contact

No recommendation

Figure 12-2 Recommended immunizations for adults. For more information and additional recommendations, visit http://www.cdc.gov/vaccines.

Sources: Centers for Disease Control and Prevention. (2012). Recommended adult immunization schedule—United States, 2012. *Morbidity and Mortality Weekly Report, 61*(4) 1–6. Centers for Disease Control and Prevention. (2011). Prevention and Control of Influenza with Vaccines: Recommendations of the Advisory Committee on Immunization Practices (ACIP), 2011 *Morbidity and Mortality Weekly Report,* 60(33);1128–1132.

Stages and Patterns of Infectious Diseases

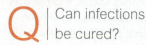 Can infections be cured?

There are different kinds of infections, and acute infections are the ones most likely to resolve on their own or be cured quickly with treatment. **Acute infections** are characterized by a short duration and a fairly typical series of stages (Figure 12-3):

- *Incubation:* Time between infection with the pathogen and the first appearance of symptoms. The immune system is able to stop some infections during this stage and clear the pathogen from the body, meaning that no disease develops.
- *Prodrome:* Initial appearance of general signs and symptoms of illness. An individual might begin to feel unwell.
- *Illness:* Signs and symptoms of the specific infection develop and become more severe.
- *Convalescence:* Acute symptoms of the infection subside. The time required for recovery depends on the severity of the infection and the underlying health of the individual.

These stages occur for many infectious diseases, including the common cold. However, infections can follow other patterns. In a **chronic infection,** the illness persists or recurs over a long period. Hepatitis can become a chronic liver infection, slowly causing *cirrhosis* (a serious condition that scars the liver) or liver cancer. Up to 10,000 Americans die from chronic hepatitis each year.[5] HIV infection can be a chronic progressive disease, meaning that the infection persists and often worsens over time, with more and more of the virus produced in the body.

In a **latent infection,** the pathogen lies dormant in the body but retains the ability to replicate. Illness can recur if immunity weakens due to aging, poor health habits, hormonal imbalance, or another infection. Chicken pox is an example of a latent infection: People can harbor the virus throughout their life without experiencing symptoms. But at some later point, if immunity weakens, they can develop shingles, a painful infection of the nerves.

Prevention and Treatment of Infectious Diseases

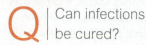 How can I keep from getting sick?

Your two best strategies for preventing infectious diseases are to keep pathogens out of your body and to maintain a strong immune system.

What can you do to avoid infectious agents? Your best defense is hand washing—do it often and do it thoroughly (Figure 12-4). If soap and water aren't available, use an alcohol-based hand sanitizer. Many common infectious diseases are transmitted through touch: An infected person transfers microbes directly (handshake) or indirectly (doorknob) to your hands. When you touch your eyes, nose, or mouth, the pathogen gains access to your body. Studies have linked good hand hygiene with reduced rates of upper respiratory and gastrointestinal illnesses.[6] However, most college students do not follow recommendations for hand washing.[7] Remember to wash your hands often—it works! (Also see the box "Hand Washing 101.")

For infections like influenza that are transmitted through airborne droplets, your best strategy is to avoid people who are sneezing and coughing or stand at least 3 feet away—6 or more feet is even better. If you're the one who is sick and sneezing or coughing, you can help stop the spread of infections by keeping your germs to yourself:

- Cover your mouth and nose with a tissue when you cough or sneeze.
- Throw out your used tissue.
- If you don't have a tissue, cough or sneeze into your upper sleeve or elbow, not your hands.
- Wash your hands often; if soap and water are not available, use an alcohol-based hand rub.

acute infection An infection that develops rapidly and lasts for a short period; characterized by incubation, prodrome (beginning of symptoms), illness, and convalescence and recovery.

chronic infection A prolonged infection that continues beyond the time when the immune system would usually clear the infection from the body.

latent infection An infection that lies dormant in the body for a period of time but may recur under certain circumstances.

Figure 12-3 Stages and patterns of infections. Acute infections follow a typical four-stage pattern and usually resolve in days or weeks. Chronic infections persist over a longer period, whereas latent infections can recur if an individual's immunity weakens.

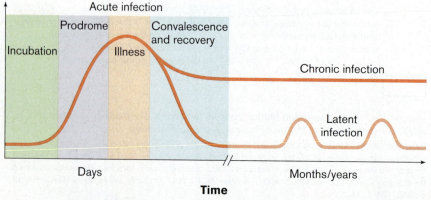

When to wash

- Before and after preparing food
- Before and after eating food
- After using the toilet
  - After changing diapers or cleaning up a child who has used the toilet
  - Before and after tending to someone who is sick
  - After blowing your nose, coughing, or sneezing
  - After handling an animal or animal waste
  - After handling garbage
  - Before and after treating a cut or wound

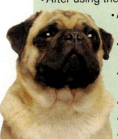

How to wash

- Wet your hands with clean running water and apply soap
- Use warm water if it is available
- Rub hands together to make a lather and scrub all surfaces
- Continue rubbing hands for 20 seconds; if you need a timer, hum the "Happy Birthday" song from beginning to end twice
- Rinse hands well under running water
- Dry your hands using a paper towel or air dryer; if possible, use your paper towel to turn off the faucet

When using hand sanitizer

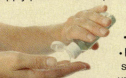

- If soap and water are not available, use alcohol-based gel (at least 60% alcohol) to clean hands
- Apply product to the palm of one hand, using the amount of product indicated on the label
  - Rub hands together
  - Rub the product over all surfaces of hands and fingers until hands are dry

Figure 12-4 Hand-washing guidelines. When and how to wash your hands may seem obvious, but the majority of people do not follow the recommendations. Consistently and thoroughly washing your hands is one of the best ways to help reduce your risk of many common infectious diseases.
Source: Centers for Disease Control and Prevention. (2010). *Clean hands save lives* (http://www.cdc.gov/handwashing/).

These strategies may sound obvious, but many people do not follow them.

To help keep your immune system strong, practice good self-care. Eat right, exercise, and get plenty of sleep.[8] Avoid behaviors like smoking and excessive drinking that hurt your body's ability to fight infection. Never inject illicit drugs; contaminated injection equipment can transmit pathogens directly into your bloodstream. If you plan to get a tattoo or piercing, go to a clean facility with a good reputation; ask about sterilization practices and be sure to follow the instructions you're given on caring for your skin.

High levels of stress and poor mental health are associated with higher rates of infectious diseases (Figure 12-5).[9] However, many of the strategies to reduce stress also help boost the immune system. For example, a study that looked at stress levels, humor, and immune function found that laughing at a humorous video reduced stress and improved the activity of immune cells.[10] Your emotional wellness can have a powerful effect on how well your body responds to infection. See the box "Keeping Yourself Well" for a summary of actions you can take to support your immune system.

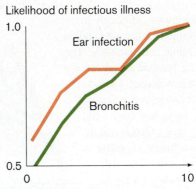

Figure 12-5 Mental health and risk of infectious disease in college students. Students who reported negative mental health—feelings of depression, anxiety, exhaustion, or hopelessness—also experienced higher rates of infectious disease.
Source: Adams, T. B., Wharton, C. M., Quilter, L., & Hirsch, T. (2008). The association between mental health and acute infectious illness among a national sample of 18- to 24-year-old college students. *Journal of American College Health, 56*(6), 657–663.

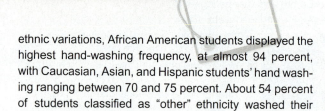

Research Brief

Hand Washing 101

Poor hand hygiene is a leading cause of infectious disease, especially in heavily populated, closely shared environments like college campuses. Researchers at a large Texas university were interested in the hand-washing behavior of students, particularly differences between the sexes and across ethnic groups. The research team conducted a total of 1,400 observations at different restrooms in academic buildings across campus, identifying who washed their hands, whether they used soap, and what their biological and ethnic background was.

The results were striking. Overall, 73 percent of the students washed their hands before exiting the restroom. Of those who washed their hands, the majority used soap (72 percent), while the remaining 28 percent used only water. Therefore, of the total sample of 1,400 students, roughly 27 percent did not wash their hands at all upon leaving the restroom; just more than half washed with soap and water; and about 1 in 5 students washed with water only.

With respect to sex differences, 76 percent of females washed their hands—a significantly higher percent than the 57 percent of male students who washed. Relevant to ethnic variations, African American students displayed the highest hand-washing frequency, at almost 94 percent, with Caucasian, Asian, and Hispanic students' hand washing ranging between 70 and 75 percent. About 54 percent of students classified as "other" ethnicity washed their hands upon exiting a restroom.

Of greatest concern is that almost half of all students (47 percent) did not wash their hands with soap. Given that using soap during hand washing has been proven to reduce the spread of infectious disease, officials may need to amplify their efforts to educate college students, as well as the public at large, about the benefits of hand washing with soap.

Analyze and Apply

- Why do you think so many college students neglect to use soap when washing their hands?
- What social pressures make you more or less likely to wash with soap after using the restroom?

Source: Anderson, J. L., Warren, C. A., Perez, E., Louis, R. I., Phillips, S., Wheeler, J., Cole, M., & Misra, R. (2008). Gender and ethnic differences in hand hygiene practices among college students. *American Journal of Infection Control, 36*(5), 361–368.

Q | I'm confused about antibiotics—when do they really work?

Antibiotics are powerful medications that have saved many lives. At the same time, they are often misused, and misuse can lead to problems. Antibiotics primarily fight bacterial infections, although they may also be prescribed for certain conditions caused by fungi and parasites. They act by killing bacteria or preventing them from reproducing. They don't work against any infections caused by viruses, including colds, flu, and most sore throats and coughs. Sometimes a person with a viral infection will develop a secondary bacterial infection as a complication; antibiotics may be prescribed to destroy the bacteria, but they won't treat the initial viral infection.

Most bacteria die when exposed to antibiotics, but some develop resistance to the drug's effects. If these resistant bacteria spread, they are more difficult to treat. Every time you take antibiotics, you increase the chances that some bacteria in your body will develop resistance.[11] So, it's important to take antibiotics no more often than necessary. In addition, when antibiotics are prescribed for an infection, you should take them for the recommended duration—not just until your symptoms disappear. Stopping treatment too soon can allow an infection to return and also contributes to the development of resistance.

Although beneficial, antibiotics also have side effects, including upset stomach, diarrhea, and, in women, vaginal yeast infections. Some antibiotics can also impair the functioning of the liver or kidneys. However, for most people, these risks are far less than the risks of not taking the antibiotic or not taking it for its full course.

antibiotic A compound that is used to treat bacterial infections by killing the bacteria or inhibiting their growth.

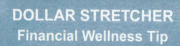

DOLLAR STRETCHER
Financial Wellness Tip

Treat most upper respiratory infections (common cold, runny nose, cough, sore throat) at home. You don't need to pay for a doctor visit, and you don't need antibiotics. Instead, rest and drink plenty of warm liquids. Most such infections are self-limiting and resolve within days. If symptoms persist or get worse, then visit your doctor.

Q | How are infections treated?

Treatment depends on the type of pathogen, the severity of the

Wellness Strategies

Keeping Yourself Well

Q | What is the best way to prevent illness?

Diligently following these guidelines will help to provide a good measure of protection against sickness.

- Get regular, moderate exercise.
- Eat a healthy diet.
- Get plenty of sleep.
- Control stress.
- Don't smoke, avoid secondhand smoke, and consume alcohol moderately, if at all.
- Wash your hands frequently and thoroughly, and use soap.
- Don't rub your eyes, touch your nose, or eat with your fingers without washing your hands first.
- Avoid people with obvious signs of illness.

- Clean shared environmental surfaces (desks, phones, doorknobs), especially if you live or work with someone who is ill.
- Handle and prepare foods safely (see Chapter 9).
- Avoid disease carriers like mosquitoes, ticks, and rodents. To protect yourself from insect bites, wear long pants and long-sleeved shirts when you hike or work outdoors; you can also apply an insect repellent (for more information, visit http://www.nlm.nih.gov/medlineplus/insectbitesandstings.html).
- Abstain from sex or consistently practice safer sex.
- Don't inject drugs.
- Keep immunizations up to date.
- Stock an emergency kit to use in case of a breakdown in public health services, such as after a natural disaster (for advice about kits, visit http://www.ready.gov).

---

infection, and the person's underlying health status. Many minor infections don't need to be treated—your immune system can successfully eliminate the pathogen. Certain symptoms, including nasal congestion and body aches, can be treated with over-the-counter medications. However, if your symptoms are unusually severe or your illness persists, check with your health care provider.

Antimicrobial drugs exist for several categories of pathogens. For bacterial infections, antibiotics may be prescribed. Specific antiviral drugs are available for a few infections, including herpes, hepatitis, influenza, and HIV. Similarly, there are drugs that specifically target fungal and protozoal infections.

Infectious Diseases on Campus

For college students, even minor infectious diseases can impact academic performance. Students should also be alert to signs and symptoms that may indicate more serious conditions.

Colds and Influenza

Q | How do you tell if you have a cold or the flu?

Colds and **influenza** ("the flu") are both caused by viruses and have some of the same symptoms, but there are differences (Table 12-1). Influenza is the more serious disease, although colds are more common and probably responsible for more lost days at school and on the job than any other infectious disease. For all the misery a cold can cause, in the vast majority of cases it will resolve without treatment—and nothing you do will shorten its duration.

There are hundreds of viruses that can cause the common cold. They are thought to be transmitted primarily by indirect contact—you touch a contaminated surface or object and then rub your eyes. Cold viruses can enter the body through the mucous membrane of the eyes. It takes about 48 hours from the time of exposure for symptoms to appear, and colds generally last 2–7 days. Weather doesn't affect your risk for a cold, although being forced indoors into more crowded conditions increases your chance for exposure. Cold viruses pass easily from person to person. Colds are more frequent in children, becoming fewer with age. Complications are fairly unusual but are more likely among older adults.

Influenza viruses are more likely to be transmitted through respiratory droplets that infected people release

influenza A highly infectious respiratory disease caused by an influenza virus; the "flu."

Mind Stretcher
Critical Thinking Exercise

Experts strongly suggest a yearly flu shot for at-risk populations, including pregnant women, young children, the elderly, and some caregivers. Would it be a prudent use of taxpayer money to *require* annual flu vaccinations for all high-risk individuals, thereby potentially preventing many cases of flu-related serious complications? Or is the current elective system just as effective? How do you think the current optional system might affect lower-income individuals?

TABLE 12-1 IS IT A COLD OR THE FLU?

SYMPTOM	COLD	FLU
FEVER	Rare	Usual; high (100°–102°F or higher); lasts 3–4 days
HEADACHE	Rare	Common
GENERAL ACHES, PAINS	Slight	Usual, often severe
FATIGUE, WEAKNESS	Sometimes	Usual; can last up to 2–3 weeks
EXHAUSTION	Never	Usual; typically at the beginning of the illness
STUFFY NOSE	Common	Sometimes
SNEEZING	Usual	Sometimes
SORE THROAT	Common	Sometimes
CHEST DISCOMFORT, COUGH	Mild to moderate	Common; can be severe
COMPLICATIONS	Sinus congestion, middle-ear infection, worsening of asthma symptoms	Bronchitis, pneumonia; worsening of chronic conditions; can be life-threatening

Source: National Institute of Allergy and Infectious Diseases. (2008). *Is it a cold or the flu?* (http://www.niaid.nih.gov/topics/Flu/understandingFlu/Pages/publications.aspx).

when they cough, sneeze, or talk. People with influenza can probably pass the virus to others up to about 6 feet away. They are contagious and able to infect others beginning about a day before symptoms develop and up to 5–7 days after becoming ill.[12] Symptoms of influenza usually come on suddenly and typically include fever, body aches, and severe fatigue. The flu typically lasts longer than a cold. It also carries a greater risk of serious complications, including pneumonia, bronchitis, and sinus and ear infections. Older adults, pregnant women, young children, and people with chronic medical conditions are more likely to have serious problems. Thousands of Americans die from influenza and its complications every year.

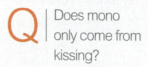

Q Does getting a flu shot really help prevent the flu?

College students are among those groups in the population who can benefit from flu vaccines. Because many students live and attend classes in close quarters with others, influenza infection can spread easily in campus settings. Also, college students often work with high-risk influenza populations, such as children, the elderly, and the chronically ill.

To be vaccinated effectively against the flu, it is important to take the type-specific vaccine. Most cases of the flu are caused by influenza A and influenza B viruses. Influenza A viruses are further divided into subtypes based on proteins on their surface (H and N); recall the H1N1 virus that caused a flu *pandemic* (worldwide outbreak of disease) in 2009–2010. Influenza viruses continually change over time—sometimes slightly, sometimes significantly—and when they do, the immune system no longer recognizes the new version of the virus. Any immunity to other strains you had from past infections or vaccinations no longer protects you, so the flu vaccine is reformulated every year to target the strains most likely to be circulating. For advice on dealing with a cold or the flu, see the box "Starve a Fever, Feed a Cold?"

Infectious Mononucleosis

Q Does mono only come from kissing?

Epstein-Barr virus (EBV), a member of the **herpes** family of viruses, is the pathogen that causes infectious mononucleosis, or "mono." Mono is transmitted through saliva and thus has earned the nickname the "kissing disease." Yet any activity that brings someone in contact with the saliva of an infected person can transfer the virus—for example, sharing a drinking glass. The primary symptoms of mono are fever, sore throat, swollen glands, and fatigue; some people also develop a swollen

herpes A family of viruses that includes those responsible for chicken pox, cold sores, mononucleosis, and genital herpes; these viruses have the ability to establish lifelong latent infections.

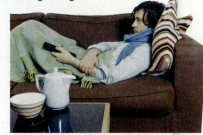

Wellness Strategies

Starve a Fever, Feed a Cold?

Q What are the best home remedies when I'm down with a rotten cold or the flu?

The adage "Starve a Fever, Feed a Cold," and its exact opposite, date back to the 1500s. Today's medical experts will tell you that neither of these is prudent advice, but it is hard for many to turn away from medical myths. Your body always needs energy, regardless of the type of infection, so make sure to eat to satisfy your appetite. Even though the common cold has no cure, there are treatments that can make the suffering more tolerable. Many of these strategies are also good for home treatment of influenza.

- *Drink plenty of liquids:* Water, juice, clear broth, or warm lemon water with honey help loosen congestion and prevent dehydration. Avoid alcohol.
- *Rest:* Colds can tire you out, but influenza is especially associated with severe fatigue and body aches.
- *Try a saltwater gargle:* Dissolve 1/2 teaspoon salt in 8 ounces of warm water and gargle to temporarily relieve a sore or scratchy throat.
- *Try saline nasal spray:* Over-the-counter saline nasal sprays can combat stuffiness and congestion. Avoid or limit use of nasal decongestant sprays, which can lead to a worsening of symptoms when the medication is discontinued.
- *Use over-the-counter cold medicines cautiously:* Decongestants may relieve some of your symptoms but will not shorten the length of your cold; some also have side effects including drowsiness and upset stomach. Choose single-ingredient products, and don't exceed the recommended dosages. Antihistamines may provide some relief from cold symptoms, but they are more appropriate for treating allergies.

- *Use pain relievers cautiously:* Aspirin, acetaminophen, or ibuprofen can all reduce a fever and bring some relief from the aches and pains, but they won't make your symptoms go away any faster. Aspirin and ibuprofen can cause stomach irritation, and if taken for a long period or in higher-than-recommended doses, acetaminophen can be toxic to your liver. Talk to your doctor before giving acetaminophen to children, and don't give aspirin to children or teens because of the risk of Reye's syndrome, a rare but potentially fatal disease.
- *Limit or avoid over-the-counter cough medicines:* Don't take a cough suppressant if you have a productive cough. Soothing your throat with warm liquids and throat lozenges and humidifying the air in your residence can be more effective than any drugs. (The Food and Drug Administration recommends that non-prescription cough medicines *not* be given to children under age 2.)

And remember, antibiotics are not effective at treating viral infections like colds and the flu.

---

spleen. Serious complications are rare, but the fatigue associated with the infection can sometimes last for several months. People who develop an enlarged spleen will be advised to avoid certain physical activities as well as contact sports to reduce the risk of rupturing the spleen.

It is estimated that 95 percent of American adults have been infected with EBV by age 40.[13] Not everyone develops symptoms, but EBV is a latent infection, so the virus remains dormant in the body (see p. 424). The infection can reactivate, but it is usually asymptomatic (without symptoms), even though it can be passed on to someone else. Because the virus can be carried in the saliva of otherwise healthy people, transmission is nearly impossible to prevent.

Meningitis

Q What is that serious infection that causes stiff neck?

Meningitis is an inflammation of the membranes that surround the brain and spinal cord, presenting symptoms that include high fever, severe headache, stiff neck, and sensitivity to bright light. The most common cause of meningitis is a viral infection, and viral meningitis usually resolves on its own after about 7–10 days. However, bacterial meningitis, which has the same symptoms, is a much more severe infection that can lead to disability or even death, although it can be treated with antibiotics. Anyone experiencing meningitis symptoms needs to see a physician immediately (Table 12-2).

meningitis Inflammation of the meninges, the membranes that surround the brain and the spinal cord.

Bacterial Skin Infections

Q What is MRSA?

The acronym *MRSA* stands for methicillin-resistant *Staphylococcus aureus.* It's a type of staph bacteria that is resistant to many antibiotics and therefore difficult to treat. MRSA used to be a common cause of hospital-acquired pneumonia and bloodstream infections,

TABLE 12-2   COMMON INFECTIONS: SYMPTOMS AND TREATMENTS

ILLNESS (PATHOGEN)	SYMPTOMS	HOME TREATMENT	WHEN TO SEEK MEDICAL CARE
COMMON COLD (over 200 different viruses)	Runny nose, nasal congestion, mild cough, sore throat, low-grade fever, sneezing	Usually resolves on its own; fluids, rest, and over-the-counter medications to treat symptoms; avoid alcohol and tobacco	Worsening symptoms after third day, difficulty breathing, stiff neck
INFLUENZA (influenza A or B virus)	Sudden-onset fever, extreme fatigue, headache, body aches, cough	Usually resolves on its own; same home treatment as for colds; prescription antivirals available	Difficulty breathing, severe headache or stiff neck, confusion, fever lasting more than 3 days; new, localized pain in ear, chest, sinuses; people at high risk for complications should contact a health care provider if they develop flu symptoms
BRONCHITIS (different viruses or bacteria)	Cough that may start out dry and later produce mucus; sore throat, fever	Usually resolves on its own; same home treatment as for colds	Shortness of breath, high fever, shaking chills (signs of pneumonia); wheezing and cough that last more than 2 weeks; people at high risk for complications should check with a health care provider
MONONUCLEOSIS (Epstein-Barr virus)	High fever, swollen glands, severe sore throat, fatigue; nausea, vomiting, and loss of appetite can occur	Usually resolves on its own; rest, fluids; avoid contact sports until symptoms resolve due to risk of spleen rupture	Fever lasting more than 3 days; symptoms lasting longer than 7–10 days; severe abdominal pain (possibly indicating ruptured spleen)
MENINGITIS (several different viruses or bacteria)	High fever, stiff and painful neck, headache; vomiting, sleepiness, confusion, seizures	Requires medical evaluation; if determined to be a viral infection, home treatment to relieve symptoms is appropriate	Immediately; bacterial meningitis requires treatment with antibiotics to avoid serious or deadly complications
STREP THROAT (*Streptococcus* bacteria)	Sudden-onset sore throat and fever; swollen glands; red and white pus on tonsils; absence of cold symptoms	A visit to health care provider is appropriate; saltwater gargles, throat lozenges, over-the-counter medications to treat symptoms	Treated with antibiotics to reduce duration of symptoms and risk of complications
BACTERIAL SKIN INFECTION (*Staphylococcus aureus* or *Streptococcus*)	Skin sore or rash; red, swollen, warm, and painful areas of skin; if infection spreads, general symptoms of fever, chills, swollen glands	A visit to health care provider is appropriate; warm compresses; keep infected area clean and dry; topical antibiotics if advised by health care provider	Usually treated with antibiotics; be alert to worsening symptoms or infection on the face
URINARY TRACT INFECTION (different bacteria)	Cloudy, bloody, or strong-smelling urine; frequent urination; pain or burning with urination; low fever; pain in lower abdomen	Requires medical evaluation; drink plenty of water; in women, drinking cranberry juice has been shown to help prevent but not treat urinary tract infections	Usually treated with antibiotics; be alert to worsening symptoms, which may indicate that the infection has spread to the kidneys

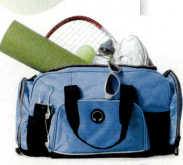

Wellness Strategies

Avoiding Infections at the Gym

Q | What infectious diseases can be transferred through the use of gym equipment?

Skin infections in serious athletes are very common. They can also affect recreational athletes and anyone who works out at a gym. These steps will reduce your risk:

- Use cleaning wipes on equipment when available. Ask the staff at your gym or exercise facility to provide them, or bring your own.
- If facility exercise mats aren't cleaned between each class, bring your own exercise mat, and clean it after each workout.
- Use clothing or a towel to act as a barrier between exercise equipment and your bare skin; if you use a towel, wash it after each workout.
- If you have skin abrasions or cuts, cover them with a sterile bandage.
- Wash your hands with soap before and after working out; hand hygiene is important in all settings.
- Shower after a workout. Wash all parts of your body with soap, including your feet. Athletes in sports with high rates of skin infection should wash with an antibacterial cleanser.

- Dry your feet, armpits, and groin area thoroughly after using a locker room or public shower. Consider wearing shower shoes in shared showering facilities—but don't skip washing your feet.
- Change all your clothes (including socks and underwear) after a workout and shower. Keep your dirty and clean clothes in separate gym bags.
- Don't borrow or share water bottles, towels, razors, bar soap, deodorant, and other personal hygiene items.
- If you notice any symptoms, see a doctor, follow the recommended treatment, and don't go back to the gym until the doctor says your infection is no longer contagious.

Sources: Zinder, S. M., Basler, R. S. W., Foley, J., Scarlata, C., & Vasily, D. B. (2010). National Athletic Trainers' Association position statement: Skin diseases. *Journal of Athletic Training, 45*(4), 411–428. American Academy of Family Physicians. (2009). *Tinea infections: Athlete's foot, jock itch, and ringworm* (http://familydoctor.org/online/famdocen/home/common/infections/common/fungal/316.html).

---

but it is now also a major agent of skin infections outside medical settings. Risk factors for the spread of MRSA include close skin-to-skin contact, skin cuts or abrasions, crowded living conditions, and contaminated items and surfaces. Places where these risk factors are common include athletic facilities, dormitories, military barracks, and day-care centers. See the box "Avoiding Infections at the Gym" for more information.

Skin infections usually start out as red, swollen, painful lumps and initially may look like pimples, boils, or insect bites. If the infection spreads, you may also experience fever and swollen glands. If you do, you should contact your health care provider for a diagnosis and appropriate treatment, because MRSA skin infections require professional care. Skin infections can also be caused by other pathogens, including *Streptococcus* bacteria. Athlete's foot, herpes, and impetigo are all examples of other common skin infections.

Sexually Transmitted Infections

Sexually transmitted infections (STIs) are among the most common infections in the United States, with an estimated 19 million new cases each year (Table 12-3). About half of all new infections occur among people ages 15–24. STIs are primarily spread through person-to-person sexual contact—vaginal, oral, or anal sex—although some can also be passed along in other ways. Some STIs can be easily treated and cured, but others are chronic, incurable, and even life threatening. All STIs are preventable.

sexually transmitted infection (STI) An infection that is primarily spread through person-to-person sexual contact.

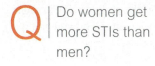

Q | Do women get more STIs than men?

Yes, women are more likely to have STIs and more likely to experience serious complications from them. Transmission of many STIs, including genital herpes and HIV, is more likely to occur from an infected male to his female partner than from an infected female to her male partner. Approximately one in five women between 14 and 49 has a genital herpes infection compared with one in nine men in the same age group.[14] Young women are also more likely than older women to contract STIs and to experience serious effects; the cervix of young women is covered with cells that are especially susceptible to STIs.

Most STIs affect both men and women, but in many cases, they cause more severe problems in women, including

TABLE 12-3 STIs IN THE UNITED STATES: A SNAPSHOT

	ESTIMATED ANNUAL INCIDENCE	ESTIMATED PREVALENCE*	OUTLOOK IF DIAGNOSED
TRICHOMONIASIS	7.4 million	n/a	Curable with antibiotics
HPV INFECTION	6.2 million	20 million	Vaccine-preventable; incurable but often resolves on its own; can cause cancer
CHLAMYDIA	2.8 million	1.9 million	Curable with antibiotics
GENITAL HERPES	1.6 million	45 million	Chronic and incurable; treatments can reduce symptoms and outbreaks
GONORRHEA	700,000	n/a	Curable with antibiotics
SYPHILIS	60,000	n/a	Curable with antibiotics
HIV INFECTION	47,000	1.2 million	Chronic and potentially fatal; treatable but incurable
HEPATITIS B	43,000	1.25 million	Vaccine-preventable; incurable but often resolves on its own; can cause fatal liver disease

*Because viral STIs can be persistent and incurable, the number of currently infected people capable of transmitting the infection (*prevalence*) greatly exceeds the annual number of new cases (*incidence*).

Sources: Centers for Disease Control and Prevention. (2010). Fact sheet: HIV in the United States (http://www.cdc.gov/hiv/resources/factsheets/us.htm). Centers for Disease Control and Prevention. (2010). HCV FAQs for health professionals (http://www.cdc.gov/hepatitis/HCV/HCVfaq.htm). Weinstock, H., Berman, S., & Cates, W. (2004). Sexually transmitted diseases among American youth: Incidence and prevalence estimates, 2000. *Perspectives on Sexual and Reproductive Health, 36*(1), 6–10. Additional data from the Kaiser Family Foundation and the Guttmacher Institute.

infertility. Having an STI during pregnancy can produce early labor, infection of the uterus, and in some cases dangerous infections in the baby.

Many sexually transmitted infections are asymptomatic, meaning that people are unaware they are infected and can pass the infection on to others. Some STIs have very minor symptoms that can be overlooked or mistaken for other conditions. Importantly, anyone who is sexually active can have an STI—even in the absence of any signs or symptoms of disease. It doesn't matter who you are, it's what you do that counts.

Trichomoniasis

Q | What's the most common sexually transmitted infection?

In terms of new STI cases each year, trichomoniasis, or "trich," is the most common. Caused by the protozoan *Trichomonas vaginalis*, **trichomoniasis** produces vaginal infections in women and infections of the urethra (urine canal) in men. Most women infected with trichomoniasis have symptoms such as vaginal discharge and painful urination, but most infected men do not have symptoms. Trichomoniasis is diagnosed through lab tests and treated with prescription medication.

If a woman develops trichomoniasis, she and her partner both need to be treated because it's likely that the partner is infected even if he or she has no symptoms. Treatment should be completed before resuming sexual activity. If untreated, trichomoniasis has two serious complications: It significantly increases the risk of HIV transmission, and, in pregnant women, it can lead to premature labor and delivery.

trichomoniasis Sexually transmitted infection caused by the protozoan *Trichomonas vaginalis*.

Women are more likely than men to contract sexually transmitted infections and to suffer serious complications from them. Infants can also be at risk for contracting infections from their mothers during pregnancy, childbirth, and breastfeeding.

Chlamydia

Q | How often should I get checked for chlamydia?

Annual screening for chlamydia is recommended for sexually active women 25 years of age and younger, as well as older women with risk factors (many sex partners or a new sex partner). Screening is also advised for all pregnant women.

Chlamydia is an STI caused by *Chlamydia trachomatis,* a bacterium that can be transmitted during vaginal, oral, or anal sex or from an infected mother to her baby during childbirth. About 70 percent of infected individuals have no symptoms, but among those who do, abnormal discharge from the vagina or penis and pain while urinating are most common.

Untreated, chlamydia can cause serious infections of the fallopian tubes in women and the urethra and epididymis (curved tube on the back of the testicle) in men. People infected through oral sex may have symptoms in the throat.

Chlamydia can be treated with antibiotics, but reinfection is possible—and even likely if a woman's partner isn't also treated. In women, untreated chlamydia is a leading cause of serious and permanent damage to the reproductive organs, which can lead to infertility. Infected infants may develop pneumonia and eye infections that can potentially cause blindness.

Gonorrhea

Q | Can a person really get gonorrhea from oral sex?

Yes, unprotected oral sex can transmit the infection, although it's not as common as infection of the reproductive or urinary tract. Among young women, as many as 25 percent of infections may be in the throat.[15] **Gonorrhea** is a bacterial infection caused by *Neisseria gonorrhoeae.* It is spread through contact with the penis, vagina, mouth, or anus; it can also be passed from mother to baby during delivery. Most women have no symptoms, and those who do may have nonspecific symptoms that are mistaken for a bladder or vaginal infection. Men can also be asymptomatic, although sometimes discharge and painful urination occur.

As with chlamydia, untreated gonorrhea can damage a woman's reproductive organs and cause infertility and chronic pelvic pain. In men, an untreated infection can harm the epididymis and also potentially lead to infertility, although the latter development is less likely than in women. If transmitted to an infant during childbirth, the bacterium can cause dangerous infections of the blood, joints, and eyes.

Gonorrhea can be treated with antibiotics, but many strains of the bacteria have developed resistance, which can make treatment more difficult. Although the infection can be cured with antibiotics, treatment does not reverse the damage, and reinfection is possible.

Fast Facts

STIs: The Sobering Reality

- One in five people in the United States has an STI.
- One in four new STI infections occurs in teenagers.
- One in four people will have an STI at some point during his or her life.
- One in 10 teenagers knows someone who is HIV-positive.
- Fifty-six percent of teenagers 12–17 years of age think STIs are a big problem for people their age.
- Many STIs have no signs or symptoms; someone without any symptoms can have an STI and transmit it to a partner.
- Anyone who has sexual contact of any kind can contract an STI.
- You do not become immune to STIs such as chlamydia and gonorrhea, so you can contract them multiple times. Infections such as herpes and HIV are chronic and incurable.
- Birth control pills do not protect against STIs.
- Douching increases the risk for several STIs as well as pelvic inflammatory disease (see below).

Pelvic Inflammatory Disease (PID)

Q | If I have chlamydia, does that mean I also have PID?

Pelvic inflammatory disease (PID) is infection and inflammation of the uterus, ovaries, fallopian tubes, and other reproductive organs in women. It is usually the result of untreated chlamydia or gonorrhea; douching and use of an intrauterine device (IUD) can also increase the risk of PID.[16] In PID, bacteria move up from the vagina and infect other reproductive organs. The infection may have no initial symptoms, or there may be severe symptoms, including sudden onset of fever and pain. Signs can include vaginal discharge, painful urination or intercourse, pain in the lower abdomen, and irregular menstrual bleeding.

PID damages the reproductive organs, and the resulting scar tissue can cause chronic pelvic pain, tubal (ectopic) pregnancy, and infertility from blocked fallopian tubes. More than 1 million women are treated for PID each year, and many others have the condition but don't know it. Each year, an estimated 100,000 women

chlamydia Sexually transmitted infection caused by the bacterium *Chlamydia trachomatis.*

gonorrhea Sexually transmitted infection caused by the bacterium *Neisseria gonorrhoeae.*

pelvic inflammatory disease (PID) Infection of the reproductive system in women, typically caused by untreated chlamydia or gonorrhea; can result in reproductive system damage and infertility.

become infertile and more than 150 women die from PID.[17] Infertility is more likely to occur as a result of prolonged or repeated bouts of PID.

If you think you have pelvic inflammatory disease, see your physician immediately: Early treatment with antibiotics can limit the damage and long-term complications. As with other sexually transmitted infections, a woman's sex partners also need to be treated.

Syphilis

Q How many stages of syphilis are there?

Syphilis has four separate but sometimes overlapping stages. **Syphilis** is caused by the bacterium *Treponema pallidum,* which can be transmitted through infected skin and mucous membranes in the genitals, lips, mouth, or anus. Syphilis can also be passed from a pregnant woman to her infant during pregnancy, giving rise to a disease called *congenital syphilis.*

Primary syphilis is the first stage, characterized by the appearance of a painless sore, called a *chancre,* at the point of infection. The sore is full of bacteria that can be transmitted to others, but it may go unnoticed. A chancre usually disappears within about 3–6 weeks regardless of whether the infection is treated.

Secondary syphilis develops 2–10 weeks later. The most common symptom is a non-itchy skin rash, usually on the palms of the hands and soles of the feet. Other signs include swollen lymph glands, headache, fatigue, sore throat, and hair loss. Symptoms of secondary syphilis usually disappear with or without treatment, although they may recur.

Latent syphilis develops in people who haven't been treated. Symptoms of the disease disappear, but the bacteria remain in the body. Early in the latent stage a person can still infect others, but this risk fades over time.

A small percentage of people with latent syphilis go on to develop the fourth stage, *tertiary syphilis.* In this stage, the syphilis bacteria damage major organs and can cause mental illness, heart disease, blindness, and death.

During pregnancy, syphilis can cause miscarriage, premature birth, stillbirth, and infant death. Babies born with syphilis (congenital syphilis) may have birth defects, seizures, development delays, and other problems. Syphilis is curable with antibiotics in all stages, but organ damage cannot be reversed. A fetus can be cured in the womb if the mother receives treatment early enough in the pregnancy.

Genital Herpes

Q Does everyone have herpes?

Not everyone has herpes, but the infection is very common, and the majority of infected people don't know their status (Table 12-4). **Genital herpes** can be caused either by herpes simplex virus type 1 (HSV 1) or, more typically, by herpes simplex virus type 2 (HSV 2). HSV 1 more often infects the lips and mouth, producing cold sores, and can cause genital herpes if transmitted through oral sex. HSV 2 is the primary cause of genital herpes and can also infect the mouth. Overall, about 50–80 percent of American adults have oral herpes (primarily from HSV 1), and about 20 percent have genital herpes (primarily from HSV 2). Read more about genital herpes in the box "Living Well with . . . Genital Herpes."

syphilis A multistage sexually transmitted infection caused by the bacterium *Treponema pallidum.*

genital herpes A chronic or latent sexually transmitted infection caused by the herpes simplex virus (HSV) and characterized by genital sores.

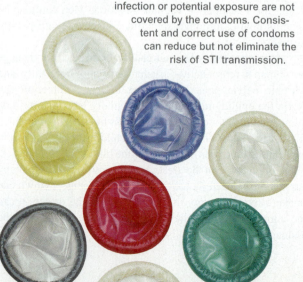

Latex condoms provide an essentially impermeable barrier to particles the size of STI pathogens and are highly effective in preventing STIs. Condoms cannot provide protection if sites of infection or potential exposure are not covered by the condoms. Consistent and correct use of condoms can reduce but not eliminate the risk of STI transmission.

Fast Facts

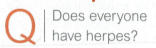

Sex Is . . .?

How do you define *sex?* Surveys of college students show changing perceptions over time.

Percentage of university students who classified behavior as sex

Behavior	1991	2007
Penile-vaginal intercourse	99.5%	97.5%
Penile-anal intercourse	81.0%	78.4%
Partner's oral contact with your genitals	40.2%	19.9%
Oral contact with a partner's genitals	39.9%	18.7%

- Which of the activities in this list can transmit microbes and cause STIs?
- What is the big take-away lesson when it comes to any of these activities?

Source: Hans, J. D., Gillen, M., & Akande, K. (2010). Sex redefined: The reclassification of oral-genital contact. *Perspectives on Sexual and Reproductive Health, 42*(2).

Living *Well* with . . .

Genital Herpes

Finding out that you have genital herpes can make you feel angry, ashamed, and worried about rejection. Remember, though, that genital herpes is a very common, manageable infection. In healthy adults, genital herpes usually doesn't cause any serious health problems. For most people, outbreaks become less frequent over time—perhaps four to five outbreaks during the first year after diagnosis and then fewer after that. Helpful strategies for living well with genital herpes include the following:

- To manage the infection, take all prescribed medications, even if the symptoms go away.
- Maintain a healthy lifestyle. Manage stress to support your immune system and reduce outbreaks (see p. 425).
- Be aware of potential triggers for outbreaks, which can vary from person to person. Some people find outbreaks linked to certain other illnesses or to hormonal changes associated with the menstrual cycle.

- Avoid sexual activity when you feel an outbreak coming on or have symptoms—but remember that you can transmit the infection even if you have no symptoms.
- During an outbreak, keep the sores clean and dry; if you touch a sore, wash your hands thoroughly. Wear loose-fitting cotton underwear and don't wear pantyhose; heat and moisture can slow healing.
- Use latex condoms during sex. Used consistently and correctly, condoms significantly reduce the risk of spreading herpes. Importantly, however, since they don't cover all potentially infectious areas, they do not completely eliminate risk.
- Tell your sexual partners so that they can be tested for herpes. Inform any new partners before you have sex.
- Find a counselor or a support group—in person or online.

TABLE 12-4 PREVALENCE OF HERPES SIMPLEX VIRUS TYPE 2 AS MEASURED BY BLOOD TESTS*

	PREVALENCE (%)
TOTAL	16.2%
AGE GROUP (YEARS)	
14–19	1.4%
20–29	10.5%
30–39	19.6%
40–49	26.1%
REPORTED NUMBER OF LIFETIME SEX PARTNERS	
1	3.9%
2–4	14.0%
5–9	16.3%
≥10	26.7%

*Over 80 percent of those whose blood test was positive for HSV 2 had never received a diagnosis of genital herpes.

Source: Centers for Disease Control and Prevention. (2010). Seroprevalence of herpes simplex virus type 2 among persons aged 14–49 years—United States, 2005–2008. *Morbidity and Mortality Weekly Report, 59*(15), 456–459 (http://www.cdc.gov/mmwr/preview/mmwrhtml/mm5915a3.htm).

Most people contract genital herpes by having sex or close skin-to-skin contact with an infected person. The main symptom of herpes is sores at the site where the virus entered the body. They may start with a tingling feeling, erupt as red bumps, and then develop into small blisters or painful open sores. Some people also experience fever, headache, muscle aches, swollen glands, and other genital or urinary symptoms.

In most people, HSV is a latent infection; the virus remains in nerve cells for life and can become active and trigger outbreaks several times a year. Recurrences often include visible sores and symptoms, but the virus can also be active without any signs. Although transmission of the virus is more likely when obvious sores are present, people with genital herpes can pass on the virus even if they have no symptoms and no idea they are infected.

There is no treatment or cure for genital herpes. There are antiviral drugs that help treat symptoms and prevent or reduce outbreaks. Using these drugs reduces but does not eliminate the chance of transmitting herpes to sexual partners. Because HSV can pass from mother to fetus and harm the baby, pregnant women who have herpes or whose sex partners have herpes should develop a plan with their physician to reduce the baby's risk of infection. Having herpes also increases the likelihood of contracting HIV from an infected partner.

Genital Warts (HPV Infection)

Q | Do genital warts go away?

For many people, genital warts clear up over time. However, they can become a chronic infection or have other serious effects.

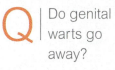

Genital warts are caused by **human papillomavirus (HPV) infection.** However, many people have genital HPV infection without having genital warts. There are more than 100 types of HPV, many of which are harmless. Of those that are sexually transmitted, some types cause genital warts and some can produce changes in cells that can lead to cancer of the cervix, vulva, vagina, penis, or anus. Genital warts can also present problems during pregnancy; in rare cases, infants born to infected mothers can develop warts in their throats.

HPV infection is very common and easily transmitted through skin-to-skin contact. Close to 30 percent of young women acquire HPV from their first male sex partner, and within 3 years of becoming sexually active, 50 percent of women have been infected.[18] Males are also infected at a high rate: In a 2-year study of heterosexually active male university students, 62 percent of the study participants acquired new HPV infections.[19]

For many people, genital HPV infection has no symptoms. Nonetheless, even in these cases, complications can develop, and the virus can be transmitted to sexual partners. When warts do appear, they may be raised or flat, small or large; they can appear anywhere on, in, or around the genitals. Women may unknowingly have warts on their cervix.

Genital warts do not turn into cancer; the types of HPV that produce the warts are different from those that cause cancer. However, an individual can be infected with both types. Therefore, the primary complication of HPV infection is cervical cancer. The cellular changes associated with cervical cancer can be detected through regular *Pap tests*—screening tests to detect the presence of cancer or precancerous changes in the cervix. Pap tests are recommended for all women starting within 3 years after they become sexually active.

Treatments for visible genital warts include creams, laser surgery, and freezing or burning, though sometimes the warts disappear without treatment. There is no treatment, however, for the underlying viral infection. So, because the virus remains in the body, the warts can come back after treatment. In about 90 percent of cases, the body's immune system clears HPV within 2 years of infection, yet sometimes HPV infections are not cleared. Lingering infections can cause genital warts, cervical cancer, and other less common but serious cancers, including those of the vulva, vagina, penis, and anus.

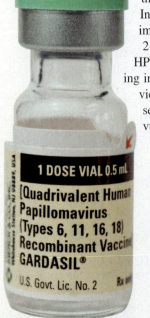

Genital HPV infection is one of the two sexually transmitted viruses for which preventive vaccines are available. There are two vaccines, Cervarix and Gardasil, that protect against the types of HPV that cause about 70 percent of cervical cancers. Gardasil also protects against the types of HPV that cause about 90 percent of cases of genital warts. The vaccines are recommended for all females when they are 11 or 12, as well as females between 13 and 26 who haven't already been fully vaccinated. Gardasil is also licensed for use in males ages 9–26 for the prevention of genital warts. The vaccines do not treat established HPV infections.

Along with the vaccine, consistent condom use can also protect against HPV infection.[20] However, condoms do not provide complete protection because not all skin surfaces that can carry the virus are covered by a condom. See the box "Preventing Sexually Transmitted Infections" for additional strategies.

Viral Hepatitis

Q | Are herpes and HIV the only incurable STIs?

Along with HPV infection, some forms of viral hepatitis can also develop into chronic, incurable infections. **Viral hepatitis** is inflammation of the liver caused by infection with one of the hepatitis viruses, the three most common forms of which are:

- *Hepatitis A virus (HAV),* which is usually transmitted through contaminated food and water. Hepatitis A usually resolves on its own, and a vaccine is available. There are about 25,000 U.S. cases per year.
- *Hepatitis B virus (HBV),* which is transmitted through semen, vaginal fluids, blood, and saliva. Hepatitis B is described in more detail below.
- *Hepatitis C virus (HCV),* which is primarily transmitted through blood. Most new U.S. infections occur through injection drug use. Hepatitis C leads to chronic infection in about 85 percent of those who contract the virus.

human papillomavirus (HPV) infection A sexually transmitted viral infection that can cause genital warts and cellular changes that lead to cervical and other cancers; can be a chronic infection.

viral hepatitis Inflammation of the liver caused by infection with one of the hepatitis viruses; can become a chronic infection.

Mind Stretcher
Critical Thinking Exercise

If you are sexually active, have you recently been screened for STIs? Have you asked whether your partner has recently been screened? Regular STI screening is important for all sexually active people, and even more so if there are or have been previous partners and no previous screenings. Where on your campus and in your community can you go for free and confidential STI screening? Do you have someone with whom you feel safe who can accompany you? The bottom line is that STI screening can save you and your partner from potentially serious personal complications and from further spreading the STI.

Wellness Strategies

Preventing Sexually Transmitted Infections

Q | What are the best practices to avoid getting an STI?

You can lower your risk of contracting an STI with the following practices and knowledge. Keep in mind, though, that no single strategy can protect you from every type of STI.

- *Don't have sex.* Abstinence from vaginal, oral, or anal sex is the best protection, though some STIs, such as genital herpes, can be spread without intercourse.
- *Be faithful.* Having multiple partners means increased risk of obtaining or spreading infection. Have sex only with each other—and no one else.
- *Limit your number of sex partners.* If you do have multiple partners, limit the number as best you can. The fewer partners you have, the less likely you are to encounter someone with an STI.
- *Use condoms correctly and every time you have sex.* A male latex condom offers the best protection, assuming that it is used correctly from start to finish.
- *Be aware that birth control will not protect you from STIs.* Birth control pills, shots, implants, and diaphragms may prevent a pregnancy, but they do not buffer against infection.
- *Talk with your sex partners about STIs and using condoms before having sex.* It's up to you to set the ground rules and to make sure that you are protected.

- *Don't assume that you're at low risk for STIs if you're a woman who has sex only with women.* Some common STIs are spread easily by skin-to-skin contact. Also, most women who have sex with women have had sex with men, too.
- *Talk frankly with your doctor and each sex partner about any STIs you or your partner has or has had.* Discuss symptoms, such as sores and discharge. Try not to be embarrassed. Your doctor is there to help you.
- *Have regular exams—get tested and insist your partners do, too.* Testing for many STIs is simple and often can be done during a checkup. The sooner an STI is found, the easier it is to treat.
- *Get vaccinated against HPV.* If you're age 26 or younger, ask if HPV vaccination is appropriate for you.
- *Be alert to symptoms.* If you experience genital or urinary symptoms, see your doctor. Don't have sex until you and your partners complete treatment.
- *Avoid using drugs or drinking too much alcohol.* These activities may lead to risky sexual behavior, such as not wearing a condom.

Source: National Women's Health Information Center. (2009). Overview. *Sexually Transmitted Infections* (http://www.womenshealth.gov/faq/sexually-transmitted-infections.cfm). Centers for Disease Control and Prevention. (2010). What patients should know when they are diagnosed with genital warts (http://www.cdc.gov/hpv/Signs-Symptoms.html).

Hepatitis B is most commonly transmitted through sex with an infected partner, through contact with the blood of an infected person, or from a mother to her infant during childbirth. Hepatitis is more easily transmitted than HIV and some other bloodborne infections, so there is some risk of infection from sharing razors or toothbrushes with an infected person. However, the virus isn't transmitted through shaking hands, coughing, or sharing utensils. There are about 43,000 new cases each year (see Table 12-3).

Symptoms of acute hepatitis B may include *jaundice* (yellowing of the skin and whites of the eyes), abdominal pain, nausea or vomiting, dark urine, and fatigue. The acute phase may last from several weeks to up to 6 months. There is no specific treatment for hepatitis B infection other than good self-care. In some people, the virus remains in the body after the acute stage of the infection, causing chronic disease. People with chronic hepatitis may exhibit no symptoms, but some develop serious and potentially fatal liver damage or liver cancer.

There is a vaccine to prevent hepatitis B. Routinely given to all infants, it is also safe for children and adults.

HIV Infection and AIDS

In the United States, someone is infected with HIV every 10 minutes, and someone dies from HIV/AIDS every 45 minutes.[21] Worldwide, the statistics are even more dramatic, with 7,400 people infected every day, half of them under age 25.[22] Although medications developed to treat the

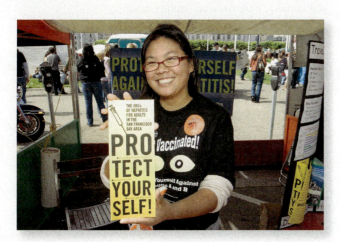

infection have dramatically extended survival and greatly improved quality of life, HIV/AIDS remains an enormous global challenge.

HIV is not equally distributed across the U.S. population. Men have higher rates of HIV infection than women (Figure 12-6). Although African Americans make up about 13 percent of the U.S. population, they account for about half of all new HIV cases. However, it's important to remember that anyone can be infected with HIV. Recent surveys indicate that nearly 40 percent of young adults engage in high-HIV-risk behavior.[23]

Q | Is there a difference between HIV and AIDS?

Human immunodeficiency virus (HIV) is the infectious agent that causes **acquired immune deficiency syndrome (AIDS).** HIV is a pathogen, and AIDS is the late stage of HIV infection—a chronic infection that slowly destroys the body's immune system. People with HIV may look and feel healthy, experiencing no symptoms for years after the initial infection. However, the virus is active in their body, infecting and destroying immune system cells as it reproduces. The specific type of blood cell that HIV destroys is called a CD4+ T cell, which is critical for the body to fight infection. Over time, HIV levels increase and CD4+ T cell levels decrease, leaving people less able to fight off other diseases and infections. Measurement of CD4+ T cell counts indicates the progress of the infection and informs treatment decisions.

If damage to the immune system is severe, a person develops AIDS. This final stage of HIV infection is diagnosed when he or she develops an *opportunistic infection*—an infection a person without HIV infection would be unlikely to contract—or has a dangerously low number of CD4+ T cells. Prior to the development of treatments, people progressed from HIV infection to AIDS within a few years. With the new medications, people may live years or even decades with HIV infection without developing AIDS.

Q | Do condoms help prevent HIV infection?

TRANSMISSION AND SYMPTOMS. Condom use does not completely eliminate risk, but it greatly reduces HIV transmission.[24] Most problems with condom effectiveness relate to improper or inconsistent use (see the box "The Dos and Don'ts of Condom Use"). HIV is found in blood, semen, and vaginal secretions and can be transmitted by sharing these body fluids. According to the Centers for Disease Control and Prevention, HIV is spread primarily in the following ways:[25]

- Not using a condom when having sex with a person who has HIV. Unprotected anal sex is riskier than unprotected vaginal sex. Unprotected oral sex can also be a risk for HIV transmission, but it is a much lower risk than anal or vaginal sex.
- Having multiple sex partners.
- The presence of other sexually transmitted infections.
- Sharing needles, syringes, other equipment, or rinse water used to prepare illicit drugs for injection.
- Being born to an infected mother—HIV can be passed from mother to child during pregnancy, birth, and breastfeeding.

Among American adolescents and adults, the three most common modes of transmission are male-to-male sexual contact, heterosexual contact, and injection drug use (Figure 12-7). Less commonly, HIV may be transmitted to health care workers through needle sticks. Before HIV blood tests, people could also be infected from a blood transfusion or an organ transplant; however, the risk is now extremely small due to rigorous screening. HIV cannot survive outside the human body and is not transmitted through air, water, or insect bites. Furthermore, there are no documented cases of transmission through saliva, tears, sweat, or closed-mouth kissing.

human immunodeficiency virus (HIV) The virus that causes HIV infection and AIDS; infects and destroys cells of the immune system.

acquired immune deficiency syndrome (AIDS) A disease of the immune system characterized by a severe reduction in the number of CD4+ cells, leaving an individual susceptible to other infections and diseases; the final stage of HIV infection.

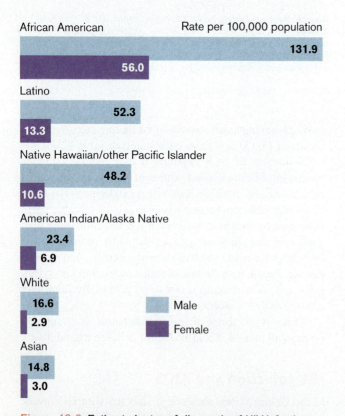

Rate per 100,000 population

African American
131.9
56.0

Latino
52.3
13.3

Native Hawaiian/other Pacific Islander
48.2
10.6

American Indian/Alaska Native
23.4
6.9

White
16.6
2.9

Asian
14.8
3.0

Male
Female

Figure 12-6 Estimated rates of diagnosis of HIV infection among U.S. adults and adolescents, by sex and race/ethnicity.
Source: Centers for Disease Control and Prevention. *HIV Surveillance Report, 2010,* vol. 22). (http://www.cdc.gov/hiv/topics/surveillance/resources/reports/). Published March 2012. Accessed March 2012.

Wellness Strategies

The Dos and Don'ts of Condom Use

Q How can I be sure I'm using condoms correctly?

Here are some key things to know when using condoms for contraception and protection against STIs.

DO

- Check the expiration date.
- Use only latex or polyurethane (plastic) condoms.
- Keep condoms in a cool, dry place.
- Put the condom on an erect (hard) penis before there is any contact with a partner's genitals.
- Use plenty of non-oil-based lubricant with latex condoms if you find that vaginal sex is uncomfortable or that condoms tend to rip or tear.
- Hold the condom in place at the base of the penis before withdrawing (pulling out) after sex.
- Throw the condom away after use.

DON'T

- Use out-of-date condoms.
- Unroll the condom before putting it on the erect penis.
- Leave condoms in hot places like your wallet and car.
- Use oil-based products such as baby or cooking oils, hand lotion, or petroleum jelly (like Vaseline) as lubricants with latex condoms. The oil quickly weakens latex and can cause breakage.
- Use your fingernails or teeth when opening a condom wrapper, because it will easily tear.
- Reuse a condom.
- Use lubricants with the spermicide nonoxynol-9 (N-9), as they may cause skin irritation or tiny abrasions that make the genital skin more susceptible to STIs.

For information on the use of condoms for pregnancy prevention—including combining condoms with other contraceptive methods and using over-the-counter emergency contraception in case of condom breakage—visit the Web sites for the American College of Obstetricians and Gynecologists' publications: http://www.acog.org/Search?Keyword=safe+sex&Topics=a1a33f40-5b12-4015-8b75-1e53e56be395) and Planned Parenthood (http://www.plannedparenthood.org).

Source: The American Social Health Association (http://www.ashastd.org/std-sti-works/condoms.html).

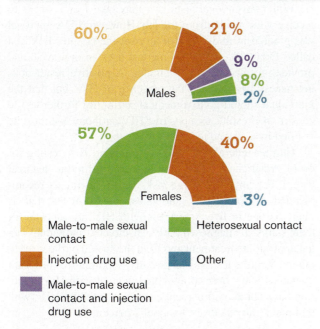

Figure 12-7 Transmission routes among U.S. adults and adolescents diagnosed with AIDS.

Source: Centers for Disease Control and Prevention. *HIV Surveillance Report, 2010*, vol. 22 (http://www.cdc.gov/hiv/topics/surveillance/resources/reports/). Published March 2012. Accessed March 2012.

To prevent the transmission of HIV, avoid or limit your risky behaviors. For specific guidelines, refer to the box "Preventing Sexually Transmitted Infections." Most important is to abstain from sex or to practice safer sex consistently. Think about your sexual behavior, and if you act in risky ways, consider how you can minimize your risk. In addition, if you inject drugs, get counseling and treatment; using clean needles and syringes reduces the risk of transmission, but it's much better to stop drug use and avoid all the associated risks.

If you do have a risky sexual encounter and believe that you were exposed to HIV, see your health care provider immediately. In some cases, HIV medications can prevent infection if they are started shortly after exposure to the virus.

Q What are symptoms of HIV and AIDS?

Most people infected with HIV are asymptomatic, although some develop nonspecific symptoms during the acute phase of the initial infection: fever, headache, fatigue, muscle aches, and enlarged lymph nodes. These symptoms typically resolve with no treatment and may be attributed to influenza or another minor illness. During this early acute phase, people are extremely infectious.

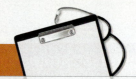

Research Brief

Unprotected Sex: How Do College Students Explain Their Behavior?

By the time young adults get to college, most have received vast amounts of information about the consequences of unprotected sex in terms of both pregnancy and STIs. Despite a lot of knowledge about the risks, many young adults still fail to practice safer sex consistently. How do they explain this inconsistency?

In a recent study, researchers asked a group of young adults to keep diaries for several weeks to track their condom use and non-use during intercourse. Once the diaries were complete, the students were interviewed to explore their decision making.

Less than 25 percent of the students used condoms or oral contraceptives consistently. Most who did use condoms saw them as a means of preventing pregnancy rather than preventing disease. Their explanations for their risky behaviors fell into several categories:

- *Biased evaluation of risk:* Students equated the degree of closeness and intimacy they felt for their partner with reduced risk for STIs.
- *Biased evaluation of evidence:* Students believed that since their pattern of behavior (unsafe sex) had not in the past resulted in pregnancy or an STI, it must not be very risky.

- *Endorsement of poor alternatives:* Some students justified their choice to not use condoms with the use of an alternative prevention strategy—even though they recognized the alternative as a poor one (withdrawal, counting on luck).
- *False justifications:* Despite stating a strong desire to avoid STIs and pregnancy, students weighted short-term benefits of not using a condom as more important than the long-term negative consequences.
- *Dismissing or ignoring risk:* Some students felt invulnerable to the negative outcomes that other people might experience ("it won't happen to me"), and others felt that the negative outcomes could be easily solved (abortion, drug treatment).

Analyze and Apply

- What would you say to yourself or a peer to dispute these false beliefs?
- What is one step you can take now to practice safer sex, assuming that you are sexually active?

Source: O'Sullivan, L. F., Udell, W., Montrose, V. A., Antoniello, P., & Hoffman, S. (2010). A cognitive analysis of college students' explanations for engaging in unprotected sexual intercourse. *Archives of Sexual Behavior*, 39, 1121–1131.

After the acute phase has passed, any symptoms that occurred resolve. Although the virus remains in the body, replicating and destroying CD4+ T cells, infected people exhibit no symptoms and likely are completely unaware of the infection. However, they are capable of infecting others.

During the late stages of HIV infection, when the immune system has been severely weakened, people may experience a variety of symptoms. These include rapid weight loss, extreme fatigue, prolonged swelling of lymph nodes, sores in the mouth or genitals, and neurological disorders. The opportunistic infections that can occur in people with full-blown AIDS include pneumonia, cancer, liver disease, and many types of otherwise unusual viral, fungal, protozoal, and bacterial infections.

Q How long do you have to wait to find out if you have HIV?

TESTING AND TREATMENT. HIV antibodies are produced 2–8 weeks following the infection (average is 25 days), therefore any HIV testing must occur at or beyond this time point, and 97 percent of infections can be detected within 3 months.[26] In very rare cases it can take up to 6 months to get an accurate test result.

With conventional testing, it may take 1 or 2 weeks to receive your results from the lab. However, FDA approval was granted in mid-2012 for an over-the-counter HIV test called OraQuick. This at-home test uses an oral swab and provides results in 20–40 minutes. A positive result does not necessarily indicate the presence of HIV, but that the individual should go to a medical setting for further test to confirm the results, as a positive HIV antibody test must be verified by a second test.

Current federal guidelines recommend HIV testing for every American ages 13–64 as part of routine medical care.[27] For anyone at high risk, yearly testing is recommended. Despite these guidelines, it's estimated that as many as one in five Americans with HIV are unaware of their status. If diagnosed early, an infected individual can get appropriate treatment and limit the spread of the virus to others. Routine testing is especially important for pregnant women. Babies born to untreated women with HIV infection have about a 25 percent chance of catching HIV; with treatment, the risk drops to about 2 percent.

Q How long until someone with HIV dies?

With treatment, people can survive many years or even decades with HIV infection. The success of treatment depends on

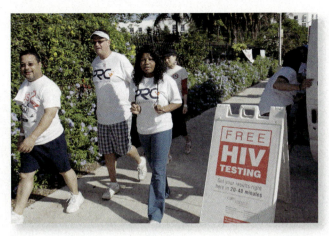

The Centers for Disease Control and Prevention recommends HIV testing at least once for all Americans ages 13–64 as part of routine medical care. For anyone at high risk, annual testing is appropriate.

many factors, including an individual's underlying health status and how early in the course of infection treatment begins. Over 30 antiviral drugs are available to treat HIV infection. These medications do not cure the infection or eliminate the virus from the body, but they do suppress the virus, sometimes to undetectable levels. A person being treated for HIV must take antiviral drugs continuously; he or she can still transmit the virus, but the risk is much lower. The medications can have side effects, sometimes serious, and HIV can also become resistant to particular medications.

Researchers have worked for many years to design a vaccine, but HIV poses significant challenges. It directly attacks the immune system—the very cells that need to be activated by a vaccine. In addition, HIV frequently mutates to produce new strains. Although a vaccine remains elusive, there has been some success in developing *microbicides*—substances that kill microbes or reduce their ability to cause infection—that can be applied to the vagina before intercourse to help lower the risk of transmission.[28] Microbicides may be particularly beneficial for women around the world who aren't able to negotiate mutual monogamy or condom use with their partners.

With no vaccine or cure on the horizon, it's important for everyone to take HIV prevention seriously.

Summary

Infectious agents are all around us and impossible to avoid. Fortunately, the body has many physical and chemical barriers to keep pathogens out and a complex immune system to tackle those microbes that do gain entry. Many infections are relatively mild and cause few problems in healthy individuals. Among the more serious infections, many can be cured with medications and self-care. On a personal level, you can help limit the impact of infectious disease by engaging in wellness behaviors that support your immune system and by taking steps to avoid the transmission of pathogens. It's also important to keep your vaccinations up to date.

Although colds, influenza, and similar infections can be challenging to avoid, infections that are sexually transmitted (STIs) have clear prevention strategies. Not having sex prevents almost all STIs, and if you are sexually active, you can greatly reduce your risk by using condoms and maintaining a mutually monogamous relationship with your partner. If diagnosed early, the bacterial STIs can be treated before serious complications occur. The viral STIs are incurable, but there are vaccines for both HPV and hepatitis. HIV/AIDS is the most serious STI, and although treatments have improved, it remains an incurable and life-threatening infection.

More to Explore

American Social Health Association
  http://www.ashastd.org
Centers for Disease Control and Prevention
  http://www.cdc.gov
Joint United Nations Programme on HIV/AIDS
  http://www.unaids.org
MedlinePlus: Infectious Diseases
  http://www.nlm.nih.gov/medlineplus/infections.html
National Institute of Allergy and Infectious Diseases
  http://www.niaid.nih.gov

LAB ACTIVITY 12-1 Infectious Disease Risk Checklist

COMPLETE IN connect

NAME _____   DATE _____   SECTION _____

Equipment: None

Preparation: None

Instructions

Indicate whether each statement is true for you always, sometimes, or never; and fill in the additional information. Any statement for which you don't check "always" indicates an area where you could change your behavior to help reduce your risk for infectious diseases.

Avoiding Pathogens

Always   Sometimes   Never

_____   _____   _____   I frequently wash my hands with soap and water for at least 20 seconds.

_____   _____   _____   I don't rub my eyes, touch my nose, or eat with my fingers without first washing my hands.

_____   _____   _____   When soap and water aren't available, I use alcohol-based hand sanitizer.

If these statements aren't always true for you, describe your typical hand hygiene practices:

_____   _____   _____   I avoid close contact with people who have colds, flu, or other infectious diseases transmitted via touch or respiratory droplets.

_____   _____   _____   I avoid disease carriers such as mosquitoes, ticks, and rodents. To avoid insect disease vectors, I use insect repellent and/or wear long sleeves and pants when necessary.

_____   _____   _____   I never inject drugs (except if medically prescribed).

_____   _____   _____   I follow food safety recommendations (see Chapter 9), including keeping foods at safe temperatures, not thawing foods on the counter, thoroughly cleaning all equipment, and using a food thermometer to check that foods are cooked to a safe temperature.

_____   _____   _____   I have a kit prepared in case of emergencies that disrupt sanitation and other public health services.

Supporting Your Immune System

Always   Sometimes   Never

_____   _____   _____   I exercise regularly.

_____   _____   _____   I eat a healthy diet.

_____   _____   _____   I get plenty of sleep.

____	____	____	I manage my stress.
____	____	____	I don't smoke, and I avoid secondhand smoke.
____	____	____	I consume alcohol moderately, if at all.
____	____	____	My immunizations are up to date, including recommended booster shots.

Check your immunization status against the recommendations in Figure 12-2 and note any vaccines recommended for you that you haven't had.

Assessing Your Risk for Sexually Transmitted Infections

Complete one of the following online assessments for STI risk. Then briefly comment on the experience.
    The Body: http://www.thebody.com/surveys/sexsurvey.html
    STD Wizard: http://www.stdwizard.org
Were you surprised by any of the questions or the results? Did you identify any risk areas that you had been unaware of?

Assessing Your Recent Experiences with Infectious Diseases

To help further identify infectious disease risks in your life, list and describe your three most recent infections. Note the symptoms and duration of your illness, and speculate on how you think you acquired the infection. For each, note one strategy you think might have reduced your risk for contracting the infection or lessened its effects on you.

Reflecting on Your Results

Are you doing all you can to prevent infectious diseases? Note at least three areas in which you could improve your behavior to reduce your risk. Then comment on what you think is holding you back. For example, if you know you should wash your hands more often, why don't you?

Planning Your Next Steps

Choose one behavior that you could change to help reduce your risk for infectious diseases, and develop at least three concrete strategies for making the change. For example, would putting hand-washing reminders in your bathroom or hand sanitizer in your backpack help improve your hand hygiene?

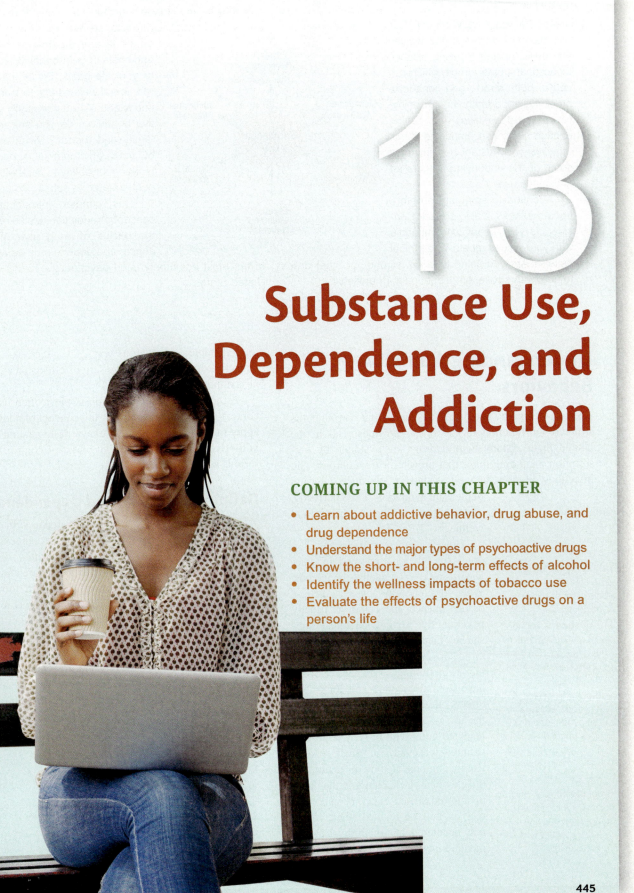

13

Substance Use, Dependence, and Addiction

For overall wellness, you need to be in control of your choices and behavior, but dependence on any substance means that you're not in control. Your physical wellness can be profoundly affected by the choices you make related to using alcohol, tobacco, and other drugs, which can cause both short- and long-term problems. Importantly, though, enjoying physical wellness—by getting enough sleep and managing stress effectively, for instance—eliminates some of the underlying triggers for substance use.

Attention to spiritual and emotional wellness is also crucial. Consider: Is your behavior compatible with your values, goals, and ethical beliefs? Are you using tobacco, alcohol, or other drugs to deal with stress, emotional pain, or anxiety?

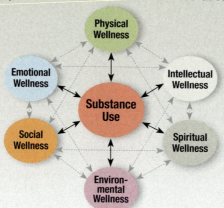

Your intellectual wellness and functioning can be significantly harmed in the short term by many drugs. Make sound choices about substance use and abuse based on a critical evaluation of the risks and costs of your behavior in terms of your life goals. Social and environmental wellness factors are also important: What potentially addictive behaviors do you see in your family and friends? What aspects of your environment support or hinder your ability to stick with your goals related to substance use?

This chapter introduces the concept of addiction. It also reviews the basics of drug use, misuse, abuse, and dependence as applied to the most commonly used psychoactive drugs in the United States.

Understanding Addictive Behaviors

The use of **drugs,** chemical substances that can alter the structure or function of the body, is widespread in the United States. Many helpful drugs are available by prescription, including those that prevent or treat chronic and infectious diseases, as well as those that reduce pain and unpleasant symptoms. Used correctly, many drugs can improve health and wellness.

However, many Americans use drugs for other reasons and in other ways—some potentially dangerous. When it comes to abuse, addiction, or dependence, the culprit is usually **psychoactive drugs,** chemical substances that affect a person's state of mind or consciousness by altering brain functioning. Psychoactive drugs have both immediate and long-term effects on wellness. In the short term, the use of many psychoactive drugs leads to **intoxication**—an abnormal mental state that, in effect, results from being poisoned by the actions of the chemical. Depending on the drug, in an intoxicated state, people may feel excited or relaxed, their mood may be altered, and their physical and mental functioning will be impaired in unpredictable or dangerous ways. Over the long term, psychoactive drugs can also have serious effects on all the wellness dimensions.

Although the term *addiction* is most often used in the context of psychoactive drugs, the concept of addiction can apply more broadly to other behaviors. In general terms, an **addictive behavior** is one that is out of control and has a serious effect on a person's life.

Defining Addiction and Dependence

Q | How do you know if someone is addicted to something? What does that mean?

While often used interchangeably in the context of drug use, the terms *addiction* and *dependence* are quite different. **Drug addiction** is a brain disease with no cure, and this stark reality makes the maintenance of sobriety a lifelong quest. While addiction may contain components of physical and psychological dependence, not all people with physical dependence on a drug go on to develop addiction. However, individuals with a drug addiction will continue to use the drug despite the negative consequences. Signs of drug addiction may include:

- Illegal drug-seeking behaviors
- Drug cravings
- Preoccupation with obtaining the drug
- Drug abuse
- Dependence and withdrawal upon stopping the drug
- Interference with normal life functions
- Relationship problems
- Legal issues

drug A chemical substance that alters the structure or function of the body.

psychoactive drug A drug that alters a person's state of mind or consciousness.

intoxication An abnormal mental state that, in effect, results from being poisoned by the actions of a chemical.

addictive behavior A behavior or habit that is out of control and has a serious effect on the person's life; characterized by craving and compulsive use of a drug.

drug addiction A chronic disease characterized by compulsive, ongoing use of a drug despite serious consequences.

Behavior-Change Challenge
Making Smoking History

You began smoking cigarettes in high school when you hung out with kids who smoked. You've recently seen some shocking TV ads, part of an antismoking campaign by the Centers for Disease Control and Prevention, showing adult smokers with terrible smoking-related health issues. Some have had heart surgery or a *tracheotomy*—the surgical opening-up of the windpipe due to a tumor or other problems. Others have suffered paralysis or lost limbs. You have tried to quit a couple of times before but not very seriously. Now, as a young adult with a baby on the way, you urgently want to quit so that you can avoid these health woes and "be there" as a positive role model for your child.

Meet James

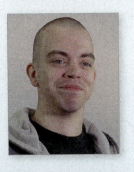

Meet James, a 25-year-old college student who plans to join the Army. He has smoked for 9 years and wants to quit smoking before boot camp. He also doesn't want to smoke around his young daughter. He doesn't smoke many cigarettes a day, but he finds it difficult to quit. In his efforts to change, he is challenged by his stressors as well as by the other smokers in his life. View the video to learn more about James and his quit-smoking plan. As you watch, consider:

- Do you think James has enough motivation and specific strategies for his program to be successful?
- What can you learn from James's experience that will help you in your own behavior-change efforts? What strategies that he adopted can you use or adapt for your own program to quit smoking?

VIDEO CASE STUDY **WATCH THIS VIDEO IN** connect

Drug dependence, in contrast, refers to a state of reliance on a drug to achieve normal physiological functioning. Examples of drug-dependent individuals include diabetics requiring daily insulin and hypertensives needing daily doses of blood pressure–lowering medicine. Abstinence from these drugs can produce withdrawal reactions. In addition, there may be a *physical dependence* (signaled, for example, by vomiting, diarrhea, or sweating) or a *psychological dependence* (manifest, for instance, in inability to concentrate, anxiety, or depression) seen with many prescribed or illicit drugs.

It isn't the amount of time spent on a behavior that defines an addiction;

drug dependence A physiological state in which real or perceived health is dependent continued use of the drug.

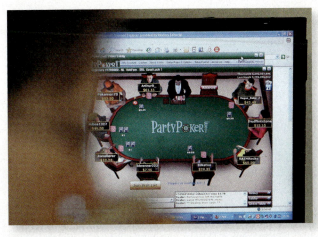

Addiction is most closely associated with use of psychoactive drugs, but any behavior that becomes the focus of a person's life and interferes with day-to-day activities is potentially addictive.

rather, it is the effect of the behavior on a person's life. Addiction is a state that pulls a person away from important responsibilities such as relationships, schoolwork, and job duties and becomes the dominant focus of the individual's life (see Lab Activity 13-1). He or she may experience health-related, financial, and/or legal problems. Despite the negative consequences, the addicted person feels out of control and unable to stop. Associated emotions may include anxiety, guilt, humiliation, hopelessness, and fear. In short, an addiction severely impairs overall functioning and wellness.

Developing Addiction

Q | Why do some people develop addictions?

There is no consensus on why addiction overtakes one person and not another. Multiple factors are involved, including the following:

- *Genes and biology:* Researchers are identifying genes and receptors that make some people more susceptible to addiction. Biological sex and underlying physical and emotional health also play a role. For drugs, it's thought that genetic heritage may account for 40–60 percent of a person's vulnerability to addiction.[1] However, it is clear that having a genetic susceptibility doesn't mean a person will become addicted.
- *Exposure:* Early and frequent exposure to a behavior or substance can increase the risk for addiction.
- *Environment:* Factors such as parental behavior, chaotic or abusive home life, and peer and community attitudes are additional influences.
- *Nature of the behavior or substance:* Behaviors or drugs that cause a rapid change in feelings—a sudden but very brief rush of pleasurable feelings—may be inherently more addicting.

Q How long does it take to become addicted to something? It varies, but addictions don't occur overnight. At first, the behavior may not be at all harmful. Yet over time, there is an increasing desire to engage in the behavior, ultimately resulting in loss of control and negative consequences. In some cases, there is a pattern of escalation, in which a person must take more and more of a substance or engage in a behavior more frequently or for longer periods in order to experience the expected positive result. Over time, an addict has to engage in the behavior just to feel normal.

Just as it takes time to become addicted, it also takes time to treat an addiction effectively. In fact, for some people, beating an addiction can take a lifetime of treatment. Treating an addiction is difficult and usually requires an individual plan developed by an experienced health care professional. Psychologists, psychiatrists, and licensed counselors are often involved in treatment for addiction, and relapses are common. Although treatment success rates are relatively low, many people do succeed in breaking addictions and developing healthier lifestyles. Anyone who experiences loss of control over a behavior—whether or not it involves drugs—should seek early treatment.

Psychoactive Drugs

There are many different and overlapping ways to group and describe drugs and drug use. Substances may be classified as prescription drugs, over-the-counter drugs, or dietary supplements depending on how they are sold and regulated.

Mind Stretcher
Critical Thinking Exercise

Have you ever thought about the difference between addiction and dependence? Most people are more likely to have a dependence (for example, on caffeine) than an addiction. On what substances might you be dependent, for medical reasons or otherwise? Does the dependence have any negative consequences? What do you think it would take to stop the dependence?

Drugs may also be grouped according to their effects, as in the case of antibiotics, stimulants, and sleeping aids.

In terms of abuse and addiction, psychoactive drugs—those that alter mental functioning—are the category of greatest concern. Psychoactive drugs may be legal or illegal depending on whether they have legitimate medical uses (as in the case of painkillers and tranquilizers) or are classified as legal for use by adults (as in the instances of alcohol and tobacco). Misuse or abuse of any drug, legal or illegal, can have serious consequences.

Q What are the most common psychoactive drugs, and who uses them? Among legal psychoactive drugs, caffeine, alcohol, and tobacco are most widely used. With respect to drugs classified as illegal, the most commonly consumed substance is marijuana (Table 13-1).

TABLE 13-1 USE OF PSYCHOACTIVE DRUGS IN THE UNITED STATES*

	PERCENTAGE OF PEOPLE AGE 18–25 YEARS OLD REPORTING USE		
	LIFETIME	PAST YEAR	PAST MONTH
ALCOHOL	84.8%	80.5%	65.8%
CIGARETTES	N/A	33.0%	21.8%
MARIJUANA	25.4%	20.6%	12.4%
COCAINE	3.2%	1.9%	0.8%
INHALANTS	13.3%	6.9%	2.8%
ECSTASY	4.9%	3.6%	1.5%
LSD	2.4%	1.6%	0.7%

*Includes nonmedical use of prescription pain relievers, tranquilizers, sedatives, or stimulants.

Source: Substance Abuse and Mental Health Services Administration. (2010). *Results from the 2010 National Survey on Drug Use and Health: Summary of National Findings.* Rockville, MD: Office of Applied Studies, Substance Abuse and Mental Health Services Administration. http://www.samhsa.gov/data/NSDUH/2k10Results/Web/HTML/2k10Results.htm#2.3.

Notably, the proportion of people who have tried a drug during their lives is much higher than the percentage of current users. Although close to 50 percent of Americans over age 12 have used an illicit drug at least once in their lives, only about 9 percent are current users, with *current* defined as within the past month. Therefore, the vast majority of Americans do not use illicit drugs.

Men are more likely to use psychoactive drugs than women, and rates of use peak among young adults (Figure 13-1). People who are unemployed are more likely to use drugs than those with either full-time or part-time employment. Overall rates of drug use haven't changed substantially over the years, although the use of particular drugs rises and falls. Alcohol consumption among people under age 21 is relatively high—a concern not only because of the immediate risks of intoxication but also because early exposure to alcohol is associated with a greater likelihood of long-term problems.

Geographically, the upper Midwest has the highest rates of overall alcohol use and binge drinking, and the Southeast has the top rates of tobacco use.[2] Caffeine consumption is high across the country.

Misuse and Abuse of Psychoactive Drugs

Q Does all drug misuse or abuse qualify as an addiction? No, it does not, but misuse and abuse can be problematic. **Drug misuse** is the intentional or unintentional use of a medication in ways other than directed or indicated, regardless of whether harm results. Examples of drug misuse include taking twice the dose of a painkiller because the first dose wasn't effective

and giving your prescription sleeping pills to someone else to try.

Drug abuse is any use of a drug that increases the risk of problems for the user or others—problems with physical health, safety, interpersonal relationships, legal status, or meeting school and job responsibilities. The problems may stem from the type or amount of the drug consumed or the situation in which it is used. Drug abuse generally encompasses the use of any illegal drug or the use of a medication with the intent of altering consciousness. Examples of drug abuse include taking LSD or a prescription stimulant to get high, smoking marijuana and then missing a class, and drinking alcohol before driving.

Q Do drugs change how our brain works? Most psychoactive drugs alter the function of *neurons,* cells in the nervous system that are responsible for conducting nerve impulses. Some drugs are chemically similar to the brain's natural chemical messengers (*neurotransmitters*), and so they can activate neurons. This activation may lead to an increased urge for more of the drugs. Other drugs trigger large increases in certain neurotransmitters.

Many drugs act on the brain's reward system,[3] which is activated when we engage in a life-sustaining behavior such as eating. This activation makes us feel good. Because we feel good, we are motivated to repeat the behavior. Drugs can also stimulate the brain's reward center in this way, but with many times the normal number of neurotransmitters. The result is a much greater reaction and one that lasts longer than normal. Over time, however, this brain-reward overload created by the drug use reduces the level of activation of the reward center under normal circumstances. Without the drug, users feel depressed and unable to enjoy activities that they used to find enjoyable. At this point, they need the drug just to bring neurotransmitter levels and brain activity back to normal. This process produces **tolerance**—the condition in which the initial dose(s) of a drug lose effectiveness over time.

Figure 13-2 summarizes key information about the major groups of psychoactive drugs, which include CNS (central nervous system) depressants, CNS stimulants,

drug misuse Intentional or unintentional use of a medication in ways other than directed or intended uses.

drug abuse A harmful pattern of drug use that persists despite negative consequences; may involve continual or intermittent use of a drug.

tolerance The condition in which the initial dose(s) of a drug lose effectiveness over time.

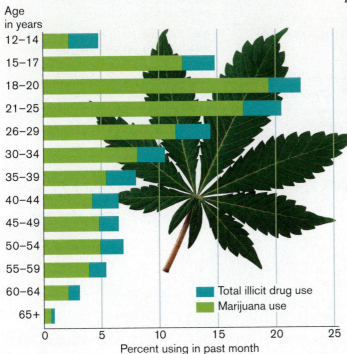

Figure 13-1 Percentage of people age 12 and older who reported any illicit drug use and marijuana use in the past month. Rates of drug use are highest among young adults and fall among older age groups. Marijuana use accounts for most of the illicit drug use in the United States.

Source: Substance Abuse and Mental Health Services Administration. (2010). *Results from the 2009 National Survey on Drug Use and Health.* Rockville, MD: Office of Applied Studies, Substance Abuse and Mental Health Services Administration.

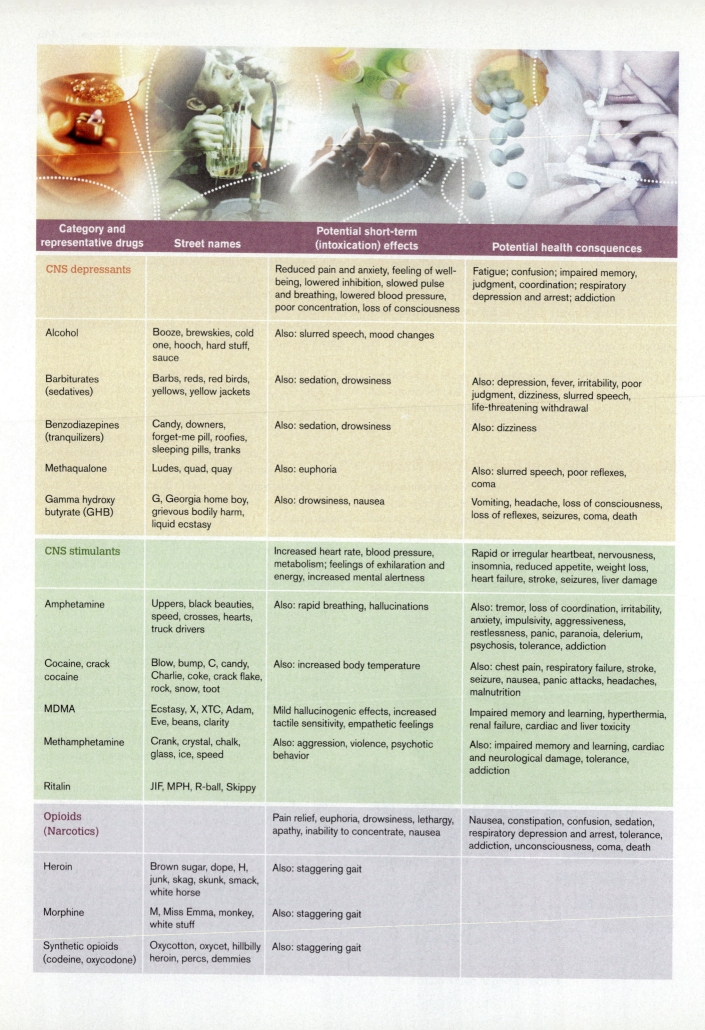

Category and representative drugs	Street names	Potential short-term (intoxication) effects	Potential health consquences
CNS depressants		Reduced pain and anxiety, feeling of well-being, lowered inhibition, slowed pulse and breathing, lowered blood pressure, poor concentration, loss of consciousness	Fatigue; confusion; impaired memory, judgment, coordination; respiratory depression and arrest; addiction
Alcohol	Booze, brewskies, cold one, hooch, hard stuff, sauce	Also: slurred speech, mood changes	
Barbiturates (sedatives)	Barbs, reds, red birds, yellows, yellow jackets	Also: sedation, drowsiness	Also: depression, fever, irritability, poor judgment, dizziness, slurred speech, life-threatening withdrawal
Benzodiazepines (tranquilizers)	Candy, downers, forget-me pill, roofies, sleeping pills, tranks	Also: sedation, drowsiness	Also: dizziness
Methaqualone	Ludes, quad, quay	Also: euphoria	Also: slurred speech, poor reflexes, coma
Gamma hydroxy butyrate (GHB)	G, Georgia home boy, grievous bodily harm, liquid ecstasy	Also: drowsiness, nausea	Vomiting, headache, loss of consciousness, loss of reflexes, seizures, coma, death
CNS stimulants		Increased heart rate, blood pressure, metabolism; feelings of exhilaration and energy, increased mental alertness	Rapid or irregular heartbeat, nervousness, insomnia, reduced appetite, weight loss, heart failure, stroke, seizures, liver damage
Amphetamine	Uppers, black beauties, speed, crosses, hearts, truck drivers	Also: rapid breathing, hallucinations	Also: tremor, loss of coordination, irritability, anxiety, impulsivity, aggressiveness, restlessness, panic, paranoia, delerium, psychosis, tolerance, addiction
Cocaine, crack cocaine	Blow, bump, C, candy, Charlie, coke, crack flake, rock, snow, toot	Also: increased body temperature	Also: chest pain, respiratory failure, stroke, seizure, nausea, panic attacks, headaches, malnutrition
MDMA	Ecstasy, X, XTC, Adam, Eve, beans, clarity	Mild hallucinogenic effects, increased tactile sensitivity, empathetic feelings	Impaired memory and learning, hyperthermia, renal failure, cardiac and liver toxicity
Methamphetamine	Crank, crystal, chalk, glass, ice, speed	Also: aggression, violence, psychotic behavior	Also: impaired memory and learning, cardiac and neurological damage, tolerance, addiction
Ritalin	JIF, MPH, R-ball, Skippy		
Opioids (Narcotics)		Pain relief, euphoria, drowsiness, lethargy, apathy, inability to concentrate, nausea	Nausea, constipation, confusion, sedation, respiratory depression and arrest, tolerance, addiction, unconsciousness, coma, death
Heroin	Brown sugar, dope, H, junk, skag, skunk, smack, white horse	Also: staggering gait	
Morphine	M, Miss Emma, monkey, white stuff	Also: staggering gait	
Synthetic opioids (codeine, oxycodone)	Oxycotton, oxycet, hillbilly heroin, percs, demmies	Also: staggering gait	

Category and representative drugs	Street names	Potential short-term (intoxication) effects	Potential health consequences
Cannabinoids		Euphoria, slowed thinking and reaction time, confusion, anxiety, impaired balance and coordination	Frequent respiratory infections, impaired lung function, cough, impaired memory and learning, increased heart rate, anxiety, panic attacks, sperm abnormalities, tolerance, addiction
Marijuana	Dope, ganja, grass, pot, joint, herb, Mary Jane, reefer, skunk, weed		Also: chronic bronchitis
Hashish	Broom, gangster, hash, hemp		
Inhalants	Laughing gas, poppers, snappers, whippets	Stimulation, loss of inhibition, slurred speech, loss of motor coordination, loss of consciousness, nausea, vomiting, headache	Cramps, weight loss, muscle weakness, memory impairment, hearing loss, bone marrow damage, depression, damage to cardiovascular and nervous systems, sudden death
Hallucinogens		Altered states of perception and feeling, nausea	Persisting perception disorder (flashbacks)
LSD	Acid, boomers, blotter, dots, yellow sunshines	Also: increased body temperature, heart rate, blood pressure, loss of appetite, sleeplessness, tremors, numbness, weakness	Also: impaired memory and learning, cardiac and neurological damage, tolerance, addiction
PCP	Angel dust, hog, love boat, ozone, peace pill, rocket fuel, wack	Also: increased heart rate and blood pressure, impaired motor function, panic, aggression, violence	Also: memory loss, numbness, nausea, vomiting, loss of appetite, depression

Figure 13-2 Effects of commonly abused classes of psychoactive drugs.

Sources: Adapted from National Institute on Drug Abuse. (2007). Commonly abused drugs (http://www.drugabuse.gov/drugpages/drugsofabuse.html). Adapted from National Institute on Drug Abuse. (2007). Selected prescription drugs with potential for abuse (http://www.drugabuse.gov/DrugPages/PrescripDrugs Chart.html).

opioids (narcotics), cannabinoids, inhalants, and halluci-nogens. Review this table to familiarize yourself with these categories, which we will regularly refer to throughout this chapter. In the following sections, we'll briefly review selected psychoactive drugs that are of special concern to college students, including marijuana. Later in the chapter, we'll take an in-depth look at two widely used psychoac-tive drugs that impair health and wellness: alcohol and tobacco.

Caffeine: A Commonly Consumed Psychoactive Drug

Caffeine, a relatively mild central nervous system stimu-lant, is the most widely used psychoactive drug. When people think of caffeine, coffee tends to come to mind. But caffeine is also found in tea, soft drinks, energy drinks, dietary supplements, and some over-the-counter medica-tions, as well as, more recently, in caffeine inhalers. The stimulant effects of caffeine are not as powerful as those from amphetamines and cocaine, but caffeine consumers can both develop tolerance and experience withdrawal, the hallmarks of physical dependence.

Q What is caffeine, and how does it keep me awake?

Although thinking about caffeine tends to bring to mind the dark, aromatic brown beans of coffee, caf-feine is a very bitter pure white crystalline powder. For habitual caffeine drinkers, caffeine is the boost needed to get their day started. Caffeine is found naturally in coffee beans, the leaves of the tea bush, kola nuts, and other plant sources.

The reason that caffeine is so good at keeping us alert is that it affects the action of the neurotransmitter adenosine, which typically makes people feel sleepy. Caffeine can bind to adenosine receptors in the brain, thereby blocking the effects of adenosine. Caffeine also enhances the action of epinephrine in the body. Together these effects result in increased heart rate and physical arousal as well as a sense of mental alertness.

Importantly, although it may seem to promote alertness in someone who is intoxicated from alcohol or other drugs, caffeine does not reduce the effects of other psychoactive drugs. In other words, consuming a caffeine-rich energy drink with alcohol doesn't make a person less intoxicated. In fact, the increased alertness from caffeine may poten-tially harm the intoxicated person by leading the individual

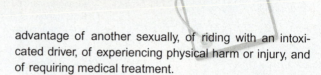

Research Brief

Energy Drinks and Alcohol: A Dangerous Mix

The consumption of a mixed beverage containing energy drinks and alcohol, referred to as ED-A, is popular among U.S. college students. Emerging research suggests that this combination of beverages enhances feelings of intoxication, thereby leading, unfortunately, to risky and potentially harmful behaviors.

To understand these effects, researchers in North Carolina sent a Web-based survey to more than 4,000 college students throughout the state. The study authors found that about one-fourth of all the students who reported drinking any alcohol in the past 30 days also indicated consuming the combination of an energy drink and alcohol. White males, fraternity or sorority members or pledges, and younger students were most likely to have used ED-A. The researchers found that when compared to drinking without using an energy drink, ED-A consumption was associated with almost twice as many days of heavy episodic drinking in the past 30 days (6.4 days versus 3.4 days) and twice as many episodes of weekly drunkenness (1.4 days per week versus 0.73 days per week). In addition, students using ED-A reported higher rates of being taken advantage of sexually, of taking advantage of another sexually, of riding with an intoxicated driver, of experiencing physical harm or injury, and of requiring medical treatment.

There is no question that irresponsible alcohol consumption during college or at any other time leads to negative consequences. What is coming to light now in regard to the latest trend of combining alcohol with energy drinks is that the negative behavioral effects of alcohol are magnified—and are therefore even more dangerous—when energy drinks are added to the mix.

Apply and Analyze

- Does your campus promote energy drinks to students? If so, how do you feel about this type of marketing?
- Should there be restrictions on who can purchase energy drinks, such as only those over 21 years? Why or why not?

Source: O'Brien, M. C., McCoy, T. P., Rhodes, S. D., Wagoner, A., & Wolfson, M. (2008). Caffeinated cocktails: Energy drink consumption, high-risk drinking, and alcohol-related consequences among college students. *Academic Emergency Medicine, 15*(5), 453–460. DOI: 10.1111/j.1553-2712.2008.00085.x.

---

to feel empowered to take on perilous risks. See the box "Energy Drinks and Alcohol: A Dangerous Mix."

Caffeine has other physical effects as well. It causes an increase in the secretion of stomach acid, which can potentially trigger heartburn and indigestion. Also, adenosine is a chemical *vasodilator,* an agent that makes blood vessels relax and open, so blocking it, as caffeine does, causes blood vessels to close and constrict. This effect is the reason for the use of caffeine in some headache medications, as constricted blood vessels decrease the throbbing blood flow to the head. Finally, when consumed at higher-than-usual levels, caffeine disrupts sleep patterns and also acts as a *diuretic,* a substance that increases the rate of urination.

Q | What product has the most caffeine?

The top sources of caffeine for American adults are coffee, soft drinks and energy drinks, and tea, although these drinks vary in the amount of caffeine they provide (Table 13-2). Researchers estimate that close to 90 percent of all Americans age 2 and older consume some caffeine, with rates highest among young and middle-aged adults.[4] Average consumption is about 200–250 milligrams per day, which is considered a moderate level. Some individuals consume much more.

Many athletes use caffeine, and studies have shown some benefit for performance in events requiring long-term endurance, short-term high-intensity effort, and repeated bouts of effort.[5] However, not everyone obtains a benefit or the same degree of benefit. The National Collegiate Athletic Association sets a limit on caffeine consumption as measured through urine testing; the level is set to allow ordinary levels of caffeine consumption but to ban high intake levels.

Q | Is caffeine addictive or even that bad?

While addiction to caffeine is possible, dependence is much more common. Also, caffeine users develop tolerance, which along with dependence creates symptoms of withdrawal if intake drops. People who habitually consume caffeine need the drug to return to a normal level of alertness and to reduce withdrawal symptoms, which include headache, irritability, anxiety, loss of concentration, and fatigue.

For most people, the equivalent of about two 8-ounce cups of coffee a day is considered a moderate and safe caffeine intake. This amount is based on the recommendation of no more than about 1.4 milligrams of caffeine per pound of body weight, or about 200 milligrams of caffeine a day for someone who weighs 150 pounds (see Table 13-2). Moderate

TABLE 13-2 COMMON SOURCES OF CAFFEINE

	SERVING SIZE	CAFFEINE (MG)
COFFEE, DRIP BREWED	6 oz	60–150
COFFEE, INSTANT	6 oz	50–90
COFFEE, ESPRESSO	1 oz	30–50
TEA, BREWED	6 oz	40–80
ENERGY DRINKS	8 oz	50–180
SOFT DRINKS	12 oz	20–70
CHOCOLATE, MILK	1 oz	2–15
CHOCOLATE, DARK	1 oz	5–35
CANDY, DARK CHOCOLATE–COATED COFFEE BEANS	10 pieces	120
VIVARIN/DEXATRIM	1 tablet	200
NODOZ	1 tablet	100
ANACIN	1 tablet	32

Source: U.S. Department of Agriculture, Agricultural Research Service. (2011). *USDA national nutrient database for standard reference,* Release 22. Nutrient Data Laboratory home page (http://www.ars.usda.gov/ba/bhnrc/ndl).

caffeine intake is associated with a number of positive health effects, including a reduced risk of type 2 diabetes [6] and improved cognitive function in Alzheimer's disease.[7]

As just described, high caffeine intake can have adverse effects. In the short term, these may include nervousness, restlessness, muscle twitching, rambling thoughts and speech, facial flushing, gastrointestinal disturbance, and sleep problems. A high dose of caffeine can also affect heart rate and rhythm, in so doing potentially posing a danger for people with underlying cardiovascular disease.

As Table 13-2 illustrates, there is a wide range of caffeine content across different products. Therefore, it's vital to check labels on beverages, supplements, and over-the-counter drugs to avoid unknowingly consuming a much larger caffeine dose than you might expect.

Marijuana

Q If marijuana is just a plant, then how is it a drug?

Marijuana is a mixture of leaves, flowers, stems, and seeds from the hemp plant, *Cannabis sativa.* This plant contains a psychoactive chemical, delta-9-tetrahydrocannabinol, or THC, making it a drug. Marijuana is mostly consumed through smoking, which allows THC to pass very rapidly from the lungs into the bloodstream and then into the brain. The drug causes intoxication that can last several hours. Like many psychoactive drugs, it also affects the brain's reward system, causing a euphoric high. As well, it affects the brain areas involved in memory, thinking, concentration, coordination, movement, and sensory and time perception.[8]

Q How does smoking marijuana affect the body?

In the short term, marijuana use produces physical, cognitive, emotional, and behavioral effects. The physical changes include an increase in heart rate; dilation of the blood vessels in the eyes, causing bloodshot eyes; reduction of the blood's capacity to carry oxygen; and enlargement of the bronchial passages. These effects impair exercise performance and may increase short-term risk of a heart attack.[9] Marijuana use also disrupts motor coordination and balance and slows reaction time.

In terms of cognitive functioning, marijuana impairs judgment, attention, the ability to form new memories, and facility at quickly shifting focus from one topic to another.

Research Brief

Marijuana and the Workplace

Researchers have documented various negative acute and chronic effects of marijuana, but there is little published information on the impact of marijuana use on cognitive function as it relates to the workplace. Recently a group of researchers identified worksites employing both users and nonusers of marijuana to study the workplace effects of cannabis use, including the drug's impact on cognitive performance, mood, and human error.

Marijuana users and non-users in this study were asked to complete laboratory tests measuring mood and cognitive function and to maintain daily diaries reporting their work performance. The tests were administered before and after individual workdays and also at the start and end of a given work week. The results of these tests indicated impairment of both cognitive function and mood in individuals identified as regular marijuana users. Marijuana use was also associated with lower alertness and slower response time. At the start of the work week, marijuana users had certain memory problems, which seemed to resolve by the end of the work week. Their ability to recall specific instances of things, however, became worse, and so did other brain functions.

Although it is difficult to know the exact cause of these cognitive impairments in the marijuana users, there are two distinct possibilities. The first possibility is that an increase in frequency of use might lead to a "hangover" effect in which there is chronic residual impairment. Another potential explanation is that the negative effects of the marijuana may be exacerbated under cognitive load and/or fatigue. These effects may also worsen with prolonged marijuana use.

Analyze and Apply

- What are some obstacles that might be encountered by researchers who seek to study the effects of drug use on workplace performance?
- What are the implications of this study's findings for work settings that involve dangerous processes and/or heavy machinery?

Source: Wadsworth, E. J. K., Moss, S.C., Simpson, S.A., & Smith, A. P. (2006). Cannabis use, cognitive performance and mood in a sample of workers. *Journal of Psychopharmacology, 20*(1), 14–23.

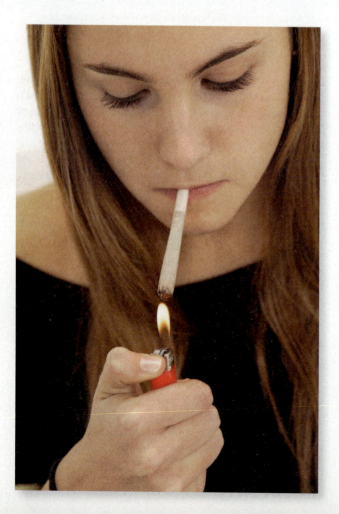

These cognitive effects can last for days or even weeks after the period of intoxication, making learning difficult. Therefore, a daily marijuana user is likely to be operating with reduced cognitive and intellectual functioning. Some users also experience more dramatic intoxication effects, including hallucinations, delusions, and loss of personal identity. For insight into how marijuana use affects job performance, see the box "Marijuana and the Workplace."

Taken together, the changes associated with marijuana use affect a person's ability to drive safely, and marijuana intoxication is associated with increased risk of being in a crash and causing a crash.[10] Further, the risk of driving under the influence of both alcohol and marijuana is greater than the risk of driving under the influence of either drug alone.[11]

The long-term effects of habitual marijuana use are more difficult to study. For example, it's hard to say if marijuana is better or worse for health than cigarettes. We know that tobacco users have enormously high rates of lung cancer, yet the evidence on long-term marijuana use is less conclusive. This inconclusiveness stems in part because of marijuana's illegal status, meaning that it is much more difficult to track users and identify negative outcomes. Also because it is illegal, people are less likely to be lifetime users, in contrast to many cigarette smokers, and are also likely to smoke smaller amounts of marijuana (fewer joints than cigarettes). However, like tobacco smoke, marijuana smoke does contain carcinogenic chemicals, and frequent users of marijuana may experience problems like daily cough, excess mucus production, more frequent acute respiratory illnesses, and a heightened risk of chronic lung disease.[12]

Chronic marijuana use has also been linked to a number of mental health problems, including increased rates of anxiety, depression, suicidal thinking, and schizophrenia. At the present time, the strongest evidence links marijuana use and schizophrenia and related disorders.[13] Marijuana can also disrupt sleep patterns.

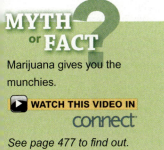

MYTH or FACT?

Marijuana gives you the munchies.

▶ **WATCH THIS VIDEO IN** connect

See page 477 to find out.

Q | Is marijuana addictive?

Long-term marijuana abuse can lead to addiction, and the need for greater psychoactive effects can progress to dependency. Problems with controlling and stopping marijuana use are most prevalent in people who start using the drug in their teens. Similarly to habitual abusers of other drugs, long-term marijuana abusers who are trying to quit complain of withdrawal symptoms such as irritability, sleeplessness, decreased appetite, anxiety, and drug craving. Withdrawal symptoms typically start and peak within a few days and tend to subside within 1 or 2 weeks following drug cessation.[14]

Marijuana is responsible for about 15 percent of all admissions to drug treatment facilities in the United States. A worrisome trend is that more than 50 percent of all marijuana treatment patients reported abusing the drug by age 14, and over 90 percent by age 18.[15]

Ecstasy (MDMA)

Q | What is Ecstasy, and what problems does it cause?

Ecstasy, also known by the abbreviation for its chemical name, MDMA, has properties of both stimulants and hallucinogens. MDMA affects several neurotransmitters, producing feelings of stimulation, emotional warmth, and well-being, as well as distortions in the user's sense of time and sensory perception. Less positive effects include nausea, involuntary teeth clenching, muscle cramps, and blurred vision.

Ecstasy consumption is associated with a range of problems, some of them potentially perilous. MDMA increases heart rate and blood pressure; it also raises body temperature, which in rare cases can lead to dehydration and kidney failure. In 2010, two known clusters of Ecstasy overdoses, associated with large-scale raves on the West Coast, resulted in several deaths.[16] MDMA also significantly reduces mental abilities, including information processing and memory formation. Some research has moreover found that heavy Ecstasy use can damage specific types of nerve cells in the brain. The drug can be addictive in some people.

The effects of Ecstasy can be hard to quantify because, as an unregulated street drug, MDMA is often sold in tablets that contain other drugs such as methamphetamine and

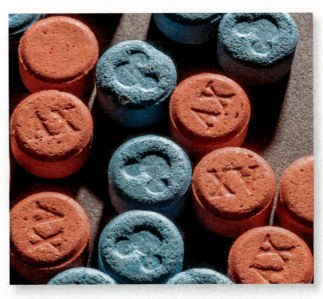

Ecstasy has both stimulant and hallucinogenic effects. It may be particularly dangerous when consumed with alcohol because it increases alertness and can mask the intoxicating effects of alcohol.

caffeine. Users also often mix MDMA with other drugs, especially alcohol. The combination of alcohol and Ecstasy may be especially dangerous because the stimulant effect of MDMA makes an alcohol-intoxicated person feel more alert, even though her or his motor skills are significantly impaired by alcohol.[17] As in the case of combining caffeine consumption with alcohol consumption, it is a real danger to be drunk and highly alert, because such a state makes a person more likely than usual to engage in high-risk behaviors.

Nonmedical Use of Prescription Drugs

Q | Are oxycodone and similar drugs still a problem?

The nonmedical use of prescription drugs remains a problem in the United States, in part because these drugs are often readily accessible at home. Some of the most commonly abused prescription drugs are pain relievers like hydrocodone and acetaminophen (Vicodin) and oxycodone (OxyContin) and the anti-anxiety/ADHD drugs methylphenidate (Ritalin), amphetamine and dextroamphetamine (Adderall), and alprazolam (Xanax). Tranquilizers, stimulants, and sedatives are also commonly abused. Although viewed by some people as safer options because they aren't street drugs, prescription drugs can be dangerous and even deadly when not used as indicated. Deaths due to overdoses on opioid drugs now represent more than a third of all poisoning deaths each year—in excess of 14,000 deaths annually.[18] The risks from these drugs are also greater when they are combined with alcohol or other drugs.

If you or someone you know has a problem with any type of psychoactive drug, get help. Resources can be found by visiting the Substance Abuse and Mental Health Services Administration (http://www.samhsa.gov) or calling its telephone hotline (1-800-662-HELP).

Alcohol

In the past month, about half of all Americans age 12 and over consumed alcohol at least one time. People use alcohol to relax, unwind, and decrease inhibitions, and alcohol consumption is widely accepted and often a part of social gatherings and celebrations. Drinking alcohol can be beneficial or harmful, depending on the situation, the individual's age and health status, and the amount consumed. Most Americans drink moderately or not at all, but problem drinking affects everyone.

National laws regulate the use of alcohol, primarily for health and safety reasons, but not a day goes by where these regulations aren't violated. Rates of drinking and driving are still remarkably high; alcohol is frequently purchased for, supplied to, or consumed by underage individuals; and many people regularly consume more alcohol than their bodies can tolerate. Although the legal drinking age is 21, people between ages 12 and 20 consume almost 20 percent of all alcohol consumed in the United States.[19] And although people who drink heavily and frequently represent only 7 percent of the population, they drink 45 percent of all the alcohol.[20]

Excessive or unsafe alcohol consumption has many dire consequences. Drunk drivers routinely kill others and themselves, and alcohol abuse frequently plays a role in domestic violence, sexual abuse, unintended pregnancies, firearm injuries, and boating accidents. Regularly drinking too much alcohol leads to a host of health problems, including the risk for alcoholism. Researchers estimate that alcohol is responsible for 85,000 deaths in the United States each year.

Alcohol may provide short-term pleasure and even excitement. However, a wise person recognizes that these transient pleasures come with real and significant risks. For wellness, you need to balance the risks and benefits of alcohol use and make wise choices. One option might be not using alcohol at all, and another is choosing to use it only moderately and in situations that do not place yourself or others at risk.

Alcoholic Beverages and Drinking Patterns

Q What is alcohol, and what counts as a drink?

The psychoactive, intoxicating substance found in all alcoholic beverages is **ethyl alcohol,** commonly referred to just as *alcohol.* The National Institute on Alcohol Abuse and Alcoholism (NIAAA) defines 1 drink as the amount of a beverage that contains 0.6 ounce (14 grams) of pure alcohol. The concentration of alcohol varies in different beverages; see Figure 13-3.

One drink is the equivalent of 12 ounces of beer, 5 ounces of table

ethyl alcohol The intoxicating psychoactive drug found in alcoholic beverages; also called *alcohol.*

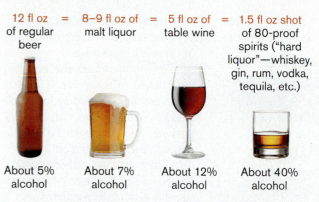

| 12 fl oz of regular beer | = | 8–9 fl oz of malt liquor | = | 5 fl oz of table wine | = | 1.5 fl oz shot of 80-proof spirits ("hard liquor"—whiskey, gin, rum, vodka, tequila, etc.) |
| About 5% alcohol | | About 7% alcohol | | About 12% alcohol | | About 40% alcohol |

Figure 13-3 A standard drink. Each drink contains about 0.6 ounce of alcohol.

Source: National Institute on Alcohol Abuse and Alcoholism. (2010). *Rethinking drinking: Alcohol and your health.* NIH Pub. No. 10-3770.

wine, or a 1.5-ounce shot of 80-proof distilled liquor. The term *proof* refers to the alcohol content of hard liquor. Proof is twice the percentage of alcohol in a beverage; so, for example, 80-proof liquor is 40 percent alcohol by volume. In contrast, most beers are 3–6 percent alcohol by volume. An additional helpful measurement is the number of drinks in a typical container:

- Regular bottle (750 milliliters) of table wine = 5 drinks
- Half-pint bottle (200 milliliters) of 80-proof liquor = 4½ drinks
- A fifth (750 milliliters) of 80-proof liquor = 17 drinks

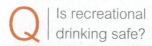

Q Is recreational drinking safe?

Whether or not "recreational" drinking is safe depends on the amount consumed and the circumstances. The National Institute on Alcohol Abuse and Alcoholism (NIAAA) has defined a daily and a weekly limit for what is called a low-risk drinking pattern (Figure 13-4). The limits are lower for women than for men because women tend to be smaller, to have higher levels of body fat, and to absorb alcohol more quickly due to lower activity of alcohol-metabolizing enzymes in the stomach (alcohol dehydrogenase or ADH). Together, these differences mean that a woman will have a higher blood alcohol concentration than a man who consumes the same amount of alcohol. Men and women who stay within both limits for alcohol consumption have much lower rates of alcohol abuse and alcoholism than those who exceed one or both of them.

However, it's important to note that low-risk drinking does not eliminate risk. Even within these limits, drinkers can have problems, especially if they drink quickly, drink unsafely, have underlying health issues, or have struggled with alcohol use in the past. For example, consuming up to the number of drinks representing the daily limit in a very short period of time can lead to intoxication.

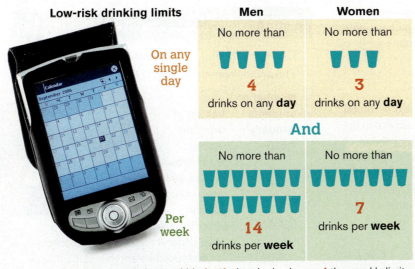

Low-risk drinking limits

Men	Women
On any single day No more than **4** drinks on any **day**	No more than **3** drinks on any **day**

And

| **Per week** No more than **14** drinks per **week** | No more than **7** drinks per **week** |

To stay low-risk, keep within **both** the single-day **and** the weekly limits.

Figure 13-4 Low-risk drinking limits.
Source: National Institute on Alcohol Abuse and Alcoholism. (2010). *Rethinking drinking: Alcohol and your health.* NIH Pub. No. 10-3770.

For the sake of health and safety, some people need to drink less or not at all. People who should never drink include:

- Women who are pregnant or trying to become pregnant
- People who plan to drive or engage in other activities that require alertness and skill
- People taking certain over-the-counter or prescription medications
- People with medical conditions that can be made worse by drinking
- Recovering alcoholics
- People younger than age 21

Individuals who exceed the limits recommended by the NIAAA are either at great risk for alcohol abuse or alcoholism or have already developed a problem with alcohol. The majority of adults either don't drink or drink at low-risk levels, but a substantial number of Americans have drinking patterns that place themselves and others at risk (Figure 13-5). Heavy drinkers who haven't yet developed a serious alcohol-related problem can reduce their risk of harmful effects by cutting back. For people with alcoholism or a serious alcohol problem, quitting is the safest strategy.

Q | What is meant by binge drinking?

The term *binge drinking* has traditionally referred to consuming a significant number of drinks—5 or more for men and 4 or more for women—in a relatively short period of time, usually within 2 hours. However, more current terminology refers to this pattern as *heavy episodic drinking (HED)*, as it isolates the incidence to a single episode. A more contemporary usage of **binge drinking** is to describe excessive drinking over an extended period of time, usually a number of days or weeks. Both HED and binge drinking can cause intoxication and drive blood alcohol concentration up to an unsafe level. HED is unquestionably a problem on college campuses, where students may party sporadically but heavily.

Students who frequently engage in HED are much more likely to drive after drinking, to be injured, to have unplanned or unprotected sex, to miss classes and get behind in school work, and to argue with their friends (Figure 13-6). Further, nondrinking students are affected by their peers who engage in HED: They may experience property damage, unwanted sexual advances, verbal insults, physical violence, and

binge drinking Excessive drinking continued over a period of days.

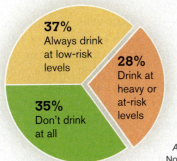

Figure 13-5 Alcohol use by U.S. adults.
Source: National Institute on Alcohol Abuse and Alcoholism. (2010). *Rethinking drinking: Alcohol and your health.* NIH Pub. No. 10-3770.

- 37% Always drink at low-risk levels
- 28% Drink at heavy or at-risk levels
- 35% Don't drink at all

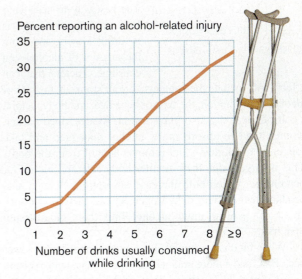

Percent reporting an alcohol-related injury

Number of drinks usually consumed while drinking

Figure 13-6 Drinking and injury rates among college students. Alcohol-related injuries are most common among students whose typical drinking pattern fits the definition of binge drinking.

Source: Wechsler, H., & Nelson, T. F. (2008). What we have learned from the Harvard School of Public Health College Alcohol Study: Focusing attention on college student alcohol consumption and the environmental conditions that promote it. *Journal of Studies on Alcohol and Drugs, 69*(4), 481–490.

interrupted sleep or studies. Binge drinking is the reason for most alcohol-related deaths among college students, with alcohol overdose and injuries being the main cause.

Short-Term Effects of Alcohol Use

The immediate effects of alcohol are determined by **blood alcohol concentration (BAC),** the amount of alcohol in the blood in terms of weight of alcohol per unit volume of blood, expressed as a percentage. BAC directly relates to the degree of intoxication. BAC depends on the amount of alcohol consumed and on individual factors such as biological sex, body weight, the rate of alcohol consumption, and whether the person has eaten.

Q I'm a big guy. Can my blood alcohol level really go up a lot?

BLOOD ALCOHOL CONCENTRATION (BAC). Depending on how much and how fast you drink, your blood alcohol certainly can rise significantly. A larger person can drink more than a smaller one before becoming significantly impaired, but any alcohol consumption has an effect on BAC (see Table 13-3). Moreover, the higher your BAC, the greater the impairment in your motor skills, judgment, and behavior. BAC is also the measure used for defining drunk driving, with the legal blood alcohol limit being 0.08 percent for anyone over 21 years. For individuals under age 21, zero tolerance laws are in effect, and a BAC of 0.02 percent or higher is considered above the legal limit for this age group.

Q What should I eat before drinking to keep my BAC down?

The best way to keep your BAC in the safe range is to drink slowly and limit the amount of alcohol you consume. Factors that can affect BAC include the contents of your stomach, the rate of alcohol consumption, the type of beverage, and body weight.

Biological sex also plays a role. As described earlier, women tend to absorb more alcohol than men and take longer to break down and remove alcohol from the body. This is largely due their smaller body size and higher fat percentage, which both increase absorption. Women also produce less alcohol dehydrogenase and therefore absorb about 30 percent more alcohol into their bloodstream than men.

When food is consumed along with alcohol, both a lower peak BAC and a more gradual increase in BAC tend to occur. Because alcohol is absorbed most efficiently in the small intestine, anything that prevents or inhibits alcohol from moving there slows the increase in BAC. With food in the stomach, the valve at the bottom of the stomach closes in order to hold food in, keeping

blood alcohol concentration (BAC) A measure of intoxication; the amount of alcohol in the blood in terms of weight of alcohol per unit volume of blood, expressed as a percentage.

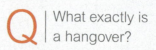
alcohol there also. Alcohol can still be absorbed from the stomach, but much more slowly. There is no conclusive evidence that any specific type of food in the stomach will dramatically alter the rate of alcohol absorption. However, the lesson is that it is important to eat something—to avoid drinking alcohol on an empty stomach.

Q What exactly is a hangover?

HANGOVERS. A hangover is the body's way of telling you that you drank too much. Most people who drink to intoxication can expect a hangover to follow. Symptoms may last from 8–24 hours and include the following:[21]

- Fatigue, lethargy, weakness, thirst
- Headache and muscle aches
- Nausea, vomiting, painful or upset stomach

TABLE 13-3 EFFECTS OF DIFFERENT LEVELS OF BLOOD ALCOHOL CONCENTRATION

BLOOD ALCOHOL CONCENTRATION (%)	TYPICAL EFFECTS
0.01–0.05	Sense of well-being, relaxation, loss of inhibitions; reduced ability to perform two tasks at the same time; impaired judgment and alertness
0.06–0.10	Pleasure, emotional arousal, numbness of feelings, nausea, sleepiness; impaired memory, self-control, motor coordination, and visual tracking
0.11–0.20	Mood swings, anger, mania, sadness, loss of balance; exaggerated emotions and inappropriate social behavior; nausea and vomiting; impaired reasoning, concentration, information processing, and depth perception
0.21–0.30	Aggression, depression, reduced response to pain and stimulation, stupor, slurred speech, inability to stand or walk; loss of temperature regulation and bowel and bladder control
0.31–0.40	Unconsciousness, slowed heart rate, difficulty breathing, coma; death possible from respiratory paralysis
0.41 AND ABOVE	Coma, death

Sources: Adapted from National Highway Traffic Safety Administration. (2005). *The ABCs of BAC.* DOT HS Publication 809 844. BCS/National Institute on Alcohol Abuse and Alcoholism. (2003). *Understanding alcohol: Investigations into biology and behavior.* NIH Pub. No. 04-4991.

- Decreased sleep, disturbed sleep patterns
- Sensitivity to light and sound, vertigo
- Depression, irritability, anxiety
- Decreased attention and concentration
- Tremors, sweating, and increased heart rate and blood pressure

Hangover symptoms may be due in part to the direct effects of alcohol, which can cause mild dehydration, electrolyte imbalance, gastrointestinal upset, low blood sugar, and sleep disturbances. A habitual drinker may experience symptoms of alcohol withdrawal after drinking stops. Different alcoholic beverages also contain other ingredients that may also contribute to hangover symptoms.

The best approach to hangovers is to avoid them by not drinking to intoxication. Coffee doesn't help sober a person up. Neither do cold showers or fresh air. The only way to sober up is to wait for your body to absorb and metabolize all the alcohol you've consumed. BAC generally peaks 30–90 minutes after drinking, though the rate of metabolism varies with the individual, but it generally takes about 2 hours per drink for the body's BAC to return to zero.[22] Thus, if you consume 3 drinks in an hour, it will take about 6 hours for your body to completely absorb and metabolize all the alcohol.

Strategies for treating hangover symptoms include replacing lost fluids by drinking nonalcoholic beverages, eating (if possible), and resting. Soup is a good choice for replacing depleted electrolytes. If you take a pain reliever, don't choose acetaminophen, because it can cause liver damage when combined with alcohol. Also keep in mind that hangovers are linked to reduced cognitive functioning and motor skills, so avoid driving or engaging in other potentially risky activities until your hangover symptoms subside.[23]

Importantly, "sleeping it off" is different from passing out. With moderate drinking, there is no worry about getting some sleep and being sober afterward. However, passing out, which can occur in someone who drinks rapidly, can prove fatal if a lethal dose of alcohol was consumed and if the signs of alcohol poisoning haven't been recognized. In this situation, the "sleeping" individual may actually be unconscious and at risk for fatal respiratory failure. See the box "Handling an Alcohol Emergency" for additional information on what to do in cases of *alcohol poisoning*—suspected alcohol overdose.

Mind Stretcher
Critical Thinking Exercise

Have you ever said or done anything under the influence of alcohol or other drugs that you regretted later? What were the consequences, and how did you deal with them? Did you change your behavior so it didn't happen again? Do you think it is right to excuse or discount things people say or do while intoxicated?

Wellness Strategies

Handling an Alcohol Emergency

Q | What should I do to help a friend who is dangerously drunk?

A fatal dose of alcohol depresses the nerves that control involuntary actions like breathing and the gag reflex. It is common for someone who drank excessive alcohol to vomit because alcohol is an irritant to the stomach. There is then the danger of choking on vomit, which can cause death by asphyxiation in a person who is not conscious because of intoxication. Never assume that someone who drinks heavily and falls asleep is OK and can be left alone.

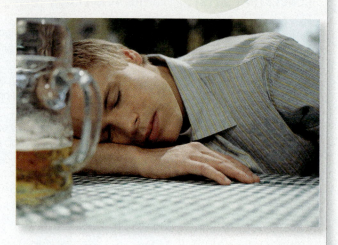

What can happen to someone with alcohol poisoning who goes untreated?

- Victim chokes on his or her own vomit
- Breathing slows, becomes irregular, or stops
- Heart beats irregularly or stops
- Hypothermia sets in
- Hypoglycemia (too little blood sugar) leads to seizures
- Untreated severe dehydration from vomiting can cause seizures, permanent brain damage, or death

What are signs and symptoms of alcohol poisoning?

- Mental confusion, stupor, or coma, or the person appears to be sleeping but cannot be wakened
- Vomiting
- Seizures
- Slow breathing (fewer than eight breaths per minute)
- Irregular breathing (10 seconds or more between breaths)
- Hypothermia (low body temperature), bluish skin color, paleness

What should I do if I suspect someone has alcohol poisoning?

- Be aware that a person who has passed out may die; don't wait for all the symptoms to be present before you act. Do not assume that the person will sleep it off or would prefer not to be disturbed.
- If there is any suspicion of an alcohol overdose, call 911. Don't try to guess the level of drunkenness.
- Roll the person on his or her side to lessen the risk of choking on vomit.
- Tell the ambulance driver or medical personnel if you believe that other drugs were also ingested.

Don't be afraid to seek medical help for a friend who has had too much to drink. Don't worry that your friend may become angry or embarrassed. Always be safe, not sorry.

Source: Adapted from National Institute on Alcohol Abuse and Alcoholism. (2010). Facts about alcohol poisoning. *College Drinking* (http://www.collegedrinkingprevention.gov/OtherAlcoholInformation/factsAboutAlcoholPoisoning.aspx).

Q | How bad is it to drink and drive?

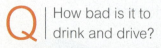

DRINKING AND DRIVING. Mixing drinking and driving is very bad. In any given year more than 30 percent of all annual traffic fatalities in the United States are due to drunk drivers.[24] The risk of being involved in a crash goes up dramatically with increasing BAC, but driving skills are impaired even at relatively low BACs (Figure 13-7). The effects of alcohol on driving skills are especially dramatic for young adults, who tend to have less driving experience and higher rates of overall risky driving. Males are also more likely to be involved in alcohol-related motor vehicle crashes than females, and weekend nights are the most dangerous time to be on the road.

Drinking and driving also carries significant legal penalties and financial costs. The impact varies by location and situation (first versus repeat offense), but even if you don't hit anyone or anything, you can expect the following expenses:

- Bail
- Cost of towing and storing your vehicle
- Court and lawyer fees, fines
- Cost of alcohol education classes
- License reinstatement fees
- Increased insurance premiums for many years

Actual costs from losses and damage often exceed $10,000. You will also lose time at work and school and possibly

Figure 13-7 Risk of motor vehicle crashes, by sex, age, and blood alcohol concentration. The risk of being in an alcohol-related vehicle crash goes up dramatically with increasing BAC, but even a low level of alcohol increases risk. Crash risk is especially high for young adults, particularly young males. Never drink and drive. To estimate your blood alcohol concentration, visit the BAC calculator (http://www.dot.wisconsin.gov/safety/motorist/drunkdriving/calculator.htm).

Source: Data from National Highway Traffic Safety Administration. (2000). *Relative risk of fatal crash involvement by BAC, age, and gender.* DOT HS 809 050.

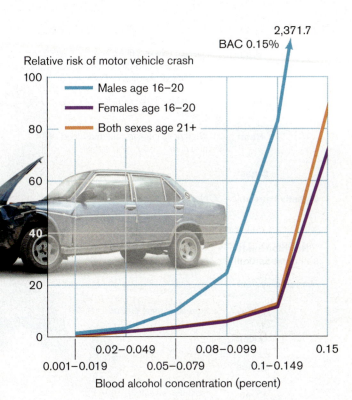

lose your job. Some jobs require a vehicle, and some companies will not hire people with open court cases or criminal records.

Long-Term Health Effects of Alcohol Use

In addition to the immediate effects related to intoxication, alcohol use over an extended period also impairs health and wellness. Alcohol use during pregnancy has long-lasting effects as well.

Q | **Isn't the liver affected by drinking alcohol?**

The liver is the main site of alcohol metabolism in the body, and even moderate drinkers can experience liver damage:

- *Fatty liver:* This condition, characterized by liver cells swollen with fat and water, can usually be reversed if alcohol use stops.
- *Hepatitis:* As described in Chapter 12, inflammation of the liver is often due to a viral infection, but it can also be caused by alcohol use. In some cases, hepatitis can lead to liver failure, liver cancer, and death.
- *Cirrhosis:* In individuals affected with the incurable disease **cirrhosis,** liver cells are replaced with scar tissue and the liver can no longer function. A liver transplant is the only treatment.

The liver is not the only organ affected by chronic alcohol use—nearly every body system is involved (Figure 13-8). Heavy drinking, particularly over time, can damage the heart and lead to high blood pressure, *cardiomyopathy* (enlarged and weakened heart), congestive heart failure, and stroke. Heavy drinking also puts more fat into the circulatory system, raising the triglyceride level and thereby increasing the risk of heart disease.

Q | **Is drinking alcohol good for my heart?**

Heavy drinking is not good for your heart or most other organs. However, moderate alcohol consumption, defined as 1–2 drinks per day for men and about 1 per day for women, has been reported to decrease the incidence of cardiovascular disease as well as all-cause mortality. This is known as a *J-curve response* because

cirrhosis A liver disease in which cells are replaced by fibrous scar tissue; can be caused by excessive long-term alcohol use.

nondrinkers have a slightly higher rate of CVD and premature death than moderate drinkers, but people who drink more than moderate amounts of alcohol have an increasingly greater risk of death.

Researchers are still studying the potential positive effects of alcohol. One potential benefit is that moderate drinkers tend to have higher levels of beneficial HDL (good cholesterol) than nondrinkers. Moderate alcohol consumption also appears to decrease the stickiness of blood cells called *platelets,* reducing the formation of clots that can potentially cause heart attacks and strokes.

Not all the news about moderate drinking is good, however. For women, moderate drinking raises the risk of breast cancer. Anyone with a family or personal history of alcohol abuse also needs to take special care. Further, occasionally engaging in HED on top of moderate intake undoes any benefit from moderate drinking. You need to evaluate the role of alcohol in your life based on your own personal risk factors and situation.

Q | **During pregnancy, how much alcohol is too much?**

No level of alcohol intake has been proven safe during pregnancy. The Centers for Disease Control and Prevention (CDC) recommends that women should not drink alcohol if they are pregnant, if they are planning to become pregnant, or if they are sexually active and do not use effective birth control. Drinking increases the risk of miscarriage and premature delivery, and it can cause a range of lifelong disorders in infants, known as

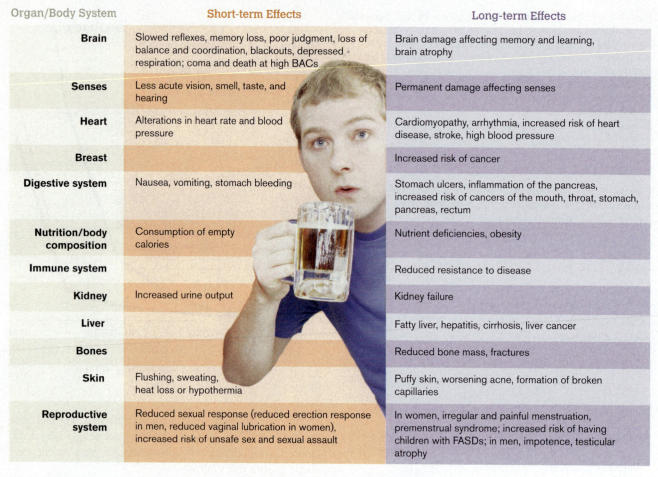

Organ/Body System	Short-term Effects	Long-term Effects
Brain	Slowed reflexes, memory loss, poor judgment, loss of balance and coordination, blackouts, depressed respiration; coma and death at high BACs	Brain damage affecting memory and learning, brain atrophy
Senses	Less acute vision, smell, taste, and hearing	Permanent damage affecting senses
Heart	Alterations in heart rate and blood pressure	Cardiomyopathy, arrhythmia, increased risk of heart disease, stroke, high blood pressure
Breast		Increased risk of cancer
Digestive system	Nausea, vomiting, stomach bleeding	Stomach ulcers, inflammation of the pancreas, increased risk of cancers of the mouth, throat, stomach, pancreas, rectum
Nutrition/body composition	Consumption of empty calories	Nutrient deficiencies, obesity
Immune system		Reduced resistance to disease
Kidney	Increased urine output	Kidney failure
Liver		Fatty liver, hepatitis, cirrhosis, liver cancer
Bones		Reduced bone mass, fractures
Skin	Flushing, sweating, heat loss or hypothermia	Puffy skin, worsening acne, formation of broken capillaries
Reproductive system	Reduced sexual response (reduced erection response in men, reduced vaginal lubrication in women), increased risk of unsafe sex and sexual assault	In women, irregular and painful menstruation, premenstrual syndrome; increased risk of having children with FASDs; in men, impotence, testicular atrophy

Figure 13-8 Potential effects of alcohol use on the body.

fetal alcohol spectrum disorders (FASDs). Infants and children with FASDs may have abnormal facial features, low body weight, shorter-than-average height, poor coordination, poor memory, difficulty paying attention, speech and language delays, poor reasoning and judgment skills, low IQ, and problems with the heart, kidneys, or bones.

Although there is no cure for FASDs, early intervention can help. FASDs are also 100 percent preventable. The more a pregnant woman drinks, the greater the risk, but no level of alcohol consumption is completely safe during pregnancy.

Alcohol Abuse and Alcoholism

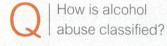

Q | How is alcohol abuse classified? — There are a number of ways to define and classify serious problems with alcohol. The APA definitions for substance abuse and dependence are often applied to alcohol.[25] **Alcohol abuse** is a pattern of drinking that results in harm to one's health, interpersonal relationships, and ability to succeed at school or work. Characteristics of alcohol abuse include the following:

- Failure to fulfill major responsibilities at work, school, or home

- Drinking in dangerous situations, such as while driving or operating machinery
- Legal problems related to alcohol, such as being arrested for drunk driving or for physically hurting someone while drunk
- Continued drinking despite ongoing relationship problems that are caused or worsened by drinking

Long-term alcohol abuse can turn into **alcohol dependence,** or *alcoholism.* The signs and symptoms of this chronic disease include a strong craving for alcohol, an inability to limit drinking, and continued use despite repeated and serious physical, psychological, and/or interpersonal problems. Alcoholics also experience physical dependence on alcohol—with tolerance to alcohol's effects and withdrawal if they stop drinking.

If you are wondering about your own drinking habits or those of someone you know, compare your pattern of consumption to the low-risk drinking

fetal alcohol spectrum disorders (FASDs) A range of birth defects that can occur in infants who were exposed to alcohol before birth.

alcohol abuse A pattern of drinking that is harmful to health, results in behavior that is harmful to others, or impairs the ability to meet school, work, and family responsibilities.

alcohol dependence Chronic, pathological use of alcohol despite repeated and serious consequences; usually characterized by tolerance and withdrawal; also known as *alcoholism.*

Wellness Strategies

Reducing Your Risk for Alcohol Problems

Q | What are some changes I can make to help myself cut down or stop drinking?

If you're considering changing your drinking habits, you need to decide whether to cut down or to quit. Discuss options with a doctor, a friend, or someone else you trust. Quitting is strongly recommended if you have tried cutting down before but can't stay within the limits you set or if you have symptoms of an alcohol disorder. If cutting down may be appropriate for you, try these strategies:

- *Keep track of how much you drink.* Use a notebook or smartphone to record when and where you drink. Making note of each drink before you drink it may help you slow down.
- *Count and measure your drinks.* Away from home, it can be hard to keep track, especially with mixed drinks, and at times you may be getting more alcohol than you think.
- *Set goals.* Decide how many days a week you want to drink and how many drinks you'll have on those days. Designate days when you don't drink, and always plan to stay within the low-risk limits.
- *Pace and space.* When you do drink, pace yourself. Sip slowly. Have no more than 1 standard drink per hour, and make every other drink a nonalcoholic one, such as water, soda, or juice.

- *Include food.* Eat some food so the alcohol will be absorbed into your system more slowly.
- *Find alternatives.* If drinking has occupied a lot of your time, then fill free time by developing new, healthy activities, hobbies, and relationships or renewing ones you've missed. If you've relied on alcohol to be more comfortable in social situations, manage moods, or cope with problems, then seek other, healthy ways to deal with those areas of your life.
- *Avoid triggers.* If certain people or places make you drink even when you don't want to, try to avoid them. If certain activities, times of day, or feelings trigger the urge, plan something else to do. If drinking at home is a problem, keep little or no alcohol there.
- *Plan to handle urges.* When you cannot avoid a trigger and an urge hits, remind yourself of your goals, call a friend, or engage in a distracting activity, such as exercise.
- *Know your "no."* You're likely to be offered a drink at times when you don't want one. Have a polite, convincing "no, thanks" ready.

For additional information and to locate professional help, visit http://rethinkingdrinking.niaaa.nih.gov/ToolsResources/Resources.asp.

Source: Adapted from National Institute on Alcohol Abuse and Alcoholism. (2010). *Rethinking drinking: Alcohol and your health.* NIH Pub. No. 10-3770.

---

pattern illustrated in Figure 13-4. Lab Activity 13-1 provides additional assistance in identifying alcohol problems. Also see the suggestions in the box "Reducing Your Risk for Alcohol Problems."

Q | Is alcoholism inherited?

Alcoholism does tend to run in families, but environmental and social influences also seem to be important contributors. Children of alcoholic parents are at greater risk of developing alcoholism, but not all of them do, and people can develop alcoholism even though no one else in their family has a drinking problem. Environmental factors that affect risk include the influence of friends, stress levels, and the ease of obtaining alcohol. If alcoholism does run in your family, carefully monitor your drinking and your responses to it.

Alcoholism is a chronic disease that can be treated but not cured, and some treatments are more effective than others. Regardless, it is important to remember that many people relapse before achieving long-term sobriety. Relapses do not mean that a person has failed or cannot eventually recover from alcoholism. If a relapse occurs, it is important for the individual to try to stop drinking again and to get whatever help is needed to abstain from alcohol. A key resource is the Center for Substance Abuse Treatment (1-800-662-HELP), which provides information about community treatment programs. Support groups including Alcoholics Anonymous

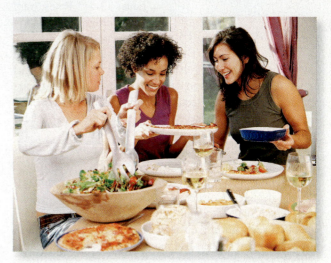

Low-risk drinking means avoiding intoxication. Men should limit their intake to no more than 4 drinks on any day and no more than 14 drinks in a week. Women should limit their intake to no more than 3 drinks on any day and no more than 7 drinks in a week.

(AA), Al-Anon (for friends and family members in an alcoholic person's life), and Alateen (for children of alcoholics) are also available in most communities.

Tobacco

According to the CDC, tobacco use remains the leading cause of preventable death in the United States, contributing to over 400,000 deaths each year and resulting in almost $100 billion in direct medical costs. Lung cancer, heart disease, and chronic obstructive pulmonary disease are just a few of the health problems linked with tobacco use and secondhand smoke.

Given the tremendous health risks associated with tobacco use, it might seem remarkable that 20 percent of adults in the United States still choose to use tobacco. Youth and adolescent use continues to exceed that of adults, and typically anyone who starts using tobacco before age 21 is more likely than others to continue using it for many years to come. Tobacco companies spend about $15 billion annually on advertising and marketing, emphasizing the excitement, allure, and prosperity that can come from using their products. In contrast, local and national public health organizations spend less than a tenth of that amount combating all these myths and trying to protect the public's health.

Giving up tobacco is one of the most difficult health behavior changes. In a recent survey, 42 percent of all cigarette smokers had stopped smoking for at least 1 day during the preceding 12 months. This is an indication of two powerful realities: first is the strong desire by current smokers to quit, and second is the difficulty of quitting.[26]

Prevalence and Patterns of Tobacco Use

Q | Everyone knows smoking is dangerous, so how many people are still doing it?

Overall, about 20 percent of U.S. adults currently smoke (Table 13-4). Rates vary across different population groups as defined by biological sex, ethnicity, and educational attainment. Although many college students report having tried cigarettes, only a small percentage are regular smokers. In fact, college graduates (bachelor's degree or higher) smoke at less than half the rate of those with less education.

One interesting pattern is that between the ages of 18 and 64, there is no significant difference in the rate of people smoking, but after age 65, the proportion of smokers sharply declines. Considering that the average life span in the United States is about 78 years and that smokers lose about 10 years off of their lives, the rates are perhaps much lower after age 65 because many chronic smokers simply don't live so long.

Despite the statistics, smoking doesn't typically start after high school. In fact, most lifetime smokers begin well before they turn 18, often due to various types of exposure, influence, and peer pressure.[27]

TABLE 13-4 PATTERNS OF SMOKING AMONG U.S. ADULTS

	PERCENT WHO ARE CURRENT SMOKERS		
	MEN	**WOMEN**	**TOTAL**
AGE			
18–24	22.8%	17.4%	20.1%
25–44	24.3%	19.8%	22.0%
45–64	23.2%	19.1%	21.1%
≥65	9.7%	9.3%	9.5%
RACE/ETHNICITY (AGE ≥18)			
White	22.6%	19.6%	21.0%
Black	24.8%	17.1%	20.6%
Hispanic	15.8%	9.0%	12.5%
American Indian/ Alaska Native	n/a	36.0%	n/a
Asian	14.7%	4.3%	9.2%
EDUCATION LEVEL (AGE ≥25)			
Less than a high school diploma	28.5%	21.8%	25.1%
GED	46.4%	44.1%	45.2%
High school diploma	27.4%	20.6%	23.8%
Some college	25.1%	21.6%	23.2%
Bachelor's degree	10.2%	9.5%	9.9%
TOTAL	21.5%	17.3%	19.3%

Source: Centers for Disease Control and Prevention. (2010). Vital signs: Current cigarette smoking among adults aged >18 years, United States, 2010. *Morbidity and Mortality Weekly Report, 60*(35), 1207–1212.

Tobacco and Nicotine

Nicotine, a naturally occurring chemical in tobacco, is both a poison and a highly addictive psychoactive drug. Nicotine affects many parts of the body, including the brain, heart, and circulatory system. During pregnancy, nicotine

nicotine Poisonous, addictive psychoactive drug in tobacco.

freely crosses the placenta. One of the attractions of nicotine is that it can produce pleasurable effects that make the user want more—a characteristic that can lead to dependency.

Q | Other than nicotine, what exactly is in a cigarette?

Cigarette smoke contains over 4,000 chemicals and more than 50 known *carcinogens,* or cancer-causing compounds. There are at least another 400 toxins in a typical cigarette. It's hard to believe that so much can fit in such a small product! Nicotine and carbon monoxide are probably the most well-known ingredients in tobacco smoke, but others include formaldehyde, ammonia, hydrogen cyanide, arsenic, and pesticides. Some of the other chemicals in tobacco may also contribute to its addictive potential.

One cigarette additive of particular concern is menthol, which gives a sensation of coolness in the mouth, throat, and lungs and which thereby may mask the harshness of cigarette smoke. Menthol may make it easier for new smokers to start and for experienced smokers to smoke more and inhale more deeply. Use of menthol cigarettes is highest among young people who have recently started to smoke and among African Americans.

Q | Why is it so easy to start smoking and so hard to quit?

Peer pressure and exposure to smoking through interactions with family members and friends who smoke increase the likelihood that individuals will try smoking. In addition, advertisers target young people, who may see smoking as a way to rebel or show their independence. Also, certain demographic features are more predictive of starting and continuing cigarette smoking. Lower educational attainment is strongly associated with smoking (see Table 13-4). The best way to keep children and adolescents from starting smoking is to model nonsmoking behavior. If they aren't exposed to smoking, they are much less likely to be tempted.

Smoking cessation has been studied by behavioral scientists for decades, and the one fact they continue to find is that quitting smoking is hard. It's unusual for chronic smokers to quit on their first attempt, in large part because of the enjoyable feelings that smoking conveys.

Like many other psychoactive drugs, nicotine activates the brain's reward system and provides a pleasurable response. Nicotine's effects occur rapidly when the drug is smoked, but they also wear off quickly. To maintain the drug's pleasurable effects and prevent withdrawal, a user seeks to continue dosing at regular intervals. Smokers who are addicted to nicotine often report that the first cigarette in the morning is the one that they crave the most and that seems the strongest or best.

Tobacco use leads to tolerance of nicotine's effects. If users stop or reduce tobacco consumption, their withdrawal symptoms include depression, irritability, anxiety, difficulty concentrating, and nicotine cravings. Dependence is also often supported by behavioral factors. The rituals associated with smoking—handling and lighting cigarettes, being in certain locations or with certain people—can make quitting especially difficult.

Nicotine is a stimulant, causing an increase in physical arousal (heart rate and blood pressure) and mental alertness. Some people associate smoking with a reduction in stress, but the only stress that smoking reduces is the stress of nicotine withdrawal. Figure 13-9 summarizes the short-term effects of smoking on the body.

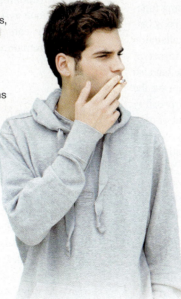

Brain
Nicotine reaches the brain within 10 seconds, triggering the reward center of the brain and causing overall nervous system stimulation; effects peak in about 10 minutes

Lungs
Smoke increases mucus production, thickens mucus, and damages cilia, preventing them from filtering foreign particles; chemicals from smoke damage cells in the lungs and are absorbed into the bloodstream and circulated throughout the body

Stomach
Smoking causes heartburn and ulcers, interferes with the absorption of several vitamins

Liver
Liver converts glycogen to glucose, increasing blood sugar levels

Kidneys
Nicotine inhibits the production of urine

Nose
Tar and toxins in smoke irritate nasal membranes, dull sense of smell

Mouth and throat
Tar and toxins in smoke irritate membranes, dull taste buds, stain teeth, cause raspy voice and bad breath

Heart and blood vessels
Nicotine increases heart rate and blood pressure and constricts blood vessels; less oxygen is delivered to cells; platelets become stickier; blood fat levels are adversely affected

Reproductive system
Smoking reduces fertility in men and women; causes impotence in men and irregular menstruation in women; in pregnant women, nicotine and tobacco chemicals pass through the placenta to the fetus

Skin
Tobacco smoke dries and damages the skin; nicotine reduces blood flow to the skin

Figure 13-9 Short-term effects of smoking.

Effects of Smoking

Cigarettes kill more Americans than alcohol, motor vehicle crashes, suicide, HIV infection, homicide, and illegal drugs combined. Most people understand that smoking causes cancer and heart disease, but it also affects the skin, senses, hormones, and reproductive system.

Q | What are the biggest health problems caused by smoking?

The list of problems caused by smoking is a long one. Smoking damages quality of life and shortens lives. Smoking is responsible for 90 percent of all lung cancer deaths in men, 80 percent of all lung cancer deaths in women, and 90 percent of all deaths from *chronic obstructive pulmonary disease (COPD),* which includes chronic bronchitis and emphysema.[28] In addition to lung cancer, smoking also produces cancers of the mouth, throat, pancreas, stomach, cervix, uterus, and kidney. As well, smoking reduces bone density and increases the risk of fractures.

Compared with nonsmokers, smokers are two to four times more likely to have coronary heart disease or a stroke. Smoking reduces the amount of oxygen in the blood, straining the cardiorespiratory system. Smoking also narrows blood vessels, raises blood pressure, damages arteries, and contributes to unhealthy blood fat levels by lowering HDL ("good") cholesterol. These effects increase the risk of cardiovascular disease.

Smoking is also very harmful to the respiratory system: It damages airways and alveoli in the lungs. It increases both the volume of mucus produced in the lungs and its thickness. At the same time, smoking destroys the cilia, which would normally move the mucus and trapped foreign material up and out of the body. The result of more and thicker mucus and lack of functional cilia is the dreaded "smoker's cough."

Tobacco use also affects athletic performance because it lowers maximal oxygen consumption and reduces lung function.[29] There is a misconception that chewing tobacco is better than smoking it because there is no smoke inhalation when tobacco is chewed. In fact, however, all forms of tobacco contain nicotine, which not only is addictive but also narrows blood vessels, thus putting additional strain on the heart. Smoking causes problems with the lungs, too, possibly even slowing lung growth, and it reduces the amount of oxygen in the blood available to muscles during activity. Anyone who wants to perform well on the court or in the field should consider quitting or not starting in the first place.

Q | Is it true that smokers get wrinkles faster?

Yes, it is, as smoke in the environment dries the skin's surface. Smoking also reduces blood flow to the skin, thereby depleting the skin of oxygen and essential nutrients. These factors lead to an increase in wrinkles, so that smokers in their 40s often have as many facial wrinkles as nonsmokers in their 60s. In addition to accelerated wrinkling, prolonged smoking causes discoloration of the fingers and fingernails on the hand used to hold cigarettes. Smoking also yellows the teeth and causes *halitosis,* or bad breath.

Q | Can smoking control my weight?

Many people believe that smoking can help control body weight, and in fact BMI tends to be lower in current smokers and higher in ex-smokers when compared with nonsmokers.[30] Although a slightly lower BMI might sound appealing, recall that smokers also develop chronic diseases and die prematurely. In addition, smokers tend to have unhealthy body fat distribution, with more fat stored in the torso, producing the "apple" shape. The more cigarettes smoked, the greater the waist-to-hip ratio.[31]

Nicotine is a stimulant, so smokers burn slightly more calories than do nonsmokers. When they quit, about 80 percent of former smokers do gain some weight, an average of less than 10 pounds. Successful quitters may put on weight because their appetite for food has increased now that their taste buds are not dulled by smoking. Their food tastes better, their hunger increases, and they eat more. Also, they are again burning calories at a normal rate.

The majority of health experts recommend that smokers focus first on quitting—the key step for health and wellness. Once they have quit, their body will adjust to life without nicotine. Most weight tends to be gained in the first 6 months after quitting; after that, many individuals start to lose the weight they gained as they adjust to being ex-smokers.

Q | Does smoking mess with getting pregnant?

Smoking appears to reduce fertility in both men and women. It also increases the risk of ectopic pregnancy (one in which the fertilized egg attaches outside the uterus), miscarriage, and preterm labor. Ultimately, smoking lowers a woman's chances of conceiving by as much as 40 percent.[32]

Smoking can also have harmful effects on the fetus, including premature birth, low birth weight, and even death.

Mind Stretcher
Critical Thinking Exercise

Do you have a friend or a family member who wants to quit smoking? What alternatives to smoking can you recommend to this individual? What health benefits from quitting do you think would resonate with this person? How much money would he or she save from quitting? Do you know a successful former smoker to whom you might refer the person for support? Quitting is tough, but having a social support system makes success more likely, so thinking of ways you can help someone quit can be a vital step toward improving that person's wellness.

Nicotine and carbon monoxide reduce the supply of oxygen to the developing fetus, adversely affecting growth and development. Babies born to smoking mothers also have higher rates of asthma, attention deficit hyperactivity disorder (ADHD), and learning problems than do those born to nonsmokers, and they are more likely to become smokers themselves in the future.[33]

Other Forms of Tobacco Use

Q | Are light cigarettes, electric cigarettes, and water pipes safe?

"Light" or "low-tar" cigarettes may contain less nicotine and tar compared to regular cigarettes, yet researchers have found that smokers usually compensate for these differences by inhaling more deeply, taking more puffs, or smoking more cigarettes. The National Cancer Institute has concluded that light cigarettes provide no benefit to smokers' health and that smokers who use them are at high risk for developing smoking-related cancers and other chronic health problems.

Electric cigarettes, or "e-cigs," are a relatively new product marketed as a safe alternative to regular cigarettes. E-cigs allow the user to inhale tobacco vapors without smoke or the usual health risks. However, to date, there are no rigorous studies to evaluate the overall benefit of e-cigs, and instead there is some evidence that e-cigs contain tobacco-specific nitrosamines (TSNAs), which are known cancer-causing agents. In fact, the state of New York is currently trying to ban e-cigs, primarily out of concern that their enticing packaging and marketing are an easy gateway to nicotine addiction.

Ultimately, there is no such thing as a safe cigarette, and the way to reduce the risk of smoking-related diseases is to quit. As recently as 2010, a new federal law was passed banning the use of the words *light, mild,* and *low* on tobacco products.

Water pipes, or *hookahs,* have recently become more popular among college students, especially athletes, who are less likely than other students to smoke standard cigarettes.[34] Because the flavored tobacco smoke from water pipes tends to be less irritating to the throat than cigarette smoke, the hookah gives the impression of being safer. However, studies comparing hookahs and cigarettes have found that water pipe use is associated with similar nicotine levels, greater carbon monoxide levels, and significantly more smoke exposure.[35]

Q | Smokeless tobacco and cigars aren't so bad, right?

Smokeless tobacco (or spit tobacco) products are not a safe substitute for smoking cigarettes, as they can also cause cancer and lead to nicotine addiction. The nicotine in smokeless tobacco is absorbed through the mucous membranes in the mouth when a user places a piece of chewing tobacco or a pinch of snuff between the cheek and gum. Use of smokeless tobacco causes *leukoplakia* (precancerous lesions in the mouth), gum recession, bone loss around the teeth, tooth decay, and bad breath. The most serious risk, though, is cancer of the mouth and pharynx. Oral cancer rates can be as much as 50-fold higher for chronic snuff dippers compared with people who do not use tobacco.

Smokeless tobacco use leads to nicotine addiction. People who use dip 8–10 times a day are exposing themselves to the amount of nicotine in 30–40 cigarettes. This may be one reason that it is so hard to give up smokeless products.

Although it's true that most cigar smokers don't inhale the smoke, that doesn't protect them from the nicotine and other chemicals in a cigar. Think about this: Some cigars have the amount of nicotine in an entire pack of cigarettes. Because of the differences in how cigars are smoked, cigar smokers usually have lower rates of lung cancer than cigarette smokers but higher rates of cancers of the mouth and throat. Cigar smokers can also become dependent on nicotine. If a cigar smoker does inhale the smoke, he or she is at increased risk for both lung cancer and chronic respiratory disease. The bottom line: Cigar smoking is not safe.

Environmental Tobacco Smoke

Q | Is secondhand smoke as bad as everyone says?

Secondhand smoke is estimated to kill up to 70,000 nonsmokers per year—which certainly seems pretty bad![36] It causes about 3,000 deaths from lung cancer, 62,000 deaths from heart disease, and nearly 3,000 infant deaths from sudden infant death syn drome (SIDS). Secondhand smoke, also referred to as **environmental tobacco smoke (ETS),** consists of sidestream smoke and mainstream smoke. **Sidestream smoke** is the smoke that comes directly from lighted tobacco products, such as cigarettes, cigars, and pipes. **Mainstream smoke** is the smoke exhaled by smokers.

Environmental tobacco smoke is classified as a known human carcinogen. In addition to

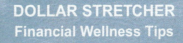

DOLLAR STRETCHER
Financial Wellness Tips

Any form of substance use can hurt your bank balance. For additional incentive to cut back or quit, calculate the weekly or monthly cost of your habit. Include not just how much you spend on the product—coffee and other caffeinated drinks, beer, cigarettes, and so on—but other costs, too, such as tooth-whitening products for nicotine-stained teeth and lost work time due to hangovers.

environmental tobacco smoke (ETS) Smoke that enters the atmosphere by a smoker's exhalation and by the burning end of a cigarette, cigar, or pipe; also called *secondhand smoke.*

sidestream smoke Smoke that enters the atmosphere from the burning end of a cigarette, cigar, or pipe.

mainstream smoke Smoke that enters the atmosphere by being exhaled by a smoker.

cancer, heart disease, and SIDS, exposure to environmental tobacco smoke is linked to these diseases and conditions:

- Bronchitis, pneumonia, and ear infections in children
- Exacerbation of asthma and other chronic respiratory problems in children
- Low birth weight
- Increased risk of cervical cancer

Despite restrictions on where people can smoke, secondhand smoke exposure is common among nonsmokers. Based on an analysis of a blood marker for smoke exposure, the CDC estimates that 88 million nonsmokers are exposed to secondhand smoke,[37] with the highest rates of exposure among children ages 4–11 years. There is no risk-free level of secondhand smoke exposure, and it's likely that future research will identify even more negative effects from exposure to ETS.

Quitting Tobacco

Quitting smoking brings with it a tremendous health improvement. Some would even say that it is lifesaving. Quitting smoking reduces a person's risk for heart disease, cancer, stroke, chronic lung diseases, and many other health problems. Women who stop smoking before pregnancy or very early in the pregnancy dramatically reduce their risk of having a low-birth-weight baby. People who quit by their 30s may avoid most tobacco-related health risks. However, even smokers who quit after age 50 substantially reduce their risk of dying early. It is *never* too late to give up smoking.

Although long-term health improvements are critical, consider some of these immediate benefits of quitting:[38]

- Your breath, clothes, and hair will smell better.
- Your sense of smell will return, and food will taste better.
- Your fingers and fingernails will slowly appear less yellow.
- Your stained teeth will slowly become whiter.
- Your children will be less likely to start smoking themselves.
- It will be easier and cheaper to find an apartment.
- You will miss fewer workdays, or you may have an easier time getting a job.
- The constant search for a place to smoke when you're out will be over.
- Friends will be more willing to be in your car or home.
- Your dating prospects will become much wider, because 80 percent of the population does not smoke.
- You will have more money (one-pack-per-day smokers spend around $2,000 per year on cigarettes).

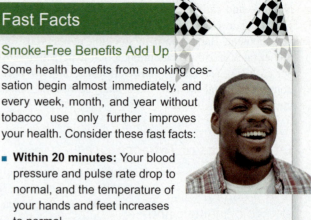

Fast Facts

Smoke-Free Benefits Add Up

Some health benefits from smoking cessation begin almost immediately, and every week, month, and year without tobacco use only further improves your health. Consider these fast facts:

- **Within 20 minutes:** Your blood pressure and pulse rate drop to normal, and the temperature of your hands and feet increases to normal.
- **Within a few hours:** Your blood carbon monoxide levels drop, and your blood oxygen levels increase, both to normal levels.
- **Within a day:** Your risk of a sudden heart attack decreases.
- **Within 48 hours:** Your senses of smell and taste begin to return to normal.
- **Within a few weeks:** Your circulation improves and your lung function increases.
- **Within a few months:** You have fewer illnesses, colds, and asthma attacks.
- **Within 1 year:** Your risk of coronary heart disease is cut in half.
- **Within 5 years:** Your risk of dying from lung cancer decreases by nearly 50 percent.
- **Quitting by age 30:** Your chance of dying prematurely from smoking-related diseases falls by more than 90 percent.
- **Quitting by age 50:** Your chance of dying prematurely from smoking-related diseases drops by more than 50 percent.
- **Quitting by age 60:** Your chance of living longer than those who continue to smoke increases.

Source: National Institutes of Health. (2011). National Cancer Institute fact sheet: Harms of smoking and health benefits of quitting (http://www.cancer.gov/cancertopics/factsheet/Tobacco/cessation).

Q | What are the most effective ways for me to quit smoking?

Some smokers quit on their own; others do better with support. A number of techniques have been shown to be effective:

- Talking with a doctor, who can provide advice and assistance
- Getting counseling, in either individual or group sessions or by telephone (call 1-800-QUIT-NOW)
- Using behavioral strategies, such as setting goals and thinking in advance about ways to overcome urges
- Using certain over-the-counter or prescription medications

In addition, review the general behavior-change strategies from Chapter 2. Identify your stage of change, and choose techniques for change that are most likely to be helpful for you.

Q | Are all patches and gums really worth it to try, and will they help me quit?

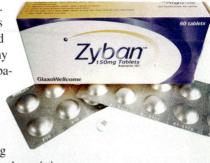

Medications can help people quit. Nicotine-replacement therapy doubles the rates of success by providing a small dose of nicotine to help reduce unpleasant feelings of withdrawal. Nicotine chewing gum, lozenges, and skin patches are available over the counter; but you need a prescription to purchase the nicotine inhaler or nasal spray. These products do not completely eliminate nicotine withdrawal because they provide a smaller dose of nicotine at a slower rate. They do reduce cravings and withdrawal symptoms. Depending on the product, you may slowly reduce the amount you are using until you are completely nicotine-free. Two other prescription medications approved for smoking cessation—bupropion (Zyban) and varenicline (Chantix)—work by affecting neurotransmitter levels and provide no nicotine.

An additional challenge for people trying to quit is breaking the habit of putting or having something in their mouth most of the time. The fact that cigarettes are often replaced by food is one of the reasons why weight gain often accompanies quitting. Therefore, finding an alternative way to occupy your hands and mouth, such as by chewing gum or using toothpicks, may also aid in the quitting process.

Regardless of the quitting method used, regular telephone contact can be helpful. After the attempt to quit has begun, weekly or monthly telephone calls from a health professional or loved one to support the attempt have proven quite successful in helping people maintain a smoke-free life. The online Smokefree.gov program includes many additional tips for putting together a step-by-step quitting program.

If you smoke, now is the time to start thinking about quitting. The first few weeks and months are usually the most difficult. By planning ahead to cope with difficult situations and triggers, you can succeed. Quitting smoking is one of the best things you can ever do for health and wellness.

Summary

Substance use and abuse in the United States are problems that have been around for generations. They are not likely to go away anytime soon. Legal psychoactive drugs—such as alcohol, tobacco, and caffeine—play a major but paradoxical role in our country's economy: Although many communities depend on the income from these products to boost their economy in the short term, they also have to bear the long-term social costs of addiction, crime, morbidity, and mortality.

People use psychoactive substances for various reasons. Using these drugs, however, carries many risks, ranging from missing class or doing something you later regret to intoxication, overdose, and death. Regular use also presents the risk of dependence. The effects of tobacco use are well known and include chronic disease and premature death for both smokers and the people around them.

Any substance or behavior that becomes the most important thing in someone's life detracts from wellness. The best way to prevent a drug problem is never to misuse or abuse drugs. Prescription drugs should be used strictly as intended and prescribed. Legal drugs like alcohol and caffeine should be consumed in moderation, and tobacco and illicit drugs should be avoided. If you experience a problem with a behavior or drug—use that has gotten out of control—seek help.

More to Explore

Alcoholics Anonymous
http://www.aa.org
Center for Internet Addiction
http://www.netaddiction.com
Narcotics Anonymous
http://www.na.org
National Council on Problem Gambling
http://www.ncpgambling.org
National Institute on Alcohol Abuse and Alcoholism
http://www.niaaa.nih.gov
National Institute on Drug Abuse
http://www.drugabuse.gov
Smokefree.gov
http://www.smokefree.gov
Substance Abuse and Mental Health Services Administration
http://www.samhsa.gov

COMPLETE IN connect

NAME	DATE	SECTION

Equipment: None

Preparation: None

Part 1: AUDIT Questionnaire for Alcohol Use

Instructions

For each question, give yourself the point total that corresponds to the answer that best describes your behavior.

QUESTIONS	0	1	2	3	4	
1. How often do you have a drink containing alcohol?	Never	Monthly or less	2–4 times a month	2–3 times a week	4 or more times a week	
2. How many drinks containing alcohol do you have on a typical day when you are drinking?	1 or 2	3 or 4	5 or 6	7–9	10 or more	
3. How often do you have 5 or more drinks on one occasion?	Never	Less than monthly	Monthly	Weekly	Daily or almost daily	
4. How often during the last year have you found that you were not able to stop drinking once you had started?	Never	Less than monthly	Monthly	Weekly	Daily or almost daily	
5. How often during the last year have you failed to do what was normally expected of you because of drinking?	Never	Less than monthly	Monthly	Weekly	Daily or almost daily	
6. How often during the last year have you needed a first drink in the morning to get yourself going after a heavy drinking session?	Never	Less than monthly	Monthly	Weekly	Daily or almost daily	
7. How often during the last year have you had a feeling of guilt or remorse after drinking?	Never	Less than monthly	Monthly	Weekly	Daily or almost daily	
8. How often during the last year have you been unable to remember what happened the night before because of your drinking?	Never	Less than monthly	Monthly	Weekly	Daily or almost daily	
9. Have you or someone else been injured because of your drinking?	No		Yes, but not in the last year		Yes, during the last year	
10. Has a relative, friend, doctor, or other health care worker been concerned about your drinking or suggested you cut down?	No	Yes, but not in the last year			Yes, during the last year	
					Total	

Results

A total score of 8 or more indicates a strong likelihood of hazardous or harmful alcohol consumption. Even if you score below 8, if you are having drinking-related problems with your academic performance, job, relationships, or health, or with the law, you should consider seeking help. Briefly describe any problems you've experienced as a result of drinking alcohol. In addition, compare your drinking pattern to the low-risk pattern described in Figure 13-4 in the chapter.

Part 2: Addictive Behavior Checklist

Instructions

Some addictive behaviors are easier to recognize than others, and some people don't notice signs that a behavior is out of control in some way. Here is a checklist of actions, thoughts, and feelings that can be associated with addictive behaviors. Choose a behavior to evaluate. Recall that many different types of behaviors can become addictive—from exercise to eating, gambling to video games, sex to shopping. Check any of the following statements that are true for you in relation to the behavior you are evaluating.

Behavior: _____

_____ I engage in this behavior fairly often.

_____ I have been engaging in this behavior for a long time.

_____ I engage in this behavior when I am stressed, worried, frustrated, angry, or in emotional pain.

_____ After engaging in this behavior, I feel bad inside—angry, guilty, or disappointed with myself.

_____ I sometimes feel panicky, restless, or irritable if I haven't engaged in the behavior in a while.

_____ I often find myself distracted from other things because I am thinking about or planning to engage in this behavior.

_____ I often reward myself with this behavior.

_____ When I engage in this behavior, I tend to lose track of time.

_____ I now engage in this behavior more often and/or for longer periods of time than I used to in order to get any satisfaction from it.

_____ I often tell myself I can stop this behavior at any time, yet I keep doing it.

_____ This behavior takes me away from healthier activities.

_____ I am often secretive about this behavior; I hide the behavior and/or lie about it to others.

_____ This behavior often leads to problems for myself and/or others.

_____ I've had others tell me this behavior is not good for me.

_____ I've lost some friends because of my involvement with this behavior.

_____ My life would be better without this behavior or if this behavior were more under control.

Results

The more items you check, the greater the chance that your behavior is a problem for you. If your answers suggest a problem, seek help from your school's counseling center or another health care provider. Professional addiction counselors can help you identify triggers, develop healthier strategies for dealing with stress and difficult emotions, and eliminate addictive behaviors.

Reflecting on Your Results

Were you surprised by the results of the AUDIT screening or by the number of yes answers on the addictive behavior checklist? Did your responses match your own impression of the role that alcohol use or other behaviors play in your life? What, if anything, in the results concerns you?

Planning Your Next Steps

If the results of these tests indicate that you could benefit from changing your behavior, state your goal for change and list at least three concrete strategies you plan to try.

Source: AUDIT test: Saunders, J. B., and others. (1993, June). Development of the Alcohol Use Disorders Identification Test (AUDIT): WHO collaborative project on early detection of persons with harmful alcohol consumption—II. Addiction, 88, 791–804.

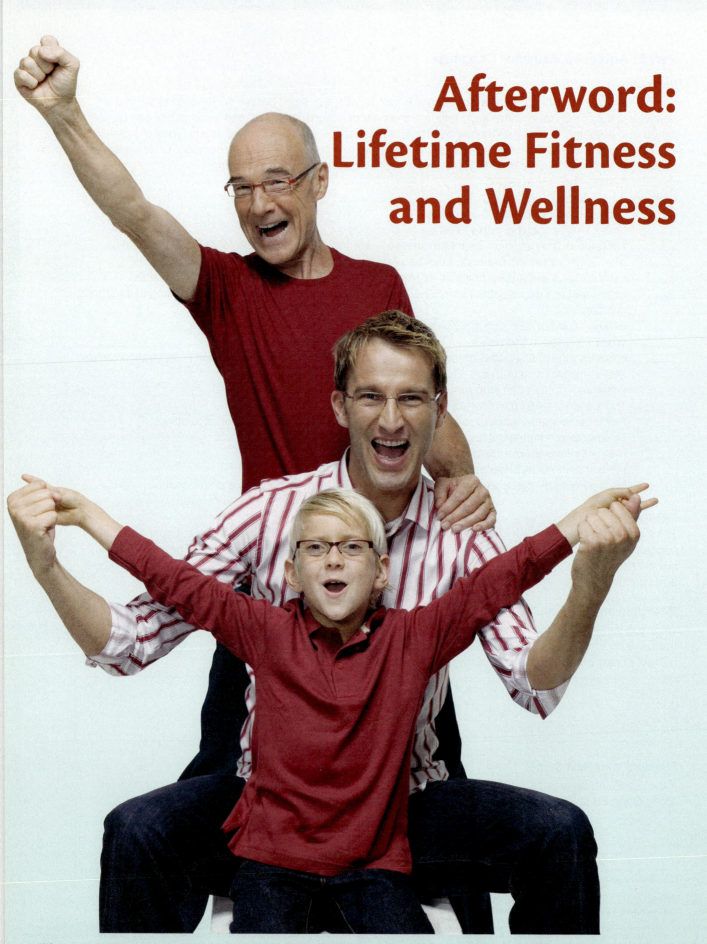

Afterword: Lifetime Fitness and Wellness

We hope you now understand that wellness is about you—every aspect of you—as well as your friends, family, community, and environment. Our goal has been to answer your questions, to introduce you to key concepts related to wellness, and to highlight important skills you can use to make positive choices and engage in successful behavior change. Our hope is that you'll also be inspired to put information into action. The priorities you set and the choices you make are the most important things you can do to help ensure a high quality of life for yourself—now and in the future. Wellness is a journey, one that continues throughout your life. The choices you make today have the potential to make your journey truly outstanding. Developing and balancing all the dimensions of wellness will help you reach your goals and become the person you want to be. We wish you a safe and wonderful journey.

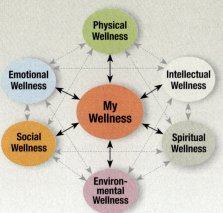

LAB ACTIVITY A-1   Wellness Reflection: How Far Have You Come?

NAME	DATE	SECTION

Equipment: None

Preparation: None

Instructions

Reflect on your experiences during your wellness course by answering the following questions.

Wellness Knowledge and Attitudes: What are some of the most surprising and relevant things you've learned about fitness and wellness? Have you learned any new skills in terms of critical analysis or consumer choices? Has what you've learned had an impact on your attitudes toward wellness? On your choices? If so, how?

Wellness Behaviors: Think about all your wellness-related behaviors. Are you more aware of them now? Are you more likely to think before you act? Have any of your habits changed during your wellness course? How and why? If possible, repeat Lab Activity 1-1 to see if your score has changed.

Lifestyle Changes: Have you engaged in a behavior-change program of any kind? If so, describe the goals and progress of your program, including the strategies you used and the key challenges you encountered. In addition, describe how you felt about the process and the change you tried to make. How successful were you? How did your efforts make you feel? Do you think you'll stick with your new behavior after the class is over? Why or why not?

Dimensions of Wellness: Think about your status for each of the wellness dimensions. What are your wellness strengths and weaknesses? How has your evaluation changed since the beginning of the course? Review the results of Lab Activity 1-2 if you completed it, and indicate what wellness strengths you've added and whether you would raise any of your wellness dimension scores.

Where Will You Go from Here? What are your major goals and aspirations? Where do you see yourself ten years in the future?

How does your current lifestyle match up to the image you have for your future? How will your current wellness strengths and positive behaviors help you achieve your goals? Could any of your current habits hold you back? List both your key strengths and positive behaviors and the areas where you need to improve. Make plans now to support your positive behaviors and make changes in any negative ones.

Appendix

Answers to Myth or Fact? Exercises

For additional information, watch the Myth or Fact? videos in Connect.

Chapter 1: Myth or Fact? People spend less money when they use cash instead of a credit card.

The answer is FACT. Financial experts report that people spend 8–18 percent more money when they use a credit card than when they pay in cash. They also make more purchases when they use credit. Why? The reasons include that it's emotionally harder to buy with cash than with plastic and that credit cards make buying so much easier—there's no need to run to the bank or an ATM.

Chapter 2: Myth or Fact? Frequently reevaluating and changing goals is a clear indication that a behavior-change program is failing.

The answer is MYTH. In a study, researchers examined whether individuals' frequent goal setting resulted in successful behavior change related to their diet and physical activity. The strategies the study participants used to work toward their goals included eating smaller portions and self-monitoring their physical activity levels. The researchers found that those who set frequent goals were more likely to practice specific strategies to accomplish those goals.

Chapter 3: Myth or Fact? It is best to work out in the morning, because morning workouts elevate your metabolism more than afternoon or evening workouts do.

The answer is MYTH. It's a common belief that morning exercise raises body metabolism more and burns more calories than does exercise at other times of the day. In fact, studies show that the time of day has *no* effect on these outcomes. Furthermore, most people have a decreased capacity for exercise in the morning. The big message is that the best time to exercise is the time that works best for you.

Chapter 4: Myth or Fact? You burn more calories running a mile than walking a mile.

The answer is FACT. Research studies show that for a given distance, running requires more energy—burns more calories—than walking does. The reason is that walking is a more efficient way of moving and hence uses fewer muscles. In contrast, running engages more muscles, using them not only to push off and to raise the body slightly from the ground but also to absorb shock. Even though walking burns slightly fewer calories than running when one is moving the same distance, many experts recommend walking (instead of running) because it places less stress on the body.

Chapter 5: Myth or Fact? Doing lots of sit-ups makes your stomach flatter.

The answer is MYTH. Many people believe that doing sit-ups and/or other abdominal exercises helps to flatten the stomach. However, a study investigating the impact of high-intensity sit-ups on fat-cell characteristics in the abdomen found that sit-ups had no effect on these characteristics and no effect with respect to flattening the stomach of study participants. Experts advise that to flatten the stomach, the best strategies are to practice a comprehensive exercise routine combining cardiovascular, resistance, and flexibility training and to modify dietary habits in ways that will promote weight loss.

Chapter 6: Myth or Fact? Static stretching before activities like sprinting or jumping decreases performance.

The answer is FACT. Recent research shows that performing static stretching before a physical activity like sprinting or jumping may have a negative effect on maximal force and torque production, running speed, and vertical jumping, thus decreasing performance. Coaches and conditioning professionals may want to rethink the recommendation to do static stretching before activities requiring high levels of strength, power, and explosiveness. Whole-body continuous movement followed by dynamic stretching or dynamic actions that mimic sports activity may be preferable before such activities.

Chapter 7: Myth or Fact? It's healthier to be 25 pounds overweight and physically active than to be at an optimal weight and sedentary.

The answer is FACT. In an important review study that analyzed the results of 24 prior relevant studies, the authors concluded that *active and fit overweight and obese individuals* had morbidity and mortality rates that were at least as low as, and in many cases much lower than, the morbidity and mortality rates of *sedentary normal-weight individuals*. So, the fact that a person is 20–30 pounds overweight doesn't necessarily mean that he or she is unhealthy or at an increased risk for chronic diseases. It depends on that person's fitness and activity level.

Chapter 8: Myth or Fact? Eating chocolate, potato chips, and other oily foods makes acne worse.

The answer is MYTH. A frequently cited 1969 study involving the ingestion of high amounts of chocolate enriched with cocoa butter, along with more recent clinical trials, fails to show an association between eating particular foods and having acne. The best strategies if you have acne are to avoid pinching and squeezing the pimples; cleaning your face once or twice daily with a mild, unscented soap; and using over-the-counter products containing benzoyl peroxide.

Chapter 9: Myth or Fact? As a general rule, avoid eating after 9 p.m., because those calories are usually stored as body fat.

The answer is MYTH. Many people, even some health and fitness professionals, erroneously believe that eating after a certain hour in the evening is not advisable because the individual is relatively inactive at that time of day and so will store the calories as fat. However, most experts say that the key factor relative to weight gain or loss is the total number of calories taken in. It really doesn't matter whether those calories are consumed early or late in the day.

Chapter 10: Myth or Fact? Ulcers are caused by stress.

The answer is MYTH. Ulcers cause pain, bleeding, and, in severe cases, perforation of the stomach wall. Many people long believed that ulcers result when stress reduces mucus production in the stomach, exposing the stomach walls to the harmful effects of digestive enzymes. Today it is known that stress does *not* cause most ulcers. Instead, the most common trigger for duodenal and gastric ulcers is infection with the *H. pylori* bacterium. Nevertheless, stress may intensify ulcer symptoms or make an ulcer worse, so controlling stress is important.

Chapter 11: Myth or Fact? Certain dogs can smell cancer.

The answer is FACT. Dogs' smelling ability is 10,000–100,000 times more sensitive than humans' sense of smell. A study investigated whether dogs' amazing power of smell might be put to use medically—specifically, to detect cancer by sniffing individuals' breath. The researchers found that specially trained dogs detected the presence of breast or lung cancer 88–97 percent of the time in individuals with these chronic diseases. As a possible explanation for this feat, experts say that dogs might be able to detect certain compounds that are present in the breath of people with cancer but not in the breath of healthy individuals.

Chapter 12: Myth or Fact? You should avoid cat litter boxes if you are pregnant.

The answer is FACT. A parasite that's commonly present in the digestive tract of cats (especially outdoor cats) may be passed on to pregnant women who handle cat litter boxes. This parasite causes a disease called toxoplasmosis. This infection can be transmitted from a pregnant woman to the developing fetus and can result in stillbirth, miscarriage, or serious postnatal consequences for infants who survive. If a pregnant woman must change or handle a litter box, she should wear gloves and a mask and, when done, should wash her hands thoroughly.

Chapter 13: Myth or Fact? Marijuana gives you the munchies.

The answer is FACT. Scientific research studies conducted since the 1960s mostly support the idea that consuming marijuana (cannabis) stimulates the appetite or gives you the munchies. This effect occurs because THC, the active ingredient in cannabis, is similar to the body chemicals that are released in the bloodstream when the stomach is empty, signaling that it's time to eat. Marijuana's appetite-stimulating potency makes cannabis a useful medicinal drug for individuals in the late stages of diseases like cancer and AIDS who have lost their desire to eat.

References

CHAPTER 1

1. World Health Organization (WHO). (1948). Preamble to the constitution of the World Health Organization. *Official Records of the World Health Organization, 2,* 100.

2. Bouchard, C., Shephard, R. J., & Stephens, T. (1994). *Physical activity, fitness, and health: International proceedings and consensus statement.* Champaign, IL: Human Kinetics.

3. U.S. Department of Health & Human Services. (2008). *2008 physical activity guidelines for Americans.* ODPHP Publication No. U0036.

4. National Center for Health Statistics (NCHS). (2011). United States life tables, 2007. *National Vital Statistics Reports, 59*(9).

5. Central Intelligence Agency (CIA). (2011). *The world factbook online.* Retrieved from https://www.cia.gov/library/publications/the-world-factbook/rankorder/2102rank.html

6. Centers for Disease Control and Prevention (CDC). (1999). Ten great public health achievements—United States, 1900–1999. *MMWR, 48*(12), 241–243.

7. U.S. Census Bureau. (2011). The older population: 2010 census briefs. Publication No. C2010BR-09.

8. National Center for Health Statistics (NCHS). (2011). Deaths: Leading causes for 2007. *National Vital Statistics Reports, 59*(8).

9. Centers for Disease Control and Prevention (CDC). (2011) Healthy People 2010 Final Review. Retrieved from http://www.cdc.gov/nchs/healthy_people/hp2010/hp2010_final_review.htm

10. Centers for Disease Control and Prevention (CDC). (2009) Healthy People 2020. Retrieved from http://www.cdc.gov/nchs/healthy_people/hp2020.htm

11. Centers for Disease Control and Prevention (CDC). (2011) Healthy People 2010 Final Review. Retrieved from http://www.cdc.gov/nchs/healthy_people/hp2010/hp2010_final_review.htm

12. Peeters, A., Barendregt, J., Willekens, F., Mackenbach, J., Al Mamun, A., & Bonneaux, L. (2003). Obesity in adulthood and its consequences for life expectancy: A life-table analysis. *Annals of Internal Medicine, 138*(1), 24–32.

13. Ibid.

14. Centers for Disease Control and Prevention (CDC). (2009). State-specific smoking-attributable mortality and years of potential life lost—United States, 2000–2004. *MMWR, 58*(02), 29–33

15. National Center for Health Statistics (NCHS). (2010). 10 Leading Causes of Injury Deaths by Age Group Highlighting Unintentional Injury Deaths, United States-2008. Publication No. CS227502.

CHAPTER 2

1. Rotter, J. B. (1966). Generalized expectancies for internal versus external control of reinforcement. *Psychological Monographs,* 80.

2. Roden, J. (2004). Revisiting the health belief model. *Nursing and Health Sciences, 6,* 1–10.

Taylor, S., and others. (2000). Psychological resources, positive illusions, and health. *American Psychologist, 55,* 99–109.

Peterson, C. (1999). Personal control and well-being. In D. Kahneman, E. Diener, & N. Schwartz (Eds.), *Well-being: The foundations of hedonic psychology.* New York, NY: Russell Sage Foundation.

Myers, D. G., & Diener, E. (1995). Who is happy? *Psychological Science, 6,* 10–18.

3. UICC (Union Internationale contre le Cancer). (2008). *Population survey of cancer-related beliefs and behaviours.* Retrieved from http://www.cancervic.org.au/site/browse.asp?ContainerID=uicc-program3

4. Harvard Center for Cancer Prevention. (1996). Harvard reports on cancer prevention; Vol. 1. Human causes of cancer. *Cancer Causes and Control, 7*(Suppl 1).

Israel, B. (2010). Cancer by the numbers: How many are caused by the environment? *Environmental Health News.* Retrieved at http://www.environmentalhealthnews.org/ehs/news/environmental-cancers

5. Epton, T. & Harris, P. (2008). Self-affirmation promotes health behavior change. *Health Psychology, 27*(6), 746–752.

Scheier, M. F., & Carver, C. S. (1992). Effects of optimism on psychological and physical well-being: Theoretical overview and empirical update. *Cognitive Therapy and Research, 16,* 201–228.

Carver, C., & Scheier, M. (2002). Optimism. In C. R. Snyder & S. J. Lopez (Eds.), *Handbook of positive psychology.* New York, NY: Oxford University Press.

Peterson, C. (2000). The future of optimism. *American Psychologist, 55,* 44–55.

6. Bandura, A. (1977). Self-efficacy: Toward a unifying theory of behavioral change. *Psychological Review, 84,* 191–215.

Bandura, A. (1997). *Self-efficacy: The exercise of control.* New York: Freeman.

7. Pekmezi, D., Jennings, E., & Marcus, B. H. (2009). Evaluating and enhancing self-efficacy for physical activity. *ACSM's Health & Fitness Journal, 13*(2), 16–21.

8. Bandura, A. (1977). *Social learning theory.* Englewood Cliffs, NJ: Prentice-Hall.

Bandura, A. (1997). *Self-efficacy: The exercise of control.* New York: Freeman.

9. Ashford, S., Edmunds, J., & French, D. P. (2010, May). What is the best way to change self-efficacy to promote lifestyle and recreational physical activity? A systematic review with meta-analysis. *British Journal of Health Psychology, 15*(2), 265–288.

10. Maddux, J. (2002). Self-efficacy: The power of believing you can. In C. R. Snyder & S. J. Lopez (Eds.), *Handbook of positive psychology.* New York, NY: Oxford University Press.

11. Williams, S. (1995). Self-efficacy, anxiety, and phobic disorders. In J. E. Maddux (Ed.), *Self-efficacy, adaptation, and adjustment: Theory, research, and application.* New York, NY: Plenum.

Maddux, J. (2002). Self-efficacy: The power of believing you can. In C. R. Snyder & S. J. Lopez (Eds.), *Handbook of positive psychology.* New York, NY: Oxford University Press.

12. Michie, S., Abraham, C., Whittington, C., McAteer, J., & Gupta, S. (2009). Effective techniques in healthy eating and physical activity interventions: A meta-regression. *Health Psychology, 28*(6), 690–701.

Artinian, N. T., and others. (2010). Interventions to promote physical activity and dietary lifestyle changes for cardiovascular risk factor reduction: A scientific statement from the American Heart Association. *Circulation, 122,* 406–441.

13. Forgas, J.P., Baumeister, R.F., & Tice, D.M. (2009). *Psychology of self-regulation.* New York, NY: Psychology Press, Taylor & Francis Group.

14. Prochaska, J. O., Redding, C. A., & Evers, K. E. (2008). The transtheoretical model and stages of change. In K. Glanz, B. K. Rimer, & K. Viswanath (Eds.), *Health behavior and health education: Theory, research, and practice* (4th ed.). San Francisco, CA: Jossey-Bass.

15. Prochaska, J., Norcross, J., & Diclemente, C. (1994). *Changing for good.* New York, NY: Morrow.

Prochaska, J. O., Redding, C. A., & Evers, K. E. (2008). The transtheoretical model and stages of change. In K. Glanz, B. K. Rimer, & K. Viswanath (Eds.), *Health behavior and health education: Theory, research, and practice* (4th ed.). San Francisco, CA: Jossey-Bass.

Hayden, J. (2009). *Introduction to health behavior theory.* Boston, MA: Jones and Bartlett.

16. Sheldon, K. M., & Kasser, T. (1998). Pursuing personal goals: Skills enable progress, but not all progress is beneficial. *Personality and Social Psychology Bulletin, 24,* 1319–1331.

Sheldon, K. M., & Elliot, A. J. (1999). Goal striving, need satisfaction, and longitudinal well-being: The self-concordance model. *Journal of Personality and Social Psychology, 76,* 482–497.

Silva, M., and others. (2010). Exercise autonomous motivation predicts three-year weight loss in women. *Medicine & Science in Sports and Exercise, 43*(4), 728–737.

17. Cantor, N., & Sanderson, C. A. (1999). Life task participation and well-being: The importance of taking part in daily life. In D. Kahneman, E. Diener, & N. Schwartz (Eds.), *Well-being: The foundations of hedonic psychology.* New York, NY: Russell Sage Foundation.

18. Locke, E. A. (2002). Setting goals for life and happiness. In C. R. Snyder & S. J. Lopez (Eds.), *Handbook of positive psychology.* New York: Oxford University Press.

19. Prochaska, J., Norcross, J., & Diclemente, C. (1994). *Changing for good.* New York, NY: Morrow.

CHAPTER 3

1. U.S. Department of Health & Human Services. (2008). *2008 physical activity guidelines for Americans.* ODPHP Publication No. U0036. Rockville, MD: Office of Disease Prevention and Health Promotion.

2. Physical Activity Guidelines Advisory Committee. (2008). *Physical Activity Guidelines Advisory Committee report, 2008.* Washington, DC: U.S. Department of Health and Human Services.

Franco, O. H., Laet, C. D., Peeters, A., Jonker, J., Mackenbach, J., & Nusselder, W. (2005). Effects of physical activity on life expectancy with cardiovascular disease. *Archives of Internal Medicine,* 2355–2360.

Sisson, S. B., Camhi, S. M., Church, T. S., Tudor-Locke, C., Johnson, W. D., & Katzmarzyk, P. T. (2010). Accelerometer-determined steps/day and metabolic syndrome. *American Journal of Preventive Medicine, 38*(6), 575–582.

3. Lacy, A. C., & Hastad, D. N. (2011). *Measurement and evaluation in physical education and exercise science* (6th ed.). San Francisco, CA: Benjamin Cummings.

4. Ibid.

5. American College of Sports Medicine. (2009). *ACSM's resource manual for guidelines for exercise testing and prescription* (6th ed.). Baltimore, MD: Lippincott Williams & Wilkins.

6. Ibid.

7. Tudor-Locke, C., Hatano, Y., Pangrazi, R. P., & Kang, M. (2008). Revisiting "How many steps are enough?" *Medicine and Science in Sports and Exercise, 40*(7 Suppl), S537–S543.

Marshall, S. J., and others. (2009). Translating physical activity recommendations into a pedometer-based step goal: 3000 steps in 30 minutes. *American Journal of Preventive Medicine, 36*(5), 410–415.

8. American College of Sports Medicine. (2009). *ACSM's resource manual for guidelines for exercise testing and prescription* (6th ed.). Baltimore, MD: Lippincott Williams & Wilkins.

9. American College of Sports Medicine. (2009). *ACSM's guidelines for exercise testing and prescription* (8th ed.). Baltimore, MD: Lippincott Williams & Wilkins.

10. Heckert, P. A. (2007). Night running walking safety tips. *Suite101.com.* Retrieved from http://walkingrunning.suite101.com/article.cfm/night_running_walking_safety_tips

11. Atanda, A. (2011). Essential Equipment. *Teens Health.* Retrieved from http://www.kidshealth.org/teen/food_fitness/exercise/sport_safety.html

12. American Academy of Orthopaedic Surgeons. (2007). *Selecting home exercise equipment.* Retrieved from http://orthoinfo.aaos.org/topic.cfm?topic=a00415

13. International Health, Racquet & Sportsclub Association. (2011). *About the industry.* Retrieved from http://www.ihrsa.org/about-the-industry

14. American Council on Exercise. (n.d.). *How to choose a health club.* Retrieved from http://www.acefitness.org/fitfacts/fitfacts_display.aspx?itemid=111

15. MayoClinic.com. (2011). *Heat and exercise: Keeping cool in hot weather.* Retrieved from http://www.mayoclinic.com/health/exercise/HQ00316

16. MayoClinic.com. (2010). *Exercise and cold weather: Tips to stay safe outdoors.* Retrieved from http://www.mayoclinic.com/health/fitness/HQ01681

17. Ibid.

18. U.S. Department of Health & Human Services. (2008). *2008 physical activity guidelines for Americans.* ODPHP Publication No. U0036.

Rockville, MD: Office of Disease Prevention and Health Promotion.

19. Cheung, K., Hume, P., & Maxwell, L. (2003). Delayed onset muscle soreness: Treatment strategies and performance factors. *Sports Medicine, 33*(2), 145–164.

Zainuddin, Z., Newton, M., Sacco, P., & Nosaka, K. (2005). Effects of massage on delayed-onset muscle soreness, swelling, and recovery of muscle function. *Journal of Athletic Training, 40*(3), 174–180.

CHAPTER 4

1. Fox, S. M., & Haskell, W. L. (1970). The exercise stress test: Needs for standardization. In M. Eliakim & H. N. Neufeld (Eds.), *Cardiology: Current topics and progress* (pp. 149–154). New York, NY: Academic Press.

2. Lanteri, C. J., & Sly, P. D. (1993). Changes in respiratory mechanics with age. *Journal of Applied Physiology, 74,* 369–378.

3. Morton, D. P., & Callister, R. (2002). Factors influencing exercise-related transient abdominal pain. *Medicine and Science in Sports and Exercise, 34*(5), 756–766.

4. Leon, A. S., Franklin, B. A., Costa, F., Balady, G. J., Berra, K. A., Stewart, K. J., Thompson, P. D., Williams, M. A., & Lauer, M. S. (2005). Cardiac rehabilitation and secondary prevention of coronary heart disease: An American Heart Association scientific statement from the Council on Clinical Cardiology (Subcommittee on Exercise, Cardiac Rehabilitation, and Prevention) and the Council on Nutrition, Physical Activity, and Metabolism (Subcommittee on Physical Activity), in collaboration with the American Association of Cardiovascular and Pulmonary Rehabilitation. *Circulation, 111*(3), 369–376.

5. Bouchard, C., An, P., Rice, T., Skinner, J. S., Wilmore, J. H., Gagnon, J., Perusse, L., Leon, A. S., & Rao, D. C. (1999). Familial aggregation of VO$_2$ max response to exercise training: Results from the HERITAGE Family Study. *Journal of Applied Physiology, 87*(3), 1003–1008.

6. Reybrouck, T., & Fagard, R. (1999). Gender differences in the oxygen transport system during maximal exercise in hypertensive subjects. *CHEST, 115*(3), 788–792.

7. Thompson, W. R., Gordon, N. F., & Pescatello, L. S. (Eds.). (2009). *ACSM guidelines for exercise testing and prescription* (8th ed., pp. 84–86). Baltimore, MD: Lippincott Williams & Wilkins.

8. Thompson, W. R., Gordon, N. F., & Pescatello, L. S. (Eds.). (2009). *ACSM guidelines for exercise testing and prescription* (8th ed., p. 190). Baltimore, MD: Lippincott Williams & Wilkins.

9. McArdle, W. D., Katch, F. I., & Katch, V. L. (2006). *Essentials of exercise physiology* (3rd ed., p. 453). Baltimore, MD: Lippincott Williams & Wilkins.

10. American College of Sports Medicine. (2004). Position stand: Exercise and hypertension. *Medicine & Science in Sports & Exercise, 36,* 533–553.

11. U.S. Department of Health and Human Services. (2008). Chapter 2: Physical activity has many health benefits. *2008 physical activity guidelines for Americans.* Retrieved from http://www.health.gov/paguidelines/guidelines/default.aspx#toc

12. Blair, S. N., Kohl, H. W., III, Paffenbarger, R. S., Jr., Clark, D. G., Cooper, K. H., & Gibbons, L. W. (1989). Physical fitness and all-cause

mortality. A prospective study of healthy men and women. *Journal of the American Medical Association, 262*(17), 2395–2401.

13. Klem, M. L., Wing, R. R., McGuire, M. T., Seagle, H. M., & Hill, J. O. (1997). A descriptive study of individuals successful at long-term maintenance of substantial weight loss. *American Journal of Clinical Nutrition, 66,* 239–246.

14. Franklin, B. (2004). MeritCare Speaker Series, Moorhead, MN.

15. American College of Sports Medicine. (2009). Position stand: Appropriate physical activity intervention strategies for weight loss and prevention of weight regain for adults. *Medicine & Science in Sports & Exercise, 41*(2), 459–471.

16. American College of Sports Medicine. (2009). *Resource manual to accompany guidelines for exercise testing and prescription* (6th ed.). Baltimore, MD: Lippincott Williams & Wilkins.

17. American College of Sports Medicine. (1998). Position stand: The recommended quantity and quality of exercise for developing and maintaining cardiorespiratory and muscular fitness and flexibility in healthy adults. *Medicine & Science in Sports & Exercise, 30*(6), 975–991.

18. U.S. Department of Health & Human Services. (2008). *2008 Physical Activity Guidelines for Americans.* ODPHP Publication No. U0036. Rockville, MD: Office of Disease Prevention and Health Promotion.

19. Thompson, W. R., Gordon, N. F., & Pescatello, L. S. (Eds.). (2009). *ACSM guidelines for exercise testing and prescription* (8th ed., pp. 166–167). Baltimore, MD: Lippincott Williams & Wilkins.

20. U.S. Department of Health and Human Services and U.S. Department of Agriculture. (2010). *Dietary guidelines for Americans, 2010.* Washington, DC: U.S. Government Printing Office. http://www.cnpp.usda.gov/dietaryguidelines.htm

21. Swain, D. P., Leutholtz, B. C., King, M. E., Haas, L. A., & Branch, J. D. (1998). Relationship between % heart rate reserve and % VO$_2$ reserve in treadmill exercise. *Medicine & Science in Sports & Exercise, 30*(2), 318–321.

22. Nieman, D. C. (2003). Current perspective on exercise immunology. *Current Sports Medicine Reports, 2*(5), 239–242.

CHAPTER 5

1. Centers for Disease Control and Prevention. (2010). *Growing stronger—Strength training for older adults.* http://www.cdc.gov/physicalactivity/growingstronger/why/index.html.

2. Andersen, J. L., Schjerling, P., & Saltin, B. (2000). Muscle, genes, and athletic performance. *Scientific American, 283*(3), 49–55.

3. Suter, E., Herzog, W., Sokolosky, J., Wiley, J. P., & MacIntosh, B. R. (1993). Muscle fiber type distribution as estimated by cybex testing and by muscle biopsy. *Medicine and Science in Sport and Exercise, 25*(3), 363–370.

4. Janssen, I., Heymsfield, S. B., Wang, Z., & Ross, R. (2000). Skeletal muscle mass and distribution in 468 men and women aged 18–88 years. *Journal of Applied Physiology, 89,* 81–88.

5. Kraemer, W. J., Nindl, B. C., Ratamess, N. A., Nicholas, A., Gotshalk, L. A., Volek, J. S., & Hakkinen, K. (2004). Changes in muscle hypertrophy in women with periodized resistance training. *Medicine and Science in Sports Exercise, 36,* 697–708.

6. Beunen, G., & Thomis, M. (2006). Gene driven power athletes? Genetic variation in muscular strength and power. *British Journal of Sports Medicine, 40,* 822–823.

7. Quinn, E. (2009). Body composition—Body fat—Body weight: Learn why body weight and body fat are not always an indication of health. About. com *Sports Medicine.* http://sportsmedicine. about.com/od/fitnessevalandassessment/a/ Body_Fat_Comp.htm.

8. Lee, D.-C., Sui, X., Artero, E. G., Lee, I.-M., Church, T. S., McAuley, P. A., Stanford, F. A., Kohl, H. W., & Blair, S. N. (2011). Long-term effects of changes in cardiorespiratory fitness and body mass index on all-cause and cardiovascular disease mortality in men. *Circulation.* 124, 2483–2490. DOI: 10.1161

9. Sui, X., LaMonte, M. J., Laditka, J. N., Hardin, J. W., Chase, N., Hooker, S. P., & Blair, S. N. (2007). Cardiorespiratory fitness and adiposity as mortality predictors in older adults. *Journal of the American Medical Association, 298*(21), 2507–2516.

10. Brown, S. P., Miller, W. C., & Eason, J. M. (2006). *Exercise physiology: The basis of human movement in health and disease* (pp. 264–66). Baltimore: Lippincott Williams & Wilkins.

11. Häkkinen, K. J. (1989). Neuromuscular and hormonal adaptations during strength and power training. A review. *Sports Medicine and Physical Fitness, 29*(1), 9–26.

12. Kelley, G. (1996). Mechanical overload and skeletal muscle fiber hyperplasia: A meta-analysis. *Journal of Applied Physiology, 81*(4), 1584–1588.

13. Tiainen, K., Sipilä, S., Alen, M., Heikkinen, E., Kaprio, J., Koskenvuo, M., & Rantanen, T. (2004). Heritability of maximal isometric muscle strength in older female twins. *Journal of Applied Physiology, 96,* 173–180.

14. Stewart, C. E. H., & Rittweger, J. (2006). Adaptive processes in skeletal muscle: Molecular regulators and genetic influences. *Journal of Musculoskeletal and Neuronal Interactions, 6*(1), 73–86.

15. Poehlman, E. T., Denino, W. F., Beckett, T., Kinaman, K. A., Dionne, I. J., Dvorak, R., & Ades, P. A. (2002). Effects of endurance and resistance training on total daily energy expenditure in young women: A controlled randomized trial. *Journal of Clinical Endocrinology Metabolism, 87*(3), 1004–1009.

16. Has, C. J., Feigenbaum, M. S., & Franklin, B. A. (2001). Prescription of resistance training for healthy populations. *Sports Medicine, 31*(14), 953–964.

17. Scully, D., Kremer, J., Meade, M. M., Graham, R., & Dudeon, K. (1998). Physical exercise and psychological well-being: A critical review. *British Journal of Sports Medicine, 32*(2), 111–120.

18. Singh, N. A., Stavrinos, T. M., Scarbek, Y., Galambos, G., Liber, C., & Fiatarone Singh, M. A. (2005). A randomized controlled trial of high versus low intensity weight training versus general practitioner care for clinical depression in older adults. *Journals of Gerontology: Biological Sciences, 60*(6), 768–776.

19. Evans, W. J., Meredith, C. N., Cannon, J. G., Dinarello, C. A., Frontera, W. R., Hughes, V. A., and others et al. (1985). Metabolic changes following eccentric exercise in trained and untrained men. *Journal of Applied Physiology,* 61, 1864–1868.

20. American College of Sports Medicine (ACSM). (2010). *Guidelines for exercise testing and prescription* (8th ed.). New York, NY: Lippincott Williams & Wilkins.

21. Connolly, D. A. J., Sayers, S. P., & McHugh, M. P. (2003). Treatment and prevention of delayed onset muscle soreness. *Journal of Strength and Conditioning Research, 17*(1), 197–298.

22. Baker, K. R., Nelson, M. E., Felson, D. T., Layne, J. E., Sarno, R., & Roubenoff, R. (2001). The efficacy of home-based progressive strength training in older adults with knee osteoarthritis: A randomized controlled trial. *The Journal of Rheumatology, 28*(7), 1655–1665.

23. Kloubec, J. A. (2010). Pilates for improvement of muscle endurance, flexibility, balance, and posture. *Journal of Strength and Conditioning Research, 24*(3), 661–667.

24. Kreider, RB. (2003). Effects of creatine supplementation on performance and training adaptations. *Molecular and Cellular Biochemistry, 244*(1–2), 89–94.

25. Husak, J. F., & Duncan, I. J. (2009). Steroid use and human performance: Lessons for integrative biologists. *Integrative and Comparative Biology, 49*(4), 354–364. DOI: 10.1093/icb/ icp015

CHAPTER 6

1. National Strength and Conditioning Association. (2008). *Essentials of strength training and conditioning* (3rd ed). Champaign, IL: Human Kinetics.

2. Weppler, C. H., & Magnusson, S. P. (2010). Increasing muscle extensibility: A matter of increasing length or modifying sensation? *Physical Therapy, 90*(3), 438–449.

Gajdosik, R. L., Allred, J. D., Gabbert, H. L., & Sonsteng, B. A. (2007). A stretching program increases the dynamic passive length and passive resistive properties of the calf muscle-tendon unit of unconditioned younger women. *European Journal of Applied Physiology, 99*(4), 449–454.

3. Ben, M., & Harvey, L. A. (2009). Regular stretch does not increase muscle extensibility: A randomized controlled trial. *Scandinavian Journal of Medicine and Science in Sport, 20*(1), 136–144.

4. Sharman, M. J., Cresswell, A. G., & Riek, S. (2006). Proprioceptive neuromuscular facilitation stretching: Mechanisms and clinical implications. *Sports Medicine, 36*(11), 929–939.

Law, R. Y., Harvey, L. A., Nicholas, M. K., Tonkin, L., DeSousa, M., & Finniss, D. G. (2009). Stretch exercises increase tolerance to stretch in patients with chronic musculoskeletal pain: A randomized controlled trial. *Physical Therapy, 89*(10), 1016–1026.

5. Smith, L. L., Burnet, S. P., & McNeil, J. D. (2003). Musculoskeletal manifestations of diabetes mellitus. *British Journal of Sports Medicine, 37,* 30–35.

6. Centers for Disease Control and Prevention. (2010). A national public health agenda for osteoarthritis 2010. Retrieved from http:// www.cdc.gov/arthritis/docs/OAagenda.pdf Steultjens, M. P., Dekker, J., van Baar, M. E., Oostendorp, R. A., & Bijlsma, J. W. (2000). Range of joint motion and disability in patients with osteoarthritis of the knee or hip. *Rheumatology, 39*(9), 955–961.

7. Battié, M. C., Levalahti, E., Videman, T., Burton, K., & Kaprio, J. (2008). Heritability of lumbar flexibility and the role of disc degeneration and body weight. *Journal of Applied Physiology, 104*(2), 379–385.

8. Children's Memorial Hospital Institute for Sports Medicine. (n.d.). Joint hypermobility syndrome. Retrieved from http://www. childrensmemorial.org/depts/sportsmedicine/ joint_hypermobility.aspx

9. Park, S. K., Stefanyshyn, D. J., Loitz-Ramage, B., Hart, D. A., & Ronsky, J. L. (2009). Changing hormone levels during the menstrual cycle affect knee laxity and stiffness in healthy female subjects. *British Journal of Sports Medicine, 37*(3), 588–598.

10. American College of Sports Medicine. (2009). *ACSM's guidelines for exercise testing and prescription.* Philadelphia, PA: Lippincott Williams & Wilkins.

11. Wallmann, H. (2009). Stretching and flexibility in the aging adult. *Home Health Care Management and Practice, 21*(5), 355–357.

12. McHugh, M. P., & Cosgrave, C. H. (2010). To stretch or not to stretch: The role of stretching on injury prevention and performance. *Scandinavian Journal of Medicine in Sports, 20*(2), 169–181.

13. Caplan, N., Rogers, R., Parr, M. K., & Hayes, P. R. (2009). The effect of proprioceptive neuromuscular facilitation and static stretch training on running mechanics. *Journal of Strength and Conditioning Research, 23*(4), 1175–1180.

14. Kokkonen, J., Nelson, A. G., Eldredge, C., & Winchester, J. B. (2007). Chronic static stretching improves exercise performance. *Medicine and Science in Sports and Exercise, 39*(10), 1825–1831.

15. McHugh, M. P., & Cosgrave, C. H. (2010). To stretch or not to stretch: The role of stretching on injury prevention and performance. *Scandinavian Journal of Medicine in Sports, 20*(2), 169–181.

Thacker, S. B., Gilcrest, J., Stroup, D. F., & Kimsey, C. D., Jr. (2004). The impact of stretching on sports injury risk: A systematic review of the literature. *Medicine and Science in Sports and Exercise, 36*(3), 371–378.

Woods, K., Bishop, P., & Jones, E. (2007). Warm-up and stretching in the prevention of muscular injury. *Sports Medicine, 37*(12), 1089–1099.

Jamtvedt, G., Herbert, R. D., Flottorp, S., and others. (2010). A pragmatic randomised trial of stretching before and after physical activity to prevent injury and soreness. *British Journal of Sports Medicine, 44,* 1002–1009.

16. Jamtvedt, G., Herbert, R. D., Flottorp, S., and others. (2010). A pragmatic randomised trial of stretching before and after physical activity to prevent injury and soreness. *British Journal of Sports Medicine, 44,* 1002–1009.

Small, K., McNaughton, L., & Matthews, M. (2008). A systematic review into the efficacy of static stretching as part of a warm-up for the prevention of exercise-related injury. *Research in Sports Medicine, 16*(3), 213–231.

17. Malliaropoulos, N., Papalexandris, S., Papalada, A., & Papacostas, E. (2004). The role of stretching in rehabilitation of hamstring injuries. *Medicine and Science in Sports and Exercise, 36*(5), 756–759.

18. Cristopoliski, F., Barela, J. A., Leite, N., Fowler, N. E., & Rodacki, A. L. (2009). Stretching exercise program improves gait in the elderly. *Gerontology, 55*(6), 614–620.

Menz, H. B., Morris, M. E., & Lord, S. R. (2005). Foot and ankle characteristics associated with impaired balance and functional ability in older people. *Journal of Gerontology: Biological Sciences, 60,* 1546–1552.

19. Carlson, C. R., Collins, F. L., Jr., Nitz, A. J., Sturgis, E. T., & Rogers, J. L. (1990). Muscle stretching as an alternative relaxation training procedure. *Journal of Behavior Therapy and Experimental Psychiatry, 21*(1), 29–38.

20. Schwellnus, M. P., Drew, N., & Collins, M. (2008). Muscle cramping in athletes—Risk factors, clinical assessment, and management. *Clinics in Sports Medicine, 27*(1), 183–194.

21. American College of Sports Medicine. (2009). *ACSM's guidelines for exercise testing and prescription.* Philadelphia, PA: Lippincott Williams & Wilkins.

22. Fletcher, I. M. (2010). The effect of different dynamic stretch velocities on jump performance. *European Journal of Applied Physiology, 109*(3), 491–498.

Behm, D. & Chaouachi, A. (2011). A review of the acute effects of static and dynamic stretching on performance. *European Journal of Applied Physiology, 111* (11), 2633-2651.

23. Mitchell, U., Myrer, J., Hopkins, J., Hunter, I., Feland, J., Hilton, S., and others. (2006). Reciprocal inhibition, successive inhibition, autogenic inhibition, or stretch perception alteration: Why do PNF stretches work? *Medicine and Science in Sports and Exercise, 38*(5), S66–S67.

24. American College of Sports Medicine. (2009). *ACSM's guidelines for exercise testing and prescription.* Philadelphia, PA: Lippincott Williams & Wilkins.

25. Ibid.

26. U.S. Department of Health and Human Services. (2008.) *2008 physical activity guidelines for Americans.* ODPHP Publication No. U0036. Rockville, MD: Office of Disease Prevention and Health Promotion.

27. Fernández-de-Las-Peñas, C., Cuadrado, M. L., & Pareja, J. A. (2007). Myofascial trigger points, neck mobility, and forward head posture in episodic tension-type headache. *Headache, 47*(5), 662–672.

28. Eltayeb, S., Staal, J. B., Hassan, A., & de Bie, R. S. (2009). Work related risk factors for neck, shoulder and arms complaints: A cohort study among Dutch computer office workers. *Journal of Occupational Rehabilitation, 19*(4), 315–322.

29. National Institute of Neurological Disorders and Stroke. (2011). Low back pain fact sheet. Retrieved from http://www.ninds.nih.gov/disorders/backpain/detail_backpain.htm.

30. Shiri, R., Karppinen, J., Leino-Arjas, P., Solovieva, S., & Viikari-Juntura, E. (2010). The association between smoking and low back pain: A meta-analysis. *American Journal of Medicine, 123*(1), 87.e7–87.e35.

31. Chou, R., Qaseem, A., Snow, V., and others. (2007). Diagnosis and treatment of low back pain: A joint clinical practice guideline from the American College of Physicians and the American Pain Society. *Annals of Internal Medicine, 147*(7), 478–491.

CHAPTER 7

1. Stehno-Bittel, L. (2008). Intricacies of fat. *Physical Therapy: Diabetes Special Issue, 88*(11), 1265–1278.

2. Hackney, K. J., Engels, H. J., & Gretebeck, R. J. (2008). Resting energy expenditure and delayed-onset muscle soreness after full-body resistance training with an eccentric concentration. *Journal of Strength and Conditioning Research, 22,* 1602–1609.

Paschalis, V., Nikolaidis, M. G., Theodorou, A. A., and others. (2010, May 27). A weekly bout of eccentric exercise is sufficient to induce health-promoting effects. *Medicine and Science in Sports and Exercise,* epub ahead of print.

3. Spaulding, K. L., Arner, E., Westermark, P. O., and others. (2008). Dynamics of fat cell turnover in humans. *Nature, 453*(7196), 783–787.

Jo, J., Gavrilova, O., Pack, S., and others. (2009). Hypertrophy and/or hyperplasia: Dynamics of adipose tissue growth. *PLoS Computational Biology, 5*(3), e1000324.

4. Bouchard, C. (1991). Heredity and the path to overweight and obesity. *Medicine and Science in Sports and Exercise, 23*(3), 285–291.

Bray, M. S. (2008). Implications of gene-behavior interactions: Prevention and intervention for obesity. *Obesity, 16*(3), S72–S78.

5. Herbert, A., Gerry, N. P., McQueen, M. B., and others. (2006). A common genetic variant is associated with adult and childhood obesity. *Science, 312*(5771), 279–283.

6. Frayling, T. M., Timpson, N. J., Weedon, M. N., and others. (2007). A common variant in the FTO gene is associated with body mass index and predisposes to childhood and adult obesity. *Science, 316*(5826), 889–894.

7. Rampersaud, E., Mitchell, B. D., Pollin, T. I., and others. (2008). Physical activity and the association of common FTO gene variants with body mass index and obesity. *Archives of Internal Medicine, 168*(16), 1791–1797.

Ruiz, J. R., Labayen, I., Ortega, F. B., and others. (2010). Attenuation of the effect of the FTO rs9939609 polymorphism on total and central body fat by physical activity in adolescents: The HELENA study. *Archives of Pediatric and Adolescent Medicine, 164*(4), 328–333.

8. Wells, J. (2007). Sexual dimorphism of body composition. *Best Practices & Research Clinical Endocrinology & Metabolism, 21*(3), 415–430.

9. Muralidhara, D. (2009). Body composition in subjects of different age and body mass index. *Journal of Physiological and Biomedical Sciences, 22*(1), 23–28.

10. U.S. Department of Health and Human Services. (2009). Mean percentage body fat by age group and sex—National Health and Nutrition Examination Survey, United States, 1999–2004. *MMWR Weekly, 57*(552), 1383. Retrieved from http://www.cdc.gov/mmwr/preview/mmwrhtml/mm5751a4.htm

Wells, J. (2007). Sexual dimorphism of body composition. *Best Practices & Research Clinical Endocrinology & Metabolism, 21*(3), 415–430.

11. Westcott, W. (2009). ACSM strength training guidelines: Role in body composition and health enhancement. *ACSM's Health & Fitness Journal, 13*(4), 14–22.

12. Mott, J. W., Wang, J., Thorton, J. C., Allison, D. B., Heymsfield, S. B., & Pierson, R. (1999). Relationship between body fat and age in four ethnic groups. *American Journal of Clinical Nutrition, 69,* 1007–1013.

13. Ibid.

14. Knutson, K. L., & Van Cauter, E. (2008). Associations between sleep loss and increased risk of obesity and diabetes. *Annals of the New York Academy of Science, 1129,* 287–304.

Cappuccio, F. P., Taggart, F. J., Kandala, N. B., Currie, A., Peile, E., Stranges, S., & Miller, M. A. (2008). Meta-analysis of short sleep duration and obesity in children and adults. *Sleep, 31*(5), 619–626.

15. George, S. A., Khan, S., Briggs, H., & Abelson, J. L. (2010). CRH-stimulated cortisol release and food intake in healthy, non-obese adults. *Psychoneuroendocrinology, 35*(4), 607–612.

Epel, E., Lapidus, R., McEwen, B., & Brownell, K. (2001). Stress may add bite to appetite in women: A laboratory study of stress-induced cortisol and eating behavior. *Psychoneuroendocrinology, 26,* 37–49.

Epel, E., McEwen, B., & Lupien, S. (2000). Cortisol reactivity to repeated stress as a function of fat distribution: Effects on cognition. *Psychoneuroendocrinology, 25*(1), S32.

16. Larson, N. I., Story, M. T., & Nelson, M. C. (2009). Neighborhood environments: Disparities in access to healthy foods in the U.S. *American Journal of Preventive Medicine, 36*(1), 74–81.

Ford, P. B., & Dzewaltowski, D. A. (2008). Disparities in obesity prevalence due to variation in the retail food environment: Three testable hypotheses. *Nutrition Review, 66*(4), 216–228.

17. American Institute for Cancer Research. (2009). *New estimate: Excess body fat alone causes over 100,000 cancers in U.S. each year.* Retrieved from http://www.aicr.org/site/News2?abbr=pr_&page=NewsArticle&id=17333&news_iv_ctrl=1102

18. Stehno-Bittel, L. (2008). Intricacies of fat. *Physical Therapy: Diabetes Special Issue, 88*(11), 1265–1278.

19. Lewis, C. E., and others. (2009). Mortality, health outcomes, and body mass index in the overweight range. A Science Advisory from the American Heart Association. *Circulation, 119,* 3263–3271.

20. American College of Sports Medicine. (2007). Position stand: The Female Athlete Triad. *Medicine and Science in Sports and Exercise, 39*(10), 1867–1882.

21. Benardot, D. (2006). *Advanced sports nutrition.* Champaign, IL: Human Kinetics.

22. Meyers, P., & Biocca, F. (1992). The elastic body image: An experiment on the effect of advertising and programming on body image distortions in young women. *Journal of Communication, 42*(3), 108–133.

23. Razak, F., Anand, S. S., Shannon, H., and others. (2007). Defining obesity cut points in a multiethnic population. *Circulation, 115*(16), 2111–2118.

World Health Organization. (2010). BMI classification. *Global database on body mass index.* http://apps.who.int/bmi/index.jsp?introPage=intro_3.html

24. Schneider, H. J., Friedrich, N., Klotsche, J., and others. (2010). The predictive value of different measures of obesity for incident cardiovascular events and mortality. *Journal of Clinical Endocrinology and Metabolism, 95*(4), 1777–1785.

25. Ashwell, M. (2009). Obesity risk: Importance of waist-to-height ratio. *Nursing Standard, 23*(41), 49–54.

26. Horowitz, J., & Klein, S. (2000). Lipid metabolism during endurance exercise. *American Journal of Clinical Nutrition, 72*(2), 558S–563S.

    Irving, B., Davis, C., Brock, D., Weltman, J., Swift, D., Barrett, E., Gaesser, G., & Weltman, A. (2008). Effect of exercise training intensity on abdominal visceral fat and body composition. *Medicine & Science in Sport & Exercise, 40*(11), 1863–1872.

27. U.S. Department of Health & Human Services. (2008). *2008 physical activity guidelines for Americans.* ODPHP Publication No. U0036.

28. Wing, R. R., & Phelan, S. (2005). Long-term weight loss maintenance. *American Journal of Clinical Nutrition, 82*(1), 222S–225S.

CHAPTER 8

1. Dietary Guidelines Advisory Committee. (2010). *Report of the Dietary Guidelines Advisory Committee on the dietary guidelines for Americans, 2010.* Retrieved from http://www.cnpp.usda.gov/DGAs2010-DGAC Report.htm

2. U.S. Department of Agriculture, Agricultural Research Service. (2009). *USDA national nutrient database for standard reference,* Release 22. Retrieved from Nutrient Data Laboratory home page, http://www.ars.usda.gov/ba/bhnrc/ndl

3. Dietary Guidelines Advisory Committee. (2010). *Report of the Dietary Guidelines Advisory Committee on the dietary guidelines for Americans, 2010.* Retrieved from http://www.cnpp.usda.gov/DGAs2010-DGAC Report.htm

4. Marriott, B., Olsho, L., Hadden, L., & Connor, P. (2010). Intake of added sugars and selected nutrients in the United States, National Health and Nutrition Examination Survey (NHANES) 2003–2006. *Critical Reviews in Food Science and Nutrition, 50,* 228–258.

5. Dietary Guidelines Advisory Committee. (2010). *Report of the Dietary Guidelines Advisory Committee on the dietary guidelines for Americans, 2010.* Retrieved from http://www.cnpp.usda.gov/DGAs2010-DGAC Report.htm

    Fardet, A. (2010). New hypotheses for the health-protective mechanisms of whole-grain cereals: What is beyond fibre? *Nutrition Research Reviews, 23*(1), 65–134.

6. Foster-Powell, K., Holt, S., & Brand-Miller, J. (2002). International table of glycemic index and glycemic load values: 2002. *American Journal of Clinical Nutrition, 76,* 5–56.

7. Dietary Guidelines Advisory Committee. (2010). *Report of the Dietary Guidelines Advisory Committee on the dietary guidelines for Americans, 2010.* Retrieved from http://www.cnpp.usda.gov/DGAs2010-DGAC Report.htm

8. World Health Organization. (2003). Obesity and overweight. *Global strategy on diet, physical activity, and health.* Retrieved from http://www.who.int/dietphysicalactivity/publications/facts/obesity/en/

9. Ibid.

10. Dietary Guidelines Advisory Committee. (2010). *Report of the Dietary Guidelines Advisory Committee on the dietary guidelines for Americans, 2010.* Retrieved from http://www.cnpp.usda.gov/DGAs2010-DGAC Report.htm

11. Bijkerk, C. J., de Wit, N. J., Muris, J. W., Whorwell, P. J., Knottnerus, J. A., & Hoes, A. W. (2009). Soluble or insoluble fibre in irritable bowel syndrome in primary care? Randomised placebo controlled trial. *British Medical Journal, 339,* 606–609.

12. Dahm, C. C., and others. (2010). Dietary fiber and colorectal cancer risk: A nested case-control study using food diaries. *Journal of the National Cancer Institute, 102*(9), 614–626.

13. American Dietetic Association. (2009). Position of the American Dietetic Association: Vegetarian diets. *Journal of the American Dietetic Association, 109*(7), 1266–1282.

14. American College of Sports Medicine, American Dietetic Association, and Dietitians of Canada. (2009). Position stand: Nutrition and athletic performance. *Medicine and Science in Sports and Exercise, 41*(3), 709–731.

15. Frank, H., and others. (2009). Effect of short-term high-protein compared with normal-protein diets on renal hemodynamics and associated variables in healthy young men. *American Journal of Clinical Nutrition, 90*(6), 1509–1516.

16. Dietary Guidelines Advisory Committee. (2010). *Report of the Dietary Guidelines Advisory Committee on the dietary guidelines for Americans, 2010.* Retrieved from http://www.cnpp.usda.gov/DGAs2010-DGAC Report.htm

17. National Cancer Institute, Risk Factor Monitoring and Methods Branch. (2010). *Food sources.* Retrieved from http://riskfactor.cancer.gov/diet/foodsources/

18. Abumweis, S. S., Barake, R., & Jones, P. J. (2008, August 18). Plant sterols/stanols as cholesterol lowering agents: A meta-analysis of randomized controlled trials. *Food and Nutrition Research.*

19. Lukert, B. P., Carey, M., McCarty, B., Tiemann, S., Goodnight, L., Helm, M., and others. (1987). Influence of nutritional factors on calcium-regulating hormones and bone loss. *Calcified Tissue International, 40*(3), 119–125.

20. Harnack, L., Stang, J., & Story, M. (1999). Soft drink consumption among U.S. children and adolescents: Nutritional consequences. *Journal of the American Dietetic Association, 99*(4), 436–441.

21. Tucker, K. L., Morita, K., Qiao, N., Hannan, M. T., Cupples, L. A., & Kiel, D. P. (2006). Colas, but not other carbonated beverages, are associated with low bone mineral density in older women: The Framingham osteoporosis study. *American Journal of Clinical Nutrition, 84*(4), 936–942.

22. Bronstein, A. C., Spyker, D. A., Cantilena, L. R., Jr., Green, J. L., Rumack, B. H., & Heard, S. E. (2008). Annual report of the American Association of Poison Control Centers' National Poison Data System (NPDS): 25th annual report. *Clinical Toxicology, 46*(10), 927–1057.

23. International Food Information Council Foundation. (2009, October 15). Functional foods fact sheet: Antioxidants. *Food Insight.* Retrieved from http://www.foodinsight.org/Resources/Detail.aspx?topic=Functional_Foods_Fact_Sheet_Antioxidants

24. Dietary Guidelines Advisory Committee. (2010). *Report of the Dietary Guidelines Advisory Committee on the dietary guidelines for Americans, 2010.* Retrieved from http://www.cnpp.usda.gov/DGAs2010-DGAC Report.htm

25. Lippi, G., Franchini, M., Favaloro, E. J., & Targher, G. (2010). Moderate red wine consumption and cardiovascular disease risk: Beyond the "French paradox." *Seminars in Thrombosis and Hemostasis, 36*(1), 59–70.

26. Dietary Guidelines Advisory Committee. (2010). *Report of the Dietary Guidelines Advisory Committee on the dietary guidelines for Americans, 2010.* Retrieved from http://www.cnpp.usda.gov/DGAs2010-DGAC Report.htm

27. Ibid.

28. Office of Dietary Supplements, National Institutes of Health. (2009). *Dietary supplement fact sheet: Vitamin D.* Retrieved from http://ods.od.nih.gov/factsheets/vitamind.asp

29. Dietary Guidelines Advisory Committee. (2010). *Report of the Dietary Guidelines Advisory Committee on the dietary guidelines for Americans, 2010.* Retrieved from http://www.cnpp.usda.gov/DGAs2010-DGAC Report.htm

30. Drewnowski, A. (2010). The Nutrient Rich Foods Index helps to identify healthy, affordable foods. *American Journal of Clinical Nutrition, 91*(4), 1095S–1101S.

CHAPTER 9

1. Dietary Guidelines Advisory Committee. (2010). *Report of the Dietary Guidelines Advisory Committee on the dietary guidelines for Americans, 2010.* Retrieved from http://www.cnpp.usda.gov/DGAs2010-DGAC Report.htm

2. Guenther, P. M., Dodd, K. W., Reedy, J., & Krebs-Smith, S. M. (2006). Most Americans eat much less than recommended amounts of fruits and vegetables. *Journal of the American Dietetic Association, 106*(9), 1371–1379.

3. Ruxton, C. H. S., Gardner, E. J., & Walker, D. (2006). Can pure fruit and vegetable juices protect against cancer and cardiovascular disease too? A review of the evidence. *International Journal of Food Sciences and Nutrition, 57*(3/4), 249–272.

4. Goldstone, A. P., de Hernandez, C. G. P., Beaver, J. D., Muhammed, K., Croese, C., Bell, G., and others. (2009). Fasting biases brain reward systems towards high-calorie foods. *European Journal of Neuroscience, 30,* 1625–1635.

5. American Dietetic Association. (2009). Position of the American Dietetic Association: Vegetarian diets. *Journal of the American Dietetic Association, 109,* 1266–1282.

6. National Heart, Lung, and Blood Institute. (2006). *Your guide to lowering your blood pressure with DASH.* NIH Publication No. 06-4082. Bethesda, MD: National Institutes of Health.

7. Smith, P. J., Blumenthal, J. A., Babyak, M. A., Craighead, L., Welsh-Bohmer, K. A., Browndyke, J. N., Strauman, T. A., & Sherwood, A. (2010). Effects of the dietary approaches to stop hypertension diet, exercise, and caloric restriction on neurocognition in overweight adults with high blood pressure. *Hypertension, 55*(6), 1331–1338.

8. Institute of Medicine. (2006). *Addressing Foodborne Threats to Health: Policies, Practices, and Global Coordination Workshop Summary.* Washington D.C.: National Academy Press.

9. Byrd-Bredbenner, C., Maurer, J., Wheatley, V., Schaffner, D., Bruhn, C., & Blalock, L. (2007). Food safety self-reported behaviors and cognitions of young adults: Results of a national study. *Journal of Food Protection, 70*(8), 1917–1926.

10. Abbot, J. M., Byrd-Bredbenner, C., Schaffner, D., Bruhn, C. M., & Blalock, L. (2009). Comparison of food safety cognitions and self-reported food-handling behaviors with observed food safety behaviors of young adults. *European Journal of Clinical Nutrition, 63*(4), 572–579.

11. U.S. Environmental Protection Agency. Mercury: Fish Consumption Advisories. (2012). Retrieved from http://www.epa.gov/mercury/advisories.htm. Last accessed January 2012.

12. U.S. Department of Agriculture National Agriculture Library. (2007). What is organic production? Retrieved from http://www.nal.usda.gov/afsic/pubs/ofp/ofp.shtml

13. Guan, T. Y., & Holley, R. A. (2003). Pathogen survival in swine manure environments and transmission of human enteric illness—A review. *Journal of Environmental Quality, 32*, 383–392.

14. Alternative Farming Systems Information Center, U.S. Department of Agriculture. (2008). *Should I purchase organic foods?* Retrieved from http://www.nal.usda.gov/afsic/pubs/faq/BuyOrganicFoodsIntro.shtml

15. Centers for Disease Control and Prevention. (2005). *Food irradiation.* Retrieved from http://www.cdc.gov/nczved/divisions/dfbmd/diseases/irradiation_food/#what

16. Sacks, F. M., and others. (2009). Comparison of weight-loss diets with different compositions of fat, protein, and carbohydrates. *New England Journal of Medicine, 360*(9), 859–873.

17. Alhassan, S., Kim, S., Bersamin, A., King, A. C., & Gardner, C. D. (2008). Dietary adherence and weight loss success among overweight women: Results from the A to Z weight loss study. *International Journal of Obesity, 32*(6), 985–991.

18. Randles, A., & Liguori, G. (2010). Does SES influence healthy eating promotions in restaurants? Abstract presented at the 2010 American Public Health Association annual meeting.

19. Artinian, N. T., and others. (2010). Interventions to promote physical activity and dietary lifestyle changes for cardiovascular risk factor reduction: A scientific statement from the American Heart Association. *Circulation, 122*, 406–441.

20. Burke, L. E., Sereika, S. M., Music, E., Warziski, M., Styn, M. A., & Stone, A. (2008). Using instrumented paper diaries to document self-monitoring patterns in weight loss. *Contemporary Clinical Trials, 29*(2), 182–193.

21. American Dietetic Association. (2009). Position of the American Dietetic Association: Weight management. *Journal of the American Dietetic Association, 109*, 330–346.

22. Wing, R. R., & Phelan, S. (2005). Long-term weight loss maintenance. *American Journal of Clinical Nutrition, 82*(1 Suppl), 222S–225S. Catenacci, V. A., and others. (2008). Physical activity patterns in the National Weight Control Registry. *Obesity, 16*(1), 153–161.

23. Larson-Meyer, D. E., Redman, L., Heilbronn, L. K., Martin, C. K., & Ravussin, E. (2010). Caloric restriction with or without exercise: The fitness versus fatness debate. *Medicine and Science in Sports and Exercise, 42*(1), 152–159.

24. International Congress on Obesity. (2010). *News release: New research finds no evidence that popular slimming supplements facilitate weight loss.*

25. Bent, S., Tiedt, T. N., Odden, M. C., & Shlipak, M. G. (2003). The relative safety of ephedra compared with other herbal products. *Annals of Internal Medicine, 138*(6), 468–471.

26. ConsumerReportsHealth.org. (2010). *Dangerous supplements: What you don't know about these 12 ingredients could hurt you.* Retrieved from http://www.consumerreports.org/health/natural-health/dietary-supplements/overview/index.htm

27. U.S. Food and Drug Administration. (2010). *"Dietary supplements" that contain undeclared prescription ingredients or other chemicals.* Retrieved from http://www.fda.gov/ForConsumers/ConsumerUpdates/ucm278980.htm

28. American Dietetic Association. (2009). Position of the American Dietetic Association: Weight management. *Journal of the American Dietetic Association, 109*, 330–346.

29. Mayo Clinic Health Information. (2012, February). Weight loss. Retrieved from http://www.mayoclinic.com/health/alli/WT00030. Last accessed April 2012.

30. U.S. Food and Drug Administration. (2010, May). Weight-loss drugs and risk of liver failure. *Consumer updates.* Retrieved from http://www.fda.gov/ForConsumers/ConsumerUpdates/ucm213401.htm

31. Smith SR, Weissman NJ, Anderson CM, Sanchez M, Chuang E, Stubbe S, Bays H, Shanahan WR. (2010). Multicenter, Placebo-Controlled Trial of Lorcaserin for Weight Management. *New England Journal of Medicine. 363*, 245–256

32. American College of Sports Medicine. (2009). Progression models in resistance training for healthy adults. *Medicine and Science in Sports and Exercise, 41*(3), 687–708.

33. National Institute of Mental Health. (2009). *Eating disorders.* Retrieved from http://www.nimh.nih.gov/health/publications/eating-disorders/complete-index.shtml

34. Borzekowski, D. L., Schenk, S., Wilson, J. L., & Peebles, R. (2010). e-Ana and e-Mia: A content analysis of pro-eating disorder Web sites. *American Journal of Public Health, 100*(8), 1526–1534.

CHAPTER 10

1. Dunser, M. W., & Hasibeder, W. R. (2009). Sympathetic overstimulation during critical illness: Adverse effects of adrenergic stress. *Journal of Intensive Care Medicine, 24*(5), 293–316.

2. Lee, H. J., Macbeth, A. H., Pagani, J. H., & Young, WS. (2009). Oxytocin: The great facilitator of life. *Progressive Neurobiology, 88*(2), 127–151.

3. Stewart, J. C., Fitzgerald, G. J., & Kamarck, T. W. (2010). Hostility now, depression later? Longitudinal associations among emotional risk factors for coronary heart disease. *Annals of Behavioral Medicine, 39*(3), 258–266.

4. Williams, R., & Williams, V. (1994). *Anger kills.* New York, NY: Harper Paperbacks.

5. Denollet, J., and Conraads, V. M. (2011). Type D personality and vulnerability to adverse outcomes in heart disease. *Cleveland Clinic Journal of Medicine.* 78 Suppl 1 S13-S19. doi: 10.3949/ccjm.78.s1.02

6. Gitau, R., Cameron, A., Fisk, N. M., & Glover, V. (1998). Fetal exposure to maternal cortisol. *Lancet, 352*(9129), 707–708.

7. Taylor, S. E. (2000). A new stress paradigm for women. *Monitor on Psychology, 31*(7).

8. Taylor, S. E., Klein, L. C., Lewis, B. P., Gruenewald, T. L., Gurung, R. A. R., & Updegraff, J. A. (2000). Biobehavioral responses to stress in females: Tend-and-befriend, not fight-or-flight. *Psychology Review, 107*(3), 411–429.

9. Lazarus, R. S., & Folkman, S. (1984). *Stress, appraisal, and coping.* New York, NY: Springer.

10. Weiner, B. (1986). *An attributional theory of emotion and motivation.* New York, NY: Springer-Verlag.

11. Lazarus, R. S., & Folkman, S. (1984). *Stress, appraisal, and coping.* New York, NY: Springer.

12. Bose, M., Olivan, B., & Laferre, B. (2009). Stress and obesity: The role of the hypothalamic-pituitary-adrenal axis in metabolic disease. *Current Opinion in Endocrinology, Diabetes, and Obesity, 16*(5), 340–346.

13. McEwen, B. S. (2000). Allostasis and allostatic load: Implications for neuropsychopharmacology. *Neuropsychopharmacology, 22*(2), 108–124.

14. Nyberg, A., Alfredsson, L., Theorell, T., Westerlund, H., Vahtera, J., & Kivimäki, M. (2009). Managerial leadership and ischaemic heart disease among employees: The Swedish WOLF study. *Occupational and Environmental Medicine, 66*(11), 51–55.

15. Mozumdar, A., Liguori, G., Fountaine, C., Braun, S., & Muenchow, E. (2008). Working status, academic activity, leisure time activity, and BMI among first and second year college students. [Abstract]. *Medicine & Science in Sports & Exercise, 40*(5), Supplement.

16. ACT. (2010). What works in student retention. *Research and policy issues.* Retrieved from http://www.act.org/research/policymakers/reports/retain.htm

17. NASPA–Student Affairs Administrators in Higher Education. (2008). *Profile of the American college student, 2008.* Retrieved from http://www.naspa.org/divctr/research/profile/results.cfm U.S. Department of Education, National Center for Education Statistics. (2009). *Digest of education statistics, 2008* (NCES 2009-020), Chapter 3.

18. Hansen CJ, Stevens LC, & Coast RJ. (2001). Exercise duration and mood state: How much is enough to feel better? *Health Psychology, 20*, 267–275

19. Hairston, K, G., Bryer-Ash, M., Norris, J, M., Haffner, S., Bowden, D. W., Wagenknecht, L. E. (2010). Sleep duration and five-year abdominal fat accumulation in a minority cohort: The IRAS family study. *Sleep, 33*(3), 289–295.

20. Capuccio, F. P., D'Elia, L., Strazzullo, P., & Miller, M. A. (2010). Sleep duration and all-cause mortality: A systematic review and meta-analysis of prospective studies. *Sleep, 33*(5), 585–592.

21. MayoClinic.com. (2009). Causes. *Insomnia* (http://www.mayoclinic.com/health/insomnia/DS00187/DSECTION=causes).

22. Cohen, D. A., Wang, W., Wyat, J. K., Kronauer, R. E., Dijk, D-J., Czeisler, C. A., & Klerman, E. B. (2010). Uncovering residual effects of chronic sleep loss on human performance. *Science Translational Medicine, 2*(14), 14ra3.

23. Benson, H., & Klipper, M. (1975). *The relaxation response.* New York, NY: HarperCollins.

24. Nidich, S. I., Rainforth, M. V., Haaga, D. A., Hagelin, J., Salerno, J. W., Travis, F., Tanner, M., Gaylord-King, C., Grosswald, S., Schneider, R. H. (2009). A randomized controlled trial on the effects of the Transcendental Meditation program on blood pressure, psychological distress, and coping in young adults. *American Journal of Hypertension 22*(12), 1326–1331.

CHAPTER 11

1. Roger, V. L., and others. (2012). Heart disease and stroke statistics 2012 update: A report from the American Heart Association. *Circulation, 125,* e2–e220.

2. Humphries, S. E., Drenos, F., Ken-Dror, G., & Talmud, P. J. (2010). Coronary heart disease risk prediction in the era of genome-wide association studies: Current status and what the future holds. *Circulation, 121*(20), 2235–2248.

   Dandona, S., Steward, A. F., & Roberts, R. (2010). Genomics in coronary artery disease: Past, present, and future. *Canadian Journal of Cardiology, 26*(Suppl A), 56A–59A.

3. American Heart Association. (2010). Heart disease and stroke statistics 2010 update: A report from the American Heart Association. *Circulation, 121,* e46–e215.

4. National Institute on Aging. (2005). *Aging hearts and arteries: A scientific quest.* NIH Publication No. 05-3738.

5. Pérez-López, F. R., Larrad-Mur, L., Kallen, A., Chedraui, P., & Taylor, H. S. (2010). Gender differences in cardiovascular disease: Hormonal and biochemical influences. *Reproductive Sciences, 17*(6), 511–531.

6. Berger, J. S., and others. (2009). Sex differences in mortality following acute coronary syndromes. *JAMA, 302*(8), 874–882.

   Regitz-Zagrosek, V. (2012). Sex and gender differences in cardiovascular disease. In S. Oertelt-Prigione & V. Regitz-Zagrosek (Eds.), *Sex and gender aspects in clinical medicine.* London: Springer-Verlag.

7. American Heart Association. (2010). Heart disease and stroke statistics 2010 update: A report from the American Heart Association. *Circulation, 121,* e46–e215.

8. Kurian, A. K., & Cardarelli, K. M. (2007 Winter). Racial and ethnic differences in cardiovascular disease risk factors: A systematic review. *Ethnicity and Disease, 17*(1), 143–152.

9. Dietary Guidelines Advisory Committee. (2010). *Report of the Dietary Guidelines Advisory Committee on the dietary guidelines for Americans, 2010.* Retrieved from http://www.cnpp.usda.gov/DGAs2010-DGAC Report.htm

   Stewart, D., Johnson, W., & Saunders, E. (2006). Hypertension in black Americans as a special population: Why so special? *Current Cardiology Reports, 8*(6), 405–410.

10. Bogers, R. P., and others. (2007). Association of overweight with increased risk of coronary heart disease partly independent of blood pressure and cholesterol levels: A meta-analysis of 21 cohort studies including more than 300,000 persons. *Archives of Internal Medicine, 167*(16), 1720–1728.

11. Roger, V. L., and others. (2012). Heart disease and stroke statistics 2012 update: A report from the American Heart Association. *Circulation, 125,* e2–e220.

12. U.S. Department of Health and Human Services. (2004). *The health consequences of smoking: A report of the Surgeon General.* Atlanta, GA: National Center for Chronic Disease Prevention and Health Promotion, Office on Smoking and Health.

13. Snow, W. M., Murray, R., Ekuma, O., Tyas, S. L., & Barnes, G. E. (2009). Alcohol use and cardiovascular health outcomes: A comparison across age and gender in the Winnipeg Health and Drinking Survey Cohort. *Age and Aging, 38*(2), 206–212.

14. Yap, S., Qin, C., & Woodman, O. L. (2010). Effects of resveratrol and flavonols on cardiovascular function: Physiological mechanisms. *Biofactors, 36*(5), 350–359.

15. Pletcher, M. J., and others. (2008). Prehypertension during young adulthood and coronary calcium later in life. *Annals of Internal Medicine, 149,* 91–99.

16. Pletcher, M. J., and others. (2010). Nonoptimal lipids commonly present in young adults and coronary calcium later in life: the CARDIA (Coronary Artery Risk Development in Young Adults) Study. *Annals of Internal Medicine, 153,* 137–146.

17. Roger, V. L., and others. (2012). Heart disease and stroke statistics 2012 update: A report from the American Heart Association. *Circulation, 125,* e2–e220.

18. Svensson, L., and others. (2010). Compression-only CPR or standard CPR in out-of-hospital cardiac arrest. *New England Journal of Medicine, 363*(5), 434–442.

19. American Cancer Society. (2012). *Cancer facts & figures 2012.* Atlanta, GA: ACS.

20. National Cancer Institute. (2012). *What is cancer?* http://www.cancer.gov/cancertopics/what-is-cancer

21. American Cancer Society. (2012). *Cancer facts & figures 2012.* Atlanta, GA: ACS.

22. Ibid.

23. Ibid.

24. U.S. Department of Health and Human Services. (2005). *National toxicology program 11th report on carcinogens.* Triangle Park, MD: National Toxicology Program.

25. American Cancer Society. (2012). *Cancer facts & figures 2012.* Atlanta, GA: ACS.

26. Singh, R., and others. (2009). Evaluation of the DNA damaging potential of cannabis cigarette smoke by the determination of acetaldehyde derived N2-ethyl-2′-deoxyguanosine adducts. *Chemical Research in Toxicology, 22*(6), 1181–1188.

    Mehra, R., Moore, B. A., Crothers, K., Tetrault, J., & Fiellin, D. A. (2006). The association between marijuana smoking and lung cancer: A systematic review. *Archives of Internal Medicine, 166*(13), 1359–1367.

27. Hu, S., and others. (2009). Disparity in melanoma: A trend analysis of melanoma incidence and stage at diagnosis among whites, Hispanics, and blacks in Florida. *Archives of Dermatology, 145*(12), 1369–1374.

28. National Institute of Diabetes and Digestive and Kidney Diseases (NIDDK). (2011). National Diabetes Information Clearinghouse: National diabetes statistics. Retrieved from http://diabetes.niddk.nih.gov/dm/pubs/statistics/index.aspx#fast

29. Ibid.

30. National Institute of Diabetes and Digestive and Kidney Diseases (NIDDK). (2011). National Diabetes Information Clearinghouse: Diabetes overview. Retrieved from http://diabetes.niddk.nih.gov/dm/pubs/overview/#types

31. Centers for Disease Control and Prevention. (2011). *National diabetes fact sheet: National estimates and general information on diabetes and prediabetes in the United States, 2011.* Atlanta, GA: CDC.

32. National Institute of Diabetes and Digestive and Kidney Diseases (NIDDK). (2007). *Type 2 Diabetes: What you need to know.* NIH Publication No. 07–6192S.

CHAPTER 12

1. Winther, B., McCue, K., Ashe, K., Rubino, J. R., & Hendley, J. O. (2007). Environmental contamination with rhinovirus and transfer to fingers of healthy individuals by daily life activity. *Journal of Medical Virology, 79*(10), 1606–1610.

2. Wood, J. P., Choi, Y. W., Chappie, D. J., Rogers, J. V., & Kaye, J. Z. (2009). *Environmental persistence of a highly pathogenic avian influenza (H1N1) virus.* Research Triangle Park, NC: Environmental Protection Agency. Pub. No. EPA/600/R-09/054.

3. Smith-McCune, K. K., Shiboski, S., Chirenje, M. Z., and others. (2010). Type-specific cervico-vaginal human papillomavirus infection increases risk of HIV acquisition independent of other sexually transmitted infections. *PLoS One, 5*(4), e10094.

4. Sadeharju, K., Knip, M., Virtanen, S. M., Savilahti, E., Tauriainen, S., Koskela, P., Akerblom, H. K., & Hyoty, H. (2007). Maternal antibodies in breast milk protect the child from enterovirus infections. *Pediatrics, 119*(5), 941–946.

5. Centers for Disease Control and Prevention. (2010). Hepatitis C FAQs for health professionals (http://www.cdc.gov/hepatitis/HCV/HCVfaq.htm).

6. Aiello, A. E., Coulborn, R. M., Perez, V., & Larson, E. L. (2008). Effect of hand hygiene on infectious disease risk in the community setting: A meta-analysis. *American Journal of Public Health, 98*(8), 1372–1381.

7. Anderson, J. L., Warren, C. A., Perez, E., Louis, R. I., Phillips, S., Wheeler, J., Cole, M., & Misra, R. (2008). Gender and ethnic differences in hand hygiene practices among college students. *American Journal of Infection Control, 36*(5), 361–368.

8. Fondell, E., Lagerros, Y. T., Sundberg, C. J., Lekander, M., Balter, O., Rothman, K. J., & Balter, K. (2010). Physical activity, stress, and self-reported upper respiratory tract infection. *Medicine and Science in Sports and Exercise, 43*(2), 272–279, February 2011. DOI: 10.1249/MSS.0b013e3181edf108.

9. Pedersen, A., Zachariae, R., & Bovbjerg, D. H. (2010). Influence of psychological stress on upper respiratory infection—A meta-analysis of prospective studies. *Psychosomatic Medicine, 72*(8), 823–832.

10. Bennett, M. P., Zeller, J. M., Rosenberg, L., & McCann, J. (2003). The effect of mirthful laughter on stress and natural killer cell activity. *Alternative Therapies in Health and Medicine, 9*(2), 38–45.

11. Costelloe, C., Metcalfe, C., Lovering, A., Mant, D., & Hay, A. D. (2010). Effect of antibiotic prescribing in primary care on antimicrobial resistance in individual patients: Systematic review and meta-analysis. *British Medical Journal, 18* (340), c2096.

12. Centers for Disease Control and Prevention. (2010). How flu spreads (http://www.cdc.gov/flu/about/disease/spread.htm).

13. Centers for Disease Control and Prevention, National Center for Infectious Diseases. (2006). Epstein-Barr virus and infectious mononucleosis (http://www.cdc.gov/ncidod/diseases/ebv.htm).

14. Centers for Disease Control and Prevention. (2010). Fact sheet: Genital herpes (http://www.cdc.gov/std/herpes).

15. Giannini, C. M., Kim, H. K., Mortensen, J., Mortensen, J., Marsolo, K., & Huppert, J., (2010). Culture of non-genital sites increases the detection of gonorrhea in women. *Journal of Pediatric and Adolescent Gynecology, 23*(4), 246–252.

16. Cottrell, B. H. (2010). An updated review of evidence to discourage douching. *MCN: The American Journal of Maternal/Child Nursing, 35*(2), 102–107.

17. National Institute of Allergy and Infectious Diseases. (2009). *Pelvic inflammatory disease* (http://www.niaid.nih.gov/topics/pelvicinflammatorydisease).

18. Winer, R. L., Fen, Q., Hughes, J. P., O'Reilly, S., Kiviat, N. B., & Koutsky, L. A. (2008). Risk of female human papillomavirus acquisition associated with first male sex partner. *Journal of Infectious Diseases, 197*(2), 279–282.

19. Partridge, J. M., Hughes, J. P., Feng, Q., Fu Xi, L., Cherne, S., O'Reilly, S., Kiviat, N. B., Koutsky, L. A. (2007). Genital human papillomavirus infection in men: Incidence and risk factors in a cohort of university students. *Journal of Infectious Diseases, 196*(8), 1128–1136.

20. Winer, R. L., Hughes, J. P., Feng, Q., O'Reilly, S., Kiviat, N. B., Holmes, K. K., & Koutsky, L. A. (2006). Condom use and the risk of genital human papillomavirus infection in young women. *New England Journal of Medicine, 354*(25), 2645–2654.

21. Centers for Disease Control and Prevention. (2010). Diagnoses of HIV infection and AIDS in the United States and dependent areas. *HIV Surveillance Report, 200,* 20 (http://www.cdc.gov/hiv/topics/surveillance/resources/reports).

National Center for Health Statistics. (2010). Deaths: Leading causes for 2006. *National Vital Statistics Reports, 58*(14).

22. Joint United Nations Programme on HIV/AIDS (UNAIDS). (2010). *UNAIDS outlook report 2010.* Geneva: UNAIDS.

23. Trepka, M. J., & Kim, S. (2010). Prevalence of human immunodeficiency virus testing and high-risk human immunodeficiency virus behavior among 18 to 22 year-old students and nonstudents: Results of the National Survey of Family Growth. *Sexually Transmitted Diseases, 37*(10), 653–659.

24. Davis, K. R., & Weller, S. C. (1999). The effectiveness of condoms in reducing heterosexual transmission of HIV. *Family Planning Perspectives, 31*(6), 272–279.

25. Centers for Disease Control and Prevention. (2010). *Basic information about HIV and AIDS* (http://www.cdc.gov/hiv/topics/basic/).

26. Ibid.

27. Centers for Disease Control and Prevention. (2006). Revised recommendation for HIV testing of adults, adolescents, and pregnant women in health-care settings. *MMWR Recommendations and Reports, 55* (RR14), 1–17.

28. Abdool, K. Q., Abdool, K. S. S., Frohlich, J. A., and others. (2010). Effectiveness and safety of tenofovir gel, an antiretroviral microbicide, for the prevention of HIV infection in women. *Science, 329*(5996), 1168–1174.

CHAPTER 13

1. National Institute on Drug Abuse. (2010). *Drugs, brains, and behavior: The science of addiction.* NIH Pub. No. 10-5605.

2. Substance Abuse and Mental Health Services Administration. (2010). *Results from the 2009 National Survey on Drug Use and Health.* Rockville, MD: Office of Applied Studies, Substance Abuse and Mental Health Services Administration.

3. National Institute on Drug Abuse. (2010). *Drugs, brains, and behavior: The science of addiction.* NIH Pub. No. 10-5605.

4. Frary, C. D., Johnson, R. K., & Wang, M. Q. (2005). Food sources and intakes of caffeine in the diets of persons in the United States. *Journal of the American Dietetic Association, 105*(1), 110–113.

5. Duchan, E., Patel, N. D., & Feucht, C. (2010). Energy drinks: A review of use and safety for athletes. *The Physician and Sportsmedicine, 38*(2), 171–179.

6. Salazar-Martinez, E., Willett, W. C., Ascherio, A., and others. (2004). Coffee consumption and risk for type 2 diabetes mellitus. *Annals of Internal Medicine, 140*(1), 1–8.

7. Prediger, R. D. (2010). Effects of caffeine in Parkinson's disease: From neuroprotection to the management of motor and non-motor symptoms. *Journal of Alzheimer's Disease, 20*(Suppl 1), S205–S220.

8. National Institute on Drug Abuse. (2010). *Research report series: Marijuana abuse.* NIH Pub. No. 10-3859.

9. Mittleman, M. A., Lewis, R. A., Maclure, M., Sherwood, J. B., & Muller, J. E. (2001). Triggering myocardial infarction by marijuana. *Circulation, 103*(23), 2805–2809.

10. Richer, I., & Bergeron, J. (2009). Driving under the influence of cannabis: Links with dangerous driving, psychological predictors, and accident involvement. *Accident Analysis and Prevention, 41*(2), 299–307.

11. Sewell, R. A., Poling, J., & Sofuoglu, M. (2009). The effect of cannabis compared with alcohol on driving. *American Journal of Addiction, 18*(3), 185–193.

12. Tetrault, J. M., Crothers, K., Moore, B. A., Mehra, R., Concato, J., & Fiellin, D. A. (2007). Effects of marijuana smoking on pulmonary function and respiratory complications: A systematic review. *Archives of Internal Medicine, 167*(3), 221–228.

13. Moore, T., Zammit, S., Lingford-Hughes, A., Barnes, T., Jones, P., Burke, M., & Lewis, G. (2007). Cannabis use and risk of psychotic or affective mental health outcomes: A systematic review. *Lancet, 370*(9584), 319–328.

14. Budney, A. J., Vandrey, R. G., Hughes, J. R., Thostenson, J. D., & Bursac, Z. (2008). Comparison of cannabis and tobacco withdrawal: Severity and contribution to relapse. *Journal of Substance Abuse and Treatment, 35*(4), 362–368.

15. National Institute on Drug Abuse. (2010). *Research report series: Marijuana abuse.* NIH Pub. No. 10-3859.

16. Centers for Disease Control and Prevention. (2010). Ecstasy overdoses at a New Year's Eve Rave—Los Angeles, California, 2010. *Morbidity and Mortality Weekly Report, 59*(22), 677–681.

17. Dumont, C. J., Wezenberg, E., Valkenberg, M. M., and others. (2008). Acute neuropsychological effects of MDMA and ethanol co-administration in healthy volunteers. *Psychopharmacology, 197*(3), 465–474.

18. Warner, M., Chen, L. H., & Makuc, D. M. (2009). Increase in fatal poisonings involving opioid analgesics in the United States, 1999–2006. *NCHS Data Brief,* No. 22. Hyattsville, MD: CDC National Center for Health Statistics.

19. Centers for Disease Control and Prevention. (2005). *Behavioral Risk Factor Surveillance System, trends data, alcohol use: Binge drinking, 2005.* Atlanta, GA: CDC.

20. Office of Juvenile Justice and Delinquency Prevention. (2005). *Drinking in America: Myths, realities, and prevention policy.* Washington, DC: U.S. Department of Justice, Office of Justice Programs, OJJDP.

21. Swift, R., & Davidson, D. (1998). Alcohol hangover: Mechanisms and mediators. *Alcohol Health and Research World, 22*(1), 54–60.

22. National Institute on Alcohol Abuse and Alcoholism. (2000). *Alcohol alert: Alcohol metabolism.* NIAAA Pub. No. 35; PH 271.

23. McKinney, A., & Coyle, K. (2004). Next day effects of a normal night's drinking on memory and psychomotor performance. *Alcohol and Alcoholism, 39*(6), 509–513.

24. Department of Transportation, National Highway Traffic Safety Administration (NHTSA). (2009). *Traffic safety facts 2008: Alcohol-impaired driving.* Washington, DC: NHTSA. Available at http://wwwnrd.nhtsa.dot.gov/Pubs/811155.PDF

25. American Psychiatric Association. (1994). *Diagnostic and statistical manual of mental disorders* (4th ed.). Washington, DC: APA.

26. Centers for Disease Control and Prevention. (2007). Cigarette smoking among adults, United States, 2006. *Morbidity and Mortality Weekly Report, 56*(44), 1157–1161.

27. Centers for Disease Control and Prevention (2005). Tobacco use, access, and exposure to tobacco in media among middle and high school students—United States, 2004. *Morbidity and Mortality Weekly Report, 54*(12), 297–301.

28. U.S. Department of Health and Human Services. *The health consequences of smoking: A report of the Surgeon General.* Retrieved from http://www.surgeongeneral.gov/library/smokingconsequences/

29. Suminski, R. R., Wier, L. T., Poston, W., Arenare, B., Randles, A., & Jackson, A. S. (2009). The effect of habitual smoking on measured and predicted VO$_2$max. *Journal of Physical Activity and Health, 6*(5), 667–673.

30. Akbartabartoori, M., Lean, M. E., & Han-key, C. R. (2005). Relationship between cigarette smoking, body size and body shape. *International Journal of Obesity, 29*(2), 236–242.

31. Barrett-Connor, E., & Khaw, K. T. (1989). Cigarette smoking and increased central adiposity. *Annals of Internal Medicine, 111*(10), 783–787.

32. Sépaniak, S., Forges, T., & Monnier-Barbarino, P. (2006). Cigarette smoking and fertility in women and men. *Gynecology, Obstetrics, and Fertility, 34*(10), 945–949.

Sepaniak, S., Forges, T., Fontaine, B., Gerard, H., Foliguet, B., Guillet-May, F., Zaccabri, A., & Monnier-Barbarino, P. (2004). Negative impact of cigarette smoking on male fertility: From spermatozoa to the offspring. *Jo1urnal of Gynecology, Obstetrics, and Biological Reproduction, 33*(5), 384–90.

33. National Cancer Institute. Smokefree.gov (n.d.). *Myths about smoking and pregnancy.* Retrieved from http://women.smokefree.gov/topic-pregnancy-myths.aspx

34. Primack, B. A., Fertman, C. I., Rice, K. R., Adachi-Mejia, A. M., & Fine, M. J. (2010). Waterpipe and cigarette smoking among college athletes in the United States. *Journal of Adolescent Health, 46*(1), 45–51.

35. Eissenberg, T., & Shihadeh, A. (2009). Waterpipe tobacco and cigarette smoking: Direct comparison of toxicant exposure. *American Journal of Preventive Medicine, 37*(6), 518–523.

36. National Cancer Institute. (2012). Health effects of exposure to environmental tobacco smoke. *Smoking and Tobacco Control Monographs,* 10. Retrieved from http://cancercontrol.cancer.gov/tcrb/monographs/10/index.html

37. Centers for Disease Control and Prevention. (2010). Vital signs: Nonsmokers' exposure to secondhand smoke—United States, 1999–2008. *Morbidity and Mortality Weekly Report, 59*(35), 1141–1146.

38. MedlinePlus.gov. (2009). Making the decision to quit tobacco. Retrieved from http://www.nlm.nih.gov/medlineplus/ency/article/002032.htm

Credits

© Arthur Turner/Alamy; Fig 7.7(left): Library of Congress, Prints & Photographs Division, [LCUSZ62-78689]; Fig 7.7(right): © Lars A. Niki, McGraw-Hill Companies; p.246: © Stockbyte/Getty Images RF; p.247: © Scott Thuen; Fig 7.8: © iStockphoto.com/DNY59; p.249(top to bottom): © Scott Thuen; © David Madison/Photographer's Choice/ Getty Images; Omron Healthcare; Life Measurement Inc.; Courtesy of GE Healthcare; p.251: © yellowdog/Cultura/age fotostock RF; Fig 7.10: © Brand X Pictures/PunchStock RF; © Photodisc/PunchStock RF; © Burke/Triolo Productions/Getty Images RF; © Stock Disc/PunchStock RF; © Blend Images/ Getty Images RF; p.253: © Nicole Hill/Rubberball/Alamy RF; p.254: © Radius Images/Getty Images RF; p.257: © Scott Thuen; p.259: © Scott Thuen.

CHAPTER 8

Opener: © Ariwasabi/Shutterstock; p.269(left): © Brella Productions; Fig 8.1(blueberries): © PhotoAlto/PunchStock RF; (donut): © Jules Frazier/Getty Images RF; Fig 8.2: © iStockphoto/webphotographer; p.270(right): © Jules Selmes/Dorling Kindersley/Getty Images; p.271: © Comstock/Jupiter Images RF; p.273: © Photodisc Collection/Getty Images RF; p.274: © Allesalltag Bildagent/age fotostock; Fig 8.3: © Brand X Pictures/PunchStock RF; p.277: © Helen Sessions/Alamy; p.278: © Chris Kerrigan /The McGraw-Hill Companies, Inc.; Fig 8.5(muffin): © Judith Collins/Alamy RF; (pear): © Stockdisc/PunchStock RF; (beans): © C Squared Studios/ Getty Images RF; (peapods): © Stockbyte/PunchStock RF; p.281: © Comstock/Jupiter Images RF; p.282: © Dorling Kindersley/Getty Images; Fig 8.6(fries): © BananaStock/ PunchStock RF; (meat): © Imagestate Media (John Foxx)/ Imagestate RF; (cheese): © Burke/Triolo Productions/Getty Images RF; (butter): © iStockphoto/Jason Lugo; (oil): © C Squared Studios/Getty Images RF; (nuts): © Burke/ Triolo Productions/Getty Images RF; (fish): © Comstock/ Jupiter Images RF; p.285: © Burke/Triolo Productions/ Getty Images RF; p.287: © The McGraw-Hill Companies, Inc. / Jill Braaten, photographer; p.288: © Brand X Pictures/ PunchStock RF; p.289: © Getty Images RF; p.291: © Image Club RF; p.294: © Creatas/PunchStock RF; p.295(left): © PRNewsFoto/Stonyfield Farm/AP Images; p.295(right): © ConAgra Foods, Inc. All Rights Reserved; p.296: © Science Photo Library/Getty Images RF; p.297: © Mike Kemp/Getty Images RF; p.298: © The McGraw-Hill Companies, Inc./ Christopher Kerrigan, photographer.

CHAPTER 9

Opener: © wavebreakmedia/Shutterstock; p.309: © Brella Productions; p.311(left): © Rick Nease/MCT/Newscom; Fig 9.3(baseball): © Richard Hutchings; (cards): © iStockphoto .com/Victor Burnside; (golf ball): © iStockphoto.com/ Onur Döngel; (mouse): © iStockphoto.com/Andrzej Burak; (dice): © Ingram Publishing/Fotosearch; (die): © C Squared Studios/Getty Images RF; p.313(left): © Jose Luis Pelaez Inc./Blend Images/Getty Images RF; p.313(right): © Beau Lark/Fancy/age fotostock; p.314: © Photodisc/PunchStock RF; p.315(top): © Wang Leng/Asia Images/Getty Images; p.315(bottom): © Davies and Starr/The Image Bank/Getty Images; p.316: © Richard Hutchings/The McGraw-Hill Companies; p.318: © John E. Kelly/Photodisc/Getty Images RF; p.320: © The McGraw-Hill Companies, Inc./Jacques

Cornell, photographer; p.321: © istockphoto.com/Diane Diederich; p.323: © Betsie Van Der Meer/Taxi/Getty Images; Fig 9.5(hands): © RF/Corbis; (raw meat): © iStockphoto.com/ Oleksii Akhrimenko; (thermometer): © iStockphoto.com/ Webking; p.325: Copyright © Foodcollection RF; p.326: Corbis Super RF/Alamy; p.329: © PhotodiscCollection/Getty Images RF; p.330: © Gerard Fritz/Photographer's Choice/ Getty Images; p.331: © David Marsden/Photolibrary/ Getty Images; p.332: © Scott Thuen; p.333: © WhitePlaid/ Shutterstock; p.334: © The McGraw-Hill Companies, Inc./Jill Braaten, photographer.

CHAPTER 10

Opener: © JGI/Tom Grill/Blend Images/Getty Images RF; p.345: © Brella Productions; Fig 10.1: © PM Images/Riser/Getty Images; p.347: © Real World People/Alamy; p.348: © Image Source/Getty Images RF; p.349: © Diego Cervo/Shutterstock; p.350: © ERproductions Ltd./Blend Images/Getty Images; p.352: © Kablonk!/photolibrary RF; p.353: © AP Photo/Elise Amendola; Fig 10.3(top to bottom): © Ingram Publishing/ age fotostock RF; © BananaStock/PunchStock RF; © Nathan Lau/Design Pics/Corbis RF; p.356: © Sean Justice/Corbis RF; p.358: © Comstock Images/Jupiter Images RF; p.360: © Joanne Rathe/The Boston Globe via Getty Images; p.363: © Asia Images Groups/Getty Images RF; p.365: © Somos RF/Getty Images; p.366: © George Doyle/Stockbyte/Getty Images RF; p.368: © Design Pics Inc./Alamy RF; p.369(top): © Eye Candy Images/Getty Images RF; p.369(bottom): © Ashley Cooper/Corbis; p.371: © B BOISSONNET/BSIP/ age fotostock; p.372(top): © Maria Teijeiro/Getty Images RF; p.372(bottom): © Rubberball/Getty Images RF; p.373: © BananaStock/PunchStock RF.

CHAPTER 11

Opener: © avava/Kalium/age fotostock RF; p.382: © Fuse/Getty Images RF; p.385: © Ingram Publishing/Fotosearch RF; p.386: © Lael Henderson/Getty Images; Fig 11.4: © iStockphoto .com/Roel Smart; p.388: © Gary S. Chapman/Photographer's Choice RF/Getty Images RF; p.389: © Thinkstock/Getty Images RF; p.392: © West Coast Surfer/moodboard/age fotostock RF; p.394: © Photodisc/Getty Images RF; p.395: © The McGraw-Hill Companies, Inc./Rick Brady, photographer; p.396: © Creatas/PunchStock RF; p.397: © Michael Hitoshi/ Getty Images RF; p.400: © Radius Images/Alamy RF; p.402: © Comstock Images/Getty Images RF; p.404: © Maria Deseo/PhotoEdit; Fig 11.7: The Skin Cancer Foundation, Inc.; p.406(right): © Deborah Jaffe/Fancy/Corbis Images RF; Fig 11.9: © Seth Joel/Digital Vision/Getty Images RF; Fig 11.10: © Britt Erlanson/Getty Images RF; p.411: © BananaStock/ Photolibrary RF.

CHAPTER 12

Opener: © Jose Luis Pelaez, Inc./Blend Images Corbis RF; p.419: © Hero/Corbis Images RF; Fig 12.1(top to bottom): CDC/ Cynthia Goldsmith; CDC/Janice Haney Carr; © Centers for Disease Control; CDC/Dr. Stan Erlandsen; © Centers for Disease Control; p.421(top): © Tetra Images/Getty Images RF; p421(bottom): CDC/James Gathany; Fig 12.4(top to bottom): © Stockbyte/PunchStock RF; © iStockphoto.com/Christian Pound; © iStockphoto.com/Ashok Rodrigues; p.428: © Stockbyte/PictureQuest RF; p.429: © Sebastian Pfuetze/

Index

Note: Key term page numbers are indicated in **boldface**.

Thank you

Academic Reviewers

Maureen Bach, Orange County Community College
Randy Bergman, Missouri Western State University
Jeff Bolender, Cedarville University
Lori Clark, Chemeketa Community College
Eric Colon-Cortes, Chemeketa Community College
Lena Marie Cool, Kalamazoo Valley Community College
Carol Lynn Fieser, Tarrant County College
Jason Fischer, St. Cloud State University
Megan Franks, Lone State College System – North Harris
Kathy Freese, Cedarville University
Robert Hess, Community College of Baltimore County – Catonsville
Sarah Hilgers, North Dakota State University
Amy Howton, Kennesaw State University
Bill Hyman, Sam Houston State University
Britt Johnson, Missouri Western State University
Kevin Kinser, Tarrant County College
Melissa Raschel Larsen, Chemeketa Community College
Karen Miller-Thornwall, Washburn University
Alicia Peterson, Longwood University
Bill Papin, Western Carolina University
Debby Singleton, Western Carolina University
Natalie Stickney, Georgia Perimeter College
Jae Westfall, Ohio State University
Lorraine Wilson, Abilene Christian University
Julie Zuleger, University of Wisconsin – Oshkosh

Connect Reviewers

Pam Anderson, Georgia Gwinnett College
Dr. Eugene Asola, Georgia Gwinnett College
Anita Behrbaum, Green River Community College
Ranae Cushing, Washburn University
Jamie Dickson, Pearl River Community College
Spencer Fee, The Ohio State University
Celeste Hajek, Washburn University
Linda-Marie Hamill, The Citadel
Candace Hendershot, University of Findlay
Lindsay Jackson, The Citadel
Julie Kaufman, Shepherd University
Amy Kim, Ohio State University
Ken Larson, Georgia Gwinnett
Michelle Lomonaco, The Citadel
Queen Martin, Prairie View A&M University
Erin Nitschke, Northern Wyoming Community College District - Sheridan College

Catherine Nolan, Moraine Valley Community College
Chad Nykamp, Oakland Community College
Christal Omni, Washburn University
Jeff Pasley, Georgia Gwinnett College
Christine Payne, University of Southern Indiana
Robert Pedrigi, Moraine Valley Community College
Karen Perell-Gerson, Georgia Gwinnett College
Jessica Priehs, Owens Community College
Mona Smith, Georgia Gwinnett College
Margaret A. Wendling, Washburn University
Traci Worby, Eastern Illinois University
Tracy Yengo, University of Wisconsin - Eau Claire

Fitness and Wellness Symposia Participants

Elliot Anderson, Snow College - Ephraim
Jana Arabas, Truman State University
Grady Armstrong, Salisbury University
Rebecca Battaglini, University of North Carolina – Chapel
Christina Beaudoin, Grand Valley State University
Claire Blakeley, Brigham Young University-Idaho
Pam Brown, University of North Carolina - Greensboro
Charles Burrage, Jr., Gainesville State College
Lena-Marie Cool, Kalamazoo Valley Community College
Mark Cullum, Harding University
Karen Dennis, Illinois State University
Donna Dey, Austin Peay State University
Judy Donahue, Ball State University
Mandi Dupain, Millersville University
Kim Eskola, University of Central Arkansas
Carol "Lynn" Fieser, Tarrant County Community College
James Fitzsimmons, University of Nevada – Reno
Megan Franks, Lone Star College-North Harris
Gail Freedman, Nova Community College – Alexandria
Richard Gibbs, Linn Benton Community College
Joyce Grohman, Atlantic Cape Community College
Jeffrey Hallam, University of Mississippi
David Harackiewicz, Central Connecticut State University
Kevin Harper, Tarrant County College – Northeast
Charles Hervey, University of Central Arkansas
David Hixson, Shepherd University
Deborah Hutchinson, Community College of Baltimore County - Essex
Bill Hyman, Sam Houston State University
Stacy Ingraham, University of Minnesota - Minneapolis
Ron Kamaka, Mount San Antonio College